Clinics in Developmental Medicine
Nos 180–181

Cover illustration

The cover depicts a three-dimensional musculoskeletal model moving from walking in crouch to walking upright. The simulations from which these images were taken were developed by Jennifer Hicks in the Department of Mechanical Engineering, Stanford University.

Clinics in Developmental Medicine Nos 180–181

The Identification and Treatment of Gait Problems in Cerebral Palsy

JAMES R. GAGE

MICHAEL H. SCHWARTZ

STEVEN E. KOOP

AND

TOM F. NOVACHECK

2009
Mac Keith Press
Distributed by Wiley-Blackwell

© 2009 Mac Keith Press
6 Market Road, London N7 9PW

Editor: Hilary M. Hart
Managing Director: Caroline Black
Project Manager: Edward Fenton
Indexer: Laurence Errington

First published in 2004 as *The Treatment of Gait Problems in Cerebral Palsy.*
Second edition 2009
Reprinted with corrections 2010.

British Library Cataloguing-in-Publication data
A catalogue record for this book is available from the British Library

ISBN: 978-1-898683-65-0

Typeset by Keystroke, 28 High Street, Tettenhall, Wolverhampton
Printed by The Lavenham Press Ltd, Water Street, Lavenham, Suffolk

Mac Keith Press is supported by Scope

CONTENTS

AUTHORS' APPOINTMENTS

A. Leland Albright, MD Professor of Neurosurgery and Pediatrics at the University of Wisconsin Health Center. Department of Neurosurgery, University of Wisconsin, Madison, Wisconsin, USA

Camilla Beattie, PT Level III Physical Therapist, Center for Gait and Motion Analysis, Gillette Children's Specialty Healthcare, St Paul, Minnesota, USA

Henry G. Chambers, MD David H Sutherland Director of Cerebral Palsy Studies; Medical Director, Motion Analysis Laboratory, Rady Children's Hospital, San Diego; Clinical Professor, Department of Orthopedic Surgery, University of California at San Diego, San Diego, California, USA

Jon R. Davids, MD Chief of Staff, Medical Director Motional Analysis Laboratory, Shriner's Hospital for Children, Greenville South Carolina; GHS Clinical Professor of Orthopaedic Surgery at the University of South Carolina School of Medicine, Columbia, South Carolina, USA

Scott L. Delp, PhD Professor, Bioengineering Department, Stanford University, Stanford, California, USA

Kaat Desloovere, PhD Clinical Motion Analysis Service and Research Manager, Laboratory for Clinical Motion Analysis, University Hospital of Pellenberg (Leuven, Belgium), Professor at the Faculty of Kinesiology and Rehabilitation Sciences, Department of Rehabilitation Sciences, Katholieke Universiteit Leuven, Leuven, Belgium

Adré J. du Plessis, MD Director of Fetal–Neonatal Neurology, Senior Associate in Neurology, Children's Hospital Boston, Massachusetts; Associate Professor in Neurology, Harvard Medical School, Boston, Massachusetts, USA

Mary Beth Dunn, MD Neurosurgery United Neurosurgery Associates, 225 North Smith Avenue, Suite 200, St Paul, Minnesota; Director of Neuro-oncology United Hospital, 333 North Smith Avenue, St Paul, Minnesota, USA

Nichola R. Fry, PhD Research Clinical Scientist, One Small Step Gait Laboratory, Guy's & St Thomas' Foundation Hospital Trust, London, UK

James R. Gage, MD Medical Director Emeritus, Gillette Children's Specialty Healthcare, St Paul, Minnesota; Professor of Orthopaedics Emeritus, University of Minnesota, Minneapolis, Minnesota, USA

George Gent, CO Certified Orthotist, Gillette Children's Specialty Healthcare, St Paul, Minnesota, USA

Martin Gough, FRCSI (Orth) Consultant Pediatric Orthopaedic Surgeon, One Small Step Gait Laboratory, Guy's & St Thomas' Foundation Hospital Trust, London, UK

H. Kerr Graham, MD, FRCS (Ed) FRACS Professor of Orthopaedic Surgery, The University of Melbourne, Murdoch Childrens Research Institute, Royal Children's Hospital, Melbourne Australia

Adrienne Harvey, PhD Senior Physiotherapist, Hugh Williamson Gait Laboratory, McMaster Child Health Research Institute Postdoctoral Fellow, The Royal Children's Hospital, Melbourne, Australia

Jennifer L. Hicks, MS Doctoral Student, Mechanical Engineering Department, Stanford University, Stanford, California, USA

Steven E. Koop, MD Medical Director, Gillette Children's Specialty Healthcare, St Paul, Minnesota; Associate Professor of Orthopaedics, University of Minnesota, Minneapolis, Minnesota, USA

Linda E. Krach, MD Director, Research Administration, Gillette Children's Specialty Healthcare, St Paul, Minnesota; Clinical Associate Professor, Department of Physical Medicine and Rehabilitation, University of Minnesota, Minneapolis, Minnesota, USA

Gary J. Kroll, CO Manager, Assistive Technology, Gillette Children's Specialty Healthcare, St Paul, Minnesota, USA

Nelleke G. Langerak, MSc Doctoral Student Biomedical Engineering, Faculty of Health Sciences, Department of Human Biology, University of Cape Town, South Africa

Anne E. McNee, MPthy Research Clinical Scientist, One Small Step Gait Laboratory, Guy's & St Thomas' Foundation Hospital Trust, London, UK

Guy Molenaers, MD, PhD Medical Director of the Cerebral Palsy Reference Centre, Laboratory for Clinical Motion Analysis, University Hospital of Pellenberg (Leuven, Belgium), Professor at the Faculty of Medicine, Department of Musculoskeletal Sciences, Katholieke Universiteit Leuven, Leuven, Belgium

Sue Murr, DPT, PCS Manager of Neurosciences Programs, Gillette Children's Specialty Healthcare, St Paul, Minnesota, USA

Tom F. Novacheck, MD Director, Center for Gait and Motion Analysis, Gillette Children's Specialty Healthcare, St Paul, Minnesota; Associate Professor of Orthopaedics, University of Minnesota, Minneapolis, Minnesota, USA

Sylvia Õunpuu, MSc Director/Kinesiologist, Center for Motion Analysis, Connecticut Children's Medical Center, Farmington, Connecticut; Assistant Professor, School of Medicine, University of Connecticut, USA

Warwick J. Peacock, MD Professor Emeritus, Department of Neurological Surgery, University of California, San Francisco, USA

Adam Rozumalski, MS Research Engineer, Center for Gait and Motion Analysis, Gillette Children's Specialty Healthcare, St Paul, Minnesota, USA

Michael Schwartz, PhD Director of Bioengineering Research, Gillette Children's Specialty Healthcare, St Paul, Minnesota; Associate Professor, Orthopaedic

Surgery Graduate Faculty, Biomedical Engineering, University of Minnesota, Minneapolis, Minnesota, USA

Adam P. Shortland, PhD Consultant Clinical Scientist, One Small Step Gait Laboratory, Guy's & St Thomas' Foundation Hospital Trust, London, UK

Sue Sohrweide, PT Level II Physical Therapist, Center for Gait and Motion Analysis, Gillette Children's Specialty Healthcare, St Paul, Minnesota, USA

Jean L. Stout, MS, PT Research Physical Therapist, Center for Gait and Motion Analysis, Gillette Children's Specialty Healthcare, St Paul, Minnesota, USA

Pam Thomason, BPhty, MPhysio Senior Physiotherapist, Service Manager, Hugh Williamson Gait Laboratory, The Royal Children's Hospital, Melbourne, Australia

Joyce Trost, PT Research Administration Manager, Gillette Children's Specialty Healthcare, St Paul, Minnesota, US

Kevin Walker, MD Pediatric Orthopaedic Surgeon, Gillette Children's Specialty Healthcare, St Paul, Minnesota; Assistant Professor of Orthopaedics, University of Minnesota, Minneapolis, Minnesota, USA

Kathryn J. Walt, PT Physical Therapist and Rehabilitation Supervisor, Gillette Childrens Specialty Healthcare, St Paul, Minnesota USA

Marcie Ward, MD Pediatric Physical Medicine and Rehabilitation, Gillette Children's Specialty Healthcare, St Paul, Minnesota; Adjunct Instructor of Physical Medicine and Rehabilitation, University of Minnesota, Minneapolis, Minnesota, USA

Beverly Wical, MD Director, Pediatric Neurology and Sleep Medicine Services; Medical Director, Epilepsy Program; Gillette Children's Specialty Healthcare, St Paul, Minnesota; Adjunct Assistant Professor of Pediatrics, University of Minnesota, Minneapolis, Minnesota, USA

PREFACE

The organization we now call Gillette Children's Specialty Healthcare was formed in 1897 by the Minnesota State Legislature. It was our nation's first public hospital for children for disabilities. Many years later Dr Arthur Gillette was asked to describe the most difficult barrier he faced while advocating for the creation of the hospital that would come to bear his name after his death. He replied that it was 'the belief that nothing could be done for the children'.

A century of care has demonstrated that belief was wrong but skepticism has persisted about the value of some of the things that were done. I imagine that if Dr Jim Gage was asked to describe the most difficult barrier he faced while advocating for a new approach for managing the disturbed walking that hampers the function of children with cerebral palsy he might reply that it was 'the belief that nothing *useful* could be done for the children'.

There was cause for doubt. Children endured multiple painful surgeries, long hospital stays, and prolonged recoveries. Too many of them experienced disappointing outcomes. This was the state of things when Dr Gage left Minnesota in 1976 to take a position as a pediatric orthopaedic surgeon at Newington Children's Hospital (near Hartford, Connecticut) and lead the cerebral palsy service. Dissatisfied with what he saw and convinced that things could be improved, Dr Gage developed an interest in the use of computer technology in the assessment of human walking. After collaboration with Dr David Sutherland of San Diego Children's Hospital, Dr Gage encouraged United Technologies Research Center to build one of the world's first fully automated motion laboratories at Newington Children's. A second laboratory followed at Gillette Children's in 1987 and Dr Gage returned to Gillette in 1990 to serve as Medical Director, a position he held until 2001.

Dr Gage's unwillingness to accept mediocrity as inevitable profoundly changed the care of children with cerebral palsy. He insisted that the baffling complexity of spastic walking could be approached by the application of basic tools: careful examination of a child, measurement by motion analysis, establishment of goals, single-event surgeries that corrected multiple problems at once, good rehabilitation, and meticulous measurement and assessment of treatment outcomes. Dr Gage solicited the involvement of individuals from multiple clinical domains including neurology, neurosurgery, physiatry, physical therapy, mechanical engineering and orthotics.

This edition of *Identification and Treatment of Gait Problems in Cerebral Palsy* contains the latest fruit of collaboration among individuals from those diverse disciplines. The book is divided into two parts: material designed to help the reader evaluate and understand a child with cerebral palsy followed by information about treatment. The early chapters in the first half of the book provide information about typical neural control and musculoskeletal development as well as normal gait. This is followed by chapters that describe the causes and consequences of cerebral palsy and the methods by which children with cerebral palsy may be evaluated. The organization of the second half of the book emphasizes the most fundamental concept of treatment: manage the child's neurologic dysfunction first and then address the skeletal and muscular consequences of that dysfunction. Many of the treatment chapters employ a standard content format. The book closes with information about the consequences of treatment.

Because human movement is difficult to describe with words, graphs, drawings and pictures the book is supplemented by two video discs. One disc is dedicated to a description of normal gait and the processes that are used to acquire information about walking. The second disc follows the chapter format of the book and contains video and other material designed to supplement the content of each chapter. Examples of the content include case studies and surgical techniques.

As evidenced by the list of authors, this book is the result of collaboration. We thank the authors for their contributions and their willingness to modify texts in order to provide readers with content that follows a logical sequence with a minimum of duplication.

In Ivan Turgenev's *Fathers and Sons*, an irritable Bazarov – discussing books and art with Anna Sergeyevna – says: 'The drawing shows me at one glance what might be spread over ten pages in a book.' This book, at heart an effort to describe human movement, would be hopelessly long and inadequate without the pictures, graphs and videos mentioned above. Key contributions have been made by Tim Trost (illustrations), Anna Bittner and Paul De Marchi (photography), Roy Wervey (video editing and motion analysis data), and Brian Hagen, Chad Halvorson, Diana Cimino and Joe Du Bord of Meditech Communications Inc. (DVD and CD). We thank them profusely!

It has been our great fortune to be Dr Gage's students and colleagues day in and day out. We hope this book will assist you in the care of the children you serve.

STEVEN E. KOOP, MD
Medical Director
Gillette Children's Specialty Healthcare

Section 1

TYPICAL MUSCULOSKELETAL DEVELOPMENT

1.1
THE NEURAL CONTROL OF MOVEMENT

Warwick J. Peacock

The only action a human can bring about is muscular contraction. This muscular contraction will cause movement that may in turn produce walking, writing or speech. However, any action must start as a thought. Thoughts arise in certain areas of the brain, which through their connections stimulate cortical motor centers. This initiation of motor actions has been recorded as an electrical potential known as the 'readiness potential', and it is located in the supplementary motor area, just anterior to the motor strip (Deecke et al. 1969). This 'readiness potential' occurs up to one second before the onset of movement, whether the movement occurs in the hand, toe, mouth, tongue or eye, and irrespective of whether the movements are complex and programmed (as in speech) or simple (Brinkman and Porter 1979, 1983, Schreiber et al. 1983, Kornhuber and Deecke 1985). Large, fast-firing neurons in the cortex, which are known as Betz cells, contribute axons to motor tracts which descend from the cortex to the brainstem (corticobulbar fibers) and spinal cord (corticospinal tracts) to connect with motor nerves that innervate muscles. The muscles, when stimulated by these motor tracts, then contract to bring about the desired purposeful movement and action.

The structural unit of the nervous system is the nerve cell or neuron, each of which is made up of a nerve cell body and a number of impulse conducting processes (Fig. 1.1.1). Gray

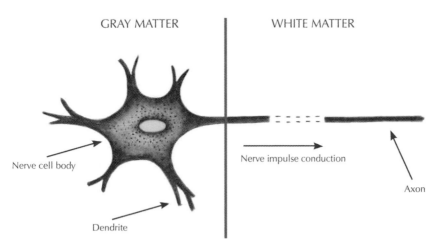

GRAY MATTER | WHITE MATTER

Nerve cell body

Nerve impulse conduction

Axon

Dendrite

Fig. 1.1.1 A neuron. The basic unit of the central nervous system is the neuron. Impulses enter the nerve cell through the dendrites and exit via the axon. Gray matter is composed of nerve cell bodies while white matter is made up of nerve processes.

matter is composed of nerve cell bodies and white matter of nerve processes. At autopsy, when the brain is examined by slicing it at various levels, the different parts of the central nervous system can be seen to be made up only of gray and white matter (Fig. 1.1.2). Gray- and white-matter areas are discrete and easily differentiated. In the cerebral hemispheres, gray matter forms the outer cerebral cortex and the deep nuclei of the basal ganglia. The nuclei of the brainstem are made up of gray matter and in the cerebellum the cortex and the deep dentate nuclei are gray matter. The spinal cord has centrally placed H-shaped gray matter.

The white matter is made up of neuronal processes arranged in bundles or tracts connecting nerve cell bodies in the gray matter of the cortex, deep nuclei or motor neurons of the spinal cord. These white-matter tracts are organized in three broad groups according

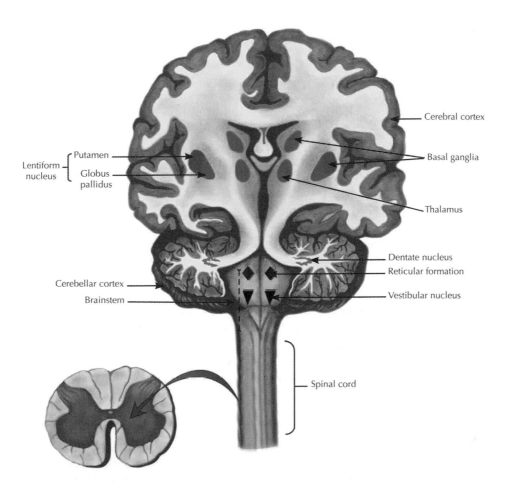

Fig. 1.1.2 Diagrammatic representation of a coronal section taken through the brain and spinal cord showing some of the major control centers.

to direction and destination. First, association tracts run backwards or forwards connecting structures on the same side such as the fronto–occipital fasciculus, which connects the frontal lobe to the occipital lobe on the same side. Second, commissural tracts such as the corpus callosum cross the midline linking corresponding areas of the two hemispheres. The third group comprises projection fibers which run up or down, connecting the cerebral hemispheres with lower levels in the brain and spinal cord, and may or may not cross. An example of the last group would be the pyramidal tract (lateral corticospinal tract), connecting the motor cortex to contralateral motor neurons of the spinal cord, or the ascending spino–cerebellar tract, carrying proprioceptive information from contracting muscles to the cerebellar cortex.

A surprisingly large number of gray- and white-matter structures can be seen by the naked eye on a freshly cut brain slice.

The motor system
The motor system is hierarchical and is made up of a chain of command centers from the cerebral cortex centers down to the motor nerves that connect with the muscles (Fig. 1.1.3). An upper motor neuron runs down from the motor cortex to connect with either bulbar or spinal lower motor neurons, which in turn leave the central nervous system via a peripheral nerve to innervate a muscle. The various components of the system are as follows.

1. Cortical motor control centers (Fig. 1.1.3) constitute the supreme command of motor activity.
2. The basal ganglia (Fig. 1.1.4) play an important role in previewing and planning movement patterns willed by the cerebral cortex, and are made up of a number of deep-seated gray-matter nuclei including the putamen, globus pallidus and caudate nucleus (comprising the corpus striatum) with the substantia nigra and subthalamic nucleus. All these structures are directly or indirectly linked to the thalamus, which is in turn connected back to the frontal lobe cortex.
3. The cerebellum (Fig. 1.1.5) is involved in assessing the degree to which a movement conforms to the instruction issued by the cortical motor centers by comparing this instruction with the information returning from peripheral sense organs for muscle length and velocity of contraction (muscle spindles) and rate of change of contraction force (Golgi tendon organs).
4. The brainstem motor (see Fig. 1.1.11) nuclei provide a background of posture and tone against which specific voluntary movements can be executed.
5. The spinal cord (Fig. 1.1.6) provides the motor neurons that connect with muscles to bring about contraction and movement. Important motor reflexes are also a feature of the cord's connections.

For the successful execution of a movement the sensory system plays an important role (Rossignol et al. 2006). First, the nervous system requires information about the position of the body parts in relationship to each other and to the surrounding environment. Secondly, input is required throughout the course of the movement about its progress so that any errors

5

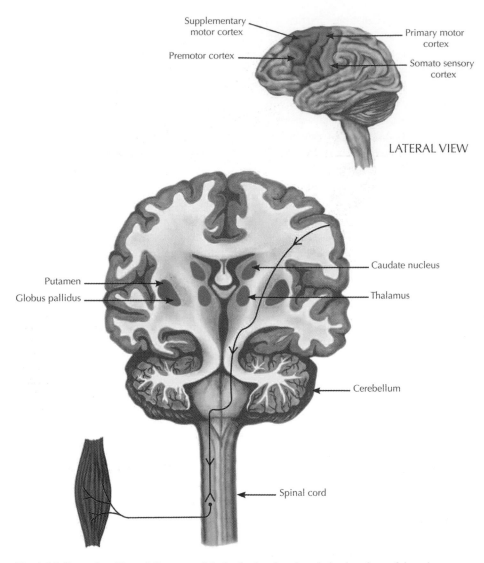

Fig. 1.1.3 Coronal and lateral diagrams of the brain showing the relative locations of the primary, premotor and supplementary motor cortices. Axons from neurons in the pyramidal system run uninterrupted from the motor cortex to synapse on lower motor neurons. Pyramidal neurons in the cortex can initiate a muscle movement since they synapse directly with lower motor neurons. However, for coordinated movement to occur, many other circuits between the motor cortex and other brain centers are required.

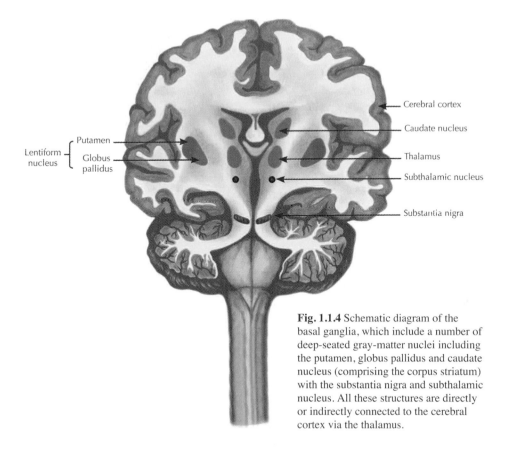

Lentiform { Putamen ⎯
nucleus { Globus ⎯
pallidus

Cerebral cortex

Caudate nucleus

Thalamus

Subthalamic nucleus

Substantia nigra

Fig. 1.1.4 Schematic diagram of the basal ganglia, which include a number of deep-seated gray-matter nuclei including the putamen, globus pallidus and caudate nucleus (comprising the corpus striatum) with the substantia nigra and subthalamic nucleus. All these structures are directly or indirectly connected to the cerebral cortex via the thalamus.

in execution can be rapidly corrected. Visual (Saitoh et al. 2007), auditory, vestibular, tactile and proprioceptive information is essential.

Overview

1. CORTICAL MOTOR CONTROL CENTERS

A thought, which will lead to a movement, may arise in any part of the cerebral cortex and an impulse is then relayed to the supplementary motor area in the anterior part of the frontal lobe (Fig. 1.1.3). Dynamic studies show that if a person simply thinks about an intended movement the supplementary motor area becomes active (Deecke et al. 1969, Roland et al. 1980). If the supplementary motor area is stimulated during awake neurosurgical procedures the patients are reported to experience an urge to move or feel that a movement is about to occur (Fried et al. 1991). The command is then passed on to the premotor cortex (Fig. 1.1.3), which is involved in the preparation for movement. The next relay is to the primary motor cortex in the precentral gyrus (Fig. 1.1.3) from where the corticospinal or pyramidal tract arises. The corticospinal fibers, which account for only 1 million of the 30 million fibers

Fig. 1.1.5 The cerebellum is involved in assessing the progress of a movement and the degree to which it conforms to the order issued by the cortical motor centers. It is attached to the rest of the brain by the cerebellar peduncles via the midbrain, pons and medulla.

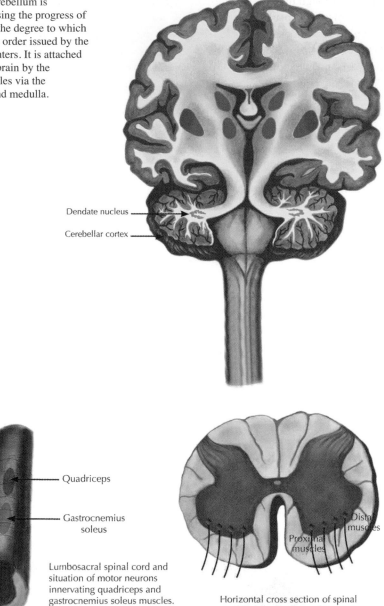

Dendate nucleus

Cerebellar cortex

L2
L3
L4
L5
S1
S2

Quadriceps

Gastrocnemius soleus

Lumbosacral spinal cord and situation of motor neurons innervating quadriceps and gastrocnemius soleus muscles.

Distal muscles

Proximal muscles

Horizontal cross section of spinal cord to show position of motor neurons innervating proximal and distal limb muscles.

Fig. 1.1.6 Longitudinal and cross-sectional views of the lumbosacral spinal cord. The longitudinal view shows the situation of the motor neurons innervating the quadriceps and the gastrocsoleus muscles. The horizontal cross-section shows the relative position of motor neurons innervating proximal and distal limb muscles.

8

running through the internal capsule, are found in the posterior third of the posterior limb of the internal capsule (Brodal 1981). These fibers become the pyramidal tracts of the medulla. The opposite half of the body is arranged in the precentral gyrus as an inverted homunculus (from Latin, diminutive of *homo* 'man'), with the leg represented superiorly near the midline and the trunk, arm and face found lower down and laterally (Fig. 1.1.7). The corticospinal tract then passes downwards as part of the deep hemispheral white matter

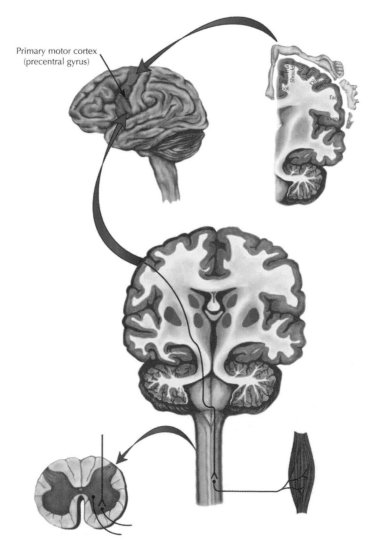

Fig. 1.1.7 Coronal and lateral diagrams of the precentral gyrus. The opposite half of the body is arranged in the precentral gyrus as an inverted homunculus (diagrammatic representation of a 'little man'). The corticospinal tract, which arises from the precentral gyrus, crosses over to the opposite side at the level of the medulla and then descends in the spinal cord to synapse with a motor neuron.

9

and through the internal capsule before forming the cerebral peduncles and entering the brainstem (Fig. 1.1.7). At the level of the medulla the corticospinal tract enters the 'pyramid', which is a prominent longitudinal bulge on the anterior aspect of the medulla, and then crosses to descend in the opposite side of the lower medulla and spinal cord. It courses down the spinal cord as the lateral corticospinal tract to synapse with a motor neuron (lower motor neuron) in the anterior horn (Fig. 1.1.7). The motor neurons in the lateral part of the anterior horn control distal muscles in the limbs, whereas the medially situated motor neurons, which are under different upper motor neuron influence, control proximal limb and trunk muscles. The axon of the lower motor neuron then exits from the spinal cord, becoming a peripheral nerve that travels out to its specific muscle and brings about a contraction leading to the intended movement. Damage to the primary motor cortex or the descending corticospinal fibers results in the loss of contralateral skilled hand function without the development of spasticity (Lawrence 1968).

2. THE BASAL GANGLIA

The basal ganglia are composed of large gray-matter nuclei found in the basal part of the cerebral hemispheres and midbrain that are involved in the appropriate planning and initiation of voluntary movement (Grillner et al. 2005). They receive a large cortical input and, after processing all the relevant information, relay back to the motor cortex. The basal ganglia form a closed loop with the cerebral cortex to bring about the desired movement but have no direct contact with lower motor neurons that are connected to muscles.

The caudate nucleus and putamen are known as the corpus striatum and work in conjunction with the globus pallidus (Fig. 1.1.8). Also included in the basal ganglia are the subthalamic nucleus and the substantia nigra. The basal ganglia store information about previously performed movements. When the cortex intends to bring about a purposeful movement the basal ganglia are called upon to provide the memory for that particular movement in relationship to the body's posture and position in space at that moment. The integrated information about the purpose and sequence of the movement is then relayed back to the cortex so that appropriate instructions can be sent from the upper to the lower motor neurons, and finally out to the group of muscles involved in performing the movement and achieving the intended goal.

Almost all cortical areas project to the caudate nucleus and the putamen. These two structures project to the globus pallidus and then, via the thalamus, the circuit is completed back to the cortex. Also hooked into the loop are the substantia nigra and the subthalamic nucleus. The main functions of the basal ganglia are the initiation and smooth performance of voluntary movements.

The two common neurological disorders that are caused by pathology in the basal ganglia are Parkinson disease, in which the substantia nigra is destroyed, and Huntington disease, in which there is marked atrophy of the caudate nucleus and putamen. In Parkinson disease there is difficulty with the initiation of movement and spontaneous movement is diminished. With Huntington disease entire motor programs are inappropriately released, as manifested by jerky, random and repetitive writhing movements, which are referred to as chorea or athetosis.

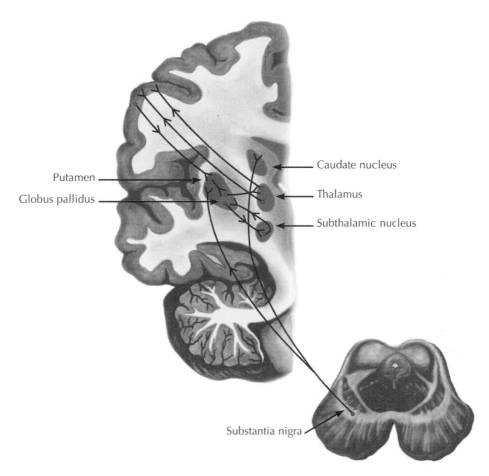

Putamen

Globus pallidus

Caudate nucleus

Thalamus

Subthalamic nucleus

Substantia nigra

Fig. 1.1.8 Diagrammatic representation of the anatomy and connections of the basal ganglia. The basal ganglia form a closed loop with the cerebral cortex and are involved in the planning and initiation of voluntary movement. The basal ganglia store motor engram (memories) which the cortex draws upon when deciding which movement will be most effective in achieving the desired goal. Neurons dive down from the cortex to connect with neurons in the putamen and caudate nucleus. The circuitry then involves the globus pallidus, the subthalamic nucleus and the substantia nigra before heading back to the cortex via the thalamus. The cortex now chooses the most appropriate motor engram to perform the desired movement.

3. THE CEREBELLUM

The cerebellum is made up of two lateral hemispheres and the midline vermis (Fig. 1.1.9). There is a folded cortex overlying central white matter with deep nuclei, the main one being the dentate nucleus. The cerebellum is extensively connected to the rest of the central nervous system via the cerebellar peduncles and is involved with the smooth execution and completion of movements and with truncal balance. There are three broad anatomical and physiological divisions to the cerebellum, which follow the stages of evolution of this organ (Brodal 1981).

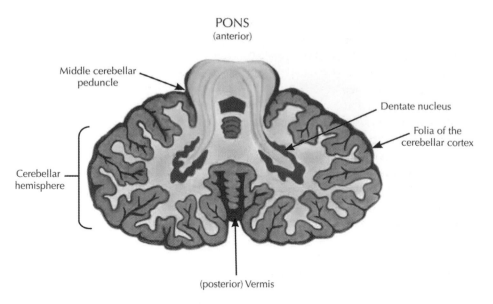

PONS
(anterior)

Middle cerebellar
peduncle

Dentate nucleus

Folia of the
cerebellar cortex

Cerebellar
hemisphere

(posterior) Vermis

Fig. 1.1.9 A cross section of the cerebellum that shows the connections via the middle cerebellar peduncle to the pons. The gray matter of the cortex and the dentate nucleus are shown. It is involved with the smooth execution and completion of movements and with truncal balance.

1. The 'vestibulocerebellum', the oldest part of the cerebellum or 'archicerebellum', is the small flocculonodular lobe which receives ipsilateral vestibular input, essential for the sense of balance, via the inferior cerebellar peduncles.
2. The midline vermis, also known as the 'spinocerebellum' or 'paleocerebellum', receives sensory input via the inferior cerebellar peduncles from the muscle spindles (which detect muscle length and velocity of contraction) and Golgi tendon organs (sensing changes in tendon force) which in turn course up the spinal cord in the spinocerebellar tracts.
3. The lateral parts of the cerebellum, called the cerebellar hemispheres, are recent additions known as the neocerebellum or pontocerebellum because of the huge input from the pontine nuclei via the middle cerebellar peduncle. Some 20 million afferent fibers are carried from pontine nuclei via the middle cerebellar peduncle to the cerebellar hemispheres.

The inferior cerebellar peduncle contains afferent fibers from the inferior olive (approximately 0.5 million in all) and from other vital peripheral sense-organs. The superior cerebellar peduncle, which contains approximately 0.8 million efferent fibers, carries information from the cerebellar nuclei to the brainstem, red nucleus and thalamus.

What is the cerebellum's role in movement? In a simplified way it can be explained as follows. At the same time that the cortical motor centers send an instruction to a group of muscles to bring about a purposeful movement they also send a message to the cerebellum (via the corticopontine and pontocerebellar tracts) informing it of the desired movement pattern (Fig. 1.1.10a). With the onset of muscular contraction, information about the pattern of the contraction is conducted back from the muscles to the cerebellum via the spino-cerebellar tracts (Fig. 1.1.10b). In the cerebellar cortex the error between what was instructed and what is being carried out is computed and this information is sent to the dentate nucleus deep in the cerebellar hemisphere. The necessary correction is then relayed to the cortical motor centers (Fig. 1.1.10c). This is followed by an adjusted command to the muscles so that the movement is carried out as originally intended. The monitoring and correcting is carried out throughout every tiny fraction of the movement until the objective is achieved.

Damage to the cerebellum causes symptoms such as loss of coordination with ongoing ipsilateral movements. Dysmetria is a common problem with cerebellar pathology and is manifested for example by the patient having difficulty picking up a pencil. The hand tends to overshoot the pencil and then rebounds back too far and only after a number of movements of decreasing amplitude does the hand achieve its goal.

4. The Brainstem Motor Nuclei

Apart from the cranial nerve motor nuclei there are a number of nuclei in the brainstem that are involved in providing a background of posture and tone in the trunk and proximal limbs so that fine distal movements, for example, of the hands, can be executed efficiently. These are the vestibular nucleus and the reticular formation (Fig. 1.1.11) and are under the control of the cortical motor centers via the corticobulbar tracts. The vestibular nucleus is also connected to the vestibular apparatus in the inner ear and is involved with balance. The reticular formation is a cluster of gray matter scattered throughout the brainstem which is involved with rhythmic activity such as heart beat, respiration and sleep–wake cycles. The pyramidal (corticospinal) tracts and the extrapyramidal tracts such as the vestibulospinal and reticulospinal (extrapyramidal) tracts are the upper motor neurons which control muscular activity. The pyramidal (corticospinal) tracts synapse with motor neurons found in the lateral part of the anterior horn that innervate distal limb muscles used for finely adjusted movements. Both the vestibulospinal and reticulospinal tracts synapse with motor neurons that lie in the medial part of the anterior horns of the spinal cord and innervate trunk and proximal limb muscles.

5. Spinal-Cord Motor Control

The majority of the neurons that control the body's skeletal muscles are to be found in the anterior horn of the spinal cord. We will not be discussing the motor neurons found in the cranial nerve nuclei, which mainly innervate the muscles of the head and neck. The fibers arising from the spinal cord (lower motor neurons) exit the spinal cord to innervate muscles and are referred to as the final common pathway. Each of these motor neurons innervates one or more muscle fibers within the same muscle. A given neuron and the group of muscle fibers it supplies are collectively known as a motor unit. All the motor neurons that innervate a specific muscle lie within a longitudinal column in the anterior horn. This column usually spans more than one spinal cord segment. For example, the longitudinal column of motor neurons innervating the quadriceps muscle extends through the L3 and L4 spinal cord segments and those for the gastrocnemii are in the L5 and S1 segments. The medial groups

(a)

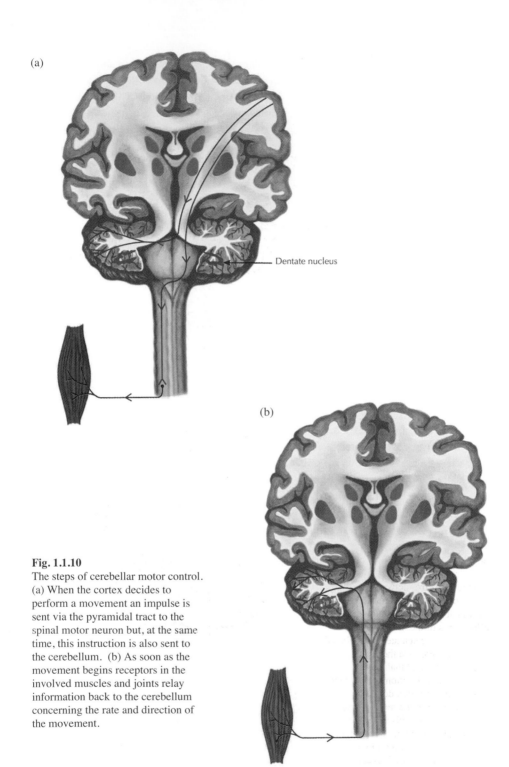

Dentate nucleus

(b)

Fig. 1.1.10
The steps of cerebellar motor control.
(a) When the cortex decides to
perform a movement an impulse is
sent via the pyramidal tract to the
spinal motor neuron but, at the same
time, this instruction is also sent to
the cerebellum. (b) As soon as the
movement begins receptors in the
involved muscles and joints relay
information back to the cerebellum
concerning the rate and direction of
the movement.

14

(c)

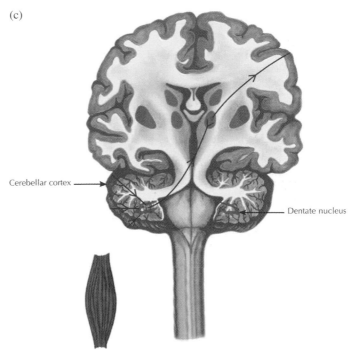

Cerebellar cortex —————→

Dentate nucleus ——

(d)

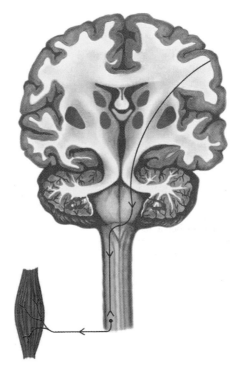

Fig. 1.1.10 continued
(c) The cerebellar cortex now
computes the error between the
instruction and the information
received about the first few
milliseconds of the movement.
A correction is calculated and relayed
back to the cortex via the cerebellar
dentate nucleus and thalamus.
(d) A revised instruction is now sent
from the motor cortex down the
pyramidal tract to the motor neurons
of the spinal cord. This monitoring and
correcting is carried out throughout
every tiny fraction of the movement
until the objective is achieved.

15

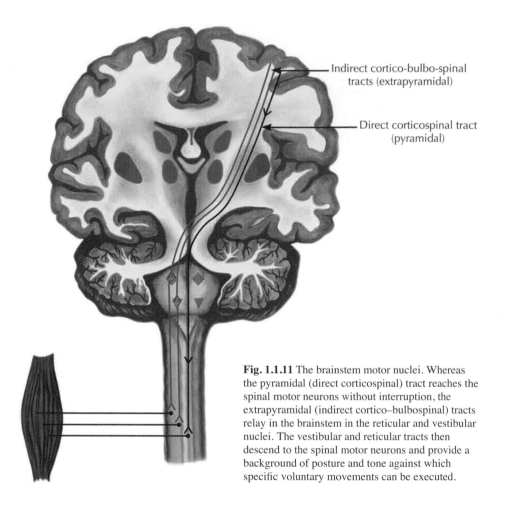

Indirect cortico-bulbo-spinal tracts (extrapyramidal)

Direct corticospinal tract (pyramidal)

Fig. 1.1.11 The brainstem motor nuclei. Whereas the pyramidal (direct corticospinal) tract reaches the spinal motor neurons without interruption, the extrapyramidal (indirect cortico–bulbospinal) tracts relay in the brainstem in the reticular and vestibular nuclei. The vestibular and reticular tracts then descend to the spinal motor neurons and provide a background of posture and tone against which specific voluntary movements can be executed.

innervate axial and proximal limb muscles while the lateral groups innervate distal limb muscles.

The spinal cord has its own intrinsic circuitry, which is best illustrated by the spinal reflex arc, also known as the stretch reflex (Fig. 1.1.12). The purpose of this reflex is to maintain a muscle at a given length. The muscle length is set for specific function and any stretch will set up a reflex to bring the muscle back to the desired length. Stretch is detected by muscle spindles within the skeletal muscle and an impulse is generated which travels to the spinal cord in the afferent or posterior nerve root. This afferent nerve fiber enters the spinal cord, where it synapses with the motor neuron, and an outgoing or efferent impulse then travels from the spinal cord via the motor or anterior root and the spinal nerve to the muscle. The muscle now contracts to return to the appropriate length. The muscle spindle afferent impulse is thus excitatory to the motor neuron. Although this stretch reflex is somewhat autonomous it is under the inhibitory influence of the upper motor neurons. Normal muscle tone is maintained by the balanced interaction between the excitatory muscle

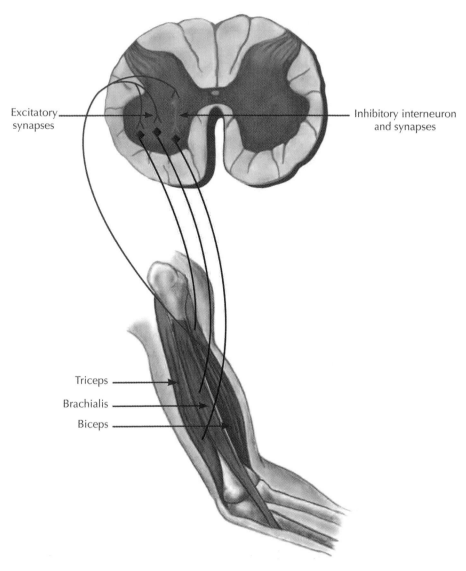

Excitatory synapses

Inhibitory interneuron and synapses

Triceps

Brachialis

Biceps

Fig. 1.1.12 Excitation and inhibition within the spinal-cord reflex. The purpose of this reflex is to maintain a muscle at a controlled length. The excitatory synapses bring about contraction in the two agonist muscles, the biceps and the brachialis, while the inhibitory synapses relax the antagonist muscle, the triceps.

spindle afferent and the inhibitory influence of the descending extrapyramidal tracts. If the upper motor neuron inhibition is reduced (by damage to upper motor neurons) velocity-dependent increases in the stretch reflex occur, producing spasticity and abnormal postures. Changes in posture are also associated with a rise in background muscle tone and, if sustained over time, may be a prelude to fixed contractures.

A muscle which brings about a movement at a joint is assisted by one or more muscles known as agonists, and opposed by one or more antagonist muscles. With flexion at the elbow, for example, when biceps is the primary muscle, brachialis would be the agonist assisting biceps while the triceps would be the antagonist. Muscle spindle afferents (neurons returning from the muscle) make connections not only with motor neurons that innervate the agonist but also with those innervating the antagonist muscles. The antagonist muscles are thereby inhibited – this is known as reciprocal inhibition – while the agonists are stimulated as part of reciprocal excitation.

Apart from the spinal reflex (discussed above), which is based on afferent input from the muscle spindle, there is another in which the afferent input is from the skin. This flexion or withdrawal response is induced by a painful cutaneous stimulus. The flexor muscles are activated to produce a withdrawal while the extensor muscles are inhibited. In the case of a painful stimulus to the foot, the hamstring muscles of the affected leg contract while the quadriceps relaxes so that the knee is flexed and the foot is lifted from the offending object. At the same time the reverse occurs in the opposite limb to maintain the upright posture.

The spinal cord also contains circuitry for certain intrinsic movement patterns (Pearson 1976, 2000). During walking and running a single limb passes through two phases: a stance phase during which the body is supported and propelled forward, and a swing phase during which the limb is advanced in order to repeat the propulsive part of the cycle (see Chapter 1.3). As the limbs move faster the timing of stance phase is decreased. In cats, if the spinal cord is transected in the thoracic region, rhythmic hindlimb movements can be elicited in the absence of corticospinal influence. If the animal is placed on a moving treadmill, the hindlimbs will begin moving with a characteristic walking pattern, which can be accelerated by increasing the speed of the treadmill. This indicates that there are central pattern generators in the spinal cord that control these basic motions (Grillner 1996).

Overview
Let us now put all these pieces together and follow the steps in the neural pathways that bring about a purposeful movement. You are about to pick up a cup of coffee and take a sip. Without your realizing it, your brain will quickly assess the size of the cup and how full it is. Does it have a handle? The size will determine how powerful the contraction will be. If it is very full, to avoid spilling the coffee, the movement of lifting will have to be performed smoothly. If the cup does not have a handle its outside temperature will influence how careful the initial contact will be. How far away is the cup and at what angle? Sight, smell, taste, temperature and weight assessment will be important to achieve your goal. All these subconscious assessments of the nature of the task contribute to what is referred to as 'anticipatory control'. Studies have shown that for hemiplegic children, use of the 'unimpaired hand' provides information about anticipatory control to the damaged hemisphere and hence to the 'impaired hand'. To this extent, practice with the 'good' hand contributes to improved use of the impaired hand (Gordon et al. 1999, Gordon and Duff 1999a, b).

The thoughts about drinking coffee will have occurred in your frontal and parietal lobes before being transferred to your supplementary motor area where the overall desire to pick up the cup and drink from it will be converted to a motor plan. The plan will now be refined in the premotor area in the frontal lobe and finally the specific motor neurons in the primary motor area in the precentral gyrus will be activated. During the preparation for this movement the basal ganglia will be brought into the planning. They will look at the intended goal and refer to memories of previous similar actions. They also will take into account time and space factors like the position of your trunk and arm and the exact site of the cup. Will you need to turn and, given the direction of the cup, how much will your shoulder need to be braced? Once all this information is computed, the motor cortex will be informed of the most efficient movement pattern to achieve the goal. The cortical motor control center will initially send an order to the brainstem motor nuclei (vestibular and reticular) to set up the appropriate background of posture and tone in the truncal and proximal limb muscles. This will be done through the corticobulbar and vestibulospinal and reticulospinal tracts (extrapyramidal) to the spinal motor neurons (medial anterior horn cells). The next step is to send instructions via the corticospinal (pyramidal) tracts to the spinal motor neurons (lateral anterior horn cells). Simultaneously, this exact set of instructions is relayed to the cerebellum where the muscles' performance will be carefully monitored. As soon as the muscles begin their contraction information is sent back to the cerebellum where the ongoing movement is compared with what was intended. The error is calculated and a proposed correction is forwarded to the cortical motor control centers. A revised command is now sent to the muscles via the upper and lower motor neurons. This constant shuttle of plans, commands, corrections, and revised commands continues until the goal is achieved. Experience of movement produces movement engrams that are immediately adaptable to most environments. It is only when conscious correction of those movements is required that the motor task is poorly performed and looks clumsy.

REFERENCES

Brinkman C, Porter R (1979) Supplementary motor area in the monkey: activity of neurons during performance of a learned motor task. *J Neurophysiol* **42**: 681–709.

Brinkman C, Porter R (1983) Supplementary motor area and premotor area of monkey cerebral cortex: functional organization and activities of single neurons during performance of a learned movement. *Adv Neurol* **39**: 393–420.

Brodal A (1981) *Neurological Anatomy in Relation to Clinical Medicine*. New York: Oxford University Press. p 294–317.

Deecke L, Scheid P, Kornhuber HH (1969) Distribution of readiness potential, pre-motion positivity, and motor potential of the human cerebral cortex preceding voluntary finger movements. *Exp Brain Res* **7**: 158–68.

Fried IKA, McCarthy G, Sass KJ, Williamson P (1991) Functional organization of human supplementary cortex studied by electrical stimulation. *J Neurosci* **11**: 3656–66.

Gordon AM, Charles J, Duff SV (1999) Fingertip forces during object manipulation in children with hemiplegic cerebral palsy. II: bilateral coordination. *Dev Med Child Neurol* **41**: 176–85.

Gordon AM, Duff SV (1999a) Fingertip forces during object manipulation in children with hemiplegic cerebral palsy. I: anticipatory scaling. *Dev Med Child Neurol* **41**: 166–75.

Gordon AM, Duff SV (1999b) Relation between clinical measures and fine manipulative control in children with hemiplegic cerebral palsy. *Dev Med Child Neurol* **41**: 586–91.

Grillner S (1996) Neural networks for vertebrate locomotion. *Scientific American* **247**: 64–9.

Grillner S, Hellgren J, Menard A, Saitoh K, Wikstrom MA (2005) Mechanisms for selection of basic motor programs – roles for the striatum and pallidum. *Trends Neurosci* **28**: 364–70.

Kornhuber HH, Deecke L (1985) The starting function of the supplementary motor area. *Behav Brain Sci* **8**: 591–2.

Lawrence DG, Kuypers HG (1968) The functional organization of the motor system in the monkey: 1. The effects of bilateral pyramidal lesions. *Brain* **91**: 1–14.

Pearson K (1976) The control of walking. *Sci Am* **235**: 72–86.

Pearson K (2000) Motor systems. *Curr Opin Neurobiol* **10**: 649–54.

Roland P, Lassen N, Skinhof E (1980) Supplementary motor area and other cortical areas in organization of voluntary movements in man. *Neurophysiol* **43**: 118–36.

Rossignol S, Dubuc R, Gossard JP (2006) Dynamic sensorimotor interactions in locomotion. *Physiol Rev* **86**: 89–154

Saitoh K, Menard A, Grillner S (2007) Tectal control of locomotion, steering and eye movements in lamprey. *J Neurophysiol* **97**: 3093–108.

Schreiber H, Lang M, Lang W, Kornhuber A, Heise B, Keidel M, Deecke L, Kornhuber HH (1983) Frontal hemispheric differences in the Bereitschaftspotential associated with writing and drawing. *Hum Neurobiol* **2**: 197–202.

1.2
MUSCULOSKELETAL GROWTH AND DEVELOPMENT

Steven E. Koop

At birth the muscles and bones of a child with cerebral palsy are like those of any child without a condition that intrinsically alters the formation of those tissues. Alterations of brain function characteristic of cerebral palsy include loss of selective motor control, abnormal muscle tone, imbalance of power between muscle agonists and antagonists, and impaired body balance mechanisms. When altered tone, power and control are imposed on the growing child's muscles and bones, the results may include reduced muscle elasticity, reduced joint range of motion, and disturbed bone and joint development. The previous chapter has described basic features of the brain and the means by which it controls locomotion. This chapter will review basic features of muscle and bone development and point to features relevant to children with cerebral palsy. When we discuss the pathophysiology of neuromuscular control in the next section, a fundamental concept will emerge: altered brain function leads to altered muscle activity and motor function which, in turn, influence the growth and development of the skeleton (Fig. 1.2.1).

Muscle

The basic element of skeletal muscle is the muscle fiber. Each muscle fiber is a mass of cytoplasm containing several nuclei enclosed in a membrane with no internal cell boundaries. Muscle fibers are supported by endomysium or supporting connective tissue. Groups or bundles of muscle fibers make up muscle fascicles, each surrounded by perimysium. Multiple groups of muscle fascicles, enclosed by enveloping epimysium, constitute a whole muscle (Fig. 1.2.2). The geometric arrangement of muscle fascicles is key to the contractile (and thus functional) properties of a muscle. Muscles may be formed by fascicles grouped in parallel, oblique (pennate), or tapering (fusiform or spindle) architecture.

One or more motor nerves control each skeletal muscle. Ultimately each muscle fiber receives innervation at a single point. A motor unit includes a single alpha motor neuron axon and all the muscle fibers it innervates. The muscle fibers of a motor unit may not be adjacent, and the number of muscle fibers in a motor unit and the number of motor units in a muscle are quite variable. A motor unit is activated (or stimulated to contract) by an electrical impulse that originates at the anterior horn cell and travels the length of the axon to the motor endplate or final point of contact with a muscle fiber. A Schwann cell specialized to facilitate the release of acetylcholine that is stored in vesicles at the nerve end covers the

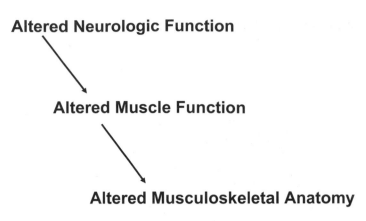

Altered Neurologic Function

Altered Muscle Function

Altered Musculoskeletal Anatomy

Fig. 1.2.1 The basic sequence of consequences of altered brain function in cerebral palsy.

end of the axon. The junctional area consists of closely interdigitated folds of axon and muscle fiber membranes. When the electrical impulse arrives at the terminal axon it permits the flow of calcium ions into the nerve cell and the increased calcium concentration prompts vesicles to fuse into the terminal membrane and release acetylcholine into the synaptic space. Acetylcholine binds to the muscle membrane and triggers depolarization of the membrane that spreads the length of the muscle fiber (known as an action potential) (Fig. 1.2.3).

The depolarization of muscle membrane reaches the interior of the fiber by a system of internal membranes. Calcium is stored along those membranes in sacs (sarcoplasmic reticula). Depolarization causes release of calcium into the muscle fiber cytoplasm and the calcium prompts chemical reactions between structural proteins that result in muscle shortening and force generation. The proteins are organized in repeating units of light and dark bands known as sarcomeres. The primary protein of the light or I-band is actin and the primary protein of the dark or A-band is myosin. The chemical reactions (which involve several other proteins) result in cross-bridges between actin and myosin that cause the thick filaments of the dark bands to slide past the thin filaments of the light bands. The sequence of muscle activation provides many points of intervention for a child with increased tone, particularly spasticity. Those interventions are described in subsequent chapters.

The immediate energy source for muscle contraction comes from the hydrolysis of adenosine triphosphate (ATP). ATP can be replenished through several mechanisms but the most efficient is the Krebs cycle. By this pathway one glucose molecule yields 38 ATP. If the intensity and duration of activity allows oxidative, or aerobic, processes to meet the energy requirements of the muscle then fatigue will be delayed. When activity is very intense or lengthy, muscle relies upon anaerobic chemical reactions to yield ATP. For example, glucose can be converted to lactic acid while yielding a small amount of energy (one glucose molecule yields two ATP). The lactic acid is later fully metabolized as energy sources are replenished at the end of exercise. The role of lactic acid as a muscle irritant that causes the soreness associated with sustained activity is debated. It is simplistic to assume muscle

Hierarchy of Skeletal Muscle Structure

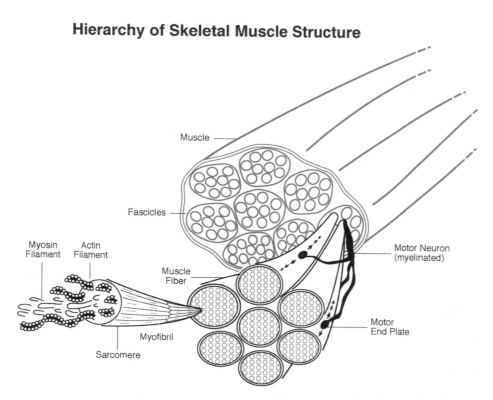

Fig. 1.2.2 The hierarchical structure of skeletal muscle. Muscle fascicles are composed of many muscle fibers. The motor unit consists of the motor neuron, the motor endplate and the muscle fibers innervated by the motor neuron. Each muscle fiber is composed of interdigitating contractile proteins, actin and myosin, structured as sarcomeres that are arranged in a series.

Neuromuscular Junction

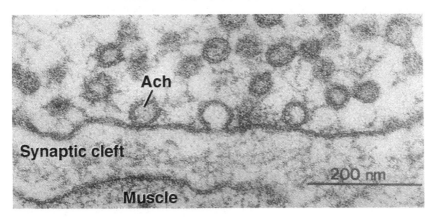

Fig. 1.2.3 An electromicrograph of the motor endplate and neuromuscular junction showing acetylcholine (Ach) vesicles fused with presynaptic membrane.

activity is sequential: utilization of available ATP comes first, followed by aerobic mechanisms, with anaerobic mechanisms last. Like any household that utilizes cash, savings, and short and long-term debt, muscle finds energy for activity by using all pathways according to circumstances.

Inappropriate muscle activation increases the use of energy resources. This is most commonly measured through quantification of oxygen utilization. Examples of inappropriate muscle activation include the increased tone of spasticity (and other tone disorders) and the increased activity of muscles coping with disturbed skeletal structures (such as joint contractures, bone torsions, and bad foot shapes). Oxygen utilization may serve as a marker of the effects of interventions in those areas.

There are different fiber types but all fibers of a single motor unit are of the same type. Fiber types have distinguishing structural and physiological features. Variations in the percentage of fiber types within a muscle are common and they are linked to the tasks of that muscle. Motor units and fiber types are recruited by the central nervous system according to size with the smallest motor units recruited first.

Muscle tension can occur passively or as the result of muscle activation. Passive muscle tension is increased as a muscle is stretched. Initial stretching yields little tension but as stretch increases the tension increases exponentially and can be many times greater than tension created by muscle activity. Excessive stretch causes muscle failure. Each muscle has an ideal length at which neurological stimulation results in maximum active muscle tension. As ideal length is approached and then passed the muscle tension or force that results from activation increases and then diminishes. Movement in the limbs of humans results from the application of tension or force to a point of muscle insertion on a bone on the opposite side of one or more joints crossed by the muscle. Torque equals the muscle force multiplied by the perpendicular distance from the line or vector of force application and the axis of rotation. Variations in torque are tied to variations in muscle force (amount activated, length at activation etc.) and variations in the moment arm or the perpendicular distance of force application.

Muscles increase in length during growth through increased tendon and muscle fiber length. While muscle lacks the discreet and specialized growth plate of immature long bones it appears that sarcomeres are added at the muscle-tendon junction. Growth in bone length and the stretching effects of everyday physical activity encourage the addition of sarcomeres and muscle length. It appears that an increase in the number of nuclei in the fibers, an increase in the number of satellite cells adjacent to muscle fibers, and hypertrophy of muscle fibers during infancy and childhood are all affected by stress that is transduced by a number of signaling molecules. Insulin-like growth factor (IGF) I and II are two of several important signaling molecules (Christ and Brand-Saberi 2002, Grefte et al. 2007).

Bone

The basic make-up of bone is 65% mineral and 35% organic. The organic component is 95% collagen (by dry weight) and 5% other proteins and proteoglycans. There are several types of collagen, but type I is the most common in bone. It is organized in fibrils with a periodicity of 64 nanometers in a quarter-stagger arrangement. Junctional areas represent sites for the deposition of hydroxyapatite crystals. The cells of bone include osteoblasts, osteocytes, and osteoclasts. Osteoblasts are cells of mesenchymal origin and are responsible for the majority of bone formation. Osteocytes are mature bone cells resident in bone lacunae and responsible for mineral homeostasis. Osteoclasts are multinucleated giant cells specialized in the breakdown of mineralized tissue.

Bone has important metabolic and mechanical functions. It serves as a calcium bank and is crucial to mineral homeostasis. Hematopoietic cells are resident within bone. Bone provides support for body segments and protection for vulnerable tissues (such as the brain, and the heart and lungs). In addition, bones serve as levers for body movement and provide origins and insertion points for muscles. Much of the content of later chapters in this book will address this bone function.

Bone formation and growth begin early in embryogenesis and continue until skeletal maturity. Bone formation continues after maturation as part of continuous remodeling of bone or as part of fracture healing. Intramembranous bone formation is the most primitive form of osteogenesis: bone trabeculae form directly with condensations of mesenchymal cells. Examples include the skull, maxilla, mandible, clavicle and scapula. Endochondral ossification is the most common bone formation of growth and development.

Condensations of mesenchymal cells act as a model for the future bone and are replaced by cartilage cells. Aging cartilage is vascularized and undergoes a primary mineralization. Osteoblasts form osteoid (unmineralized bone matrix) along the mineralized cartilage. Early mineralization of osteoid yields woven bone, immature bone that has not been organized in response to stress application. Remodeling yields lamellar bone, mature bone that has been formed and remodeled into stress-responsive layers.

Cortical bone is lamellar bone organized into osteons, cylindrical structures of layered bone organized around a central canal. The appearance of a saguaro cactus is an apt visual analogy. Cortical bone makes up the tubular walls of long bone and the outer shell of other bones. It comprises approximately 80% of skeletal mass. Cancellous, or trabecular, bone is organized into scaffold-like lattices. It makes up the ends of long bone and much of the inner structure of flat and cuboidal bones. It is often lamellar but lattices can be made of immature woven bone. Factors that affect the mechanical properties of bone include the geometry of bone (tubular, flat, cuboid), type of bone (woven or lamellar, cortical or cancellous, child or adult), and status of mineralization. Other factors include the rate and type of load application (compression, tension, bending and twisting).

Centers of ongoing bone formation by endochondral ossification exist in the bones of children. These are located near the ends of long bones as plate-like cartilage structures (physes or 'growth plates') or along the edges of flat bones (such as the apophyseal cartilage of the ilium). Articular cartilage in children may also be considered a type of 'growth plate'. Through ongoing endochondral bone formation at these sites, and intramembranous bone formation along bone surfaces, the skeleton of a child grows in size.

The growth of the body is commonly described by graphs that portray the progressive acquisition of stature and mass. A more pertinent graph for considering skeletal growth and the impact of stress application on bone portrays growth velocity. Such a graph demonstrates both speed of growth at a given age and growth potential (represented by the area remaining under the curve before skeletal maturity). Growth occurs in three phases. Between birth and approximately 3 years of age the speed of growth is extraordinary but it is steadily decelerating. From age 3 years to the onset of puberty, growth occurs at a slowly decelerating linear rate. At puberty (18 months later for males) growth velocity increases for 18–24 months, achieves a peak velocity, and then decreases until the skeleton is mature (Fig. 1.2.4).

Bone is affected by its mechanical environment, created by passive and active muscle tension, weight-bearing, and other forces. The mature skeleton responds according to Wolff's law, by which bone changes in response to mechanical stresses (Wolff 1896). The cellular and molecular means of this response remain poorly understood. The response of the immature skeleton to stress is even more complicated but key to understanding the skeletal problems of children with cerebral palsy. Three features of the immature skeleton are important: the presence of growth cartilage within bone, the relatively large amounts of cartilage tissue in epiphyses and periarticular areas (such as the acetabulum), and the structural characteristics of immature bone tissue. The contribution of these features is strongly affected by the growth potential that remains for a child. Examples of the consequences of these factors in children without cerebral palsy can be seen in fracture patterns (torus and greenstick fractures and growth plate injuries) and problems such as infantile hip instability and secondary dysplasia.

The Heuter–Volkmann principle states that (within physiological limits) compressive forces stimulate the growth of articular, epiphyseal, and/or physeal cartilage (Heuter 1862, Volkmann 1862). Atypical forces have different effects. Excessive compression forces suppress growth cartilage activity. Reduction of usual compressive forces has the opposite effect. Arkin and Katz (1956) showed that immature rabbit long bones subjected to bending or rotational stress will develop an angular or torsional deformity. These observations are fundamental to understanding the effects of delayed motor skills or the effects of increased and unbalanced muscle tone on a child's growing bones. Dr James Gage describes these bone growth principles in the following fashion for the orthopaedic residents who work at Gillette: 'What they are saying is that if you put a twist on a growing bone, it takes the twist, which is why the growing bone follows the *Star Wars* principle, "May the force be with you!" However, if you prefer the older literature, the words of Alexander Pope also apply: "Just as the twig is bent, the tree's inclin'd."'

An example of the immature skeleton's response to normal stress application is the resolution of fetal femoral anteversion. Anteversion is the term used to describe the shape of the femur in the coronal plane. If an anatomic specimen is placed on a tabletop, resting on the three points of the greater trochanter and the posterior aspect of the femoral condyles, the line segment representing the femoral neck is inclined above the plane of the table. At birth an infant has approximately 45° of anteversion. As the central nervous system matures a child progresses through the developmental milestones of crawling, standing, and walking. The growth-responsive proximal femur is subjected to stresses applied by the anterior hip capsule and the stresses of weight bearing and muscle activity during walking. Anteversion decreases rapidly in the first three to four years of life and shows further resolution until puberty. This pattern of torsion resolution follows the growth potential described by the three phases of the growth-velocity graph.

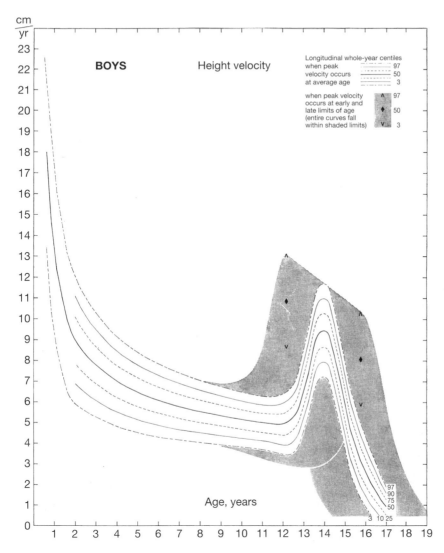

Fig. 1.2.4 The phases of skeletal development of a child as portrayed by the growth velocity of increasing stature.

The pertinence of the relationship between muscle activity and skeletal growth potential is found in the musculoskeletal problems of cerebral palsy. Altered central nervous system function, often resulting in increased and unbalanced muscle tone, sets off a cascade of bone and muscle responses leading to problems familiar to every clinician. Muscle architecture can change with alterations in muscle use associated with spasticity. Muscle cells in children with cerebral palsy demonstrate decreased resting sarcomere length and nearly a doubling of the modulus of elasticity when compared to other children. The resulting loss of elasticity or 'stiffness' combines with altered spontaneous limb movement (part of disturbed motor milestones) to reduce muscle length and limit joint motion (contracture) (Lieber and Friden 2000, Christ and Brand-Saberi 2002, Friden and Lieber 2003, Tidball 2005). The bones to which the muscles are attached change their growth. Infantile bone shapes, which would be expected to change with the emergence of normal motor skills, fail to resolve. The femur is an example of this. Infantile femoral anteversion fails to resolve and may increase in the presence of persistent medial hip rotation. Some bones develop torsions under the persistent influence of increased muscle tone or torsional stresses. The tibia is an example of this, often developing internal or external torsion (see Chapter 5.6). Other examples include tarsal bones, particularly the calcaneus (see Chapter 3.2). Lastly, the joints bridged by the altered muscles are affected. Persistent imbalance of muscle activity can lead to bone dysplasia, subluxation and dislocation. Altered bone shapes change the effect of muscles, leading to lever arm dysfunction, which will be discussed more completely in Chapter 2.3 (Fig. 1.2.5).

Because the hip joint (femur and pelvis and associated muscles) has such a prominent place in the musculoskeletal problems of cerebral palsy it will be described in more detail. At birth an infant's hip range of motion reflects its position in utero. The hip is flexed, abducted, and externally rotated. The femur has anteversion of approximately 40°. With typical brain function the infant moves through motor milestones that reflect increasingly sophisticated muscle control. Crawling and walking promote extension and internal rotation of the hip and the stresses of muscle activity and body mass are applied to the femur. The infantile hip flexion contracture disappears and internal rotation increases. Anteversion

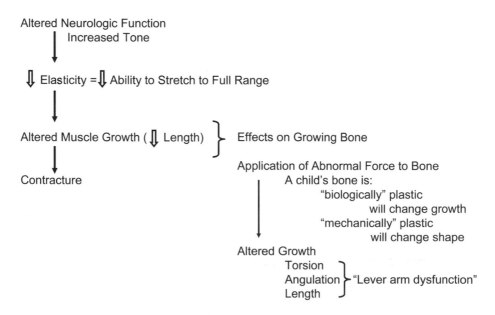

Fig. 1.2.5 The cascade of muscle and bone consequences that follow altered brain function in cerebral palsy.

decreases in response to stresses applied to the proximal femur by the anterior hip capsule during extension (Somerville 1957). Muscles, ligaments, ground reaction forces and limb segment masses combine to create the net joint reaction force that, during growth and development, is the key factor in the ultimate structure of the hip joint.

Altered motor function in cerebral palsy leads to a different outcome for the hip. Increased muscle tone and altered milestones lead to reduced muscle elasticity, decreased muscle growth, and failure to resolve the normal infant hip flexion contracture. Because spasticity seems to affect hip adductors and flexors more than abductors and extensors the muscle changes of cerebral palsy result in atypical, unbalanced application of stress to the femoral head and acetabulum. Infantile anteversion fails to resolve or actually increases. Anteversion is associated with coxa valga, which further reduces the mechanical effect of the hip abductors. The lateral portion of the acetabulum experiences increased compression stress and displays reduced growth (seen as an increased acetabular angle in radiographs). Simultaneously the medial portion of the femoral head experiences compression stresses that inhibit growth and lead to a loss of sphericity. The femoral begins to lose contact with the medial wall of the acetabulum, which thickens because of a loss of compression stresses. Ultimately the femoral head may dislocate and its articular surface deteriorate (Figs 1.2.6, 7).

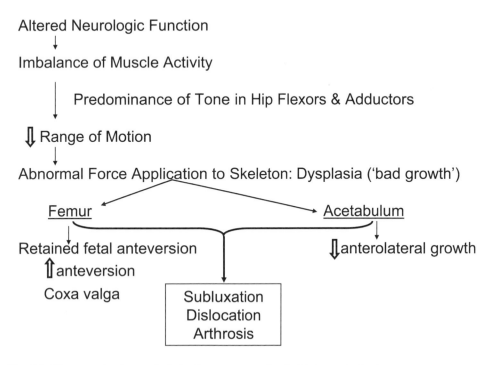

Fig. 1.2.6 The cascade of musculoskeletal consequences for the hip in cerebral palsy.

29

Fig. 1.2.7 The evolution of hip dysplasia in cerebral palsy.

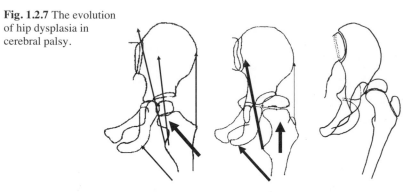

Normal   **Cerebral Palsy**

Understanding this cascade and accurately placing a child in the sequence of events will assist in formulating a treatment plan. Tone reduction has a primary place in all treatment strategies because of the impact of increased tone (particularly spasticity) on bone growth. The method of tone reduction will vary with the nature of the central nervous system problems and the age of the child. Systemic medications, intramuscular and intrathecal medications, and selective dorsal lumbar rhizotomy, all have a role in the right circumstance. Early spasticity reduction will minimize bone and joint problems. Spasticity that persists into the juvenile years may require simultaneous plans to reduce the spasticity and address the bone and joint dysplasias that have evolved (and which will not improve spontaneously due to reduced remaining growth potential). Bone interventions to restore joints and the lever functions of the skeleton are key to the best functional outcomes. But we have learned that persistent tone in the presence of growth will be followed by recurrent bone deformity that will erode early functional gains after skeletal procedures and, perhaps, necessitate secondary bone surgeries.

REFERENCES

Arkin AM, Katz JF (1956) The effects of pressure on epiphyseal growth; the mechanism of plasticity of growing bone. *J Bone Joint Surg* **38A**: 1056–76.
Christ B, Brand-Saberi B (2002) Limb muscle development. *Int J Dev Biol* **46**: 905–14.
Friden J, Lieber RL (2003) Spastic muscle cells are shorter and stiffer than normal cells. *Muscle Nerve* **27**: 157–64.
Grefte S, Kuijpers-Jagtman MM, Torensma R, Von den Hoff JW (2007) Skeletal muscle development and regeneration. *Stem Cells Dev* **16**: 857–68.
Heuter C (1862) Anatomische Studien an den extremitatengelenken Neugeborener und Erwachsener. *Virchows Archiv* **25**: 572–99.
Lieber RL, Friden J (2000) Functional and clinical significance of skeletal muscle Architecture. *Muscle Nerve* **23**: 1647–66.
Somerville EW (1957) Persistent foetal alignment of the hip. *J Bone Joint Surg* **39B**: 106–13.
Tidball JG (2005) Mechanical signal transduction in skeletal muscle growth and adaptation. *J App Physiol* **98**: 1900–8.
Volkmann R (1862) Chirurgische Erfahrungen uber Knochenverbiegungen und Knochenwachsthum. *Arch Pathol Anat* **24**: 512–40.
Wolff J (1896) *The Law of Bone Remodeling*. Berlin, Heidelberg, New York: Springer. (Translation of 1892 German edn.)

1.3
NORMAL GAIT

James R. Gage and Michael H. Schwartz

Locomotion is an important animal trait. Quadrupeds are inherently fast and stable. Their center of mass is located just under the trunk, inside the base of support. A long stride is possible because the body is interposed between the front and back limbs. In fast running animals such as cougars, the flexors and extensors of the vertebral column are actually used to augment stride length and power. Thus when galloping, the back is rolled into flexion as the animal brings the hindlimbs past the planted forelimbs. Once weight is transferred to the hindlimbs, the spine and hips are powerfully extended as the shoulders flex to swing the forelimbs far forward in preparation for contact (Fig. 1.3.1).

Humans employ bipedal gait that is less efficient and less stable than quadrupedal gait. Bipeds are unstable because their center of mass is located above their base of support. In the human, the center of mass is located just in front of the S2 vertebra. In order to remain upright, the center of mass must be maintained in balance over the base of support. Since this is more easily obtained in quadrupeds, it may be one of the reasons why ambulation is delayed for a significant period after birth in bipeds as opposed to quadrupeds. In addition, speed and stride length are constrained by the fact that the trunk musculature is not used as extensively in gait and the body is not interposed between the limbs in the line of progression. In fact, however, pelvic rotation is used to partially interpose the pelvic width into the line of progression during gait. Bipedal gait does have the significant advantage of freeing the upper extremities for other use (Fig. 1.3.2).

Gait is a complex activity. It requires (1) a control system, (2) an energy source, (3) levers providing movement, and (4) forces to move the levers.

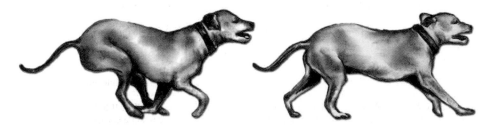

Fig. 1.3.1 A dog uses the power of its spinal extensors when running, and its center of gravity is located inside its base of support.

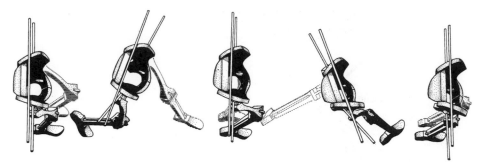

Fig. 1.3.2 Pelvic rotation in human gait. Although not as efficient as quadrupedal gait, bipedal gait does have the significant advantage of freeing the upper extremities for other use. This is an illustration of the transverse rotations of the pelvis, lower extremities, and feet. Small sticks have been attached to the pelvis and femurs and the actual rotations amplified threefold to emphasize that the lower extremities rotate through a greater range than the pelvis. Notice that the pelvis rotates with and acts to elongate the swinging limb, thus allowing a longer stride than would otherwise be possible. (From Inman et al. 1981, by permission.)

The control system

Central nervous system control of locomotion has been covered in detail in Chapter 1.1. Control of locomotion is initiated from the pyramidal region of the motor cortex, and the controlling system needs to have complete integration of sensory and motor function if it is to perform properly. Furthermore, the complexity of the central locomotor control system requires interaction between several other brain regions and the spinal cord in what could best be described as a pyramidal hierarchy. This hierarchical system of motor control begins with the cerebral cortex and ends with the final common pathway (the motor neuron) (Fig. 1.3.3). The components of this system include (1) the motor cortex, (2) the basal ganglia, (3) the thalamus and hypothalamus, (4) the midbrain, (5) the cerebellum, and (6) the brainstem and spinal cord.

The energy source

Energy is required for walking. Since this ultimately depends on the delivery of metabolic fuel and oxygen to the muscles by the cardiovascular system and the oxidation of that fuel in the muscles, energy production and utilization have a finite limit. We measure that limit by a parameter known as the VO_2 max. This is defined as the rate of oxygen usage (liters/minute) under maximal aerobic metabolism. For short-term metabolic debt we can depend on anaerobic glycolysis, but for sustained activity locomotion must be carried out aerobically, i.e. without oxygen debt. As such, energy conservation is critical to normal performance. Therefore speed and distance traveled are dependent upon (1) the rate of energy production and transport to the muscles (VO_2 max), and (2) the extent to which energy is conserved. Conservation of energy is a major problem in individuals with neuromuscular disorders such as cerebral palsy.

THE CONTROL SYSTEM
FOR LOCOMOTION

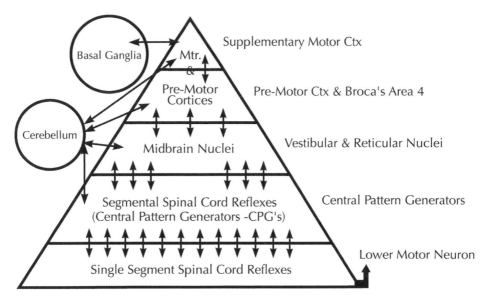

Fig. 1.3.3 The hierarchical system of motor control. Motor control is extremely complex. Motion is initiated in the supplementary motor cortex; but in order for a coordinated movement to occur, many other circuits in the basal ganglia, cerebellum and spinal cord need to be involved (see Chapter 1.1). Ctx, cortex.

The levers

Movement of the body is generated by moments. A moment is a force couple, which is defined as force acting on a lever about an axis of rotation, which produces an angular acceleration about that axis. Moments arise from the effects of two components: (1) a force, and (2) a lever-arm. Moments will be discussed in detail when we come to pathological gait (Chapter 2.4)

The forces

Our muscles are the physiologic motors that generate the forces that allow us to move. In so doing they produce internal moments around the joint centers. However, when we stand or perform any activity in which our muscles resist the force of gravity, ground reaction and/or inertial forces are created. These forces, which are external to the body, also act on skeletal levers to produce external joint moments. Walking then is a trade-off between the internal moments generated by the muscles and the external moments generated by the ground reaction and inertial forces (Fig. 1.3.4).

Muscles and their function were discussed in Chapter 1.2. They are well designed for function with respect to their shape, internal architecture, power, endurance, speed, and type of contraction.

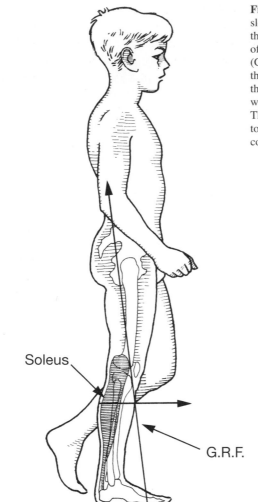

Fig. 1.3.4 Mid-stance. By using the soleus to slow the forward momentum of the shank, the ground reaction force is brought in front of the knee. The ground reaction force (GRF) acting on the lever arm of the foot thereby generates an extension moment on the knee that provides the needed stability without the necessity of other muscle action. This extension moment is generally referred to as a 'plantarflexion/knee extension couple'.

Soleus

G.R.F.

Muscle power relates primarily to its cross-sectional area and secondarily to factors such as pennate structure, fiber type, and degree of fatigue. Muscle power, which is computed as force times contractile velocity, is optimal when the muscle is contracting at about one-third of its maximal velocity (Lieber 1986).

A muscle's pennate structure also determines its power and range since the pennates function as internal levers within the muscle. Isometric stabilizers such as the gluteus medius have relatively horizontal pennates within their structure, which act to greatly amplify the muscles' force production at the expense of speed and range of motion (Rab 1994).

As a child grows, muscle strength and overall body mass both increase. Since muscle power is related to cross sectional area, it can be estimated by multiplying π times the square

34

of the muscle's radius. It is equal to roughly 16–30 Newtons per square centimeter of cross-sectional area. However, weight or mass is a function of volume, which is cubic. For example, the mass of a cubic volume of water which measures 2 cm on a side would be 2 × 2 × 2 = 8 cubic centimeters × density of water. The implication of this is that as a child grows, her/his mass increases as a function of the cube, but strength increases only as a function of the square. In other words, young children are relatively Herculean for their weight, i.e. they have a much greater power-to-mass ratio than adults.

A muscle's tension also affects its power. Studies have shown that if a muscle is stretched just prior to contraction it will contract with greater power (Cavagna et al. 1968, Vredenbregt and Rau 1973, McClay et al. 1990). It is interesting to note that during normal gait, inertial and/or ground reaction forces stretch most of the major muscle groups of the lower extremity muscles just prior to the onset of their contraction. The hamstrings in terminal swing are just one example of this.

Muscle forces can be much more easily understood if we always picture them as moment generators. As stated previously, muscles produce internal moments that resist the external ground reaction and/or inertial forces. In every case, the lever arm upon which the muscle is acting is the bone and the axis about which it is acting is the joint center. If the muscle is acting perpendicular to the axis of rotation, the moment of force produced is always equal to the muscle force times its distance from the axis of joint rotation (Fig. 1.3.5).

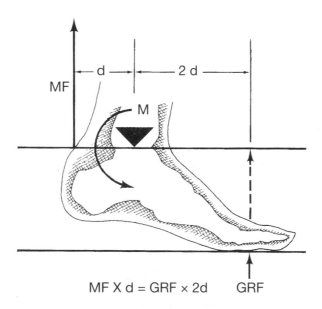

MF X d = GRF × 2d   GRF

Fig. 1.3.5 The relationship between the external moment produced by the ground reaction force (GRF) and the internal moment (MF = muscle force) produced by the muscles. In each case they act on a skeletal lever (d and 2d) and their fulcrum is the joint center. Since the lever arm of the GRF is twice as long as that of the muscles (MF), its magnitude is only half as much: d (MF) = 2d (GRF) and dividing through by d: MF = 2 (GRF), where d is the moment arm of the MF.

35

As a simple example of force moments, think of two children on a teeter-totter (see-saw). Each child is creating a moment around the axle to which the teeter-totter is attached, and since the moments are in opposite directions, they are tending to balance each other (Fig. 1.3.6). A lighter child can balance a heavier one so long as she sits further from the center of the teeter-totter because she has a 'mechanical advantage'. In the same way, the length of the lever arm on which a muscle is acting is frequently spoken of as its 'mechanical advantage'. Inman et al. (1981) pointed out that particular joint positions are assumed in daily activities because they allow the maximum moment for the muscles acting on that joint. Because muscles can exert maximum power at only one fiber length the skeleton has provided certain compensatory mechanisms:

1. As the muscle shortens and becomes weaker, the effective lever arm of the muscle lengthens. Since the magnitude of a moment is given as force $\times$ distance, the effect of this phenomenon is to produce a moment with a relatively constant magnitude. Quadriceps action at the knee is an example of this since the patella acts to amplify knee motion in mid-range where the muscle has a strong mechanical advantage, but not in terminal extension where the muscle is working near end-range (Fig. 1.3.7).
2. A muscle that passes over two joints can be maintained at a favorable resting length by simultaneous and related movements of the other joint over which the muscle passes. For example, the hamstrings in sitting undergo little change in length since the hip and knee are flexing simultaneously with elongation at the former joint and shortening at the latter.

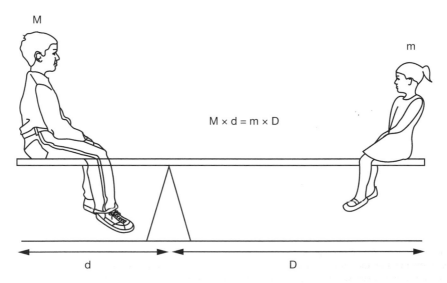

Fig. 1.3.6 The relationship between an older boy and a young girl on a teeter-totter is exactly the same as that of the muscle and the ground reaction forces at each of the lower extremity joints. The pivot point or fulcrum is always the joint center. M, boy's weight in Newtons; d, his lever arm (distance to the fulcrum) in meters; m, girl's weight in Newtons; D = her lever arm (distance to the fulcrum) in meters.

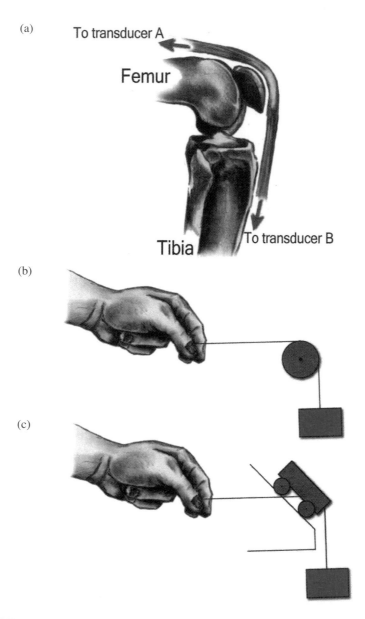

(a)

To transducer A

Femur

To transducer B

Tibia

(b)

(c)

Fig. 1.3.7 Diagram showing how the motion of the patella affects the excursion of the knee.
(a) Schematic drawing of the knee joint; (b) rope running over a fixed pulley; (c) model that
magnifies movement by the same principle as the patellar–femoral joint. In (b) for every 1 cm
movement of the hand there will be 1 cm of movement of the weight, whereas in (c) for every 1 cm
of movement of the hand there will be 2 cm of movement of the weight because as the rope is pulled,
the cart will move up the incline. Consequently the force exerted by the hand must be twice the that
of the weight, because the work (force $\times$ distance) done on the weight cannot be more than the work
done by the hand (Adapted from Alexander 1992, by kind permission of Professor R. McNeill
Alexander.)

Types of muscle contraction

Muscles work in one of three modes.

1. Concentric contraction (shortening contraction), in which the muscle does positive work. All accelerators work in this mode. The iliopsoas acting in pre-swing and initial swing is an example of this type of contraction.
2. Eccentric or lengthening contraction, in which the muscle does negative work. All decelerators and/or shock absorbers work in this mode. Alexander (1992) cites studies that indicate that the efficiency of negative work by a muscle is greater than that of positive work (Rab 1994). The energy efficiency of negative work may be part of the explanation as to why it is the most frequent type of contraction in normal gait. The soleus contracting in mid-stance is an example of this type of contraction.
3. Isometric contraction, in which the muscle length is static. Stabilizers work in this mode. Most of these are postural, antigravity muscles. The gluteus medius during the period of single limb support is an example of this type of contraction.

Assessing muscle function with electromyography

The electrical activity , which can be measured through the skin or by indwelling fine-wire electrodes, indicates motor-unit activation and provides an indirect indicator of muscle function. The use of EMG for clinical gait analysis interpretation varies from one laboratory to another, but plays an important role. The goal of interpretation is often centered on determining: (1) the timing of muscle action (including coordination with kinetic moment graphs), (2) evidence of spasticity and other types of hypertonia, (3) evidence of selective motor control and muscle coordination, and (4) information on individual muscles via fine-wire techniques to assess whether a muscle is appropriate for surgical transfer. EMG can also be used to assess muscle fatigue (by frequency analysis and determination of the ability to sustain recruitment) and relative intensity by changes of amplitude within a muscle, but not actual force.

The EMG signal represents the activation of multiple motor units within the detection area of an electrode. Each signal contains two types of information that are important in gait: timing of muscular action and relative intensity. The amplitude of the signal reflects the total number of motor units firing and the rate the motor units are firing. Differences of amplitude within a single muscle represent changes in the recruitment of motor units, the rate motor units are recruited, rate the motor units are firing, and/or the type of motor units recruited. Because muscle force is proportional to the number of motor units recruited and the rate of firing, a muscle generating increased force may exhibit an increased amplitude. However, as noted earlier, the type and speed of muscle contraction and fiber length determined by joint position also directly define the force the muscle fibers can produce. These changes can occur without a change in the number or rate of firing of active motor units which is the content of the EMG signal. In addition, the muscle force used for a particular torque varies with the lever arm available at each joint position. Dynamic EMG therefore identifies the amount of muscular effort, but does not indicate the actual muscle force associated with that effort (Perry 1992, pp. 381–411).

Meaningful comparisons between muscles within a subject or between subjects require normalization and quantification. Normalization provides a common frame of reference relative to variables such as time or effort of contraction and removes electrode sampling differences. Quantification transforms the amplitude into numerical values. Normalization to the gait cycle is likely the single most common normalization for EMG in gait analysis. Additional normalization and quantification schemes are used when the raw signal is rectified or integrated for comparison across subjects and often include normalization to a dynamic maximum (Fig. 1.3.8) (Winter 1984, Yang and Winter. 1984, den Otter et al.

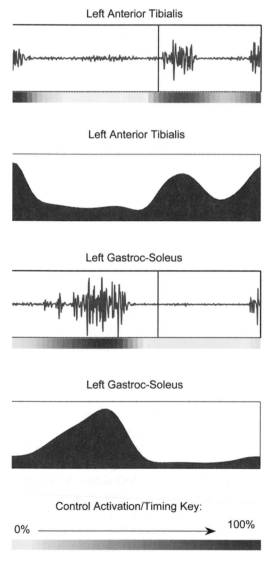

Fig. 1.3.8 Muscle activity. Surface EMG signals: example of dynamic EMG of the tibialis anterior and gastrocnemius of a patient. In this illustration, the EMG signal of the patient is presented as a raw EMG signal, and a rectified smoothed EMG of the normal (or typical EMG) for that particular muscle is shown under it. In the Gillette Motion Analysis Laboratory, rather than printing out the rectified smoothed EMG, the patient's EMG is presented in raw form with the 'normal' or typical EMG for most walkers presented as a control bar underneath the raw signal. The bottom bar demonstrates the control activation timing key, in which absence of activity is indicated by yellow and strong activity of a muscle indicated in red.

39

2004, Schwartz et al. 2008). For interpretation of an EMG profile for an individual patient it is important to understand the techniques used for data collection and processing (type of electrodes, methods of normalization and quantification).

The prerequisites of normal gait

Normal gait has five attributes or prerequisites that are frequently lost in pathological gait (Perry 1985). These are (1) stability in stance, (2) sufficient foot clearance during swing, (3) appropriate swing phase pre-positioning of the foot, (4) an adequate step length, and (5) energy conservation.

Stability in stance is challenged by two major factors: (1) the body is top-heavy, such that the center of mass lies above the base of support, just in front of the S2 vertebra; and (2) walking continually alters segment alignment. As an individual walks, the center of mass (CoM), which remains within the base of support while standing, moves forward with each step from one base of support to another. This means that the body must constantly alter the position of the trunk in space in order to maintain balance over the base of support and/or to maintain balance when moving.

Therefore stability in stance involves much more than a stable foot. In addition to having the stance foot stable on the floor, the major lower-extremity joints must function to (1) allow advancement of the limb in swing, (2) maintain balance, (3) provide propulsion, and (4) ensure appropriate position of the structures above.

Clearance in swing requires (1) appropriate position and power of the ankle, knee and hip on the stance side; (2) adequate ankle dorsiflexion, knee flexion and hip flexion on the swing side; (3) stability of the stance foot; and (4) adequate body balance.

Pre-position of the foot in terminal swing necessitates (1) appropriate body balance; (2) stability, power and proper position on the stance side; and (3) adequate ankle dorsiflexion, balance between inverters and everters of the foot, appropriate knee position, and proper foot position.

An adequate step-length demands that there is (1) adequate body balance; (2) a stable and properly positioned stance side; (3) adequate hip flexion and knee extension on the swing side; and (4) neutral dorsiflexion, inversion and eversion of the foot on the swing side.

Finally, *energy conservation* requires that when possible (1) joint stability is provided by the ground reaction force (GRF) in conjunction with ligaments instead of muscles; (2) the center of mass excursion is minimized in all planes; and (3) muscle forces are optimized. Optimizing muscle forces involves the following:

- eccentric muscle forces (as opposed to concentric) are used to the greatest extent possible during gait
- 'stretch energy' in tendons and muscles is returned as kinetic energy, since in normal gait muscles tend to be 'pre-stretched' before they fire concentrically
- biarticular muscles serve to transfer energy from one segment to another
- walking is accomplished in a manner that minimizes the forces in our muscles (Alexander 1992).

Development of normal gait

In a toddler, ambulation begins without these prerequisites. Initially, the knees are relatively stiff and the child walks with a wide base of support. Gradually, as the toddler develops balance and equilibrium, gait evolves toward the adult pattern. Sutherland et al. (1980, 1988) pointed out that although walking usually starts at about one year of age, children do not develop an adult, heel-toe gait until at least 3½ years of age. The problem is that as the child matures, central nervous system development and musculoskeletal growth progress in tandem; so how do you separate their effects? Scaling step-length, cadence, step-width, and single-limb stance as dimensionless variables solves this problem (Hof 1996). Hof (1996) and Vaughan (2003) have both concluded that these dimensionless gait parameters are invariant after 80 months of age.

A number of authors have studied energy expenditure as a function of walking speed and found that if the curve of energy cost is plotted on the ordinate versus speed on the abscissa, the curve is parabolic. As such it exhibits a minimum value at a particular speed (Fig. 1.3.9) (Rose et al. 1994). Ralston (1958) is credited with the hypothesis that if a person is allowed to walk at her/his natural rate, s/he will select a speed that allows minimum

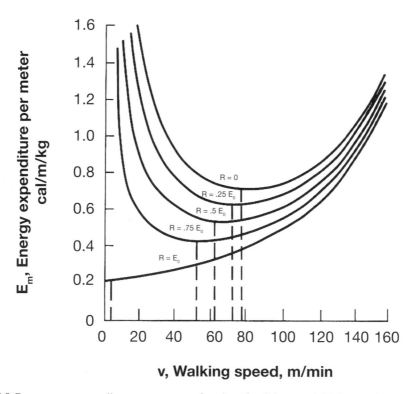

Fig. 1.3.9 Gross energy expenditure per meter as a function of walking speed (V) for a typical subject walking naturally at different speeds. The lower curves show that as increasing amounts of energy (R) are subtracted from the gross energy expenditure per minute, the optimal speed corresponding to minimal E_m becomes smaller and smaller. (From Rose et al. 1991, by permission.)

41

energy expenditure. Corcoran and Brengelmann (1970) later confirmed this. Winter (1991) noted that with increasing linear velocity, the angular velocities of the hip, knee, and ankle increase in nearly identical proportions. In addition, he noted that the timing of the power patterns during the gait cycle is identical at all walking speeds, and only the gain increases with cadence. Both these observations give evidence to a finely tuned proprioceptive feedback system. The other inference which can be drawn from Ralston's (1958) hypothesis is that any deviation of gait from the norm will interfere with this mechanism and therefore increase energy cost.

The gait cycle

A complete gait cycle or stride begins when one foot strikes the ground and ends when the same foot strikes the ground again.

Temporal Gait Measurements

Further characterization of the gait cycle can be done with temporal measurements such as walking velocity, cadence, step-length, and stride-length. Step-length is defined as the longitudinal distance between the two feet. Thus the right step-length is measured from the point of contact of the trailing left foot to the point of contact of the right foot. One stride-length is the distance covered during a complete gait cycle and represents the sum of the right and left step-lengths. That is, stride length extends from the initial contact of one foot to the following initial contact of the same foot. Walking velocity is equal to step-length × cadence.

Elements of the Gait Cycle

Stance

The gait cycle can be described according to phases, tasks and periods (Perry 1992, pp. 1–19). The cycle is divided into two major phases, *stance* and *swing*. Within these phases it is possible to further subdivide stance into the instant of initial contact (IC), followed by the periods of loading response (LR), mid-stance (MSt), terminal-stance (TSt), pre-swing (PSw), and concluding with the instant of foot-off (FO) (Fig. 1.3.10). Similarly, swing can be subdivided into initial swing (ISw), mid-swing (MSw), and terminal-swing (TSw). Using this scheme, the three tasks that must be accomplished during the cycle are weight acceptance, single limb support, and limb advancement. Weight acceptance occurs during IC and LR, single limb support during the MSt and TSt, and limb advancement during PSw, ISw, MSw, and TSw (Fig. 1.3.11).

During normal walking, foot-off occurs at approximately 60% of the cycle. Therefore stance represents approximately 60% of the gait cycle and swing 40%. Opposite FO and opposite IC occur at approximately 10% and 50% of the cycle respectively. This means that during walking there are two periods of 'double support' when both feet are on the ground, and that each of these periods constitutes about 10% of the cycle. The first double-support period occurs immediately after initial contact and the second just prior to foot-off. Loading response is a period of deceleration when the shock of impact is absorbed. The initial double-support period is followed by a period of single support, comprising about 40% of the cycle.

42

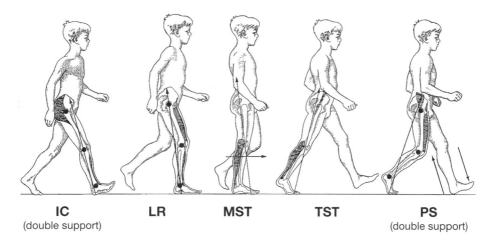

IC   **LR**   **MST**   **TST**   **PS**

(double support)   (double support)

Fig. 1.3.10 The stance phase of gait. Stance phase constitutes roughly 60% of the cycle and is divided into five subphases: initial contact (IC), loading response (LR), mid-stance (MST), terminal stance (TST), and pre-swing (PS).

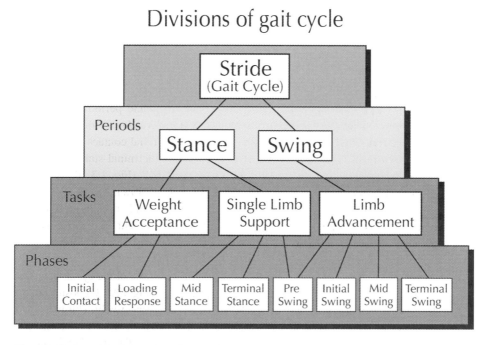

Fig. 1.3.11 The gait cycle consists of one stride, which is subdivided into two periods, stance and swing. The tasks that must be accomplished during a single cycle include weight acceptance, single-limb support, and limb advancement. These occur during the phases shown in the bottom row. (From Perry 1992, by permission.)

43

During this period, the opposite limb is going through its swing phase. Thus in walking, single support on the stance side must be equal to the period of swing of the opposite limb. In late stance there is a second period of double support called pre-swing which begins at approximately 50% of the gait cycle and lasts until foot-off on the stance side. Therefore loading response is equivalent in time and is, in fact, the same event as pre-swing on the opposite side.

Since normal gait is symmetrical, it is important to remember these relationships in order to form a mental picture of where the opposite limb is in the cycle. The period of single support can be subdivided into mid-stance and terminal stance. During mid-stance, the body's center of mass is climbing to its zenith, and passes over the base of support. In terminal stance the center of mass has passed in front of the base of support and is accelerating as it falls forward and toward the unsupported side. During this period of acceleration an amount of energy equivalent to that lost earlier in the gait cycle must be added back into the cycle if steady-state walking is to be maintained. Notice that in walking the activity of muscles tends to be concentrated at the beginning and end of the swing and stance phases, since one of their principal actions seem to be to redirect the body's center of mass during the periods of double support (Fig. 1.3.12) (Vaughan 2003, Kuo 2007).

Swing
Swing phase constitutes about 40% of the gait cycle. The purpose of swing is to (1) advance the limb, (2) provide foot clearance, (3) allow variation in cadence, and (4) conserve energy.

During swing phase, the limb behaves like a compound pendulum. As a result, our speed and cadence depend largely on the mass distribution of the shank (Hicks et al. 1985, Tashman et al. 1985) (Fig. 1.3.13). That is, we tend to select a walking speed at which our limb swings with only a small amount of extraneous muscle action. If the period of the swinging leg could not be altered, variation of cadence during gait would be impossible. In order to accelerate cadence, the swinging compound pendulum must be accelerated early in swing and then decelerated in the latter part of swing. Thus swing must consist of three periods: a period in which the rate of swing is increasing (ISw), a transition period (MSw), and a final period in which the rate of swing is decreased (TSw) (Fig. 1.3.14).

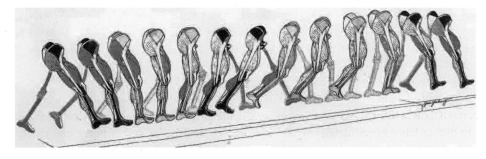

Fig. 1.3.12 A schematic of the complete gait cycle. Muscle activity is denoted by the intensity of color. Note that most of the muscles are active at the beginning and end of swing and stance phases. (From Inman et al. 1981, by permission.)

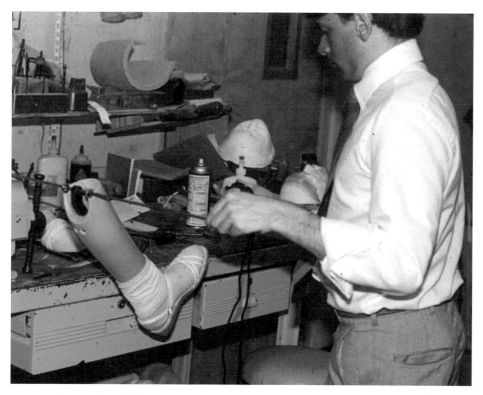

Fig. 1.3.13 A simple experiment that can be done using an above-knee prosthesis with a single-axis knee. The leg acts like a pendulum and its period is dictated by its mass moment of inertia. Since the lower-extremity functions as a compound pendulum in gait, the period of the pendulum (in this case the shank) will be equal to the cadence of the individual to whom it belongs. Given that the cadence of swing is usually found to be much lower than normal in these experiments, a strong argument could be made to bring the mass moment of inertia closer to the fulcrum by minimizing the weight distally and/or adding weight proximally.

Running is differentiated from walking by the fact that the two periods of 'double support' are replaced by two periods of 'double float' when neither foot is on the ground. To accommodate the periods of 'double float' during running, the period of time spent in stance must always be shorter than the time spent in swing (Fig. 1.3.15 a, b).

COMPONENTS OF THE GAIT CYCLE

As mentioned earlier, the stance phase of walking can be broken down into five separate parts (IC, LR, MSt, TSt, PSw) and swing phase into three (ISw, MSw, TSw). Each of these sub-phases has a specific purpose and is marked by particular events in the gait cycle. Consequently, we now need to spend a bit of time looking at the purpose and mechanism of each of these periods.

There is a coordinated flow of muscle activity in normal walking during stance and swing, which in general starts proximally and flows distally (Fig. 1.3.16). During walking

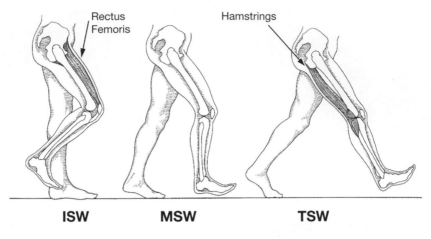

ISW   **MSW**   **TSW**

Fig. 1.3.14 Swing phase consists of three periods known as initial swing (ISW), mid-swing (MSW), and terminal swing (TSW). Mid-swing is a switching period when no muscles are active. During running or fast walking, the rectus femoris decelerates the shank in initial swing and the hamstrings decelerate it in terminal swing.

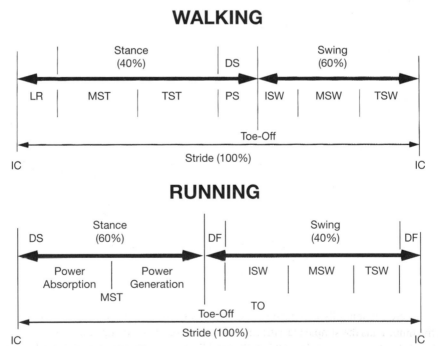

Fig. 1.3.15 (a, b) Walking (above) versus running (below). Walking features two periods of double support (DS) when both feet are on the ground. In running these are replaced by two periods of double float (DF) when neither foot is on the ground. Thus, in walking, stance always occupies more than 50% of the gait cycle, whereas stance is always less than 50% in running. LR, loading response; MST, mid-stance; TST, terminal stance; PS, pre-swing; ISW, initial swing; MSW, mid-swing; TSW, terminal swing; IC, initial contact; TO, toe-off.

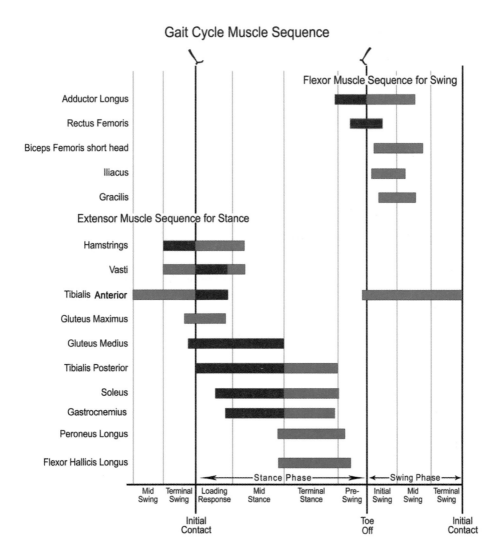

Fig. 1.3.16 Perry's concept of muscle flow, which starts proximally and flows distally. According to Perry (1988), there are two periods of transition when this sequential activation is initiated, which are terminal swing and pre-swing. The former is the transition from swing-to-stance and the latter from stance-to-swing.

muscles are sequentially activated in response to the stance and swing demands imposed on the limb. Thus the simple classification of muscle action as acting at the hip, knee, ankle or foot is inadequate since, in walking, the total limb requirements require a subtle overlap of muscle functions.

The following graphs provide a functional synopsis of the different gait periods and describe critical elements of joint kinematics (position and motion), joint kinetics (moment and power), and muscle activity during each of the subphases of gait (Figs 1.3.17–21).

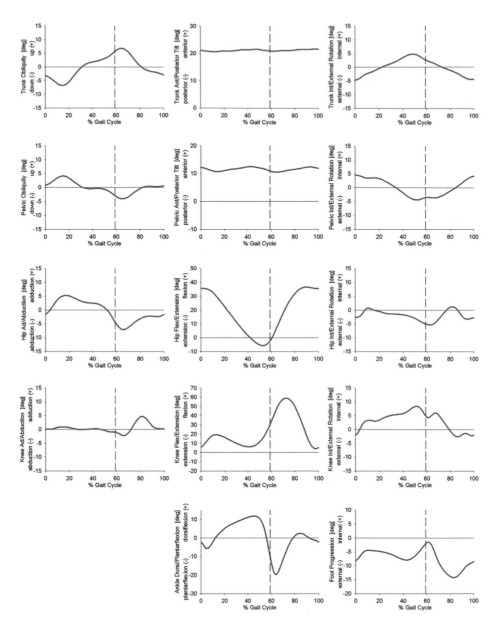

Fig. 1.3.17 An example of kinematics. Three-dimensional joint rotations are shown at typical walking speed (left column = coronal, middle column = sagittal, and right column = transverse planes).

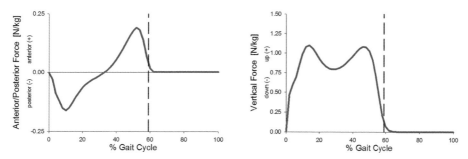

Fig. 1.3.18 Ground reaction forces. Anterior/posterior and vertical components of the ground reaction force are shown at a typical walking speed. Each line represents the average of trials within the corresponding group.

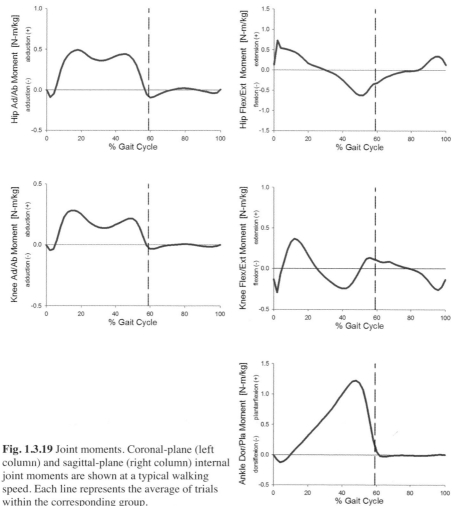

Fig. 1.3.19 Joint moments. Coronal-plane (left column) and sagittal-plane (right column) internal joint moments are shown at a typical walking speed. Each line represents the average of trials within the corresponding group.

Fig. 1.3.20 Joint power. The total power generated/absorbed at the hip, knee, and ankle is shown at a typical walking speed.

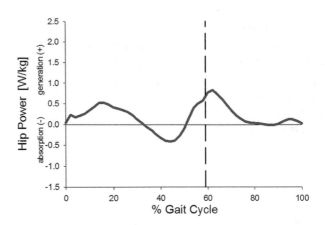

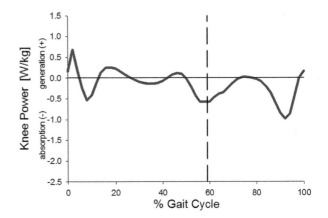

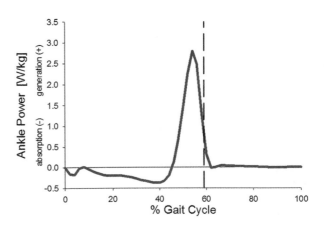

Further details, including definitions and derivations of the joint kinematics and kinetics, can be found in the electronic supplement to this chapter. It should be noted that the muscle activations and functions are taken partly from Perry's data, with some modifications based on our work and the work of others (Anderson and Pandy 2003, Schwartz et al. 2008).

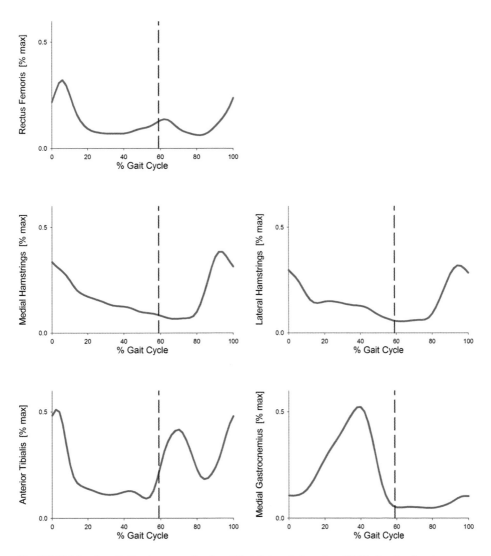

Fig. 1.3.21 Muscle activity. An example of rectified, integrated, surface EMG signals of rectus femoris, medial and lateral hamstrings, tibialis anterior, and medial gastrocnemius at typical walking speed.

Terminal swing (Fig. 1.3.22)

The swinging leg is decelerated in preparation for landing and stance phase during TSw. The pelvis levels in the coronal plane, and rotates internally to provide adequate step length. The foot also rotates internally, from its maximum external orientation, in order to be properly positioned for landing.

Eccentric hamstring activity generates hip-extension and knee-flexion moments, the latter of which decelerates the extending knee with notable knee-power absorption. The tibialis anterior, which has already lifted the foot out of plantarflexion in early swing, turns on again in order to stabilize the foot at heel contact and prevent a foot-slap.

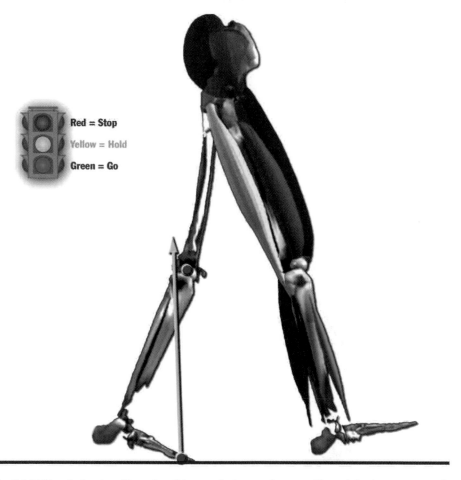

Red = Stop

Yellow = Hold

Green = Go

Fig. 1.3.22 Terminal swing. The color of the muscle denotes the type of its activity (green, concentric contraction; red, eccentric contraction; and yellow, isometric contraction). The illustration illustrates rapid gait. Note that the hamstrings are yellow (isometric) because they are acting like elastic straps to slow the rate of extension of the knee and accelerate the rate of extension of the hip. That is, they are absorbing or harnessing the kinetic energy of the shank and transferring it up to the hip. This is one of the body's methods of energy conservation.

Initial contact (Fig. 1.3.23)

This is the instant that the lead foot contacts the floor. Since the trailing foot is still on the ground, this initiates the beginning of double support. In normal walking IC is made with the heel and as such the ground reaction force passes posterior to the ankle and knee joints and close to hip joint.

Because the control system anticipates the forces that the ground reaction will deliver, the hip-extensors, vasti, ankle-dorsiflexors and toe-extensors are all active and ready to absorb the force of impact. The gluteus maximus opposes the flexor moment at the hip produced by ground reaction forces, while the hamstrings inhibit knee hyperextension and assist in controlling the flexion moment at hip.

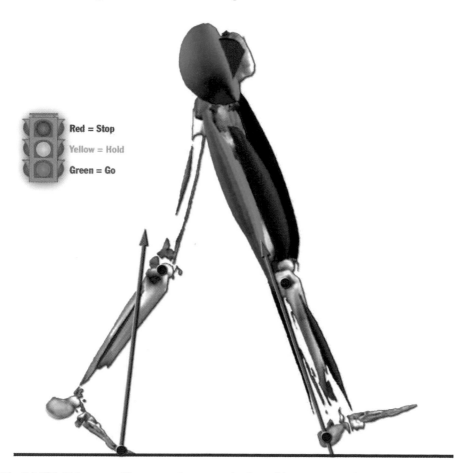

Red = Stop

Yellow = Hold

Green = Go

Fig. 1.3.23 Initial contact. The same color convention is used (green, concentric contraction; red, eccentric contraction; and yellow, isometric contraction). The quadriceps and anterior tibial musculature are working eccentrically to limit (decelerate) knee flexion and ankle plantarflexion respectively. The hamstrings are contracting concentrically as hip-extensors. Although the hamstrings are biarticular muscles, they are able to work here as accelerators of the lower extremity at the hip because the vasti are preventing their action at the knee.

53

Loading response – the period of 1st rocker (Fig. 1.3.24)

This phase begins when the foot touches the floor and lasts until the beginning of single support (foot-off on the contralateral side). During LR, the opposite limb is in pre-swing, and therefore is rapidly *unloading*.

The purpose of LR is shock absorption or weight acceptance. The body has been accelerated by gravity as it fell from its zenith at mid-stance to its nadir at loading response. As a result, the total force on the limb as it impacts the floor is about 120% of body weight. The ankle and knee play critical roles in this process.

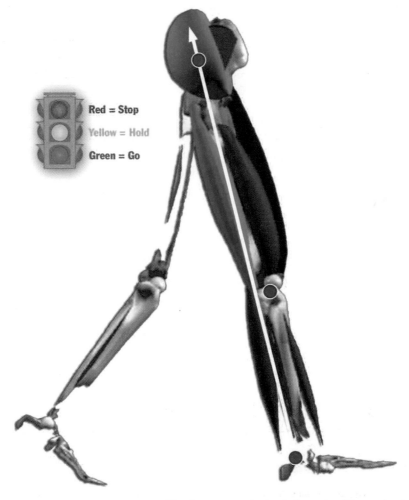

Red = Stop

Yellow = Hold

Green = Go

Fig. 1.3.24 Loading response. The purpose of loading response is shock absorption. The vasti and tibialis anterior muscles are acting eccentrically during the period of first rocker as shock absorbers at the knee and ankle respectively. The gluteus maximus and hamstrings continue to work as accelerators at the hip (green, concentric contraction; red, eccentric contraction; and yellow, isometric contraction).

The ankle and foot during LR, MSt and TSt have been described in terms of three rockers, which have the effect of producing a wheel-like rolling motion under the foot. (Fig. 1.3.25) (Perry 1992, pp. 19–47). First rocker (heel rocker) begins at IC and extends through LR. In normal gait the fulcrum (or pivot point) of this rocker is the heel. Posterior protrusion of the heel creates a lever equal to 25% of the foot's total length. Because the ground reaction force acting on this lever is passing through the heel, its immediate effect is to thrust the entire foot towards the floor. The external moment about the ankle is resisted by the controlled, eccentric contraction of the pre-tibial muscles (tibialis anterior, extensor digitorum longus, and peroneus tertius) at the ankle while the joint undergoes a slight plantarflexion motion ($\approx 3°$). Modest ankle power absorption can be noted as a result of this eccentric action (Fig. 1.3.20).

At the knee, the vastus medialis, lateralis, and intermedius also contract eccentrically, producing an internal knee extension moment and power absorption throughout most of LR. It is worth noting that the rectus femoris is not active at this time (Nene et al. 1999, 2004, Arnold et al. 2005).

There are large stabilizing moments in both the sagittal and coronal planes at the hip during LR. These are associated with activation in the gluteus maximus and medius. In the sagittal plane, the hip begins to extend under this action. In the coronal plane, the abductors hike the pelvis to its high point at the end of LR.

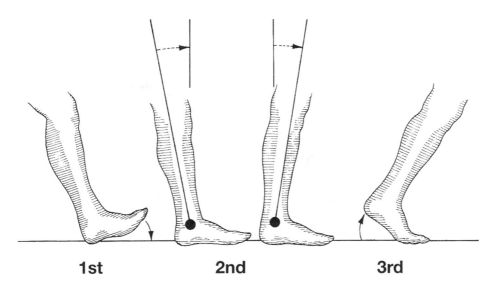

1st **2nd** **3rd**

Fig. 1.3.25 The foot and ankle in stance: three foot rockers. The first two are deceleration rockers and so their respective muscles are acting eccentrically, i.e. undergoing a lengthening contraction with energy absorption (negative work). Third rocker is an acceleration rocker and so the plantarflexors must act concentrically, i.e. produce positive work. Notice that the point of application of the ground reaction force is forced to move forward with each successive rocker thus allowing the center of mass to move forward with it.

Mid-stance – the period of 2nd rocker (Fig. 1.3.26)

This period constitutes the first half of single limb support. It begins with FO of the contralateral limb and ends with heel-rise on the ipsilateral side. During mid-stance, the opposite limb is in mid-swing. The muscles of the stance limb act to allow smooth progression over the stationary foot. At the same time, they control the position of the ground reaction force relative to the hip and knee, thereby contributing to energy conservation.

The MSt period corresponds to second rocker (ankle rocker), during which the rocker's fulcrum has moved from the heel to the center of the ankle joint as the tibia hinges forward on the stationary foot. This is accomplished via eccentric contraction of the ankle

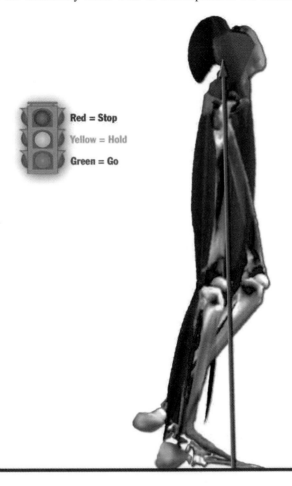

Red = Stop

Yellow = Hold

Green = Go

Fig. 1.3.26 Mid-stance. The purpose of midstance is energy conservation. Since the ground reaction force (GRF) is now anterior to the knee joint center, the forefoot acts like a lever to push the knee back into extension so that the knee is stabilized by the posterior capsule thereby obviating the need muscle action of the vasti. The only muscle action that is required to accomplish this is eccentric action of the soleus.

plantarflexors (principally the soleus), which act to retard forward motion of the tibia. This, in turn, allows the GRF to pass in front of the knee so that it acts to produce an external extension moment at that joint via the lever-arm of the forefoot. Once the knee joint has been stabilized by the GRF, the action of the quadriceps is no longer needed. Consequently, the vastus muscles are quiescent during mid-stance.

As the body moves forward over the planted foot, the ground reaction force moves posterior to the hip. When this occurs, the hip also becomes stable, because the anterior capsule (Bigalow's ligament) passively limits further hip extension. Consequently, hip extensor activity ceases during the latter half of mid-stance. By controlling the position of the ground reaction force referable to the joints above, mid-stance contributes to energy conservation.

Terminal stance – the period of 3rd rocker (Fig. 1.3.27)
The purpose of terminal stance is propulsion. Towards the end of mid-stance, the combined action of the plantarflexors acts to arrest the forward progression of the tibia. The gastrocnemius and long toe-flexors join the soleus to produce enough force to arrest dorsiflexion and subsequently initiate active ankle plantarflexion. This forces the fulcrum of the pivot forward to the metatarsal heads as the heel rises off the ground – the event that marks the onset of terminal stance. This also begins the 3rd rocker (forefoot rocker). The rocker's fulcrum now has moved from the ankle to the metatarsal heads, and the action of the plantarflexors has switched from eccentric to concentric. By the end of TSt, the peak plantarflexion moment has been reached, and significant ankle power is generated. The knee also reaches its peak knee-flexion moment, however, because there is limited knee motion, knee power is inconsequential.

Extension at the hip continues, but this extension is slowing, with corresponding hip power absorption on the hip power graph. The pelvis reaches its most external orientation.

It is important to note that during TSt, the opposite limb is in TSw. The coordination of the propulsive action of TSt and the pre-positioning action of TSw are felt to be critical for an efficient redirection of the body CoM during the double support phase.

The tibialis posterior and peroneals are also active to stabilize the foot against eversion and inversion forces respectively. Since weight bearing is now occurring mainly on the forefoot, the long toe flexors act to stabilize the metatarsal-phalangeal joints thereby adding toe support to augment forefoot support.

The deceleration of the first two rockers must be balanced by the acceleration produced by the third. The combined actions of the muscles of the posterior calf generate a significant amount of the total propulsive force needed for walking (Neptune et al. 2001, 2004). In particular, the gastrocnemius, which is made up primarily of fast-twitch fibers, acts as an accelerator to begin active plantarflexion of the ankle. This provides the necessary power to advance the limb and flex the knee. The accelerative force of 3rd rocker peaks at the end of terminal stance and then falls rapidly to zero by the end of pre-swing (Õunpuu et al. 1991).

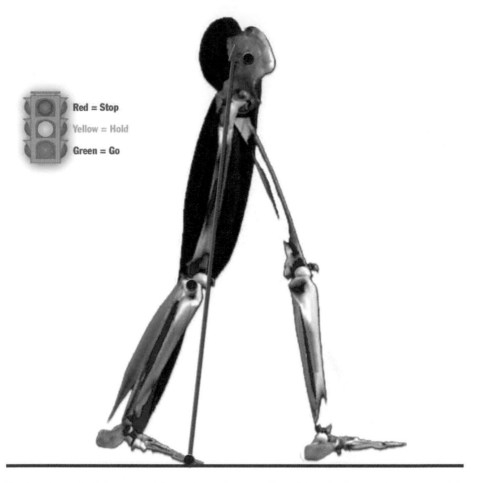

Fig. 1.3.27 Terminal stance. The color of the calf has now changed from red to green (green, concentric contraction; red, eccentric contraction; and yellow, isometric contraction). Since the gastrocnemius has now joined the soleus, their resultant force is sufficient to drive the ankle into plantarflexion. The force generated by the triceps surae in terminal stance accounts for about 50% of the total propulsive power needed in walking. Note too that the ground reaction force has now moved behind the hip joint thereby generating a hip extension moment that renders the joint stable against the ilio–femoral (Bigalow's) ligament. Consequently gluteus maximus activity is no longer required for stability.

Pre-swing (Fig. 1.3.28)

Pre-swing on the stance leg begins when the swinging foot strikes the ground, and two limbs once again support the individual. The purpose of pre-swing is to prepare the stance limb for swing by transferring weight from the trailing limb to the front limb. Residual body weight on the trailing limb has moved forward to the forefoot; and the GRF is now well behind the knee, thus creating a strong flexion moment.

The gastrocnemius–soleus complex is just completing its activity and the force it has imparted to the trailing limb is driving it forward and upward. Rapid plantarflexion is

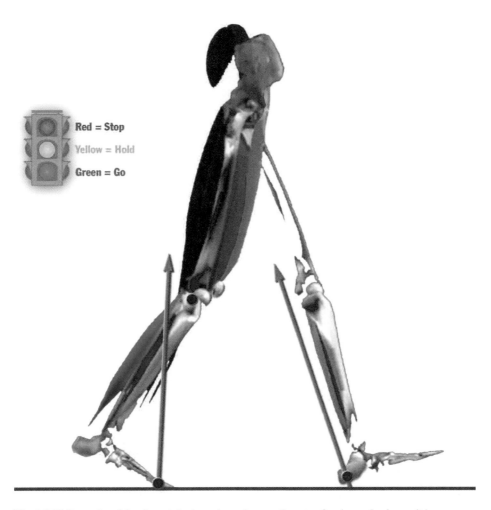

Red = Stop

Yellow = Hold

Green = Go

Fig. 1.3.28 Pre-swing. Muscle activity here depends upon the rate of cadence. In slow gait knee flexion has to be augmented, whereas in rapid gait it has to be restrained. Augmentation is brought about by concentric action of the sartorius, gracilis, and/or short head of biceps femoris. Restraint is accomplished by relatively isometric action of the rectus femoris, which acts like an isometric strap to decelerate the knee and transfer the kinetic energy of the shank proximally to augment hip flexion. Rapid gait is pictured here (green, concentric contraction; red, eccentric contraction; and yellow, isometric contraction).

occurring, the plantarflexion moment is diminishing, and the ankle power burst is coming to an end. The anterior tibialis is just beginning its activity, which will have a significant role in ISw. In addition to plantarflexion, the gastrocnemius also provides knee flexion at this time.

At the upper end of the femur, the hip-flexors and the superficial adductors (adductor longus, brevis and gracilis) are pulling the hip into flexion with an associated increase in hip-flexor moment and hip power. It is worth noting that, in normal gait at typical free speed, the rectus femoris is not (or is at most minimally) active at this time. The hip-flexors, in

59

addition to their direct action at the hip, also have the effect of producing knee flexion through induced acceleration (Perry 1992, pp. 116–22, Neptune et al. 2001, Kimmel and Schwartz 2006).

Thus the knee, driven from both the ankle and hip, begins to flex rapidly. At normal speed and cadence, the knee flexion produced by these forces drives the knee into about 60° of flexion in swing, which is just enough to clear the swinging foot.

Initial swing (Fig. 1.3.29 a, b)
This period begins at foot-off and ends as the swinging limb passes the stance limb. At normal walking speed the limb swings in a largely passively manner, with little muscle

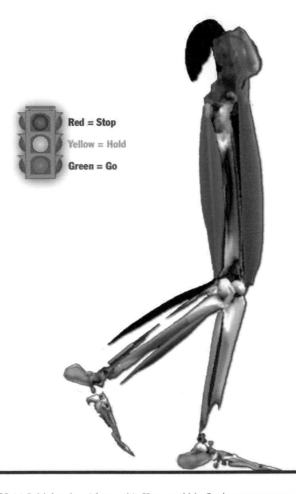

Red = Stop

Yellow = Hold

Green = Go

Fig. 1.3.29 (a) Initial swing (slow gait). Knee and hip flexion are augmented by concentric action of the sartorius and gracilis. The short head of the biceps can also work concentrically to augment knee flexion during slow gait (green, concentric contraction; red, eccentric contraction; and yellow, isometric contraction).

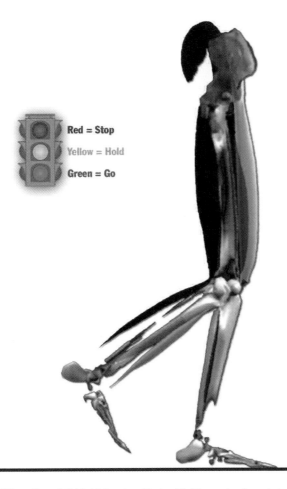

Red = Stop

Yellow = Hold

Green = Go

Fig. 1.3.29 continued (b) Initial swing (fast gait). The rectus femoris is working as an isometric strap to restrain knee flexion and augment hip flexion. In a sprinter the periods of gastrocnemius and rectus femoris activity are probably less than 0.1 second, which demands a great deal of precision from the control system; therefore it is not surprising that these biarticular muscles almost always function abnormally in spastic diplegia.

activity except the tibialis anterior, which works as an accelerator to lift the foot out of plantarflexion. When gait is faster or slower than normal, muscle activity is required to modify the rate of cadence.

Mid-swing (Fig. 1.3.30)
Mid-swing is a switching period between the muscle activity that occurs in initial swing and the muscle activity in terminal swing, so there is limited muscle activity – the main job of the muscles is to get out of the way of the properly launched swing leg. The tibialis anterior does remain on, supporting the foot near a neutral position against the pull of the gravitational external moment.

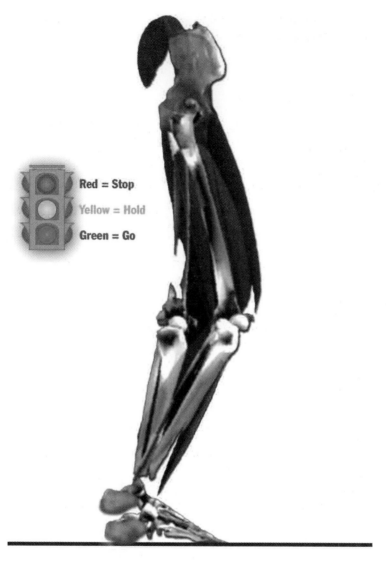

Fig. 1.3.30 Mid-swing is the switching period between acceleration and deceleration or vice versa. Inertial forces are propelling the limb, so very little muscle action is necessary.

Conclusion

Gait is an elegant and complex activity, critical to human function. In this chapter, we have given a basic description of the normal gait pattern, as well as some insight into the neurological control and muscle activity governing the movement. Further details, including numerous video and animated examples, can be found in the electronic supplement to this chapter. A thorough understanding of normal gait is essential before delving into the myriad of pathological changes that occur in cerebral palsy. Too often in the past, basic ignorance of normal gait principles has led to treatment strategies that either were ineffective or even worsened the gait pathology.

REFERENCES

Alexander RM (1992) *Walking. The Human Machine*. London: Natural History Museum Publications. p 59–73.

Anderson FC, Pandy MG (2003) Individual muscle contributions to support in normal walking. *Gait Posture* **17**: 159–69.

Arnold AS, Anderson FC, Pandy MG, Delp SL (2005) Muscular contributions to hip and knee extension during the single limb stance phase of normal gait: a framework for investigating the causes of crouch gait. *J Biomech* **38**: 2181–9.

Cavagna GA, Dusman B, Margaria R (1968) Positive work done by a previously stretched muscle. *J Appl Physiol* **24**: 21–32.

Corcoran PJ, Brengelmann GL (1970) Oxygen uptake in normal and handicapped subjects, in relation to speed of walking beside velocity-controlled cart. *Arch Phys Med Rehabil* **51**: 78–87.

den Otter AR, Geurts ACH, Mulder T, Duysens (2004) Speed related changes in muscle activity from normal to very slow speeds. *Gait Posture* **19**: 270–8.

Hicks R, Tashman S, Cary JM, Altman RF, Gage JR (1985) Swing phase control with knee friction in juvenile amputees. *J Orthop Res* **3**: 198–201.

Hof AL (1996) Scaling gait data to body size. *Gait Posture* **4**: 222–3.

Inman VT, Ralston HJ, Todd F (1981) Muscle. In: Lieberman JC, editor. *Human Walking*. Baltimore, MD: Williams and Wilkins. p 93.

Kimmel SA, Schwartz MH (2006) A baseline of dynamic muscle function during gait. *Gait Posture* **23**: 211–21.

Kuo AD (2007) The six determinants of gait and the inverted pendulum analogy: a dynamic walking perspective. *Hum Move Sci* **26**: 617–56.

Lieber RL (1986) Skeletal muscle adaptability. I: Review of basic properties. *Dev Med Child Neurol* **28**: 390–7.

McClay IS, Lake MJ, Cavanagh PR (1990) Muscle activity in running. In: Cavanagh PR, editor. *Biomechanics of Distance Running*. Champaign, IL: Human Kinetics Books. p 177–8.

Nene A, Mayagoitia R, Veltink P (1999) Assessment of rectus femoris function during initial swing phase. *Gait Posture* **9**: 1–9.

Nene A, Byrne C, Hermens H (2004) Is rectus femoris really a part of quadriceps? Assessment of rectus femoris function during gait in able-bodied adults. *Gait Posture* **20**: 1–13.

Neptune RR, Kautz SA, Zajac FE (2001) Contributions of the individual ankle plantar flexors to support, forward progression and swing initiation during walking. *J Biomech* **34**: 1387–98.

Neptune RR, Zajac FE, Kautz SA (2004) Muscle force redistributes segmental power for body progression during walking. *Gait Posture* **19**: 194–205.

Õunpuu S, Gage JR, Davis RB (1991) Three-dimensional lower extremity joint kinetics in normal pediatric gait. *J Pediatr Orthop* **11**: 341–9.

Perry J (1985) Normal and pathologic gait. In: Bunch WH, editor. *Atlas of Orthotics*, 2nd edn. St Louis, MI: C.V. Mosby. p 76–111.

Perry J (1988) *Gait analysis instructional course; normal muscle control sequence during walking*. Paper presented at the Annual Meeting of the American Academy of Cerebral Palsy and Developmental Medicine, Toronto, Canada.

Perry J (1992) *Gait Analysis: Normal and Pathological Function*. Thorofare, NJ: Slack.

Rab GT (1994) Muscle. In: Rose J, Gamble JG, editors. *Human Walking*. Baltimore, MD: Williams and Wilkins. p 101–22.

Ralston HJ (1958) Energy-speed relation and optimal speed during level walking. *Int Zeitsch Angewand Physiol Einschliess Arbeitsphysiol* **17**: 277–83.

Rose J, Ralston HJ, Gamble JG (1994) Energetics of walking. In: Rose J, Gamble JG, editors. *Human Walking*, 2nd edn. Baltimore, MD: Williams and Wilkins. p 45–72.

Schwartz MH, Rozumalski A, Trost JP (2008) The effect of walking speed on the gait of typically developing children. *J Biomech* **41**: 1639–50.

Sutherland DH, Olshen R, Cooper L, Woo SL (1980) The development of mature gait. *J Bone Joint Surg Am* **62**: 336–53.

Sutherland DH, Olshen RA, Biden EN, Wyatt MP (1988) *The Development of Mature Walking*. Philadelphia: J.B. Lippincott.

Tashman S, Hicks R, Jendrejczyk D (1985) Evaluation of a prosthetic shank with variable inertial properties. *Clin Prosthet Orthot* **9**: 23–5.

Vaughan CL (2003) Theories of bipedal walking: an odyssey. *J Biomech* **36**: 513–23.

Vredenbregt J, Rau G (1973) Surface electromyography in relation to force, muscle length and endurance. In: Desmedt JE, editor. *Electromyography and Clinical Neurophysiology*. Basel: Karger. p 607–22.

Winter DA (1984) Biomechanics of human movement with applications to the study of human locomotion. *Crit Rev Biomed Eng* **9**: 287–314.

Winter DA (1991) *Kinematics. The Biomechanics and Motor Control of Human Gait: Normal, Elderly, and Pathological*, 2nd edn. Waterloo, Ontario: University of Waterloo Press. p 17–31.

Yang JF, Winter DA (1984) Electromyographic amplitude normalization methods: improving their sensitivity as diagnostic tools in gait analysis. *Arch Phys Med Rehabil* **65**: 517–21.

Section 2

GAIT PATHOLOGY IN INDIVIDUALS WITH CEREBRAL PALSY

INTRODUCTION AND OVERVIEW

James R. Gage

Now that we have reviewed typical function and development, it is time to turn our attention to the gait disorders and problems encountered in an individual with cerebral palsy. The complexity of control of normal locomotion as well as the complex mechanisms of muscle and bone growth should have led us to expect that there would be a great many places in which things could go awry. Now, as we concentrate on the pathology of cerebral palsy, we will see that is indeed the case.

Cerebral palsy is a movement disorder produced by an injury to the immature brain. It is, by definition, a static encephalopathy, but the manifestations of that injury are by no means static. Furthermore, the brain injuries are in no way homogeneous.

As I said in the preface to the first edition of this book, locomotion begins in the brain with the wish/thought to relocate, i.e. to move from one place to another. So we must begin our study of gait problems in cerebral palsy with the brain, because that is where things have gone wrong. The location and degree of the brain lesion determine the type of tone present, the degree to which selective motor control and balance are impaired, and the extent of growth deformity which results. The background information necessary to understand the nature and effects of brain injury in cerebral palsy are provided in the excellent chapters by Drs du Plessis, Peacock and Albright. From there we move on to a discussion as to how the cerebral injury affects the musculoskeletal system in a growing child. By that time it will be apparent that the problems relating to gait, which include musculoskeletal deformity, abnormal muscle tone, inadequate balance, and impaired motor control, are all in some way secondary to the brain injury. With the concepts of cause and effect of gait disorders firmly in hand, we can move on to a discussion of the classification and natural history of the condition.

2.1
MECHANISMS AND MANIFESTATIONS OF NEONATAL BRAIN INJURY

Adré J. du Plessis

Cerebral palsy is caused by a wide spectrum of developmental and acquired abnormalities of the immature brain. In earlier years, the cause of cerebral palsy remained unknown in more than half of all cases (Hagberg et al. 1989a). In 1862, William Little associated cerebral palsy with 'abnormal parturition' and 'difficult labors'. Subsequent epidemiologic studies challenged the importance of intrapartum asphyxia in the overall prevalence of cerebral palsy (Nelson and Ellenberg 1986, Blair and Stanley 1988), and emphasized instead the role of antenatal factors. In these reports, perinatal factors such as intrapartum asphyxia were implicated in only 8%–30% (Blair and Stanley 1988, Hagberg et al. 1989a, 1996, 2001) of cerebral palsy cases. However, even at these lower rates, the absolute number of children affected is high and the debilitating consequences are lifelong.

In recent years, major developments in basic neuroscience, medical care and neuro-diagnostic technology have advanced our understanding of the mechanisms of brain injury in early life and their clinical manifestations. Sophisticated neuroimaging techniques, such as magnetic resonance imaging (MRI) with its superb tissue resolution, have facilitated the accurate early-life diagnosis of the etiologies, mechanisms and timing of cerebral abnormalities underlying cerebral palsy (Huppi and Barnes 1997, Inder et al. 1999a, c, Rutherford et al. 2006). Improved obstetric and neonatal care has influenced the rate, etiologic spectrum, and clinical subtypes of cerebral palsy. In spite of, or perhaps because of, the decreased mortality of sick newborn infants, the overall incidence of cerebral palsy has remained unchanged or increased in recent decades (Hagberg et al. 1989a, b). This is particularly true of infants born preterm, whose risk of cerebral palsy is up to 30-fold greater than that of full-term infants (Stanley 1992, Pharoah et al. 1996). The increased survival of preterm infants has translated into an increase in the clinical subtypes of cerebral palsy more commonly seen in ex-preterm infants, e.g. spastic diplegia (Dale and Stanley 1980, Volpe 1994). This chapter focuses on the motor manifestations of neonatal brain injury, particularly as these relate to gait. However, associated non-motor complications, such as cognitive, behavioral, epileptic and visual dysfunction, may play an important role in the child's level of function, and hence in decisions regarding the optimal management of motor dysfunction. In recent years, our understanding of the mechanisms underlying these non-motor sequelae has been advanced through more sophisticated outcome testing, as well as the application of quantitative and functional neuroimaging.

Experimental neuroscience has elucidated many of the fundamental mechanisms of perinatal and neonatal brain injury, and in so doing has stimulated the development of experimental agents that prevent or arrest brain injury in animal models. These developments have fueled expectations for future effective neuro-protection in the newborn human infant at risk for cerebral palsy. Thus the importance of intrapartum and neonatal causes of cerebral palsy goes far beyond medico–legal culpability, and lies in the exciting possibility that some of these injuries may be preventable in future.

A broad spectrum of etiologies mediate neonatal brain injury in preterm and term infants. However, the focus here is on the mechanisms and manifestations of the most common cause, namely cerebrovascular injury. Other etiologies such as trauma, infection, and metabolic dysfunction are discussed in detail elsewhere (Volpe 2008). Although there is overlap in the cerebrovascular brain lesions affecting infants at these two ends of the gestational age spectrum, there are sufficient differences to warrant their separate discussion.

Brain injury in the preterm infant

The intrinsic vulnerability of the preterm infant's brain to ischemic and hemorrhagic injury is related to both the anatomic–structural and functional immaturity of the cerebral vessels.

VULNERABILITY OF THE PREMATURE CEREBRAL VASCULATURE

The *anatomic underdevelopment* of the cerebral arterial and venous systems of the preterm infant is illustrated in Figure 2.1.1. Between mid-gestation and term, arterial branches of the surface vessels penetrate the cerebral wall and grow toward the ventricles. Since the extent of arterial growth into the white matter is proportional to the gestational age, the periventricular white matter of the infant born preterm lies in an end-zone relatively deficient in arterial supply. Immature vessels may be extremely thin in certain regions (e.g. the involuting germinal matrix) and they are easily ruptured. Consequently, germinal matrix hemorrhage (GMH, previously called grade I intraventricular hemorrhage) is common in the preterm infant. Since this structure is situated adjacent to the lateral ventricles, extension of the hemorrhage through the ependymal lining results in *intraventricular hemorrhage* (IVH). Two grades of GMH-IVH are distinguished depending on whether the intraventricular *blood* (not cerebrospinal fluid) causes distention of the ventricle (grade III) or not (grade II). The terminal vein is a major venous conduit draining large areas of the cerebral hemisphere. This vessel courses along the lateral margin of the lateral ventricle and through the germinal matrix, an anatomic relationship that predisposes to obstruction of venous drainage. When the terminal vein is compressed by hemorrhagic distention of the germinal matrix or lateral ventricle, widespread venous ischemia may develop in the cerebral hemisphere.

The *physiologic immaturity* of the cerebral vasculature in preterm infants manifests as defective intrinsic regulation of cerebral blood flow, with the tenuous pressure-flow autoregulation being particularly important. In the mature brain, pressure-flow autoregulation maintains steady cerebral blood flow over a wide range of blood pressure changes, i.e. the autoregulatory plateau (Fig. 2.1.2). In the preterm infant the autoregulatory plateau is narrow and shifted to the left. Furthermore, the normal blood pressure in preterm

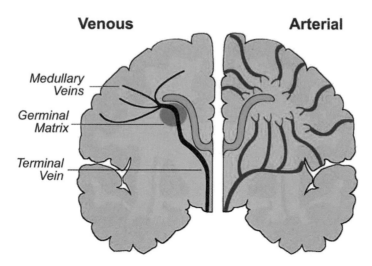

Venous   **Arterial**

Medullary
Veins

Germinal
Matrix

Terminal
Vein

Fig. 2.1.1 The *anatomic underdevelopment* of the cerebral arterial and venous systems in the preterm infant. Incomplete *arterial* ingrowth into the periventricular white matter leaves end-zones of deficient arterial supply vulnerable to ischemia. Immature vessels in the involuting *germinal matrix* are extremely fragile and easily ruptured, often into the lateral ventricles. The course of the *terminal vein* through the germinal matrix and along the lateral margin of the lateral ventricle predisposes it to obstruction following germinal matrix–intraventricular hemorrhage with subsequent venous ischemia and hemorrhagic infarction.

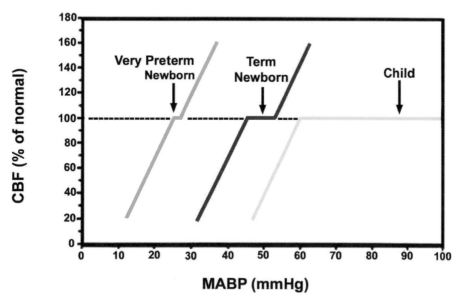

Fig. 2.1.2 Pressure-flow autoregulation at different ages. Compared to term infants and adults, the autoregulatory plateau in the preterm infant is narrow and shifted to the left. The normal blood pressure (arrows) in preterm infants approaches the lower limit of the autoregulatory plateau. CBF, cerebral blood flow; MABP, mean arterial blood pressure.

infants may be perilously close to the lower limit of this autoregulatory plateau. Finally, the already narrow autoregulatory plateau is particularly vulnerable to insults such as hypoxia–ischemia, which render the cerebral vasculature pressure-passive. In this condition, fluctuations in systemic blood pressure are transmitted directly into the immature cerebral microvasculature. Recent studies suggest a high prevalence of fluctuating cerebral pressure passivity in sick preterm infants (Soul et al. 2007).

VULNERABILITY OF THE IMMATURE OLIGODENDROCYTE

Superimposed on this vascular predisposition to injury is a developmental vulnerability of the immature oligodendrocyte (Back et al. 1998, 2001, Kadhim et al. 2001). The ultimate responsibility of the oligodendrocyte lineage is myelination of the developing central nervous system. During the critical period of high risk for injury to the immature white matter (i.e. 24–32 gestational weeks), the developing oligodendrocyte is particularly vulnerable to oxidative stress (Oka et al. 1993, Yonezawa et al. 1996) This vulnerability is in part due to a mismatch between development of critical anti-oxidant enzymes (e.g. catalase, superoxide dismutase and glutathione peroxidase) and development of pro-oxidant pathways (e.g. accumulation of iron for oligodendrocyte differentiation) (Ozawa et al. 1994, Iida et al. 1995, Back and Volpe 1997). The propensity of the immature white matter to hypoxia–ischemia during this phase of development provides a potent trigger for the generation of particularly noxious free radicals. Although most oligodendrocytes are in a premyelination phase of development between 24 and 32 weeks of gestation, injury at this stage will disrupt subsequent myelination and result in abnormal and incomplete white-matter development.

CARDIORESPIRATORY VULNERABILITY IN THE PRETERM INFANT

In the sick preterm infant, instability of the immature cardiorespiratory system is common, causing fluctuations in systemic blood pressure and circulating oxygenation. Cardiovascular dysfunction results from immaturity at a number of levels, including inefficient myocardial function, autonomic reflex immaturity, and major changes in cardiac afterload after preterm birth (Friedman and Fahey 1993, Evans 2006). Delayed closure of normal fetal pathways (e.g. patent ductus arteriosus and foramen ovale) after birth further compromises early postnatal hemodynamics in the sick preterm infant. Even minor routine handling of these infants (e.g. a diaper change or positioning for X-ray studies) may precipitate sharp fluctuations in blood pressure. If the cerebral circulation is pressure-passive, increases in pressure may rupture small vessels, the most fragile of which are in the germinal matrix. Conversely, fluctuations in perfusion pressure may cause repeated ischemia in the arterial end zones of the periventricular white matter. The immature oligodendrocytes in these areas may be poorly equipped to deal with the free radicals generated by such ischemia–reperfusion events. Taken together, these features – of the immature systemic and cerebral vasculature and the immature cerebral parenchyma – underlie the occurrence and topography of brain injury in the preterm infant.

A. Primary arterial ischemic injury to the white matter (periventricular leukomalacia)
During hypotensive episodes, hypoxic–ischemic insults in the arterial end-zones may cause the classic lesion of immature white matter, i.e. periventricular leukomalacia (PVL). The pathology of this lesion is infarction with necrosis of all cell types and of axonal pathways coursing adjacent to the ventricles in these regions. These foci of infarction are usually bilateral and situated dorsolateral to the external angle of the lateral ventricle (Banker and Larroche 1962). The two most common locations for PVL (Fig. 2.1.3) along the length of the ventricle are (1) the peritrigonal area of the parietal white matter, and (2) the white matter adjacent to the frontal horns. These two foci have different clinical manifestations (see below) but in severe cases may occur together. If the insult is large enough, the ultrasound features of PVL evolve through a focal echo dense phase and a later cystic phase (Fig. 2.1.4). Surrounding the areas of focal infarction, more diffuse and relatively selective oligodendrocyte loss occurs. Recently this pattern of pancellular infarction with later cystic transformation has become rare (Khwaja and Volpe 2008), while a more diffuse form of white matter injury is increasingly recognized, resulting from selective loss of immature oligodendrocytes, cells ultimately responsible for myelination of the white matter tracts. Unlike the focal (infarction) form of PVL, diffuse white matter injury is commonly missed by routine cranial ultrasound screening protocols used for sick preterm infants

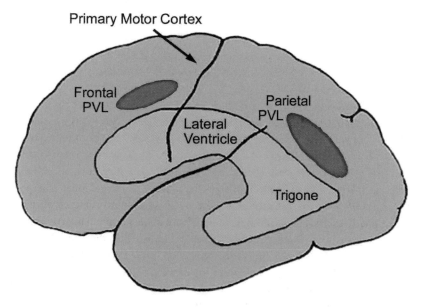

Fig. 2.1.3 Common locations for periventricular leukomalacia (PVL) in the parietal and frontal white matter of the preterm infant. Lesions in these locations have different clinical sequelae described in the text. In severe cases these lesions become confluent along the periventricular white matter. By brain ultrasound these lesions evolve through an initial echodense phase and a later cystic phase.

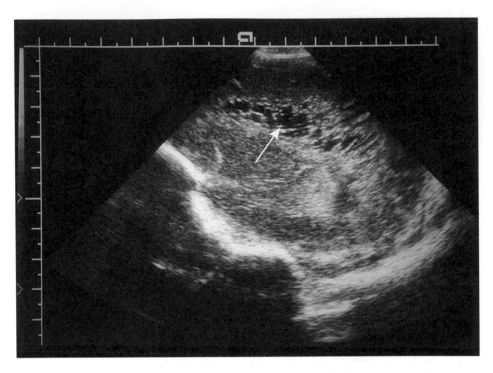

Fig. 2.1.4 Cystic periventicular leukomalacia. Parasagittal cranial ultrasound view showing extensive multicystic injury to the periventricular white matter (arrow).

(Inder et al. 1999c, 2005). Consequently, the diagnosis of diffuse white-matter injury is often delayed until follow-up brain-imaging shows loss of white matter volume, diffuse hypomyelination, and atrophic ('ex vacuo') ventriculomegaly (Fig. 2.1.5).

Although white-matter injury has long been recognized as the principal form of parenchymal brain injury in the preterm infant, recent work has emphasized the structural and functional importance of neuronal injury and its consequences in survivors of pre-term birth (discussed below) (Inder et al. 1999b, 2005, Counsell et al. 2007, Srinivasan et al. 2007).

B. Cerebral parenchymal complications of intraventricular hemorrhage
Periventricular hemorrhagic infarction develops when GMH-IVH impairs drainage through the terminal vein, causing venous stasis and ischemia through large areas of the hemisphere. Characteristic of venous ischemia, this lesion typically undergoes hemorrhagic transformation. Cerebral perfusion studies (Volpe et al. 1983) suggest that the area of ischemia may be far more extensive than the lesion seen by ultrasound. Periventricular hemorrhagic infarction tends to be unilateral or obviously asymmetric, which influences the clinical manifestations of this lesion. The incidence and mortality of this lesion has decreased modestly over time, except among the very smallest preterm infants, most of whom are now surviving (Bassan et al. 2006).

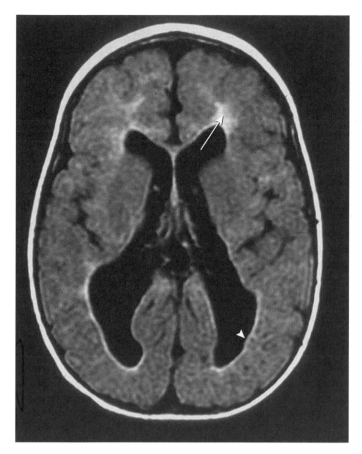

Fig. 2.1.5 Diffuse (non-cystic) periventricular leukomalacia. Axial T1-weighted MRI with atrophic ventriculomegaly, gliosis (arrow), and severe white matter loss particularly in the parieto–occipital regions (arrowhead).

Posthemorrhagic hydrocephalus is another major complication of IVH that results when extravasated blood obstructs the cerebrospinal fluid pathways. The onset of posthemorrhagic hydrocephalus is usually after one or more weeks of life, with later-onset ventricular distention likely mediated by an inflammatory arachnoid response in the posterior fossa. With progressive ventricular distention, there is distortion and compression of periventricular white matter structures (Quinn et al. 1992, Guzzetta et al. 1995, Del Bigio and Kanfer 1996, Del Bigio et al. 1997). In addition to injuring axonal tracts coursing alongside the distending ventricles, compression of the immature arterial and venous structures (see above) may cause ischemic injury to the white matter (Shirane et al. 1992, Chumas et al. 1994, Da Silva et al. 1994, 1995).

C. Cerebellar injury in the preterm infant
Injury to the cerebellum of preterm infants has been underrecognized until recently (Johnsen et al. 2005, Messerschmidt et al. 2005). This predilection is particularly evident in the very low-birthweight infant (<750 g) in whom the incidence by cranial ultrasound may approach 20% (Limperopoulos et al. 2005). Cranial ultrasound through the anterior

73

fontanelle is poorly sensitive to cerebellar injury; prior to use of a posterior fossa ultrasound-imaging approach through the mastoid foramen (Fig. 2.1.6), cerebellar injury was rarely diagnosed in the neonatal period. These lesions have a prominent hemorrhagic component and are likely a form of germinal matrix hemorrhage in the immature cerebellum; others have suggested that these lesions are primary infarctions with secondary hemorrhagic transformation (Johnsen et al. 2005). The majority of cerebellar injuries are associated with neonatal supratentorial injury, with one-quarter being isolated (Limperopoulos et al. 2005). Since the development of the cerebellum is prolonged into early childhood, it is not surprising that these early hemorrhagic lesions may be associated with marked cerebellar hypoplasia at follow-up imaging (Fig. 2.1.7).

Inflammatory cytokines and injury to the immature brain. Although this discussion is focused almost exclusively on cerebrovascular mechanisms of brain injury in the newborn, recent data suggesting a role for pro-inflammatory substances warrant brief review. In recent years a number of epidemiologic (Alexander et al. 1998, Nelson et al. 1998, Grether et al. 1999) and animal studies (Yoon et al. 1996, 1997, 2000, Cai et al. 2000) have demonstrated an association between maternal, fetal and neonatal infection (Yoon et al. 1996, 1997, 2000, Dammann and Leviton 1997, Baud et al. 1999), and injury (Martinez et al. 1998) to the

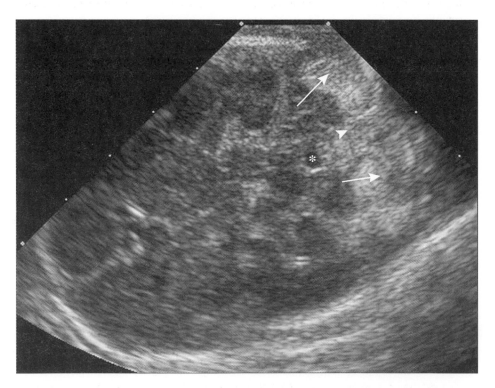

Fig. 2.1.6 Bilateral cerebellar hemorrhage. Cranial ultrasound mastoid view showing hemorrhagic injury in both cerebellar hemispheres (arrows) and vermis (arrowhead). Asterisk indicates 4th ventricle.

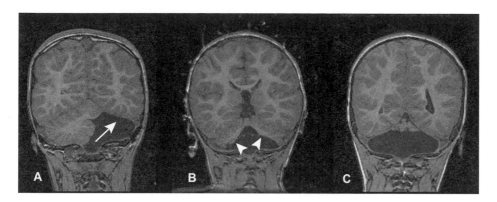

Fig. 2.1.7 Long-term structural outcome of different severity grades of cerebellar hemorrhage in ex-preterm infants. Coronal T1-weighted studies. (A) Marked unilateral hemispheric atrophy (arrow). (B) Bilateral inferomedial hemispheric and vermian injury (arrows). (C) Almost complete destruction of the cerebellum.

immature brain. One postulated mechanism of injury is the toxic effect of inflammatory cytokines on the immature oligodendrocyte (Selmaj and Raine 1988). However, circulating cytokines may also have important effects on the systemic and cerebral circulations that predispose to cerebral ischemia. Furthermore, cerebral ischemia may trigger the release of cytokines from certain cell types as part of the cascade of injury. In summary, the precise relationship or causal pathway(s) between infection, cytokines, ischemia and brain injury in the newborn infant is extremely complex and its understanding awaits further study (Stanley et al. 2000).

CLINICAL–PATHOLOGIC CORRELATION OF BRAIN INJURY IN THE PRETERM INFANT
The relationship between the topography of the various brain lesions in the preterm infant and their long-term clinical sequelae is depicted in Figures 2.1.8 and 9. The superimposed homunculus cartoon in Figure 2.1.8 shows the cortical origin and white matter pathways of motor fibers to the face, trunk and extremities. *Periventricular leukomalacia* is typically bilateral and occurs most frequently toward the posterior aspects of the ventricles in the peritrigonal white matter, as well as in the white matter adjacent to the frontal horns of the lateral ventricles (Figs 2.1.3, 8). In severe cases these regions of injury may be confluent. Since the axons conducting input to the lower extremities course through the frontal regions, injury in this location produces the typical clinical picture of *spastic diplegia*, in which the most prominent motor impairment is in the legs, but may also involve the trunk, arms, and face to a lesser extent. PVL confined to the parietal white matter is associated with cognitive and visual deficits (described below) but tends to cause less severe motor dysfunction.

Periventricular hemorrhagic infarction (PVHI) is usually unilateral but may involve extensive areas of the hemisphere. This lesion has a poor prognosis, previously associated with a 90% long-term prevalence of severe neurodevelopmental impairment. More recent data suggest a modest improvement in functional outcome, although two-thirds of survivors still demonstrate long-term motor and/or cognitive impairment (Bassan et al. 2007). Severity

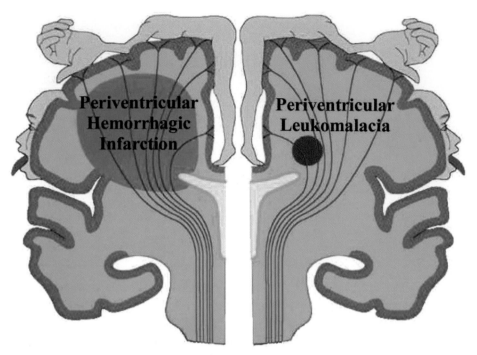

Fig. 2.1.8 Location of common brain lesions in the preterm infant and their motor sequelae. Diagram of cerebral hemispheres (coronal view) with superimposed homunculus to demonstrate the cortical origin and white matter pathways of motor fibers to the face, trunk and extremities. *Periventricular leukomalacia* (typically bilateral) in the frontal regions as shown here involves pathways to the lower extremities and results in the typical clinical picture of *spastic diplegia*. *Periventricular hemorrhagic infarction* (usually unilateral) affects pathways to the arms, legs and even the face, producing the typical form of hemiparesis seen in surviving preterm infants (contrast with arterial stroke in term infants, Fig. 2.1.11).

scores based on the neonatal ultrasound studies may assist in predicting the severity of long-term outcome (Bassan et al. 2007). The diffuse lesion of periventricular hemorrhagic infarction affects fibers supplying the upper and lower extremities, and possibly also the face. This topography of injury underlies the typical picture of preterm infants who survive periventricular hemorrhagic infarction, i.e. *hemiparesis* involving the upper and lower extremity more or less equally. The clinical picture of hemiparesis in ex-preterm infants differs from that in (usually term) infants with middle cerebral artery stroke (see below). *Post-hemorrhagic hydrocephalus* manifests as progressive ventricular distention that may distort or compress the adjacent axonal tracts directly, or cause regional periventricular ischemia and secondary injury to these pathways. Similar to the primary arterial ischemic lesion of PVL, this lesion tends to affect pathways to the lower extremities earlier and more severely, although in advanced cases the arms and face may also be affected.

Cerebellar injury in the preterm infant is associated with a high prevalence of pervasive neurodevelopmental sequelae (Limperopoulos et al. 2007). Severe motor impairment

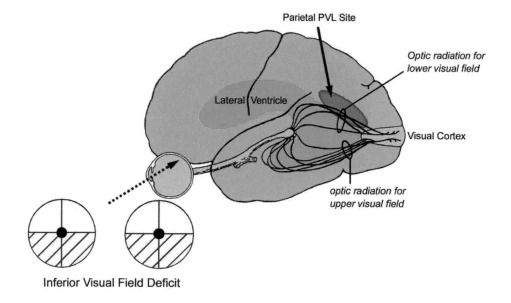

Parietal PVL Site

Optic radiation for
lower visual field

Lateral Ventricle

Visual Cortex

optic radiation for
upper visual field

Inferior Visual Field Deficit

Fig. 2.1.9 Visual-field deficits in the preterm infant. Diagram of cerebral hemispheres (sagittal view) showing the course of the optic radiations for the lower visual field through the white matter superolateral to the occipital horns of the lateral ventricles. As shown in Figure 2.1.3, this is a high-risk region for periventricular leukomalacia (PVL), which may result in lower visual-field deficits.

develops in up to 50% of these infants, most commonly with hypotonia and ataxia, particularly of the trunk and gait.

The clinical correlates of these different lesions in the preterm infant's brain have been discussed separately. However, the clinical picture is often difficult to ascribe to one mechanism alone, and in these cases more than one lesion type is likely to be present. For example, coexisting PVL (usually bilateral) and periventricular hemorrhagic infarction (usually unilateral) will result in combined hemiparesis and spastic diplegia, a picture sometimes called *spastic triplegia*.

A number of other, *non-motor manifestations* of brain injury in preterm infants may indirectly impact motor function and management strategies. Cognitive and learning deficits become evident in 25 to 50% of ex-preterm infants after school entry (Msall et al. 1991, McCormick et al. 1993, Robertson et al. 1994, Botting et al. 1998, Saigal et al. 2000). Not surprisingly, these deficits are more prevalent among children who suffer severe bilateral lesions, in which case there is also marked motor impairment of the upper extremities. These cognitive and learning deficits may be related to injury of the visual and auditory association pathways in the parietal white matter. As discussed above, these areas are particularly prone to injury in PVL and posthemorrhagic hydrocephalus. In addition, these intellectual deficits as well as later epilepsy may also reflect disturbances in later cortical development following earlier white-matter injury (Inder et al. 1999b, 2005). Fortunately, later epilepsy in this population is uncommon (Amess et al. 1998) and in general relatively easily controlled (Kwong et al. 1998).

Follow-up of ex-preterm infants with cerebellar injury has shown an unexpectedly high prevalence of significant language (expressive and receptive), cognitive, and behavioral disturbances (Limperopoulos et al. 2007). Autism-spectrum features develop in almost 40% of these infants, particularly those with injury to the cerebellar vermis (Limperopoulos et al. 2007). Together these non-motor disturbances suggest a form of developmental 'cerebellar cognitive-affective disorder', described in older subjects (Schmahmann and Caplan 2006), and may contribute to the high prevalence of long-term cognitive, learning, and behavioral dysfunction seen in survivors of preterm birth (Tyson and Saigal 2005).

Visual deficits in survivors of preterm birth may result from a variety of causes (e.g. retinopathy of prematurity). Here we consider cerebral visual dysfunction due to injury in the posterior visual pathways (Cioni et al. 1996, Jacobson et al. 1996), specifically the optic radiations. As shown in Figure 2.1.9, the optic radiations for the lower visual field course through the peritrigonal white matter around the superolateral aspects of the occipital horns of the lateral ventricles. As discussed above, this is a particularly high-risk area for PVL and injury in these regions may thus result in cerebral visual dysfunction, particularly in the lower visual fields. Since spastic diplegia is the most common motor abnormality in preterm infants with PVL, such inferior field defects may compound the already compromised gait. Since the motor dysfunction usually dominates the clinical picture, cerebral visual impairment may go unrecognized unless specific testing is performed. Visual function in the preterm infant differs from that seen in term infants as discussed below.

Brain injury in the term infant

VULNERABILITY TO BRAIN INJURY IN THE TERM INFANT
The cerebrovascular system. By term gestation the *anatomic maturation* of the cerebrovascular system approximates that of the adult. In the term infant with systemic hypotension, the brain regions most vulnerable to ischemia are those situated in the watershed areas of the three main cerebral artery (anterior, middle and posterior) territories. The most prominent watershed areas (Fig. 2.1.10) are in the parasagittal cortex and subcortical white matter along the superior convexity of the cerebral hemispheres. Parasagittal cerebral injury is usually bilateral and most intense in the parieto–occipital regions, i.e. an end-zone for all three major cerebral arteries.

At term the *functional maturation* of the cerebral vasculature has advanced the efficacy and robustness of cerebral pressure-flow autoregulation. Compared to the tenuous plateau of the preterm infant, the autoregulatory plateau is wider and shifted rightward. However, although autoregulatory function has improved in the term infant, the cerebral vasculature may still be rendered pressure-passive by even moderate hypoxic–ischemic insults. In the asphyxiated term infant, the loss of autoregulatory function in combination with compromised myocardial function predisposes to cerebral injury (see below).

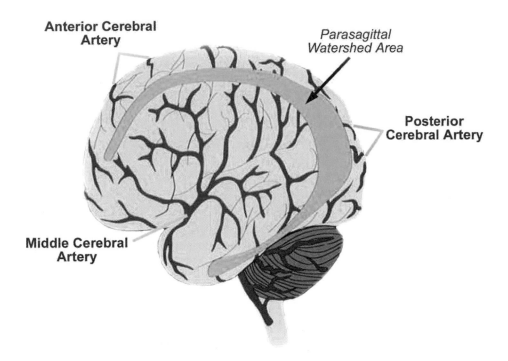

Anterior Cerebral Artery

Parasagittal Watershed Area

Posterior Cerebral Artery

Middle Cerebral Artery

Fig. 2.1.10 Diagram of cerebral hemisphere (sagittal view) showing watershed areas between the supply territories of the anterior, middle, and posterior cerebral arteries.

Vulnerability of the developing neuron. By term gestation, the oligodendrocyte lineage has passed through its most vulnerable developmental phases. In the term infant, the most intense cellular and regional maturation events in the brain involve the developing neuron. Synaptogenesis and organizational events are occurring most rapidly in specific regions of cortex, deep gray matter and brainstem (see below). The rapid developmental activity in these areas is highly demanding of constant glucose and oxygen supply; if this supply becomes inadequate, the developmental demands render these regions particularly susceptible to ischemic insults. At a cellular level, a critical feature of neuronal vulnerability in these rapidly developing regions is the high density of neuronal glutamate receptors, particularly NMDA receptors (Johnston 1995). When activated by glutamate, these NMDA ionophores allow calcium influx into the cytoplasm for the activation of enzymes critical for neuronal development. Activity of these NMDA receptors is highly regulated and very dependent on consistent energy supply. During cerebral hypoxia-ischemia, control of calcium influx through these receptors is lost, allowing sustained calcium influx to toxic levels in the neuronal cytoplasm. In so doing, cerebral hypoxia–ischemia transforms glutamate receptors from important mediators of normal brain development into potentially lethal mediators of neuronal cytotoxicity. During hypoxia–ischemia, this form of neuronal toxicity is maximally expressed in areas of greatest glutamate receptor density, i.e., the basal ganglia (especially the caudate and putamen), thalamus, brainstem nuclei, and specific

79

areas of cerebral cortex (e.g. hippocampus, sensorimotor cortex). To summarize, it is the confluence of the above vascular, cellular and regional factors that determines the severity and distribution of cerebral injury in the term infant.

CEREBROVASCULAR INJURY IN THE TERM INFANT
The principal cerebrovascular lesions in the term infant result from global hypoxia–hypoperfusion insults to the entire brain (e.g. perinatal asphyxia) and focal infarction following embolic occlusion of a cerebral artery.

Global cerebral hypoxic–ischemic insults
During the development of intrauterine asphyxia, the impaired oxygen and glucose supply triggers certain compensatory hemodynamic responses in the systemic and cerebral circulations of the fetus. These responses are aimed at so-called 'brain sparing'. Specifically, these adaptive mechanisms redirect fetal blood supply to the brain at the expense of organs such as the kidney, liver and heart. Within the brain, blood supply is redirected toward the most actively developing areas, which at term include the basal ganglia-thalamus, brainstem and sensorimotor cortex. Decompensation of these adaptive mechanisms can occur in two broad ways, each with its characteristic topography of injury. If the impairment in fetal oxygenation is brief, these adaptive responses may effectively preserve cerebral integrity with little detriment to other organs. However, when the insult is either too prolonged or too severe, these intrinsic attempts at brain protection fail. With prolonged but incomplete asphyxia, end-organ damage develops in the liver, kidney and heart, while in the brain the areas most affected are the watershed areas of the parasagittal cortex (Fig. 2.1.10) and white matter. Conversely, when asphyxia is severe (e.g. with placental abruption, maternal cardiac arrest or uterine rupture) but rapidly reversed, the hemodynamic compensatory mechanisms fail from the outset. In these situations, the severe disruption of cerebral oxygen and substrate supply results in injury that is most marked in regions with the greatest metabolic demand, i.e. the basal ganglia–thalamus, brainstem (Fig. 2.1.11, left) and the primary sensorimotor cortex. With rapid delivery and effective resuscitation, these infants may show minimal injury to other end organs and other less demanding brain regions.

Arterio–occlusive stroke in the term newborn infant
Cerebral infarction, or stroke, due to embolic occlusion of one or more cerebral arteries is another important cause of cerebral palsy that originates in most cases during the perinatal or early neonatal period (Fig. 2.1.11, right). A definite etiology is seldom identified, and the assumption is that emboli generated by involuting placental or fetal vessels enter the cerebral circulation through fetal vascular pathways such as the foramen ovale and ductus arteriosus, prior to their closure in early life. Rarely, a hypercoagulable state or congenital heart defect is identified. Focal strokes may also complicate perinatal asphyxia and occur in twin-to-twin transfusion syndromes.

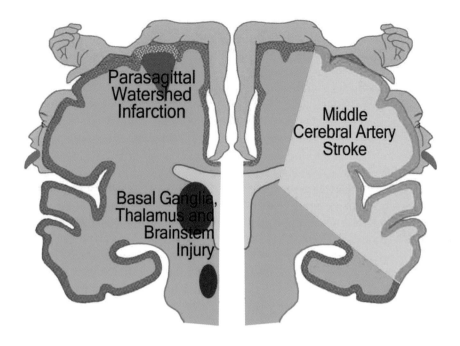

Fig. 2.1.11 Location of brain lesions in the term infant and their motor sequelae. Diagram of cerebral hemispheres (coronal view) with superimposed homunculus to demonstrate the cortical origin of motor fibers to the face, trunk and extremities. (A) Left, regions of injury following global cerebral ischemia, with parasagittal watershed injury in the distribution of the trunk and proximal upper-extremity regions of representation (see also Fig. 2.1.10), as well as selective neuronal necrosis in the basal ganglia and thalamus. (B) Right, distribution of injury in the most common vaso-occlusive lesion, i.e. middle cerebral artery stroke.

CLINICAL–PATHOLOGIC CORRELATION OF BRAIN INJURY IN THE TERM INFANT

For the purposes of this discussion, the long-term clinical correlates are considered in the context of the distinct mechanisms and topographies of injury outlined above.

Parasagittal cerebral injury resulting from watershed ischemia between the anterior and middle cerebral arteries affects the motor cortex, particularly regions innervating the upper extremities (especially proximal muscles) and trunk (Figs 2.1.10, 11, left), usually with lesser involvement of areas representing the pelvic girdle and leg muscles. This topography of injury results in a characteristic type of spastic quadriparesis involving the arms more than the legs, i.e. the reverse of spastic diparesis in the preterm infant (see above). The *gradient* of weakness (i.e. arm more than leg), which resembles that in hemiplegia following middle cerebral artery stroke, has led to the term 'bilateral hemiplegia', a confusing and inappropriate term for the motor deficits after parasagittal injury. Because the parasagittal watershed area is particularly broad in the important association areas of the parietal cortex, *cognitive/intellectual deficits* are common after this form of injury, as are distinct learning disabilities (Yokochi 1998). *Visual function* following parasagittal cerebral injury in infants

81

is not well described. In adults, however, watershed injury in this area causes visual neglect, disordered tracking and difficulties interpreting complex diagrams (Balint's syndrome). Because of the cortical involvement, epilepsy is particularly common following this form of brain injury.

Basal ganglia–thalamic injury (Fig. 2.1.11, left) typically occurs during severe but brief insults (see above). Following more severe insults, injury may extend to include the tegmental brainstem nuclei. The typical long-term clinical picture is one of fluctuating but predominantly rigid muscle tone, with varying degrees of underlying spasticity. Superimposed on this fluctuating tone are different types of involuntary movements, presumably reflecting the predominant basal ganglia nuclei injured in each case (Rutherford et al. 1992). For reasons that are poorly understood, increasing rigidity and dyskinetic features may emerge after years of predominant spasticity (Burke et al. 1980, Saint Hilaire et al. 1991). This form of injury is associated with prominent oromotor dysfunction especially if brainstem nuclei are also involved. As a consequence, speech is often markedly dysarthric and the common feeding difficulties often require gastrostomy tube placement (Roland et al. 1988, Pasternak et al. 1991). Cognitive function in these children spans a wide range but many appear to have cognitive function that is *relatively* preserved (Kyllerman et al. 1982, Rosenbloom 1994), compared to the motor dysfunction. Specific learning disabilities may occur (Lou et al. 1989). In cases with cognitive impairment, these deficits may be due to thalamic injury.

Another cause of extrapyramidal cerebral palsy results from the acute bilirubin toxicity (or kernicterus) in severe neonatal jaundice (Connolly and Volpe 1990). After decades of steady decline in the incidence of this condition, kernicterus appears to be resurfacing (Ebbesen 2000). In this condition neuronal injury is widespread but is particularly prominent in the basal ganglia, brainstem and cerebellum (Ahdab-Barmada and Moossy 1984, Connolly and Volpe 1990). The long-term features of chronic bilirubin encephalopathy include often severe retrocollis and opisthotonus, athetosis, and gaze abnormalities (Connolly and Volpe 1990). The athetosis in this condition often fluctuates (Hayashi et al. 1991), and may be triggered by attempted skilled movements. In addition, neuronal injury in the cochlear nuclei and auditory nerve results in high-frequency hearing loss (Byers et al. 1955). Over 50% of affected children have cognitive function in the normal range (Byers et al. 1955).

Focal arterio–occlusive injury or stroke has long-term sequelae that are influenced by the particular arterial territory involved. The acute presentation of the vast majority of strokes is with focal neonatal seizures in the first days of life (Clancy et al. 1985, Levy et al. 1985), while motor deficits may remain relatively subtle over the first 6 months or more. In fact, imaging studies suggest that hemiparesis may develop in only one-quarter of infants with unilateral strokes (Bouza et al. 1994a, b, Dall'Oglio et al. 1994, de Vries et al. 1997, Estan and Hope 1997, Rutherford et al. 1998, Mercuri et al. 1999). Since strokes most commonly involve the left middle cerebral artery, right hemiparesis is more common (Volpe 2001). Unlike the hemiparesis that follows PVHI in the pre-term infant, hemiparesis in the term infant tends to affect arm and face more than leg (Fig. 2.1.11, right); unlike the upper-extremity weakness in parasagittal injury which is

82

predominantly proximal, in focal stroke the distal upper extremities are more impaired. Hemiparesis is virtually assured when occlusion of the proximal middle cerebral artery segment causes injury of the entire territory including the basal ganglia, white matter, posterior limb of the internal capsule and cortex (de Vries et al. 1997). Conversely, when injury is confined to the proximal penetrating branches or more distal branches, functionally significant hemiparesis is rare (de Vries et al. 1997). Even when motor deficits become manifest, their functional severity is often less than would be expected for the volume of cerebral injury on imaging studies. This has been ascribed to the incompletely understood phenomenon of 'plasticity' in the immature brain (Stiles 2000). Cognitive function in neonatal stroke survivors is normal in 50%, and 18% have an IQ over 100 (Fennell and Dikel 2001). Lesions of either hemisphere may impair non-verbal function, often with dissociation of verbal and performance IQs (Fennell and Dikel 2001). Children with a left hemisphere lesion are at greater risk for impairment of syntactic awareness and sentence repetition (Fennell and Dikel 2001), while receptive vocabulary appears to be intact. Conversely, right hemisphere lesions are associated with decreased mathematical ability, possibly due to the associated visual-spatial dysfunction (Fennell and Dikel 2001). Later epilepsy has been reported in 10%–60% of children after unilateral neonatal strokes (Sran and Baumann 1988, Wulfeck et al. 1991, Koelfen et al. 1995, Sreenan et al. 2000). The presence of epilepsy may be a more powerful predictor of impaired cognitive function than the laterality of the lesion.

Visual dysfunction in unilateral lesions, e.g. periventricular hemorrhagic infarction and unilateral stroke, may cause contralateral homonymous hemianopia, which impairs the child's ability to appreciate both learning material and obstacles in the affected field. Fortunately this complication appears to be relatively rare (Black 1980, 1982).

Summary
The mechanisms and manifestations of brain injury leading to cerebral palsy have been presented as discrete entities for the purposes of this discussion. More often than not varying degrees of more than one mechanism may be operative in a causal pathway (Stanley et al. 2000). Likewise, the long-term manifestations of injury to the immature brain may reflect the combined effects of more than one lesion. Furthermore, although the ultimate manifestations of each injury type are generally those discussed above, it is important to note that although the injury underlying cerebral palsy is static, the manifestations may evolve over time. For example, infants who ultimately develop spastic diplegia may initially evolve through phases of hypotonia and dystonia (Bax 1992). Likewise, infants destined for an extrapyramidal form of cerebral palsy may initially evolve through hypotonic or spastic phases before manifesting extrapyramidal features as late as the second decade of life (Burke et al. 1980, Saint Hilaire et al. 1991). The reasons for this changing clinical picture after a static insult remain poorly understood but raise intriguing questions about the interaction between brain injury and development, and potential avenues for future intervention.

83

REFERENCES

Ahdab-Barmada M, Moossy J (1984) The neuropathology of kernicterus in the premature neonate: diagnostic problems. *J Neuropathol Exp Neurol* **43**: 45–56.

Alexander JM, Gilstrap LC, Cox SM, McIntire DM, Leveno KJ (1998) Clinical chorioamnionitis and the prognosis for very low birth weight infants. *Obstet Gynecol* **91**: 725–9.

Amess PN, Baudin J, Townsend J, Meek J, Roth SC, Neville BG, Wyatt JS, Stewart A (1998) Epilepsy in very preterm infants: neonatal cranial ultrasound reveals a high-risk subcategory. *Dev Med Child Neurol* **40**: 724–30.

Back S, Volpe J (1997) Cellular and molecular pathogenesis of periventricular white matter injury. *MRDD Res Rev* **3**: 96–107.

Back SA, Gan X, Li Y, Rosenberg PA, Volpe JJ (1998) Maturation-dependent vulnerability of oligodendrocytes to oxidative stress-induced death caused by glutathione depletion. *J Neurosci* **18**: 6241–53.

Back SA, Luo NL, Borenstein NS, Levine JM, Volpe JJ, Kinney HC (2001) Late oligodendrocyte progenitors coincide with the developmental window of vulnerability for human perinatal white matter injury. *J Neurosci* **21**: 1302–12.

Banker B, Larroche J (1962) Periventricular leukomalacia in infancy. *Arch Neurol* **7**: 386–410.

Bassan H, Feldman HA, Limperopoulos C, Benson CB, Ringer SA, Veracruz E, Soul JS, Volpe JJ, du Plessis AJ (2006) Periventricular hemorrhagic infarction: risk factors and neonatal outcome. *Pediatr Neurol*, 35: 85–92.

Bassan H, Limperopoulos C, Visconti K, Mayer DL, Feldman HA, Avery L, Benson CB, Stewart J, Ringer SA, Soul JS, Volpe JJ, du Plessis AJ (2007) Neurodevelopmental outcome in survivors of periventricular hemorrhagic infarction. *Pediatrics* **120**: 785–92.

Baud O, Emilie D, Pelletier E, Lacaze-Masmonteil T, Zupan V, Fernandez H, Dehan M, Frydman R, Ville Y (1999) Amniotic fluid concentrations of interleukin-1beta, interleukin-6 and TNF-alpha in chorioamnionitis before 32 weeks of gestation: histological associations and neonatal outcome. *Br J Obstet Gynaecol* **106**: 72–7.

Bax M (1992) Cerebral palsy. In: Aicardi J, editor. *Diseases of the Nervous System in Childhood*. London: Mac Keith Press. p 330–74.

Black PD (1980) Ocular defects in children with cerebral palsy. *Br Med J* **281**: 487–8.

Black P (1982) Visual disorders associated with cerebral palsy. *Br J Ophthalmol* **66**: 46–52.

Blair E, Stanley FJ (1988) Intrapartum asphyxia: a rare cause of cerebral palsy. *J Pediatr* **112**: 515–9.

Botting N, Powls A, Cooke RW, Marlow N (1998) Cognitive and educational outcome of very-low-birthweight children in early adolescence. *Dev Med Child Neurol* **40**: 652–60.

Bouza H, Dubowitz LM, Rutherford M, Pennock JM (1994a) Prediction of outcome in children with congenital hemiplegia: a magnetic resonance imaging study. *Neuropediatrics* **25**: 60–6.

Bouza H, Rutherford M, Acolet D, Pennock JM, Dubowitz LM (1994b) Evolution of early hemiplegic signs in full-term infants with unilateral brain lesions in the neonatal period: a prospective study. *Neuropediatrics* **25**: 201–7.

Burke RE, Fahn S, Gold AP (1980) Delayed-onset dystonia in patients with 'static' encephalopathy. *J Neurol Neurosurg Psychiatry* **43**: 789–97.

Byers R, Payne R, Crothers B (1955) Extrapyramidal cerebral palsy with hearing loss following erythroblastosis. *Pediatrics* **15**: 248.

Cai Z, Pan ZL, Pang Y, Evans OB, Rhodes PG (2000) Cytokine induction in fetal rat brains and brain injury in neonatal rats after maternal lipopolysaccharide administration. *Pediatr Res* **47**: 64–72.

Chumas P, Drake J, Del Bigio M, da Silva M, Tuor U (1994) Anaerobic glycolysis preceding white-matter destruction in experimental neonatal hydrocephalus. *J Neurosurg* **80**: 491–501.

Cioni G, Fazzi B, Ipata AE, Canapicchi R, van Hof-van Duin J (1996) Correlation between cerebral visual impairment and magnetic resonance imaging in children with neonatal encephalopathy. *Dev Med Child Neurol* **38**: 120–32.

Clancy R, Malin S, Laraque D, Baumgart S, Younkin D (1985) Focal motor seizures heralding stroke in full-term neonates. *Am J Dis Child* **139**: 601–6.

Connolly AM, Volpe JJ (1990) Clinical features of bilirubin encephalopathy. *Clin Perinatol* **17**: 371–9.

84

Counsell SJ, Dyet LE, Larkman DJ, Nunes RG, Boardman JP, Allsop JM, Fitzpatrick J, Srinivasan L, Cowan FM, Hajnal JV, Rutherford MA, Edwards AD (2007) Thalamo–cortical connectivity in children born preterm mapped using probabilistic magnetic resonance tractography. *Neuroimage* **34**: 896–904.

Dale A, Stanley FJ (1980) An epidemiological study of cerebral palsy in Western Australia, 1956–1975. II: Spastic cerebral palsy and perinatal factors. *Dev Med Child Neurol* **22**: 13–25.

Dall'Oglio AM, Bates E, Volterra V, Di Capua M, Pezzini G (1994) Early cognition, communication and language in children with focal brain injury. *Dev Med Child Neurol* **36**: 1076–98.

Dammann O, Leviton A (1997) Maternal intrauterine infection, cytokines, and brain damage in the preterm newborn. *Pediatr Neurol* **42**: 1–8.

Da Silva MC, Drake JM, Lemaire C, Cross A, Tuor UI (1994) High-energy phosphate metabolism in a neonatal model of hydrocephalus before and after shunting. *J Neurosurg* **81**: 544–53.

Da Silva MC, Michowicz S, Drake JM, Chumas PD, Tuor UI (1995) Reduced local cerebral blood flow in periventricular white matter in experimental neonatal hydrocephalus: restoration with CSF shunting. *J Cereb Blood Flow Metab* **15**: 1057–65.

de Vries LS, Groenendaal F, Eken P, van Haastert IC, Rademaker KJ, Meiners LC (1997) Infarcts in the vascular distribution of the middle cerebral artery in preterm and fullterm infants. *Neuropediatrics* **28**: 88–96.

Del Bigio MR, Kanfer JN (1996) Oligodendrocyte-related enzymes in hydrocephalic rat brains. *Soc Neurosci* **22**: 482.

Del Bigio MR, Kanfer JN, Zhang YW (1997) Myelination delay in the cerebral white matter of immature rats with kaolin-induced hydrocephalus is reversible. *J Neuropath Exp Neurol* **56**: 1053–66.

Ebbesen F (2000) Recurrence of kernicterus in term and near-term infants in Denmark. *Acta Paediatr* **89**: 1213–7.

Estan J, Hope P (1997) Unilateral neonatal cerebral infarction in full term infants. *Arch Dis Child Fetal Neonatal Ed* **76**: F88–93.

Evans N (2006) Assessment and support of the preterm circulation. *Early Hum Dev* **82**: 803–10.

Fennell EB, Dikel TN (2001) Cognitive and neuropsychological functioning in children with cerebral palsy. *J Child Neurol* **16**: 58–63.

Friedman AH, Fahey JT (1993) The transition from fetal to neonatal circulation: normal responses and implications for infants with heart disease. *Semin Perinatol* **17**: 106–21.

Grether JK, Nelson KB, Dambrosia JM, Phillips TM (1999) Interferons and cerebral palsy. *J Pediatr* **134**: 324–32.

Guzzetta F, Mercuri E, Spano M (1995) Mechanisms and evolution of the brain damage in neonatal post-hemorrhagic hydrocephalus. *Childs Nerv Syst* **11**: 293–6.

Hagberg B, Hagberg G, Olow I, von Wendt L (1989a) The changing panorama of cerebral palsy in Sweden. V. The birth year period 1979–82. *Acta Paediatr Scand* **78**: 283–90.

Hagberg B, Hagberg G, Zetterstrom R (1989b) Decreasing perinatal mortality–increase in cerebral palsy morbidity. *Acta Paediatr Scand* **78**: 664–70.

Hagberg B, Hagberg G, Olow I, van Wendt L (1996) The changing panorama of cerebral palsy in Sweden. VII. Prevalence and origin in the birth year period 1987–90. *Acta Paediatr* **85**: 954–60.

Hagberg B, Hagberg G, Beckung E, Uvebrant P (2001) Changing panorama of cerebral palsy in Sweden. VIII. Prevalence and origin in the birth year period 1991–94. *Acta Paediatr* **90**: 271–7.

Hayashi M, Satoh J, Sakamoto K, Morimatsu Y (1991) Clinical and neuropathological findings in severe athetoid cerebral palsy: A comparative study of globo–luysian and thalamo–putaminal groups. *Brain Dev* **13**: 47–51.

Huppi PS, Barnes PD (1997) Magnetic resonance techniques in the evaluation of the newborn brain. *Clin Perinatol* **24**: 693–723.

Iida K, Takashima S, Ueda K (1995) Immunohistochemical study of myelination and oligodendrocyte in infants with periventricular leukomalacia. *Pediatr Neurol* **13**: 296–304.

Inder TE, Huppi PS, Warfield S, Kikinis R, Zientara GP, Barnes PD, Jolesz F, Volpe JJ (1999a) Periventricular white matter injury in the premature infant is followed by reduced cerebral cortical gray matter volume at term. *Ann Neurol* **46**: 755–60.

Inder TE, Huppi PS, Zientara GP, Jolesz FA, Holling EE, Robertson R, Barnes PD, Volpe JJ (1999b) The postmigrational development of polymicrogyria documented by magnetic resonance imaging from 31 weeks postconceptional age. *Ann Neurol* **45**: 798–801.

Inder T, Huppi PS, Zientara GP, Maier SE, Jolesz FA, di Salvo D, Robertson R, Barnes PD, Volpe JJ (1999c) Early detection of periventricular leukomalacia by diffusion-weighted magnetic resonance imaging techniques. *J Pediatr* **134**: 631–4.

Inder TE, Warfield SK, Wang H, Huppi PS, Volpe JJ (2005) Abnormal cerebral structure is present at term in premature infants. *Pediatr* **115**: 286–94.

Jacobson L, Ek U, Fernell E, Flodmark O, Broberger U (1996) Visual impairment in preterm children with periventricular leukomalacia – visual, cognitive and neuropaediatric characteristics related to cerebral imaging. *Dev Med Child Neurol* **38**: 724–35.

Johnsen SD, Bodensteiner JB, Lotze TE (2005) Frequency and nature of cerebellar injury in the extremely premature survivor with cerebral palsy. *J Child Neurology* **20**: 60–4.

Johnston M (1995) Developmental aspects of NMDA receptor agonists and antagonists in the central nervous system *Psychopharmacol Bull* **30**: 567–75.

Kadhim H, Tabarki B, Verellen G, De Prez C, Rona AM, Sebire G (2001) Inflammatory cytokines in the pathogenesis of periventricular leukomalacia. *Neurology* **56**: 1278–84.

Khwaja O, Volpe JJ (2008) Pathogenesis of cerebral white matter injury of prematurity. *Arch Dis Child Fetal Neonatal Ed* **93**: F153–61.

Koelfen W, Freund M, Varnholt V (1995) Neonatal stroke involving the middle cerebral artery in term infants: clinical presentation, EEG and imaging studies, and outcome. *Dev Med Child Neurol* **37**: 204–12.

Kwong KL, Wong SN, So KT (1998) Epilepsy in children with cerebral palsy. *Pediatr Neurol* **19**: 31–6.

Kyllerman M, Bager B, Bensch J, Bille B, Olow I, Voss H (1982) Dyskinetic cerebral palsy. I. Clinical categories, associated neurological abnormalities and incidences. *Acta Paediatr Scand* **71**: 543–50.

Levy SR, Abroms IF, Marshall PC, Rosquete EE (1985) Seizures and cerebral infarction in the full-term newborn. *Ann Neurol* **17**: 366–70.

Limperopoulos C, Benson CB, Bassan H, Disalvo DN, Kinnamon DD, Moore M, Ringer SA, Volpe JJ, du Plessis AJ (2005) Cerebellar hemorrhage in the preterm infant: ultrasonographic findings and risk factors. *Pediatrics* **116**: 717–24.

Limperopoulos C, Bassan H, Gauvreau K, Robertson RL Jr., Sullivan NR, Benson CB, Avery L, Stewart J, Soul JS, Ringer SA, Volpe JJ, duPlessis AJ (2007) Does cerebellar injury in premature infants contribute to the high prevalence of long-term cognitive, learning, and behavioral disability in survivors? *Pediatrics* **120**: 584–93.

Little W (1862) On the influence of abnormal parturition, difficult labour, premature birth and asphyxia neonatorum on mental and physical conditions of the child, especially in relation to deformities. *Trans Obstet Soc Lond* **3**: 293–344.

Lou HC, Henriksen L, Bruhn P, Borner H, Nielsen JB (1989) Striatal dysfunction in attention deficit and hyperkinetic disorder. *Arch Neurol* **46**: 48–52.

Martinez E, Figueroa R, Garry D, Visintainer P, Patel K, Verma U, Sehgal PB, Tejani N (1998) Elevated amniotic fluid interleukin-6 as a predictor of neonatal periventricular leukomalacia and intraventricular hemorrhage. *J Matern Fetal Investig* **8**: 101–7.

McCormick MC, McCarton C, Tonascia J, Brooks-Gunn J (1993) Early educational intervention for very low birth weight infants: results from the Infant Health and Development Program. *J Pediatr* **123**: 527–33.

Mercuri E, Rutherford M, Cowan F, Pennock J, Counsell S, Papadimitriou M, Azzopardi D, Bydder G, Dubowitz L (1999) Early prognostic indicators of outcome in infants with neonatal cerebral infarction: a clinical, electroencephalogram, and magnetic resonance imaging study. *Pediatr* **103**: 39–46.

Messerschmidt A, Brugger PC, Boltshauser E, Zoder G, Sterniste W, Birnbacher R, Prayer D (2005) Disruption of cerebellar development: potential complication of extreme prematurity. *Am J Neuroradiol* **26**: 1659–67.

Msall ME, Buck GM, Rogers BT, Merke D, Catanzaro NL, Zorn WA (1991) Risk factors for major neurodevelopmental impairments and need for special education resources in extremely premature infants. *J Pediatr* **119**: 606–14.

Nelson KB, Ellenberg JH (1986) Antecedents of cerebral palsy. Multivariate analysis of risk. *N Engl J Med* **315**: 81–6.

Nelson KB, Dambrosia JM, Grether JK, Phillips TM (1998) Neonatal cytokines and coagulation factors in children with cerebral palsy. *Ann Neurol* **44**: 665–75.

Oka A, Belliveau MJ, Rosenberg PA, Volpe JJ (1993) Vulnerability of oligodendroglia to glutamate: pharmacology, mechanisms, and prevention. *J Neurosci* **13**: 1441–53.

Ozawa H, Nishida A, Mito T, Takashima S (1994) Development of ferritin-positive cells in cerebrum of human brain. *Pediatr Neurol* **10**: 44–8.

Pasternak JF, Predey TA, Mikhael MA (1991) Neonatal asphyxia: vulnerability of basal ganglia, thalamus, and brainstem. *Pediatr Neurol* **7**: 147–9.

Pharoah PO, Platt MJ, Cooke T (1996) The changing epidemiology of cerebral palsy. *Arch Dis Child Fetal Neonatal Ed* **75**: F169–73.

Quinn M, Ando Y, Levene M (1992) Cerebral arterial and venous flow-velocity measurements in post-hemorrhagic ventricular dilation and hydrocephalus. *Dev Med Child Neurol* **34**: 863–9.

Robertson C, Sauve RS, Christianson HE (1994) Province-based study of neurologic disability among survivors weighing 500 through 1249 grams at birth. *Pediatr* **93**: 636–40.

Roland E, Hill A, Norman M, Flodmark O, MacNab A (1988) Selective brainstem injury in an asphyxiated newborn. *Ann Neurol* **23**: 89–92.

Rosenbloom L (1994) Dyskinetic cerebral palsy and birth asphyxia. *Dev Med Child Neurol* **36**: 285–9.

Rutherford MA, Pennock JM, Murdoch-Eaton DM, Cowan FM, Dubowitz LM (1992) Athetoid cerebral palsy with cysts in the putamen after hypoxic–ischaemic encephalopathy. *Arch Dis Child* **67**: 846–50.

Rutherford MA, Pennock JM, Counsell SJ, Mercuri E, Cowan FM, Dubowitz LMS, Edwards AD (1998) Abnormal magnetic resonance signal in the internal capsule predicts poor neurodevelopmental outcome in infants with hypoxic–ischemic encephalopathy. *Pediatrics* **102**: 323–8.

Rutherford M, Srinivasan L, Dyet L, Ward P, Allsop J, Counsell S, Cowan F (2006) Magnetic resonance imaging in perinatal brain injury: clinical presentation, lesions and outcome. *Pediatr Radiol* **36**: 582–92.

Saigal S, Burrows E, Stoskopf BL, Rosenbaum PL, Streiner D (2000) Impact of extreme prematurity on families of adolescent children. *J Pediatr* **137**: 701–6.

Saint Hilaire MH, Burke RE, Bressman SB, Brin MF, Fahn S (1991) Delayed-onset dystonia due to perinatal or early childhood asphyxia. *Neurology*, 41: 216–22.

Schmahmann JD, Caplan D (2006) Cognition, emotion and the cerebellum. *Brain* **129**: 290–2.

Selmaj KW, Raine CS (1988) Tumor necrosis factor mediates myelin and oligodendrocyte damage in vitro. *Ann Neurol* **23**: 339–46.

Shirane R, Sato S, Sato K, Kameyama M, Ogawa A, Yoshimoto T, Hatazawa J, Ito M (1992) Cerebral blood flow and oxygen metabolism in infants with hydrocephalus. *Childs Nerv Syst* **8**: 118–23.

Soul JS, Hammer PE, Tsuji M, Saul JP, Bassan H, Limperopoulos C, DiSalvo DN, Moore M, Akins P, Ringer SA, Volpe JJ, Trachtenberg F, du Plessis AJ (2007) Fluctuating pressure-passivity is common in the cerebral circulation of sick premature infants. *Pediatr Res* **61**: 467–73.

Sran SK, Baumann RJ (1988) Outcome of neonatal strokes. *Am J Dis Child* **142**: 1086–8.

Sreenan C, Bhargava R, Robertson CM (2000) Cerebral infarction in the term newborn: clinical presentation and long-term outcome. *J Pediatr* **137**: 351–5.

Srinivasan L, Dutta R, Counsell SJ, Allsop JM, Boardman JP, Rutherford MA, Edwards AD (2007) Quantification of deep gray matter in preterm infants at term-equivalent age using manual volumetry of 3-tesla magnetic resonance images. *Pediatr* 119: 759–65.

Stanley FJ (1992) Survival and cerebral palsy in low birthweight infants: implications for perinatal care. *Paediatr Perinat Epidemiol* **6**: 298–310.

Stanley F, Blair E, Alberman E (2000) *Cerebral Palsies: Epidemiology and Causal Pathways*. London: Mac Keith Press.

Stiles J (2000) Neural plasticity and cognitive development. *Dev Neuropsychol* **18**: 237–72.

Tyson JE, Saigal S (2005) Outcomes for extremely low-birth-weight infants: disappointing news. *J Am Med Assoc* **294**: 371–3.

Volpe JJ (1994) Brain injury in the premature infant – current concepts. *Prev Med* **23**: 638–45.

Volpe J (2001) *Neurology of the Newborn* 4th edn. Philadelphia: W.B. Saunders. p 217–76.

Volpe JJ (2008) *Neurology of the Newborn* 5th edn. Philadelphia: Saunders Elsevier.

Volpe JJ, Herscovitch P, Perlman JM, Raichle ME (1983) Positron emission tomography in the newborn: extensive impairment of regional cerebral blood flow with intraventricular hemorrhage and hemorrhagic intracerebral involvement. *Pediatrics* **72**: 589–601.

Wulfeck BB, Trauner DA, Tallal PA (1991) Neurologic, cognitive, and linguistic features of infants after early stroke. *Pediatr Neurol* **7**: 266–9.

Yokochi K (1998) Clinical profiles of subjects with subcortical leukomalacia and border-zone infarction revealed by MR. *Acta Paediatr* **87**: 879–83.

Yonezawa M, Back S, Gan X, Rosenberg P, Volpe J (1996) Cystine deprivation induces oligodendroglial death: rescue by free radical scavengers and by a diffusible glial factor. *J Neurochem* **67**: 566–73.

Yoon BH, Romero R, Yang SH, Jun JK, Kim IO, Choi JH, Syn HC (1996) Interleukin-6 concentrations in umbilical cord plasma are elevated in neonates with white matter lesions associated with periventricular leukomalacia. *Am J Obstet Gynecol* **174**: 1433–40.

Yoon BH, Jun JK, Romero R, Park KH, Gomez R, Choi JH, Kim IO (1997) Amniotic fluid inflammatory cytokines (interleukin-6, interleukin-1beta, and tumor necrosis factor-alpha), neonatal brain white matter lesions, and cerebral palsy. *Am J Obstet Gynecol* **177**: 19–26.

Yoon B, Romero R, Park J, Kim C, Kim S, Choi J, Han T (2000) Fetal exposure to an intra-amniotic inflammation and the development of cerebral palsy at the age of three years. *Am J Obstet Gynecol* **182**: 675–81.

2.2
THE PATHOPHYSIOLOGY OF SPASTICITY

Warwick J. Peacock

Spasticity is one of the major problems in patients who have an upper motor lesion in the brain or spinal cord. Pathology in the nervous system produces some negative features such as loss of power, decreased fine-motor control or a sensory deficit, but also positive features. These positive or release effects manifest as spasticity, involuntary movements or epileptic seizures. The site of the lesion rather than the pathology determines the combination of positive and negative features that produce the characteristic clinical picture. For example, a lesion in the cervical spinal cord produces negative effects such as weakness and loss of fine-motor control as well as the positive feature of increased muscle tone (spasticity) in all four limbs frequently associated with muscle spasms, whereas a lesion in the left cerebral hemisphere in an adult causes weakness in the right face, arm and leg with loss of speech (negative features). However, the weakness of the right arm and leg is associated with spasticity (positive feature). The spasticity in this case is not accompanied by muscle spasms and, in addition, right-sided focal motor seizures (also a positive feature) may appear some time later.

The clinical feature of spasticity is an elevation in muscle tone evidenced by a velocity-dependent increase in resistance to passive movement. The examiner experiences a clasp-knife feel to this resistance. Brisk tendon reflexes and clonus are also present.

Lance (1980) offered us a definition of spasticity: 'Spasticity is a motor disorder characterized by a velocity-dependent increase in tonic stretch reflexes, with exaggerated tendon jerks resulting from hyperexcitability of the stretch reflex, as one component of the upper motoneuron syndrome.'

In a healthy individual at rest, 'background muscle tone' is electrically silent. However, in subjects with upper motor neuron disorders associated with spasticity, an 'electrically active' excessive 'background muscle tone' may be observed.

Although spasticity could be considered to be a compensation for weakness, the increased muscle tone it produces may interfere with a movement pattern once that movement program is being executed.

In addition to the increased muscle tone due to an exaggeration of the stretch reflex, there is evidence to show that structural changes occur within the muscle cells causing intrinsic muscle stiffness (Olsson et al. 2006). It is well recognized that spasticity in a growing child frequently leads to deformities such as muscle contractures and joint dislocations.

Does damage at any site in the nervous system produce spasticity or are there very specific sites where a lesion will lead to spasticity? To answer this question, let us review the five different areas of the central nervous system involved in movement and see which one of these, when damaged, will lead to spasticity: (1) the pyramidal and extrapyramidal systems, (2) the corpus striatum, (3) the cerebellum, (4) the brainstem motor nuclei, and (5) the spinal cord.

The pyramidal and etxrapyramidal systems
All movements start as a thought in a remote area of the cerebral cortex and then the supplementary motor area and other cortical control centers become involved (Deecke et al. 1969). An order is then issued from the motor cortex via upper motor neurons, which are both pyramidal and extrapyramidal, to initiate appropriate muscular contraction and achieve the desired goal (Fig. 2.2.1). Fibers in the pyramidal tract descend through the cerebral hemisphere via the internal capsule and enter the brainstem where

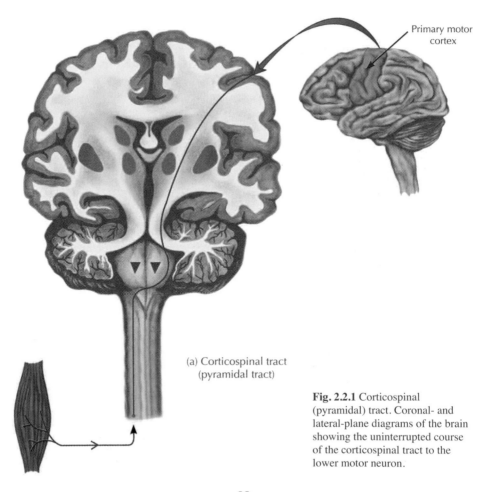

Primary motor cortex

(a) Corticospinal tract (pyramidal tract)

Fig. 2.2.1 Corticospinal (pyramidal) tract. Coronal- and lateral-plane diagrams of the brain showing the uninterrupted course of the corticospinal tract to the lower motor neuron.

they gather together as the pyramid on the anterior aspect of the medulla oblongata. At the level of the pyramid the majority cross to the opposite side. The pyramidal fibers continue down the spinal cord as the crossed lateral corticospinal tract or as the much smaller uncrossed anterior corticospinal tract. The extrapyramidal tracts do not pass through the medullary pyramid and include descending cortical fibers to brainstem nuclei, such as the vestibular and reticular nuclei. From these two nuclei the vestibulospinal and reticulospinal tracts arise which descend down the spinal cord to influence lower motor neuron activity.

The basal ganglia are first consulted for advice about the best strategy to achieve this goal based on memory of previous similar movements and the position of the body at that time (Fig. 2.2.2). The cerebellum is informed of the motor plan and asked to monitor it throughout its course (Fig. 2.2.3). The brainstem motor nuclei are instructed to provide the correct background posture and tone to enable the movement to be carried out (Fig. 2.2.4). The cortical motor control centers then issue their order to the motor

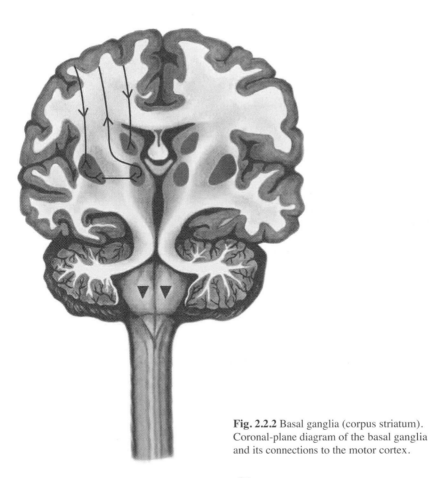

Fig. 2.2.2 Basal ganglia (corpus striatum). Coronal-plane diagram of the basal ganglia and its connections to the motor cortex.

91

Fig. 2.2.3 Cerebellar system. Coronal-plane diagram of the cerebellum showing its afferent connections to the muscle and its afferent and efferent connections to the motor cortex.

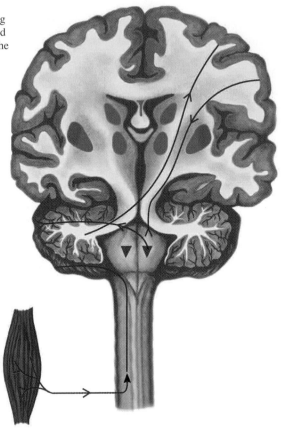

neurons in the spinal cord via the pyramidal tracts. Through the lower motor neurons the muscles are made to bring about the appropriate sequence of contractions. The final order is delivered via the corticospinal (pyramidal) tract.

The spasticity seen in a patient with a stroke or in a child with cerebral palsy is often attributed to damage to the corticospinal or pyramidal tract. This is incorrect. This recently evolved and highly specialized tract controls mainly the distal limb muscles and would be involved in discrete movements such as writing, using a knife and fork and for speaking. Damage to the corticospinal tract alone only produces loss of fine motor control in distal limb muscles without spasticity (Hepp-Reymond et al. 1974, Kuypers 1981). However, it is uncommon for the corticospinal tract to be injured in isolation. Many other motor tracts, such as the cortico–bulbospinal (extrapyramidal) tracts, surround the pyramidal tract along its course and are also damaged. It is the involvement of these other tracts that lead to the increase in muscle tone. Precisely which tracts these are we will have to work out by a process of elimination. What we can say with certainty is that isolated injury to the corticospinal or pyramidal tract alone does not produce spasticity.

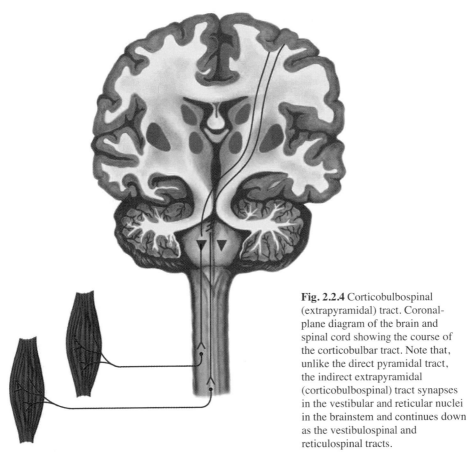

Fig. 2.2.4 Corticobulbospinal (extrapyramidal) tract. Coronal-plane diagram of the brain and spinal cord showing the course of the corticobulbar tract. Note that, unlike the direct pyramidal tract, the indirect extrapyramidal (corticobulbospinal) tract synapses in the vestibular and reticular nuclei in the brainstem and continues down as the vestibulospinal and reticulospinal tracts.

We will first review the other possibilities before returning to the cortico–bulbospinal tract.

Corpus striatum

The corpus striatum is made up of large clusters of gray-matter nuclei situated deep within the cerebral hemispheres. The caudate nucleus, the putamen and the globus pallidus can be seen by the naked eye on a cross section through the cerebral hemisphere, while the substantia nigra can similarly be seen when the midbrain has been sectioned. These structures play a role in the planning and initiation of any movement. What happens to muscle tone when structures in the corpus striatum are damaged as in Huntington disease or Parkinson disease?

Huntington disease is inherited in an autosomal dominant pattern with the pathological substrate being atrophy of the caudate nucleus and putamen (Fig. 2.2.5). The characteristic clinical feature is a movement disorder involving choreiform movements that are purposeless, involuntary and jerky. They are almost imperceptible at first but slowly increase

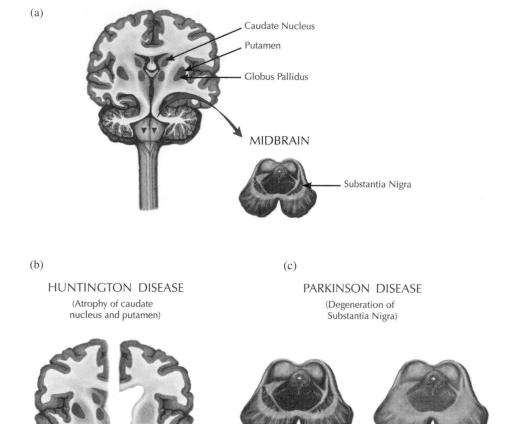

(a)

Caudate Nucleus

Putamen

Globus Pallidus

MIDBRAIN

Substantia Nigra

(b)

HUNTINGTON DISEASE
(Atrophy of caudate
nucleus and putamen)

Normal   Huntington
              Disease

(c)

PARKINSON DISEASE
(Degeneration of
Substantia Nigra)

Normal   Parkinson Disease

Fig. 2.2.5 Corpus striatum. Schematic drawings of (a) the healthy basal ganglia, (b) atrophy of the caudate nucleus and putamen in Huntington disease, and (c) degeneration of the substantia nigra in Parkinson disease.

in amplitude until the patient becomes incapacitated. What is thought to be happening is that somehow the movement patterns stored in the corpus striatum are inappropriately released, so that they are no longer under voluntary control. As far as muscle tone is concerned, it fluctuates but does not have the characteristic features of spasticity.

With Parkinson disease there is loss of neurons in the substantia nigra in the midbrain. The unfortunate individuals who are affected experience a tremor at rest and have difficulty initiating movement. They have an expressionless face and a short, stepping gait. Muscle tone in the extremities is described as rigid. Rigidity is often considered to be the same as spasticity. It is not. In rigidity the tone is elevated but does not have a clasp-knife quality to it. Rather, when a limb is moved against this rigidity, a resistance is encountered, which is the same throughout the range of the movement and is likened to the feel of bending a lead pipe. Rigidity is not muscle spindle dependent and is therefore not relieved by cutting the excitatory muscle spindle afferents in the posterior roots.

In Huntington disease the involuntary movement patterns are released whereas in Parkinson disease involuntary movements are lost. However, spasticity does not result in either case. Thus, we can conclude that spasticity is not a feature of pathology in the corpus striatum.

Cerebellum

The cerebellum is made up of the two cerebellar hemispheres and the midline vermis. The cerebellum is attached to the brainstem via three peduncles on each side. It has a highly folded cortex and deep-seated nuclei of which the dentate is the most important.

When the midline vermis is damaged the main clinical feature is an ataxic gait with loss of balance. If the lateral lobes are affected the patient loses the ability to perform rapidly repetitive alternating movements in the ipsilateral limbs. With involvement of either the vermis or the lateral lobes there is no increase in muscle tone; rather, muscle hypotonia may be noted. Consequently, spasticity is not caused by a lesion in the cerebellum.

Spinal cord

Although damage to the spinal cord can produce spasticity, it occurs because the spinal cord motor neurons are disconnected from the higher centers in the brain. Poliomyelitis (the myelitis referring to the spinal cord), which is characterized by destruction of the anterior horn cells (the nerve cell body of the spinal motor neurons), does not produce spasticity. Rather, it causes a flaccid paralysis of the affected muscles leading to marked wasting. Thus, although spasticity can arise from spinal-cord injury, the cause of that spasticity is really the severing of connections between the brain and spinal cord. Nevertheless, it is these spinal lesions that produce the most intractable, disabling and painful spasticity.

The brainstem motor nuclei

Muscle tone, especially in the lower limbs, is controlled by brainstem nuclei, especially the reticular and vestibular nuclei. (Although there are subdivisions of these nuclei and other centers in the brainstem that are involved with the maintenance of posture and tone, for the purpose of this chapter only the major parts of these two nuclei will be discussed.) The reticulospinal tract originates in the reticular nucleus of the brain stem and descends down the spinal cord where its fibers synapse with motor neurons that innervate muscles. The effect of this tract is to inhibit muscle tone (Houk and Rymer 1981). In addition, the cerebral cortex is connected to the reticulospinal nucleus via a bundle of fibers, which excite the nucleus, increasing its inhibitory influence on the motor neurons in the cord. When the reticular nucleus or the reticulospinal tract is damaged the inhibitory influence is lost and muscle tone rises resulting in what we call spasticity. The vestibular nucleus, via the vestibulospinal tract, is connected to, and excites the motor neurons in the spinal cord. The vestibular nucleus is involved with balance and antigravity support and brings about contraction in the antigravity or extensor muscles in the lower limbs. The cortical connections with the vestibular nucleus inhibit its activity and thus reduce antigravity or extensor activity in the lower limbs.

When the spinal cord or lower brainstem is damaged, both the reticulospinal and vestibulospinal nuclei are disconnected from the spinal motor neurons (lesion A, Fig. 2.2.6). The loss of reticulospinal inhibition leads to increased firing of the spinal motor neurons with resultant increased muscle tone or spasticity. The loss of vestibulospinal excitation leads to decreased firing of the motor neurons responsible for lower limb extensor muscle contraction so the patient tends to develop a flexed posture and flexor spasms.

When the cerebral hemisphere is damaged (lesion B, Fig. 2.2.6), there is loss of excitation of the reticular nucleus by the cerebral cortex so that its inhibitory influence on the spinal motor neurons is reduced. Muscle tone rises because there is less firing of the

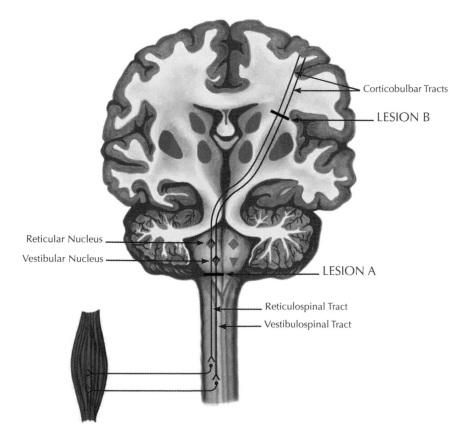

Fig. 2.2.6 Coronal-plane diagram showing two different lesions producing different types of spasticity. Note *lesion A* in the brainstem or spinal cord is distal to the brainstem nuclei, and *lesion B* in the cerebral hemisphere is proximal to the brainstem nuclei (see text for explanation).

reticular nucleus. At the same time, the inhibitory influence of the cortex on the vestibular nucleus is lost so that the vestibular nucleus fires more vigorously, resulting in increased antigravity or extensor activity in the lower limbs.

The natural history of spasticity

Acute cerebral injury is often accompanied by an initial flaccid weakness followed by increased reflex excitability, reaching a maximum within a few months. Over the next few years, this reflex excitability may subside as changes within the muscle itself occur such as muscle wasting and contracture. These features were carefully documented in the detailed studies of adults suffering from strokes by an American physician/physiologist, Richard Herman (1970), and by Thilmann et al. (1991). Hufschmidt and Mauritz (1985) subsequently demonstrated an increase in the 'viscoelastic' resistance to passive muscle stretch as the time from the stroke elapsed. This was accompanied by an increase in the work done to stretch the muscle passively. Importantly, viscous resistance is also velocity-dependent but, naturally, is electromyographically silent. Examples of increased viscoelastic stiffness in children were first demonstrated by Dietz, Quintern and Berger, this increased mechanical resistance being accompanied by little or no electromyographic activity (Dietz et al. 1981, Dietz and Berger 1995).

CO-CONTRACTION

When dealing with spastic gait, it is important to ask whether the disturbance is pathologically abnormal, whether it is due to developmental delay, or whether it is simply altered by the physiological task. An interesting study by Leonard et al. (1991) compared the electromyographic (EMG) and joint patterns of infants and toddlers with and without cerebral palsy. Initially, both groups had similar patterns of co-contraction during supported walking, this being accompanied by joint synchronies (e.g. simultaneous flexion of the hip, knee and ankle joints). Children without cerebral palsy eventually developed fluid patterns of unsupported walking (characterized by less co-contraction and associated with physiological joint asynchrony, e.g. hip flexion, knee extension, ankle dorsiflexion), which are typical of mature gait patterns, whereas children with cerebral palsy retained the co-contraction pattern of unsupported walking.

An additional problem is the fact that the faster one walks, the greater the duration of EMG in both the stance and swing phases of gait (Detrembleur et al. 1997): that is, the faster the speed of walking, the greater the degree of physiological 'wrap-around' of EMG activity that occurs. Since gait is usually assessed at a self-selected speed, care must be taken to ensure that EMG patterns are not interpreted as pathological on the basis of the speed of walking. Many children with diplegia have a tendency to rush or run when intending to walk, which would favor a 'wrap-around' pattern of EMG discharge. This phenomenon could be termed 'task-dependent co-contraction.' A fundamental stimulus to walking fast is the combination of weakness and instability of the stance limb. However, it is clear that the child with diplegia has active co-contraction of the leg muscles in both the supine and vertical positions, and even on waking from sleep. In other words, the spasticity is there before the first step is taken.

97

It is thus possible to have excessive electromyographic activity associated with co-contraction from a variety of causes: (1) as the result of delayed maturation in healthy children (Sutherland et al. 1988), (2) as a consequence of increasing the speed of walking, which induces wrap-around EMG and co-contraction (Detrembleur et al. 1997), or (3) pathologic co-contraction as a feature of abnormal motor planning (Leonard et al. 1991).

Summary

Spasticity is due to lesions affecting the reticular and vestibular nuclei in the brainstem. (1) If the damage is below these nuclei, the absence of the influence of the reticulospinal tract will cause an increase in muscle tone, brisk reflexes and clonus due to loss of inhibition of the spinal motor neurons. Loss of the influence of the vestibulospinal tract (which normally induces contraction of the extensors or antigravity muscles of the legs) will result in a flexed posture and flexor spasms. (2) Damage above the reticular and vestibular nuclei reduces the cortical influence on these two nuclei. There is thus loss of the cortical excitation of the intact reticular nucleus so there is still some, but less inhibition of the spinal motor neurons. The degree of of spasticity is less than would be seen in spinal-cord injury. The inhibitory cortical influence on the intact vestibular nucleus (which brings about contraction of antigravity muscles) is lost, resulting in excessive lower-limb extension.

REFERENCES

Deecke L, Scheid P, Kornhuber HH (1969) Distribution of readiness potential, promotion positivity, and motor potential of the human cerebral cortex preceding voluntary finger movements. *Exp Brain Res* 7: 158–68.

Detrembleur C, Willems P, Plaghki L (1997) Does walking speed influence the time pattern of muscle activation in normal children? *Dev Med Child Neurol* 39: 803–7.

Dietz V, Berger W (1995) Cerebral palsy and muscle transformation. *Dev Med Child Neurol* 37: 180–4.

Dietz V, Quintern J, Berger W (1981) Electrophysiological studies of gait in spasticity and rigidity. Evidence that altered mechanical properties of muscle contribute to hypertonia. *Brain* 104: 431–49.

Hepp-Reymond M, Trouche E, Wiesendanger M (1974) Effects of unilateral and bilateral pyramidotomy on a conditioned rapid precision grip in monkeys (Macaca fascicularis). *Exp Brain Res* 21: 519–27.

Herman R (1970) The myotatic reflex. Clinico–physiological aspects of spasticity and contracture. *Brain* 93: 273–312.

Houk J, Rymer JC (1981) Neural control of muscle length and tension. In: Brookhart JM, Mountcastle VB, Brooks VB, Geiger SR, editors. *The Nervous System*, vol. II. Bethesda, MD: Williams and Wilkins. p 257–323.

Hufschmidt A, Mauritz KH (1985) Chronic transformation of muscle in spasticity: a peripheral contribution to increased tone. *J Neurol Neurosurg Psychiatry* 48: 676–85.

Kuypers H (1981) Anatomy of the descending pathways. In: Brookhart JM, Mountcastle VB, Brooks VB, Geiger SR, editors. *The Nervous System*, vol. II. Bethesda, MD: Williams and Wilkins. p 597–666.

Lance JW (1980) Pathophysiology of spasticity and clinical experience with baclofen. In: Feldman RG, Young RR, Koella WP, editors. *Spasticity: Disordered Motor Control*. Chicago, London: Year Book Medical. p 185–203.

Leonard CT, Hirschfeld H, Forssberg H (1991) The development of independent walking in children with cerebral palsy. *Dev Med Child Neurol* 33: 567–77.

Olsson MC, Kruger M, Meyer LH, Ahnlund L, Gransberg L, Linke WA, Larsson L (2006) Fibre type-specific increase in passive muscle tension in spinal-cord injured subjects with spasticity. *J Physiol* 577: 339–52.

Sutherland D, Olshen R, Biden EN, Wyatt MP, editors (1988) *The Development of Mature Walking*. London: Mac Keith Press. p 153–62.

Thilmann AF, Fellows SJ, Garms E (1991) The mechanism of spastic muscle hypertonus. Variation in reflex gain over the time course of spasticity. *Brain* 114: 233–44.

2.3
BASAL GANGLIA INJURY AND RESULTING MOVEMENT DISORDERS

Leland Albright

Basal ganglia

STRUCTURAL ANATOMY AND PHYSIOLOGY

The basal ganglia consist of five nuclei deep within the cerebral hemispheres – the caudate and putamen (together termed the corpus striatum or simply 'the striatum'), the globus pallidus, subthalamic nucleus (STN) and substantia nigra pars compacta (SNpc) – which participate in the control of movement (Fig. 2.3.1 a, b). The caudate and putamen arise from the same fetal tissue (telencephalon) and their cellular composition is nearly identical. The globus pallidus has an external segment (GPe) and an internal segment (GPi). The GPi and SNpc function essentially as part of the same nucleus. The thalamus is anatomically adjacent to the basal ganglia, but it is not considered part of them.

In the past, it was thought that movement was regulated by parallel, independent systems – the pyramidal and extrapyramidal systems. Lesions of the pyramidal system resulted in weakness and spasticity; lesions of the extrapyramidal system resulted in bradykinesia, tremor, chorea and dystonia. The term 'extrapyramidal' is inaccurate, however, because (1) other brain structures (e.g. the cerebellum) also regulate movement, (2) the basal ganglia are not independent of the pyramidal system but rather, are extensively connected with it, and (3) the basal ganglia affect cognition and behavior in addition to movement. Although the basal ganglia affect movement, neither their input nor their output is directly connected to the spinal cord. The basal ganglia receive input from nearly all the cortical areas; their output goes to frontal lobes and brainstem.

Connections between cortex and basal ganglia are arranged topographically and somatotopically. The cortex and basal ganglia are connected by two neural circuits, a direct circuit and an indirect one (Fig. 2.3.2). Cortical output to the basal ganglia is downward into the striatum, where the excitatory neurotransmitter glutamate is released. Neurons in the striatum also receive input from neurons that release acetylcholine, and from neurons in the substantia nigra that release dopamine. Some dopaminergic pathways end on D1 receptors which are excitatory and some end on D2 receptors which are inhibitory. Two pathways exit the putamen and end up in the thalamus before heading back up to the cortex, (1) a direct pathway from the putamen through the internal globus pallidus to the thalamus, and (2) an

Fig. 2.3.1 (a) Axial fast spin echo-inversion recovery MRI demonstrating normal basal ganglia. Caudate nucleus, 1; putamen, 2; globus pallidus, 3; thalamus, 4. (b) Coronal fast spin echo-inversion recovery MRI demonstrating normal basal ganglia. Caudate nucleus, 1; putamen, 2; internal globus pallidus, 3 (the lamina visible just lateral to internal globus pallidus separates it from external globus pallidus); thalamus, 4; subthalamic nucleus, 5.

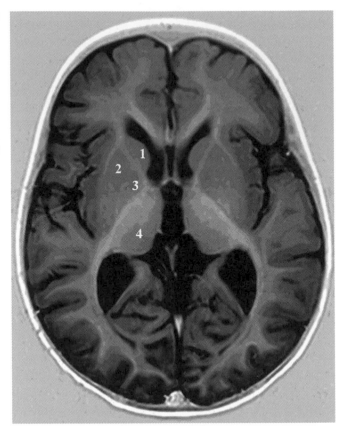

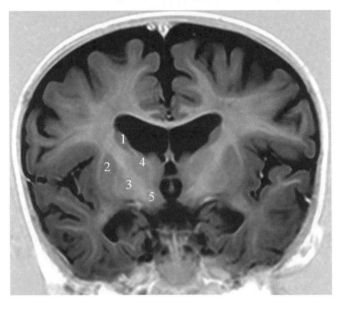

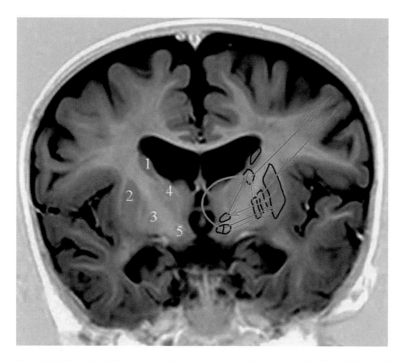

Fig. 2.3.2 Functional interconnections of cortex and basal ganglia. Nuclei in the diagrammed hemisphere correspond to numbers in the opposite hemisphere except for number 5, where the small medial inferior nuclei are the subthalamic nucleus superiorly and the substantia nigra (SN). The SN has a medial pars reticulata and a lateral pars compacta. Excitatory impulses descend from the cortex to the putamen and caudate, then via either the direct or indirect pathway to the thalamus and back to the cortex. Excitatory impulses are shown in green and represent pathways releasing glutamate. Inhibitory impulses are shown in blue and represent pathways releasing GABA. The two pathways from the SN pars compacta transmit dopamine to the putamen and terminate on inhibitory D2 receptors and excitatory D1 receptors.

indirect pathway from the putamen through the external globus pallidus to the subthalamic nucleus to the internal globus pallidus, then to the thalamus. The direct pathway has a total of two inhibitory synapses and is relatively excitatory on the thalamus. The indirect pathway has a total of three inhibitory synapses and its overall effect on the thalamus is inhibitory. If the output of the two circuits is synchronized and normal, their input to the thalamus is inhibitory, its output up to the cortex is excitatory, and the resulting movement is normal.

The basal ganglia work synergistically with the cerebellum to regulate movement, so that when a thought to move arrives at the motor cortex, the resultant movement is appropriate. The ways in which all the pathways interact to regulate movement is unknown. One hypothesis is that they select a pattern of movement based on the intended movement, on experience from previous movements, and on current sensory input, then feed that pattern to the motor cortex and suppress other potential movements (Mink 1996). Other hypotheses involve 'scaling' of movement by varying the extent of stimulation or inhibition of the GPi, and phasic adjustments of the GPi output (Montgomery 2007).

PATHOPHYSIOLOGY

Abnormalities in the cortical–basal ganglia–cortical circuits result in both hypokinetic and hyperkinetic movement disorders, depending on the site of injury and the resultant disorder of neurotransmitters. Lesions affecting the putamen usually cause dystonia – generalized dystonia if the insult is bilateral (as is usually the case in cerebral palsy) and hemidystonia if secondary to a unilateral injury such as a stroke or trauma. Output from the putamen, both in the direct and in the indirect pathways, releases the inhibitory neurotransmitter GABA, so the development of hyperkinetic and disordered movement is not surprising. Although clinically dystonia is a hyperkinetic movement disorder, microelectrode recording in people with dystonia has revealed a *decrease* in the mean discharge rate of neurons in the GPi, with considerable variation from patient to patient (Vitek 2002). The decreased discharge rates are associated with uncontrolled changes in synchronization of neuronal populations in GPi, resulting in increased cortical excitability. Dystonia does not result from changed discharged rates alone, however: GPi neurons in dystonia discharge in irregular bursts separated by intermittent pauses. Neurophysiologic studies suggest that the pathophysiology is different in primary and secondary dystonia. In primary dystonia the abnormality seems to be an increase in inhibitory output from the striatum to GPi and GPe; in secondary dystonia the putamen is typically abnormal and unable to increase its output. The reason why some dystonic movements are transient and others are sustained is unknown.

Abnormalities in the caudate in Huntington disease cause reductions in choline acetyltransferase, glutamic acid and GABA, and result in chorea. Lesions in the substantia nigra pars compacta reduce dopamine, serotonin and norepinephrine and result in Parkinsonism. It appears that *increased* mean discharge rates of GPi neurons are associated with hypokinetic movement disorders, e.g. Parkinsonism.

Movement disorders related to basal ganglia

DYSTONIA

Dystonia is the third most common pediatric movement disorder (after spasticity and tics). It is a hyperkinetic movement disorder characterized by intermittent or sustained involuntary muscle contractions that result in twisting and abnormal postures or repetitive movements (Sanger et al. 2007). Dystonia contracts muscle agonists and antagonists simultaneously, a feature readily evident on electromyography. During dystonic muscle contractions, spasticity cannot be evaluated because the simultaneous contraction of agonists and antagonists prevents evaluating resistance to passive muscle stretch at different velocities.

Dystonic movements may be either stereotypical, i.e. more sustained muscle contractions that cause repeated, similar muscle postures (e.g. torticollis to the same side), or random transient muscle contractions that migrate from one body region to another. When the contractions are stereotypical and chronic over months or years, they may result in contractures. Random dystonic movements are more common, however, and contractures are relatively uncommon in dystonia.

Muscle tone in dystonia, particularly dystonic cerebral palsy (CP), often varies widely: children are described as sometimes being 'loose as noodles' and at other times 'as stiff as a board'. When a child with dystonia attempts to move a dystonic limb, the dystonia often spreads to cause muscles contractions in other limbs. Dystonia is often misdiagnosed as athetosis; the two may coexist in fact, but the distinction is important, primarily because the treatments – whether oral medications or neurosurgical operations – and the response to those treatments, are so different (Video 2.3.1 on Interactive Disc, a child and an adult with dystonia).

Dystonia is classified by age at onset (childhood or later), by site of involvement, and by etiology. *Sites of involvement* range from focal (where only one body part is affected, as in torticollis or writer's cramp) to segmental (where adjacent body regions are affected, e.g. cervical and upper extremity) to hemidystonia (affecting one side of the body) to generalized, the most common form in childhood. Dystonic CP may also, rarely, affect both lower extremities with minimal or no dystonia elsewhere (Fig. 2.3.3).

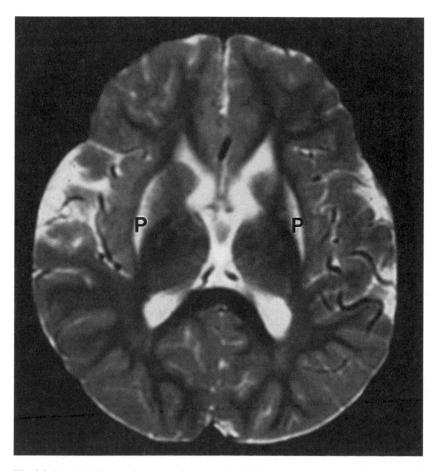

Fig. 2.3.3 Axial MR scan demonstrating putaminal (P) changes associated with dystonic CP.

103

Dystonia may be classified by *etiology* into at least two categories – primary and secondary. *Primary* dystonia develops with no evident structural or disease-related cause. It may be associated with GAG deletions in *DYT* genes (Klein and Ozelius 2002). The most common form of primary dystonia, early limb onset, is associated with the *DYT-1* gene; mixed early-onset dystonia is associated with the *DYT-6* gene. Conventional 1.5 Tesla magnetic resonance (MR) scans are normal in primary dystonia, but recently 3T MR scans have demonstrated subtle white-matter changes (Garraux et al. 2004). Children with primary dystonia are born after normal pregnancies and develop normally initially. During childhood, usually between 5–10 years of age but occasionally before 5 years, dystonia begins in one body region – often a foot or ankle – and progresses slowly over a few years to involve more of the body, ultimately to become generalized in 60% of cases. Primary dystonia may be associated with a positive family history, such as torticollis in a parent and writer's cramp in an aunt.

One rare form of primary dystonia can mimic cerebral palsy: dopa-responsive dystonia (DRD, Segawa's disease) (Mink 2003). This disorder, which is associated with the DYT-5 gene, may begin in early childhood (1–2 years of age) with dystonia and spasticity in the lower extremities and worsens to become generalized. The disorder is exceedingly rare, however, and often remains undiagnosed for several years. MR scans are normal. Because treatment of DRD with levo-dopa (e.g. Sinemet) can completely ameliorate the dystonia, any child with dystonia who does not have a known diagnosis or a history consistent with cerebral palsy (preterm birth, intraventricular hemorrhage, low birthweight, etc.) should be given a therapeutic trial of levo-dopa for 2–3 months to exclude this treatable disorder.

Some authors consider *heredo-degenerative dystonia* to be a separate category of dystonia whereas others consider it in the secondary dystonia category. Heredo–degenerative dystonias are associated with hereditary disorders such as Wilson disease or glutaric aciduria, and with degenerative disorders such as pantothenate-kinase deficiency (PKAN, Hallervorden–Spatz disease). MR scans often reveal abnormalities that are characteristically associated with the various disorders. The heredo–degenerative dystonias are typically not postural/stereotypical, but rather have nearly continuous contractions of varying muscle groups. They are usually progressive and are ideally treated by operations that can be adjusted as the disease/dystonia worsens, operations such as intrathecal baclofen or deep brain stimulation.

Secondary dystonia is by far the most common form of dystonia, encompassing perhaps 90% of all cases in children, and is secondary to structural brain lesions – most commonly those associated with cerebral palsy. The lesions are in the basal ganglia – most often, the putamen, with the globus pallidus and thalamus affected less frequently (Video 2.3.1 on Interactive Disc). Dystonic CP is generalized more often than segmental or hemidystonic, and, least commonly, focal. Dystonic CP may begin in infancy or throughout childhood, rarely after 18 years, and usually has its final distribution at its onset, although the severity of muscle contraction in that distribution may worsen over a few years (in contradistinction to spasticity which stays stable or improves in the early childhood years). Dystonia secondary to trauma or stroke is more likely to be hemidystonic, with an onset months to years after the injury; the mean interval in one series was 4.1 years (Chuang et al. 2002).

The severity of dystonia is often graded with two validated scales, the Burke–Fahn–Marsden (BFM) scale and the Barry–Albright Dystonia (BAD) scale (Burke et al. 1985, Barry et al. 1999). The Unified Dystonia Rating Scale and the Global Dystonia Rating Scale have also been used. The BFM scale was developed to grade primary dystonia in adults, the BAD scale to grade secondary dystonia in children. The BFM scale grades dystonia in nine body regions (eyes, mouth, speech/swallowing, neck, right arm, left arm, trunk, right leg, left leg) according to a 'provoking factor' of 0–4. The BAD scale grades dystonia on a 0–4 scale in eight body regions (eyes, face, neck, trunk, upper extremities, lower extremities).

ATHETOSIS

Athetosis is an involuntary hyperkinetic movement disorder characterized by writhing movements of distal muscles – perioral muscles, hands/fingers, and often the feet and toes – but it can be generalized and involve the entire body. Intellect is often normal. Athetosis is far less common now than it was 40 years ago, when it developed in infants with severe untreated ABO incompatability that caused red cell lysis and hyperbilirubinemia. Bilirubin lodged in the basal ganglia to cause the classic marbled appearance, *status marmoratus*. There are no validated classification scales or grading scales for athetosis. In the absence of such, the Abnormal Involuntary Movement Scale (AIMS) can be used. MR scans of people with athetosis may be normal or may show abnormalities in the caudate and thalamus. Some neurologists have considered athetosis to be a variant of dystonia but the two are distinct movement disorders – the distribution of muscles involved is different, the MR scan features are different, and the response to intrathecal baclofen is markedly different (Fig. 2.3.2; Video 2.3.2 on Interactive Disc, woman with athetosis).

CHOREA

Chorea is a hyperkinetic movement disorder characterized by brief irregular sudden muscle contractions, particularly at rest. Chorea may diminish during voluntary movement, and, like all other movement disorders, disappears during sleep. The contractions vary in duration from 200 to 1000 msec. The amplitude of the contraction also varies, from small jerks of the hand or fingers to larger movements of more proximal muscles. Chorea affects the upper extremities most often and can be focal or generalized. Chorea is occasionally the only movement disorder in people with CP but more commonly is associated with athetosis or dystonia. Huntington chorea, the prototypical form of generalized chorea, is associated with atrophy of the caudate nucleus. *Ballism* is the term applied to exaggerated large muscle contractions that cause jerking, flailing movements, particularly of proximal portion of the upper extremities, and is considered to be a severe form of chorea. Such flailing may injure either the individual or caregivers (Fig. 2.3.3; Video 2.3.3 on Interactive Disc, a man, a young girl and a child with chorea).

MYOCLONUS

Myoclonus is the term used to describe brief, irregular lightning-like muscle contractions (similar to definition of chorea) but the duration of myoclonic contractions is shorter: myoclonic muscle jerks are less than 10–30 msec in duration – too brief to be voluntary –

whereas choreiform movements are greater than 200 msec. Like dystonia, myoclonus may be focal, segmental or generalized. It may occur at rest or only during voluntary movement. Myoclonus is relatively uncommon in people with CP.

RIGIDITY
Rigidity is the term used to describe the sustained, non-velocity-dependent, increased resistance to passive stretch of both muscle agonists and antagonists. Rigidity is not associated with hyperkinesia and is classically seen in Parkinson disease where it often has a cogwheel feel. Rigidity as a movement disorder does not occur in childhood except in the extraordinarily rare childhood Parkinsonism. Rigidity secondary to musculoskeletal contratures may of course develop as a consequence of chronic spasticity, but that is obviously not a movement disorder.

OTHER MOVEMENT DISORDERS
Mixed movement disorders are common in children with CP. The most common associations are dystonia with spasticity, and chorea with athetosis. Some children with CP have spasticity, dystonia, chorea and athetosis. Their treatment is more complex and the outcomes harder to predict than if the disorders occur singly. Ataxia (gait incoordination) is associated with lesions of the cerebellum or cerebellar-outflow pathways (dentate–rubro–cerebellar) and, as an isolated movement disorder, is never associated with basal ganglia lesions or hypertonia. Tics are lightning-like muscle contractions associated with Tourette syndrome and are never associated with basal ganglia lesions or cerebral palsy.

REFERENCES

Barry MJ, Van Swearingen JM, Albright AL (1999) Reliability and responsiveness of the Barry-Albright Dystonia Scale. *Dev Med Child Neurol* **41**: 404–12.
Burke RE, Fahn S, Marsden CD, Bressman SB, Moskowitz C, Friedman J (1985) Validity and reliability of a rating scale for the primary torsion dystonias. *Neurology* **35**: 73–7.
Chuang C, Fahn S, Frucht S (2002) The natural history and treatment of acquired hemidystonia: review of 33 cases and review of the literature. *J Neurol Neurosurg Psychiatry* **72**: 59–67.
Garraux G, Bauer A, Hanakawa T, Wu T, Kansaku K, Hallett M (2004) Changes in brain anatomy in focal hand dystonia. *Ann Neurol* **55**: 736–9.
Klein C, Ozelius LJ (2002) Dystonia: clinical features, genetics and treatment. *Curr Opin Neurol* **15**: 491–7.
Mink JW (1996) The basal ganglia: focused selection and inhibition of competing motor programs. *Prog Neurobiol* **50**: 381–425.
Mink JW (2003) Dopa-responsive dystonia in children. *Curr Treat Options Neurol* 5: 279–82.
Montgomery EB Jr (2007) Basal ganglia physiology and pathophysiology: a reappraisal. *Parkinson Rel Dis* **13**: 45–65.
Sanger TD, Delgado MR, Gaebler-Spira D, Hallett M, Mink JW (2007) Classification and definition of disorders causing hypertonia in childhood. *Pediatrics* **111**: 89–97.
Vitek JL (2002) Pathophysiology of dystonia: a neuronal model. *Mov Disord* **17**: S49–62.

2.4

CONSEQUENCES OF BRAIN INJURY ON MUSCULOSKELETAL DEVELOPMENT

James R. Gage and Michael H. Schwartz

In the first section of this book we discussed the neurological control system, the mechanisms which guide musculoskeletal growth and development and normal gait. The beginning of this section dealt with the mechanisms and consequences of brain injury. If our intent is to derive a rational means of treating gait disturbances in cerebral palsy, we now need to spend some time looking at how the brain injury affects the pathophysiology of typical gait.

Brain injury early in life profoundly affects musculoskeletal growth and development and, of course, gait itself. Normal gait has several attributes (see Chapter 1.3). Because of the neuromuscular problems that occur in cerebral palsy, all of these attributes are lost in varying degrees. When looking at pathological gait, it is important to remember that what we are seeing is a combination of cause and effect. For example, look at a typical brain injury, such as the one illustrated in Chapter 2.1 (Fig. 2.1.8), which typically results from periventricular leukomalacia secondary to preterm birth. This type of brain damage can interfere with gait in several specific ways: (1) loss of selective control of muscles, particularly in the distal part of the limb, (2) difficulties with balance, and (3) abnormal muscle tone (usually spasticity). We refer to these abnormalities of gait as the *primary effects of the brain injury*. Primary effects arise at the moment of brain injury and as a direct result of the injury. In general they are permanent, and to a large extent cannot be corrected.

The principles of normal musculoskeletal growth and development were discussed in Chapters 1.2 and 1.3 where it was explained that in a growing child the activities of daily activity impose forces upon the skeleton that, in large part, govern its growth. The primary effects of the brain injury impose abnormal forces on the skeleton, with the result that neither bone nor muscle grows normally. These changes, which we refer to as the *secondary effects of the brain injury*, are not immediate because muscles and bones grow slowly over time. Consequently, musculoskeletal deformities emerge slowly over time, and in direct proportion to the rate of skeletal growth.

A child who is trying to walk with impaired motor control as well as dynamic and structural musculoskeletal deformities does not have an easy task, and s/he must learn to cope with the resultant problems. For example, a child with hemiplegia and spasticity of the rectus femoris on the affected side might have difficulty getting the affected knee to bend and, as a result, might demonstrate foot drag during the swing phase of gait. The child might cope with this problem in one of several ways: (1) vaulting on the stance limb, (2) circumduction of the limb on the swing side, and/or (3) hyperflexion of the hip on the swing side. While these mechanisms may solve the problem, they are in themselves gait abnormalities. We refer to these coping mechanisms as the *tertiary effects of the brain injury*.

Pathological gait, then, is a mixture of *primary*, *secondary* and *tertiary* abnormalities. It is important to discriminate between these different types of abnormalities, for as we said earlier, the primary abnormalities of gait usually are permanent, the secondary abnormalities can frequently be corrected, and the tertiary abnormalities (coping responses) will disappear spontaneously once they are no longer required. This fact provides us with the foundation of our treatment program for gait problems in cerebral palsy, which is perhaps best expressed in the words attributed to Reinhold Niebuhr, 'God, give us grace to accept with serenity the things that cannot be changed, courage to change the things which should be changed and the wisdom to distinguish the one from the other.'[1]

Our task then is to sort out the primary, secondary, and tertiary abnormalities of gait, determine which ones can and should be corrected, and have the wisdom to leave the rest of the pathology alone. The remainder of this book will be dedicated to the successful execution of that task.

Gait abnormalities

THE PRIMARY ABNORMALITIES OF GAIT
As detailed in Chapter 2.1, injuries to specific brain centers will generate fairly specific types of functional loss. For example, injury to the cerebellum will produce a specific abnormality of gait that we refer to as ataxia. Consequently, although injury to different brain control centers may generate different types of functional loss, they all contribute in different ways to the three primary abnormalities of gait: (1) loss of selective motor control, (2) impaired balance, and (3) abnormal tone.

Selective motor control
The degree to which selective motor control is impaired depends a great deal on the site and the extent of the injury. For example, in a child with mixed tone there is injury to the basal ganglia or its connections to the cortex. As pointed out in Chapters 1.1 and 2.3, the basal ganglia contain 'motor memories' of previous similar movement patterns. Consequently, *injury to the basal ganglia usually results in severe loss of selective motor control*, which affects all four extremities to some degree. For this reason it is probably more appropriate to consider all children with mixed tone as having quadriplegic involvement.

A child who presents with spastic diplegia typically has an injury, which we refer to as *periventricular leukomalacia*. This lesion occurs in the descending tracts of the corona

---

1 *Simpson's Contemporary Quotations*, compiled by James B. Simpson. 1988.

radiata, and involves both the pyramidal and extrapyramidal fibers, which pass through that area on their way to the lower extremities. The neurological injury is typically bilateral and occurs most frequently in the white matter adjacent to the frontal horns of the lateral ventricles, as well as toward the posterior aspects of the ventricles in the peritrigonal white matter (see Chapter 2.1). The basal ganglia are not involved in this injury. Consequently, these children present with pure spasticity for reasons explained earlier (see Chapters 2.1 and 2.2).

Since the pyramidal tracts are distributed primarily to the distal end of the extremities, loss of selective motor control is more severe in the distal portion of the limb than the proximal. As such, the child with spastic diplegia typically demonstrates fairly good selective motor control at the hip, limited control of the knee, and poor control of the ankle and foot. In addition from a control standpoint, biarticular muscles are more severely involved than those that are monoarticular. The specific reason why this is true is not entirely clear, but may relate to the composition and function of the muscles. Consequently, an axiom to remember in treating cerebral palsy is that *the distal, biarticular muscles are involved primarily and more severely than those that are monoarticular and/or proximal*. The classification system that we developed for hemiplegia is based on this premise (see Chapter 2.6) (Winters et al. 1987). This maxim also has implications in the treatment of cerebral palsy. Look, for example, at the triceps surae. It is made up of a monoarticular muscle (the soleus) and a pair of biarticular muscles (the medial and lateral gastrocnemius). The axiom above predicts that the biarticular gastrocnemii should be more severely involved than the monoarticular soleus, and in fact, this has been shown to be true (Rose et al. 1993, Delp et al. 1995). Yet tendo-Achilles lengthening, a procedure commonly used to correct contracture of this muscle, lengthens both equally – often to the great detriment of the patient. A similar situation exists with the iliopsoas at the hip. The psoas is biarticular and the iliacus monoarticular. In the past a recession of the iliopsoas tendon from the lesser trochanter to the capsule was often done to correct contracture of this muscle (Bleck 1971). However, this is analogous to tendo-Achilles lengthening at the ankle because the iliacus, which usually is not contracted, is lengthened along with the contracted psoas. For that reason, we feel that intramuscular lengthening of the psoas alone is a better procedure (Novacheck et al. 2002).

Balance

Disequilibrium is another of the primary problems of cerebral palsy. Balance and equilibrium are abnormal in cerebral palsy, particularly in the anterior–posterior plane. Winter (1991) stated that the body is an unstable pendulum, since two-thirds of the mass of the head, arms and trunk (HAT) is located at about two-thirds of the body's height above the ground. He then demonstrated that the hip is the center for balance control since the forces and/or postural compensations necessary to maintain the HAT segment balanced over the lower limbs are much smaller when applied at the hip than would be the case if they were applied more distally in the limb (Fig. 2.4.1). The situation is not unlike that of a seal balancing a ball on its nose, with the ball representing the trunk, the seal the lower limbs and the seal's nose the hip joint (Fig. 2.4.2). When we reflect on this a bit, we immediately

Fig. 2.4.1 Moments about the supporting hip. (a) In order for an individual to maintain erect posture, the upper body (head, arms and trunk, or HAT) must remain balanced over the lower extremities throughout the gait cycle. (b) Winter (1991) has shown that an external unbalancing moment (ground reaction force and/or inertia) is always counteracted by an internal balancing moment of equal magnitude. Thus the total inertial moment of HAT is always close to zero. (Reproduced from Winter 1991, fig. 6.12, p. 79, by kind permission of Dr D. Winter and Waterloo Biomechanics.)

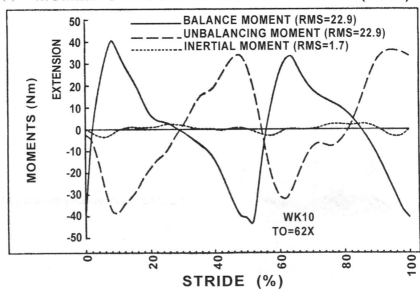

realize that the task of the seal is quite complex, as is the task of maintaining balance while walking. An inebriated man, with alcohol-induced ataxia, can maintain balance and walks only with great difficulty, and it is doubtful if an inebriated seal could balance a ball on his nose at all. The point of this is that if an individual is to maintain balance without the use of balance aides (such as crutches or a walker), good selective motor control and normally functioning muscles are mandatory. This is probably also the case in cerebral palsy. From this we would infer that the child with diplegia who can walk without aids has reasonably normal muscle function and fairly good selective motor control around his/her hips, whereas the child who needs balance aids to walk probably does not.

Hagberg et al. (1972) likened the falling of a child with abnormal equilibrium reactions to a 'felled pine tree'. Almost all children with diplegia or quadriplegia have significant balance problems and many require aids such as walkers or crutches for ambulation. For example, in our experience, most children with hemiplegia are able to ride a bicycle, whereas children with diplegia or quadriplegia usually cannot. Horstmann and Bleck (2007) pointed out that, because of lateral instability, a child with balance instability will frequently lean to the side of the single stance limb when attempting to stand on one foot, which is often mistaken for hip abductor weakness (positive Trendelenburg sign). They suggested that

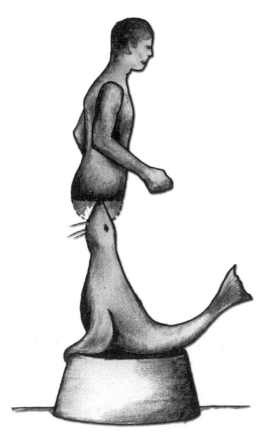

Fig. 2.4.2 A seal balancing the head and trunk. If one equates the ball that a seal commonly balances with the head and trunk, the seal's nose with the hip joint, and the seal itself with the lower extremities, the feat is not unlike the one that we perform daily when we stand and/or walk.

after 6 years of age balance can be quickly be assessed by asking the child to hop on one foot. If s/he can do this, balance reactions are close to normal. If the child is unable to hop, s/he should be asked to stand on one foot for at least 10 seconds. A typical child of 5 years of age or more can do this, even though many children with diplegia who can walk independently will fail this test on one or both sides. Children who have spastic diplegia with fairly minimal involvement still have deficient equilibrium reactions to some degree. These often become apparent when balance is stressed, for example, when avoiding an object and/or rapidly changing direction. Liao et al. (1997) studied a group of eight children with cerebral palsy and compared them to 16 sex- and age-matched non-disabled children. They concluded that the children with cerebral palsy walked at a slower speed and with greater physiological cost than the non-disabled children. They felt that dynamic balance significantly correlated with walking function. In a larger and more recent study, they tested balance reliability of children with cerebral palsy compared to non-disabled children using a variety of testing methods including the Smart Balance System, which measured postural sway and the Bruininks–Oseretsky Test of Motor Proficiency (BOTMP) (Liao et al. 2001). They concluded that postural stability in center-target condition and the one-leg standing test are reliable tests in children with cerebral palsy, but that further study is needed to establish more reliable balance tests for children in general. Although sophisticated force platforms for testing balance now exist, Bleck (1987, pp. 32–3) pointed out that equilibrium reactions can easily be tested clinically by gently pushing the child from side to side and anteriorly and posteriorly. Children with normal equilibrium will easily maintain their balance and if necessary make a stepping response to regain their equilibrium, whereas the child with deficient equilibrium reactions will topple over (Fig. 2.4.3). Bleck feels that if a child has adequate side to side but poor fore and aft equilibrium reactions, crutches will be required for support. If lateral equilibrium reactions are also deficient, a walker will be required. However, he contends that even children with spastic diplegia who walk without aids generally have poor posterior equilibrium reactions and so may fall backwards with very little provocation (Bleck 1987, pp. 124–5).

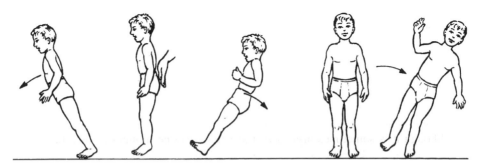

Fig. 2.4.3 Standing equilibrium reactions. Lack of normal equilibrium is easily demonstrated by pushing forward, backward, and/or from side to side. The child will fall down as opposed to demonstrating a normal stepping response. (From Bleck and Horstmann 2007, by permission of Mac Keith Press.)

112

There is an argument in the literature over whether or not deficient equilibrium reactions can be improved by training and/or therapy (Liao et al. 1997, Shumway-Cook et al. 2003, Woollacott et al. 2005). Following surgery in which the limbs have been realigned, tone reduced, and/or stance phase stability restored, it is certainly common to see a child discard crutches or aids as s/he becomes accustomed to the new positions of her/his limbs in space. However, this does not necessarily mean that the child's underlying balance mechanisms have improved. Providing the child with a better base of support has been shown to be helpful in improving balance, and in this regard orthotics are very helpful (Butler et al. 1992, Burtner et al. 1999). However, Bleck states: 'Of all the motor problems in cerebral palsy, deficient equilibrium reactions interfere the most with functional walking' (Bleck 1987, pp. 124–5). After 30 years of working with these children, the senior author concurs with this statement and would add that the neurological injury, which underlies the equilibrium disorder, is permanent.

Abnormal tone

Abnormal tone is a universal finding in cerebral palsy. Athetosis describes only one type of abnormal tone emanating from injury to the basal ganglia. Dystonia, chorea, and/or rigidity are also abnormal muscle tones that may arise as a result of basal ganglia injury. To better understand the mechanism by which these abnormal tones arise, please see Chapters 2.1–2.3. It is fairly clear now that spastic muscle tone arises as a result of injury to the extra-pyramidal system (the cortical connections to the vestibular and/or reticular brain stem nuclei, the nuclei themselves, and/or the tracts emanating from them). Injury to the pyramidal system (Broca's area 4 and/or the pyramidal tracts) was once thought to produce spasticity. However, it has now been shown that damage to these structures in isolation only produces loss of fine-motor control in distal limb muscles without spasticity (Hepp-Reymond et al. 1974, Kuypers 1981).

Of the abnormal muscle tones present in cerebral palsy, spasticity is the most common. As stated in Chapter 2.2, spasticity arises as a result of loss of central nervous system inhibition. Its 'hallmark feature' is the fact that it is velocity-dependent: that is, the higher the rate of muscle stretch, the more resistance to movement that is encountered.

There are several ways in which spasticity interferes with function in cerebral palsy: (1) it acts like a brake on the system and this drag on movement increases energy consumption, (2) it inhibits voluntary control of movement, (3) it interferes with the stretch on muscles that normally occurs during activity and so inhibits growth, (4) it contributes to bony deformity of the growing skeleton by inducing excessive torques on long bones during gait, (5) it inhibits muscle stretch during activity, which is the primary mechanism for muscle growth, thereby contributing to the development of muscle contractures.

Although it is sometimes argued that spasticity can be thought of as a beneficial compensation for weakness, the increased muscle tone induces abnormal movement patterns and frequently leads to deformities such as muscle contractures and joint dislocations. At the present time spasticity is the only type of abnormal tone, or for that matter the only primary abnormality, which we can significantly alter surgically. Albright and co-workers have claimed some success in the treatment of dystonia with the intrathecal baclofen pump, however, which is discussed in detail in Chapter 5.3 (Albright 1996, 2007, Albright et al. 1996, 2001). The ability to alter tone, and in particular reduce spastic tone, has represented a major advance in the treatment of cerebral palsy. In fact, to the mind of the senior author, it is the most significant treatment advance that he has seen in his 30 years of practice.

Abnormalities of tone arising from injury to the basal ganglia (athetosis, dystonia, chorea, and/or rigidity) are always associated with severe loss of selective motor control. As such it is difficult to determine whether abnormal muscle tone emanating from basal ganglia injury is a problem in itself or whether the abnormal tone merely represents a symptom of the problem, i.e. the underlying injury to the control system in the basal ganglia.

THE SECONDARY ABNORMALITIES OF GAIT

As stated earlier, the secondary abnormalities arise as a result of the abnormal forces imposed on the skeleton by the effects of the primary brain injury. By definition, therefore, the secondary abnormalities are anomalies of muscle and/or bone growth.

As was pointed out earlier, these skeletal deformities emerge slowly over time, and in direct proportion to the rate of skeletal growth. There are two types of secondary abnormalities: (1) muscle contractures and (2) abnormal bone growth, which can take a variety of forms. Unlike the primary abnormalities of cerebral palsy, which are usually permanent, the secondary abnormalities are frequently amenable to correction. To understand why and how they arise, however, one first needs to understand the normal growth process, which is covered in Chapter 1.2.

Muscle growth

The mechanism and nature of muscle growth was discussed earlier (see Chapter 1.2). If we accept that the stretch necessary for daily muscle growth is incurred during the play activities of a typical child, it becomes apparent that muscle growth in a child with cerebral palsy will be abnormal for the following reasons:

1. The primary problems of cerebral palsy (loss of selective motor control, impaired balance, and abnormal tone) prevent normal play activities.
2. A spastic muscle will not allow stretch to the same degree as one with normal tone. As a result a muscle that initially has dynamic contracture secondary to the spasticity itself will eventually develop true contracture as muscle growth fails to keep pace with growth of the bone.
3. From a standpoint of motor control and spasticity, the distal biarticular muscles are the most severely involved. Therefore it is reasonable to assume that these muscles would be the ones that are most prone to contracture.

Bone growth

Growth of the long bones occurs by means of epiphyseal plates or, in the case of cartilaginous bone, appositionally via the periosteum. Skeletal growth was discussed extensively in Chapter 1.2, so we will not reiterate the discussion here. However, recall that it is the forces, which act upon bone during growth, that determine its ultimate shape. The

Heuter–Volkmann principle (Heuter 1862) and the postulates of Arkin and Katz (1956), which were discussed in Chapter 1.2, simply tell us how epiphyseal growth typically responds to those external forces. In simple terms, what they are saying is that if you put a twist on a growing bone, it will take the twist. Or, in the words of the British satirical poet Alexander Pope, 'Just as the twig is bent, the tree's inclin'd' (Epistle to Cobham, 1, 149).

The implications of this are that following the onset of cerebral palsy, future bone growth is likely to be abnormal. However, it was some time before we realized that the errors of bone modeling imposed by the primary abnormalities of cerebral palsy work in two directions: that is, bones not only fail to mold or model normally as they grow; they also fail to remodel normally. The best example of this is femoral anteversion. Persistent fetal alignment as described by Somerville (1957) and the mechanism by which it remodels were described in Chapter 1.2. In a child with cerebral palsy, however, there are several reasons why this process of femoral remodeling fails.

1. The age of standing and/or walking is delayed, such that by that time the child starts to walk much of the proximal femur has ossified and so is much less malleable.
2. The rate of remodeling is directly proportional to the rate of growth, which is greatest in the 1st year of life and decreases steadily thereafter. Consequently, by the time the child starts walking the rates of both growth and remodeling have slowed significantly.
3. Remodeling of the proximal femur is dependent on the pressure of Bigalow's ligament against the femoral head and neck, which is greatest when the hip is in full extension. However, a child with cerebral palsy typically stands and walks with hips and knees in some flexion.

As a result of this, children with cerebral palsy retain what Somerville (1957) termed *persistent fetal alignment*.

Because of the abnormal forces imposed on the skeleton during walking, however, forward or future modeling of the long bones of the lower extremity also is abnormal. For example, Arnold et al. (1997, 1999) pointed out that internal rotation gait may be a mechanism by which the strength of the hip abductors is restored; and Delp et al. (1999) showed that in flexion the gluteus minimus is a strong internal rotator of the hip. Accordingly, in a child who walks with her/his hips in flexion, the gluteus minimus exerts a strong internal rotation torque on the proximal femur, which with time and growth, would tend to increase anteversion. In fact, Fabry et al. (1973) showed this to be the case.

Lever-arm dysfunction

In Chapter 1.3 and in the accompanying Normal Gait DVD describing normal gait, we introduced the concept of levers, forces and moments. There it was pointed out that the rotations of joints are accomplished by moments. Forces acting on skeletal levers produce these moments. We have coined the term *lever-arm dysfunction* to describe the alteration in the leverage relationships necessary for normal gait. In particular, lever-arm dysfunction describes a set of conditions in which internal and/or external lever arms become distorted because of bony or positional deformities. In this chapter, we will concentrate on those deformities that are common in the lower extremities of children and adults with cerebral palsy. These include torsional deformities of long bones (femurs and/or tibias), hip subluxation or dislocation, foot deformities and positional anomalies such as crouch gait.

Clinicians and engineers in the field of gait analysis have been slow to recognize the role and importance of lever-arm dysfunction. There is a tendency to think of muscles as force generators. However, modern research into the functional micro- and macro-anatomy of muscle tissue makes it clear that muscles are actually highly optimized generators of rotation (Zajac and Gordon 1989, Lieber 1997). It is also common to think of the power generating capacity of muscles as being directly related to muscle force. But again, since power is the result of both force and motion, the force that a muscle produces cannot generate or absorb power without a concomitant joint motion. To fully understand the pathogenesis and treatment of the gait disorders common in cerebral palsy, it is necessary to think of muscles as generators of rotation. This thought process will naturally lead to the analysis of muscle moments, which in turn points directly at the issue of lever-arm dysfunction.

Lever-arm dysfunction, once recognized, can usually be corrected. The details of many such corrections will be found in the later chapters and in the surgical examples on the Interactive Disc, which deal with treatment. For example, the flexible lever-arm dysfunction created by a severe pes valgus might be remediable with an appropriate foot orthosis and/or with appropriate surgery to stabilize the foot (Chapter 5.8). Torsional deformities of long bones are easily corrected with derotational osteotomies (Chapter 5.6). Hip subluxation and dislocation can be remedied in a number of ways (Chapter 5.7). Crouch gait can be treated by conventional single-event multilevel surgery, or by a combination of distal femoral extension osteotomies and patellar tendon advancement (Chapter 5.11). In other words, once lever-arm dysfunction is recognized, correction of the problem is generally straightforward. However, it is the recognition/understanding of the problem that often poses a challenge. To understand this lever arm dysfunction, one first needs to understand the mechanics of levers and moments.

LEVERS

A lever is a 'simple machine' used to harness forces to produce rotations. The basic elements common to all levers are the lever itself (a rigid member), the fulcrum or pivot point, and finally the external forces – sometimes divided into load (force of the object to be moved or overcome) and effort (force that does the moving or overcoming) (Fig. 2.4.4a-c). These simple elements can be arranged to provide a variety of mechanical consequences. Bones form the levers of the human body and joints generally act as the fulcra. Though the distinction between load and effort is somewhat arbitrary, it is generally more 'natural' to think of body weight (i.e. gravity), ground reaction forces, and inertial forces of motion as the load, while muscle forces supply the effort against these loads.

The purpose of a lever is to produce either a mechanical advantage over the load or a rapid motion of the load. The mechanical advantage of a lever is the ratio of the load to the effort,

Mechanical advantage = Load/Effort.

This ratio, in turn, can be expressed in terms of the relative lever arms (*d*) of the load and effort,

Mechanical advantage = d_{effort}/d_{load}

There is an inherent compromise between goals of mechanical advantage and rapid motion. That is, to achieve a mechanical advantage inherently involves losing the capacity for rapid motion. In contrast, rapid motion of loads requires effort in excess of the load.

In 1st-class levers, the effort and the load are on opposite sides of the fulcrum (Fig. 2.4.4a). This type of lever is commonly exemplified by a teeter-totter (or see-saw). In a balanced teeter-totter, the weight of one individual (load) multiplied by his/her distance from the fulcrum (lever arm) is equal to the weight of another individual (effort) times his/her distance from the fulcrum (lever arm). The mechanical advantage of 1st-class levers can be *either* greater than or less than one, depending on the ratio of lever arms. An example of a biomechanical 1st-class lever is the pelvis during single leg support. The body weight is the load; the hip-abductor force, primarily supplied by the gluteus medius, is the effort; and the hip joint acts as a fulcrum (Fig. 2.4.4a).

Second-class levers can be used to slowly move large loads (mechanical advantage > 1.0). An everyday example of a 2nd-class lever system is a *wheelbarrow,* which has a fulcrum where the wheel meets the ground, a load in the container portion, and an upward effort applied at the end of the handles. A biomechanical example of a 2nd-class lever is the foot at toe off. In this case, the load is the body weight acting at the ankle, the triceps surae force is the effort, and the foot acts as the lever (Fig. 2.4.4b).

In a 3rd-class lever, the fulcrum is at one end, the effort is adjacent to the fulcrum, and the load is at the other end of the lever (Fig. 2.4.4c). A *catapult* is an example of a 3rd-class lever. In the body, an excellent example of a 3rd-class lever can be found in the forearm. There, the action of the biceps brachii on the radius supports a weight carried in the hand with a fulcrum at the elbow. These types of levers can produce very rapid motions (such as a pitched baseball) at the cost of large effort demands. In general the bones, joints, ligaments and muscles comprising the skeletal system represent combinations of all three types of levers.

As we learn to view the body as a system of levers, which moves via rotation of joints, it becomes more natural for us to think of muscles as generators of moments rather than forces. It is therefore important to understand a bit more about what a moment is, and in particular how both the magnitude and direction of a moment result from bony and muscular organization. A moment consists of both a magnitude and a direction. The direction of a moment depends on the relative orientation of the force and the center of rotation. The magnitude is the product of the force and the lever arm, which is the perpendicular distance from the center of rotation to a point on the line-of-action of the force.

$$M = F \times d$$

This equation can be understood better by considering the simple problem of tightening a bolt with a wrench. One applies a force to the end of the wrench and rotation of the bolt

Fig. 2.4.4 The three classes of levers. (a) First-class levers have the fulcrum in the middle and the load and effort at opposite ends. The common example of a 1st-class lever is a teeter-totter (see-saw). A biomechanical example is the pelvis during single limb support. The load is the body weight, the effort is the hip abductor force, and the fulcrum is the hip joint. First-class levers can have a mechanical advantage either greater or less than one depending on the relative lengths of the two lever arms.

(a)

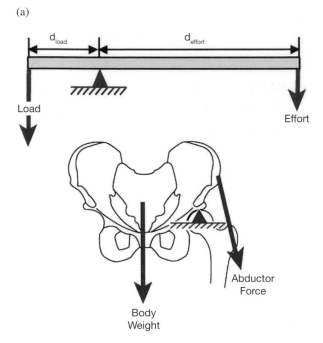

Fig. 2.4.4 continued
(b) Second-class levers have the fulcrum at one end, the load in the middle, and the effort at the other end. A common example of a 2nd-class lever is the wheelbarrow. The foot during push-off is a good biomechanical example. Here the fulcrum is the metatarsal heads, the load is the body weight acting through the ankle joint, and the effort is the force of the ankle plantarflexors. The advantage of a 2nd-class lever system is that large loads can be supported with small efforts.

(b)

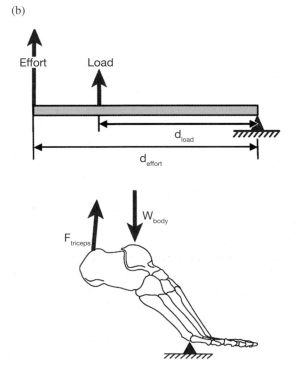

(c)

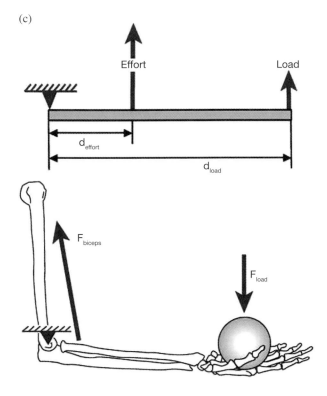

Effort   Load

d_{effort}

d_{load}

F_{biceps}

F_{load}

Fig. 2.4.4 continued
(c) Third-class levers have the fulcrum at one end, the effort in the middle, and the load at the opposite end. Although now usually seen only in pictures, the medieval catapult is an excellent example. In the body, the best example would be the forearm when throwing a ball. In this case, the ball is the load, the effort is the force of the elbow flexors, and the fulcrum is the elbow joint. The advantage of 3rd-class lever systems is speed. However, this speed comes at the expense of the need for a relatively large effort. (Reproduced from Paley 2002, by permission.)

occurs. The direction of rotation depends on the direction in which the force is applied. The magnitude depends on the magnitude of the force applied to the wrench, the length of the wrench handle, and the *angle of application* of the force (Fig. 2.4.5).

To gain a better idea of how muscles and lever arms are at work during normal gait, begin by considering the normal function of the ankle and foot. The action of the ankle in stance was described in terms of three rockers in Chapter 1.3 (see Fig. 1.3.25). Recall that during normal gait, the foot acts as a 2nd-class lever during 1st rocker. The heel is the fulcrum and the foot is the lever. The load is the body's weight acting at the ankle, and the effort is the force of the pretibial muscles preventing an uncontrolled foot slap against the ground. Posterior protrusion of the heel creates a lever arm for the body's weight equal to ≈25% of the foot's total length. The immediate effect of the load (body weight) is to cause a moment about the heel (fulcrum) that rotates the toes toward the floor.

Second rocker begins when the entire plantar surface of the foot is in contact with the floor. The foot becomes a 1st-class lever, with the fulcrum moved from the heel to the ankle joint. The ground reaction force is the load acting on the lever arm of the forefoot and the soleus acting on the lever arm of the heel provides the effort. This is an example of a 1st-class lever (Fig. 2.4.4a).

During 3rd rocker, the gastrocnemius and other plantarflexors have joined the soleus to create a propulsive force. The fulcrum of the foot lever has now moved forward to the

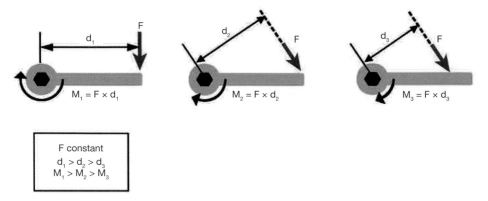

Fig. 2.4.5 Moments and lever arms. The magnitude of a moment (M) is the product of force (F) × length of the lever arm (d). A lever arm is defined as the perpendicular distance between the force and the center of rotation. A change in either the position or the orientation of the applied force will cause a change in the magnitude of the moment. To create the largest moment, the force must be perpendicular to the lever. (Reproduced from Paley 2002, by permission.)

metatarsal heads, and the heel rises off the ground. Consequently, the foot again acts as a 2nd-class lever, with the effort from the plantarflexors acting on the heel end, the load (body weight) in the middle at the ankle, and the metatarsal heads acting as the fulcrum (Fig. 2.4.3b).

In a neuromuscular condition such as cerebral palsy, the various elements of the body's leverage systems; the levers, fulcra, and forces, become distorted. We call this condition 'lever-arm dysfunction'. Five distinct types of dysfunction exist: (1) short lever arm, (2) flexible lever arm, (3) malrotated lever arm, (4) abnormal pivot or action point, and (5) positional lever-arm dysfunction.

Short lever arm
Some examples of a short lever arm include coxa breva and coxa valga. The way in which coxa breva shortens a lever arm is straightforward. To better understand how coxa valga results in lever arm dysfunction, recall that the lever arm is defined as the *perpendicular* distance from the center of rotation (hip joint center) to the line of action of the muscle (Fig. 2.4.6). Thus, even though the femoral neck may be of appropriate length, the effective abduction lever is reduced because of the change in the line-of-action. Because the abduction moment is the abductor force multiplied by the lever arm, the effect of a shortened lever arm is to reduce the magnitude of the internal abduction moment (effort) in exact proportion to the shortening of the lever arm itself. If no postural compensation occurs, an increased hip abductor force is required because the external moment of the body weight (load) is unchanged. Often the abductors cannot meet this demand. Consequently, it is common to see postural adjustments, such as shifting the upper trunk over the stance limb, which has the effect of moving the body's center of mass closer to the fulcrum, thereby reducing the load (Fig. 2.4.7). If shifting the trunk cannot sufficiently compensate, pelvic drop (Trendelenburg sign) is seen with each single leg stance. This example indicates how an

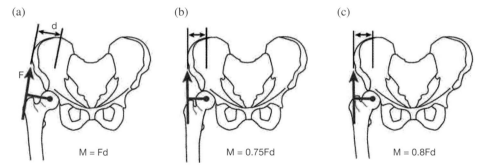

(a)	(b)	(c)
M = Fd	M = 0.75Fd	M = 0.8Fd

Fig. 2.4.6 Hip-abductor moments. (a) Demonstrates the abduction moment acting on a normal hip. The lever arm 'd' is the perpendicular distance from the hip joint center to the abductor muscle. The moment generated about the hip is equal to the muscle force times the length of the lever. A moment of Fd is generated in this case. (b) Shows a hip joint that has excessive valgus. In this example, the lever arm is shortened by 25% because the gluteus medius insertion has been drawn closer to the hip joint center by the effect of the valgus. The result is that, even though the muscle force is unchanged, the magnitude of the moment has been reduced by 25%. (c) Shows the effect of a coxa breva that can occur following a fracture in an adult or avascular necrosis of the capital femoral epiphysis in a growing child. Again, the effect of the femoral neck shortening is to draw the gluteus medius closer to the center of the hip joint (by 20% in this example). As a result the magnitude of the moment has been reduced to 80% of normal despite normal muscle strength. (Reproduced from Paley 2002, by permission.)

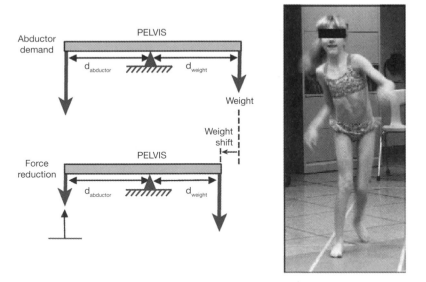

Fig. 2.4.7 Gait compensation for a short hip-abduction lever. (a) If the location of the body weight (load) is unchanged, a higher force will be demanded of the hip-abductors. If this effort cannot be supplied, a compensatory posture will be found that reduces the lever arm of the external force, thereby reducing the demand on the hip-abductors. Trendelenburg gait is an example of this sort of compensation. (b) The girl in the photograph has an upper body shift and a pelvic drop (Trendelenburg sign) during single limb stance. (Reproduced from Paley 2002, by permission.)

121

'effective' hip-abductor insufficiency can arise in a patient with normal muscle strength and control.

Flexible lever arm

Flexible lever-arm dysfunction has been likened to attempting to pry up a rock with a rubber crowbar. Rather than moving the rock, the work done on the end of the crowbar merely causes a bending deformation. In a child with spastic diplegia the classic example of this is flexible pes valgus (Figs 2.4.8, 9), which is thought to be a significant factor in promoting crouch gait since it results in substantial loss of the normal plantarflexion / knee-extension couple that provides a large portion of the support necessary for upright posture. These children have a 'midfoot break', which results in excessive dorsiflexion during mid-stance. Relative contracture of the triceps surae imposes additional stress on

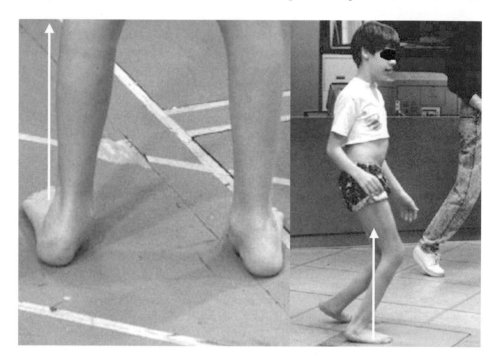

Fig. 2.4.8 Flexible lever-arm dysfunction. (a) During terminal stance the heel normally moves into relative varus and the arch lifts as the plantar fascia is winched around the metatarsal heads. These actions render the foot rigid so that it is an excellent lever for push-off. In pes valgus, the hindfoot remains in valgus and the forefoot in abduction and supination/varus throughout stance. As such the foot is externally rotated to the knee axis and there is excessive motion in the midfoot. This means that the lever arm is not only mal-directed (it is not in the plane of progression); it is also flexible – like a crowbar made of rubber. (b) Boy with spastic diplegia and severe pes valgus. It is apparent that no plantarflexion/knee-extension couple can be generated since the ground reaction force is always behind the knee axis. This means that the entire task of sustaining lower extremity extension falls to the hip and knee extensors. Unfortunately, in an adult there is not enough power in these two muscle groups to assume this burden and so crouch gait invariably occurs. (Reproduced from Paley 2002, by permission.)

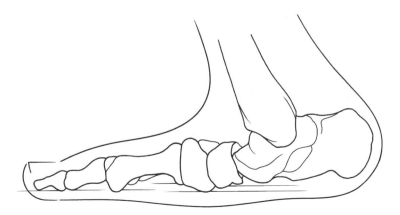

Fig. 2.4.9 Schematic drawing of a 'midfoot break'. The hindfoot, including the talus, is forced into equinus by excessive triceps surae force. An excessive ground reaction force then pushes the forefoot into relative dorsiflexion, abduction and supination on the hindfoot. In the face of these forces the tibialis posterior and spring ligament are unable to sustain the longitudinal arch, with the result that the navicular subluxates dorsally and laterally on the talus.

the midfoot in 2nd rocker. Because these children also have inherent weakness of the tibialis posterior, which supports the longitudinal arch, collapse of the arch occurs with resultant dorsal–lateral subluxation of the navicular on the talus. Consequently, the foot is not rigid enough to transmit the force and, as a result, bends as the loading increases. It is also common to see an abduction deformation of the forefoot, which further reduces the effectiveness of the foot lever, as will be discussed in the malrotated lever section below. Treatment options for this and other foot pathologies are described in Chapter 5.8.

Malrotated lever arm
The most common examples of malrotated levers in the body are excessive (or un-remodeled) femoral anteversion, and excessive tibial torsion. In the case of cerebral palsy, as described earlier, this occurs partly because of failure to remodel fetal anteversion. There is often both femoral anteversion and external tibial torsion, a combination often referred to as the 'malignant malalignment syndrome' (Fig. 2.4.10). To understand the consequences of this type of lever-arm dysfunction, it is necessary to visualize its effects in both the sagittal and transverse planes.

Consider tibial torsion (for now, in the absence of anteversion). In the sagittal plane, it can be seen that the relative length of the knee-extension lever arm of the ground reaction force has been reduced. In the transverse plane, the rotated position of the foot due to the torsion can be seen (Fig. 2.4.11). From this perspective, it can be noted that valgus and external rotation moments about the ankle/knee have been introduced as well. Hence, malrotated levers produce two effects: (1) reduction of the magnitude of the primary or intended moment, and (2) introduction of secondary moments. The effect of tibial torsion has been quantified using simulation techniques, and has been shown to significantly reduce the capacity of muscles to extend the knee and hip. More detail can be found in Chapter 5.6.

Fig. 2.4.10 Young man with 'malignant malalignment syndrome'. This condition features internal femoral torsion (femoral anteversion) in conjunction with external tibial torsion and/or pes valgus. The result is that the foot and knee are not aligned to the plane of progression and the normal plantarflexion/knee-extension couple cannot occur.

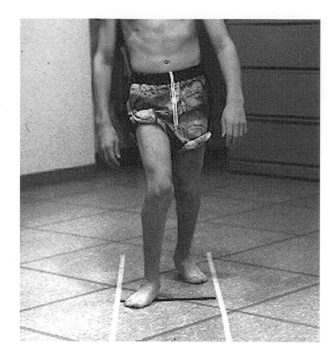

a.

$$M_{flex/ext} = F_z * D$$
$$M_{var/val} = 0$$
$$M_{iR/eR} = 0$$

b.

$$M_{flex/ext} = F_z * d$$
$$M_{var/val} = F_z * h$$
$$M_{iR/eR} = F_x * h$$

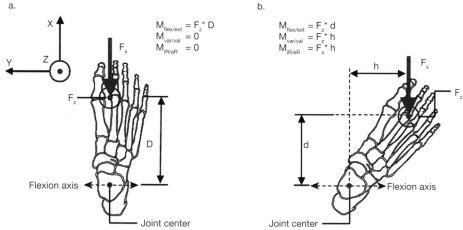

Fig. 2.4.11 Malrotated lever-arm dysfunction, external tibial torsion. Malrotated lever arms most commonly occur in the long bones of the lower extremity (femoral anteversion, tibial torsion). (a) Normal anatomy and alignment. Note the relative length of the extension moment $F_z * D$ and that the varus-valgus and rotational moments are zero. (b) External tibial torsion causes the ground reaction force to move posterior and lateral to its normal position. This has the effect of shortening the extension moment lever arm. This means that the knee extension moment is reduced. In addition, valgus and external rotation moments are introduced that will generate valgus and external rotation forces at the foot, shank, and knee. In a growing child these abnormal forces acting over time will produce pes planovalgus, further external tibial torsion, and genu valgum. M, moment; F, force; D/d/h denote various lever arms. (Reproduced from Paley 2002, by permission.)

124

Lever-arm dysfunction affects both the external moments from gravity and ground reaction forces, and internal moments from muscles. With femoral anteversion, the specific effect would depend on the relative positions of the hip and knee during gait. For example, if an individual with 45° of excessive anteversion were to walk with the knee directed anteriorly, the insertion point of the gluteus minimus referable to the hip-joint center would have to be rotated externally by the same 45°. This would reduce the abduction moment on the hip by an amount proportional to the reduction of length of the abduction lever arm. In addition, it would introduce a hip-extension moment of approximately equal magnitude (Fig. 2.4.12).

Note that the introduction of secondary moments and the reduction of primary moments can occur without any change in the *magnitude* of the muscle forces. Hence, a lever of proper length can cause pathology solely as a result of its improper orientation. From our earlier discussions on the mechanism of bone growth, it should be remembered that growing bone is plastic and remodels in accordance with the stresses that are imposed on it. Therefore the long-term effect of malrotated lever-arm dysfunction in a growing child is to generate further deformity of the long bones and feet.

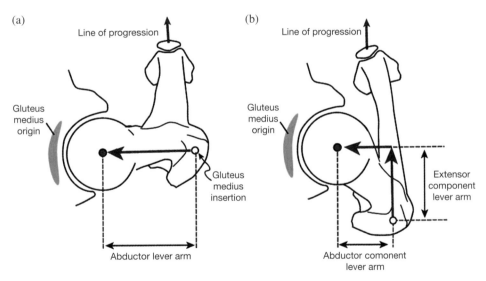

Fig. 2.4.12 Malrotated lever arm, femoral anteversion. (a) Just as tibial torsion generates lever arm dysfunction at the foot, so femoral anteversion will generate lever arm dysfunction at the hip. This figure depicts a transverse view of normal anatomy at the hip. The gluteus medius insertion point is directly lateral to the hip and as such the moment produced by this muscle would be only abduction. The product of the extension and external rotation moments would be zero. Panel (b) shows the situation when severe femoral anteversion is present. By internal rotation of the entire limb, the individual is able to neutralize some of the anteversion. However, the portion that is not neutralized with internal rotation of the limb has the effect of carrying the gluteus medius insertion point posteriorly. The result of this would be that the abduction moment of the gluteus medius is reduced in magnitude and hip extension and internal rotation moments are introduced, which are not normally present. (Reproduced from Paley 2002, by permission.)

The treatment of a malrotated lever arm is straightforward. The malrotation must be surgically corrected, either acutely via osteotomy and internal fixation of the affected bone or slowly via a derotation component in an Ilizarov frame. More details on the identification and treatment of femoral anteversion and tibial torsion are described later in this book (Chapter 5.6).

Unstable fulcrum

A good example of an unstable fulcrum is hip subluxation or dislocation (Fig. 2.4.13). In this case, even in the presence of an adequate force and lever, an effective moment cannot be generated. Because the hip is subluxated, there is no stable fulcrum. As a result, a normal hip-abductor muscle would not produce abduction, but rather upward subluxation of the femoral head. There is an element of similarity between the effect of a flexible lever and that of an unstable fulcrum, but the underlying causes are substantially different.

Treatment would depend on the integrity of the joint and the length of time the condition had been present. For example, a hip subluxation or dislocation in a child with cerebral palsy can usually be corrected with open reduction plus appropriate femoral and acetabular osteotomies. However, in an adult with cerebral palsy and concurrent degenerative joint disease, a total hip replacement might be required to remedy this situation.

Positional lever-arm dysfunction

Positional lever-arm dysfunction is a bit more difficult to understand. One of the best examples of it is seen in the effect of a crouch gait. As was discussed in Chapter 1.4, in normal erect gait the hamstrings function primarily as hip-extensors during the first half of stance phase. This is possible, despite the fact that the hamstrings are biarticular muscles,

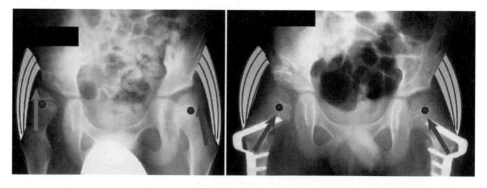

Fig. 2.4.13 (a) Unstable fulcrum, hip subluxation. Hip subluxation or dislocation provides an excellent example of the effect of an unstable fulcrum. In this illustration it can be seen that the right hip joint is severely subluxated and unstable. Consequently, contraction of the hip-abductors will not produce abduction, but rather upward translation of the femoral head and neck. On the opposite side the femoral head is stable in the acetabulum, but the severe coxa valga has the effect of shortening the abduction lever arm (short lever-arm dysfunction). (b) After bilateral varus–derotational femoral osteotomy and a right acetabuloplasty, both hips are stable and normal hip-abduction lever arms have been restored. Dots denote center of rotation and arrows are the weight-bearing vectors. (Reproduced from Paley 2002, by permission.)

126

because the distal joint (the knee) is locked (initially by the action of the vasti and later by the effect of the plantarflexion/knee-extension couple). Because of this, the concentric action of the hamstrings is able to augment hip extension without flexing the knee. Waters and colleagues demonstrated the effectiveness of the hamstrings as hip extensors (Waters et al. 1974). Perry and Newsam also pointed out their function in cerebral palsy (Perry and Newsam 1992). However, much of this knowledge has not been assimilated by the orthopaedic community at large. Now, however, there is further evidence from the modeling community that shows the hamstrings act as knee extensors during stance (Arnold 1999). This is a result of induced accelerations arising from a coupled, closed, kinematic chain.

During crouch gait, however, the situation changes dramatically. A number of factors change with this posture, including the position of the ground reaction force and gravity relative to the knee and hip, which now cause significant external flexion moments at both joints. The internal moment arms of muscles crossing the hip and knee also change because of the flexed posture. Finally, the coupled dynamics of the lower extremity change because of the relative positions and orientations of the joints and body segments. The results of these changes are twofold: (1) the patellar–femoral pressures increase, and (2) the quadriceps (including the rectus femoris) and hamstrings are called on for more assistance to resist the external flexion moments. However, in addition to being a knee extensor, the biarticular rectus femoris is also a hip-flexor. And the hamstrings, in addition to their action as hip extensors, are knee-flexors. Thus with rectus femoris and hamstring activity, even larger extension moments are required at the hip and knee to resist their collapse into flexion. The result is a vicious cycle in which the hip and knee flexion moments get progressively larger and the extension moments become progressively more inadequate. The situation has been analyzed using advanced modeling techniques (Hicks et al. 2008). The findings of Hicks and colleagues quantify the extent by which crouch alters the dynamic function of muscle groups. Further details related to treatment of crouch gait can be found in Chapter 5.11.

Since the problem can arise from a variety of causes, the treatment of positional lever-arm dysfunction is complex. In contrast, in a neuromuscular condition such as cerebral palsy, crouch gait can be secondary to poor balance, loss of selective motor control, abnormal muscle tone, muscle weakness, and/or other types of lever-arm dysfunction discussed earlier in this chapter. In contrast, in paralytic conditions such as myelo-meningocele or poliomyelitis, the problem often emanates from distal weakness of the triceps surae, which in turn produces an inadequate plantarflexion/knee-extension couple during mid-stance. It is important to remember that this particular type of lever-arm dysfunction often arises, in part, as a consequence of the other types of lever-arm dysfunction that were discussed earlier. Since the treatment of positional lever-arm dysfunction is complex and relates directly to the treatment of crouch gait, we will discuss it more completely when we come to crouch gait in the treatment section of this book.

In summary, pathological gait is complex; and even within the narrower framework of spastic diplegia can come about from multiple etiologies. These include the primary abnormalities (inadequate selective motor control, balance deficiencies and spasticity), the secondary deformities (muscle contracture and lever-arm dysfunction), and even the coping responses, which arise in response to the individual's need to circumvent these constraints. It follows, then, that the treatment of gait problems in cerebral palsy must also be complex because it requires the examiner first to structure an accurate problem list and then to determine how best to address each of the items using the tools at hand. However, there is no shortcut of which we are aware, and unless this is done routinely with each case in question, consistent outcomes can not be achieved.

REFERENCES

Albright AL (1996) Intrathecal baclofen in cerebral palsy movement disorders. *J Child Neurol* **11** (Suppl 1): S29–35.

Albright AL (2007) Intrathecal baclofen for childhood hypertonia. *Childs Nerv Syst* **23**: 971–9.

Albright AL, Barry MJ, Fasick P, Barron W, Shultz B (1996) Continuous intrathecal baclofen infusion for symptomatic generalized dystonia. *Neurosurgery* **38**: 934–9.

Albright AL, Barry MJ, Shafton DH, Ferson SS (2001) Intrathecal baclofen for generalized dystonia. *Dev Med Child Neurol* **43**: 652–7.

Arkin AM, Katz JF (1956) The effects of pressure on epiphyseal growth. *J Bone Joint Surg Am* **38**: 1056–76.

Arnold AS (1999) *Quantitative descriptions of musculoskeletal geometry in persons with cerebral palsy: guidelines for the evaluation and treatment of crouch gait.* (D. Phil. Dissertation.) Department of Biomedical Engineering, Northwestern University, Evanston, IL.

Arnold AS, Komattu AV, Delp SL (1997) Internal rotation gait: a compensatory mechanism to restore abduction capacity decreased by bone deformity. *Dev Med Child Neurol* **39**: 40–4.

Bleck E (1971) Postural and gait abnormalities caused by hip-flexion deformity in spastic cerebral palsy. Treatment by iliopsoas recession. *J Bone Joint Surg Am* **53**: 1468–88.

Bleck EE (1987) *Orthopaedic Management in Cerebral Palsy.* London: Mac Keith Press.

Burtner PA, Woollacott MH, Qualls C (1999) Stance balance control with orthoses in a group of children with spastic cerebral palsy. *Dev Med Child Neurol* **41**: 748–57.

Butler PB, Thompson N, Major RE (1992) Improvement in walking performance of children with cerebral palsy: preliminary results. *Dev Med Child Neurol* **34**: 567–76.

Delp SL, Statler K, Carroll NC (1995) Preserving plantar flexion strength after surgical treatment for contracture of the triceps surae: a computer simulation study. *J Orthop Res,* **13**: 96–104.

Delp SL, Hess WE, Hungerford DS, Jones LC (1999) Variation of rotation moment arms with hip flexion. *J Biomechan* **32**: 493–501.

Fabry G, MacEwen GD, Shands AR (1973) Torsion of the femur. A follow-up study in normal and abnormal conditions. *J Bone Joint Surg Am* **55**: 1726–38.

Hagberg B, Sanner G, Steen M (1972) The dysequilibrium syndrome in cerebral palsy. Clinical aspects and treatment. *Acta Paediatr Scand Suppl,* **226**: 1–63.

Hepp-Reymond M, Trouche E, Wiesendanger M (1974) Effects of unilateral and bilateral pyramidotomy on a conditioned rapid precision grip in monkeys (Macaca fascicularis). *Exp Brain Res* **21**: 519–27.

Heuter C (1862) Anatomische Studien an den Extremitatengelenken Neugeborener und Erwachsener. *Virchows Arch* **25**: 572–99.

Hicks JL, Schwartz MH, Arnold AS, Delp S (2008) Crouched postures reduce the capacity of muscles to extend the hip and knee during the single-limb stance phase of gait. *J Biomechan* **41**: 960–7.

Horstmann HM, Bleck EE (2007) *Orthopaedic Management in Cerebral Palsy.* London: Mac Keith Press. p 26–7.

Kuypers H (1981) Anatomy of the descending pathways. In: Brookhart JM, Mountcastle VB, Brooks VB, Geiger SR, editors. *The Nervous System,* vol. II. Bethesda, MD: Williams and Wilkins. p 597–666.

Liao HF, Jeng SF, Lai JS, Cheng CK, Hu MH (1997) The relation between standing balance and walking function in children with spastic diplegic cerebral palsy. *Dev Med Child Neurol* **39**: 106–12.

Liao HF, Mao PJ, Hwang AW (2001) Test–retest reliability of balance tests in children with cerebral palsy. *Dev Med Child Neurol* **43**: 180–6.

Lieber RL (1997) Muscle fiber length and moment arm coordination during dorsi- and plantarflexion in the mouse hindlimb. *Acta Anat (Basel)* **159**: 84–9.

Novacheck T, Trost J, Schwartz M (2002) Intramuscular psoas lengthening improves dynamic hip function in children with cerebral palsy. *J Pediatr Orthop* **22**: 158–64.

Paley D (2002) *Principles of Deformity Correction*. Berlin, Heidelberg, New York: Springer.

Perry J, Newsam C (1992) Function of the hamstrings in cerebral palsy. In: Sussman M, editor. *The Diplegic Child: Evaluation and Management*. Rosemont, IL: American Academy of Orthopaedic Surgeons. p 299–307.

Rose SA, DeLuca PA, Davis RB 3rd, Õunpuu S, Gage JR (1993) Kinematic and kinetic evaluation of the ankle after lengthening of the gastrocnemius fascia in children with cerebral palsy. *J Pediatr Orthop* **13**: 727–32.

Somerville EW (1957) Persistent foetal alignment of the hip. *J Bone Joint Surg Br* **39**: 106.

Shumway-Cook AS, Hutchinson S, Kartin D, Price R, Woollacott M (2003) Effect of balance training on recovery of stability in children with cerebral palsy. *Dev Med Child Neurol* **45**: 591–602.

Waters RL, Perry J, McDaniels JM, House K (1974) The relative strength of the hamstrings during hip extension. *J Bone Joint Surg Am* **56**: 1592–7.

Winter DA (1991) *The Biomechanics and Motor Control of Human Gait: Normal, Elderly, and Pathological*, 2nd edn. Waterloo, Ontario: University of Waterloo Press. p 35–52, 75–85.

Winters TF, Jr., Gage JR, Hicks R (1987) Gait patterns in spastic hemiplegia in children and young adults. *J Bone Joint Surg Am* **69**: 437–41.

Woollacott M, Shumway-Cook A, Hutchinson S, Ciol M, Price R, Kartin D (2005) Effect of balance training on muscle activity used in recovery of stability in children with cerebral palsy: a pilot study. *Dev Med Child Neurol* **47**: 455–61.

Zajac FE, Gordon ME (1989) Determining muscle's force and action in multi-articular movement. *Exerc Sport Sci Rev* **17**: 187–230.

2.5
MUSCLE STRUCTURE AND FUNCTION IN CEREBRAL PALSY

Adam P. Shortland, Nicola R. Fry, Anne E. McNee and Martin Gough

Our current knowledge of muscle deformity and weakness in spastic cerebral palsy (SCP) is based largely on our clinical observations of children as they grow. It is commonly understood that very young children have few significant muscle deformities, but that as they develop their musculotendinous units do not lengthen at the same rate as their neighboring long bones, and muscle contractures result. Our inferences of muscle deformity are born from the passive range of motion examinations that we conduct in our clinic rooms and assessment centers. But the musculotendinous unit is the sum of parts: the muscle fibers, the muscle belly and the tendon all contribute to its length (Fig. 2.5.1). In the clinical setting, we do not routinely assess the contributions of these elements to musculotendinous length.

In a general sense deformity need not concern the measurement of length alone. Its meaning may encompass any changes in muscle morphology and structure that are deviant from the norm. Changes in muscle shape, internal architecture and composition alter passive and active muscular performance, particularly the ability of muscle to generate force and power through range. It has long been recognized that weakness is an important negative feature of the upper motor neuron syndrome, but the origin of weakness in SCP and the contribution of altered muscular structure have not been fully explored.

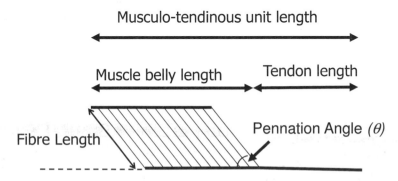

Fig. 2.5.1 A simple diagrammatic representation of the gross structure of a unipennate muscle.

Muscle is a highly malleable tissue. It responds rapidly to mechanical stress and hormonal activity, as well as changes in amount and magnitude of activity. The potential for adaptation in muscle derives from the rapid turnover of proteins in the muscle cell.

In this chapter we describe some of the deficits in muscle morphology and structure present in children and young adults with SCP. Imaging techniques that elucidate features of muscle properties and performance are then discussed. We place the structural muscular deficits in the context of other impairments in SCP, and we demonstrate the potential for improving muscular performance in this group of patients.

Muscle morphology, architecture and function

Most of the muscles in the normal lower limb are pinnate, i.e. the muscle fibers attach to the aponeuroses (internal tendons) of the muscle belly at an angle (the angle of pinnation) (Fig. 2.5.2). Because of this, the length of the muscle fibers can be much shorter than the length of the muscle belly and particularly in the extensors. This means that the contribution made by fiber length to musculotendinous length in pinnate muscles may be small. But why is it advantageous for the extensors of the limb to have short fibers?

Any discussion of muscle architecture rightly begins with a description of the dynamics of the sarcomere. The sarcomere is the fundamental structural unit of muscular contraction. Within the sarcomere there are overlapping (interdigitating) protein filaments. Mechanical linkages (crossbridges) are formed between these proteins and it is the reconfiguration of these crossbridges, regulated by action potentials and fuelled by adenosine triphosphate (ATP), that causes the filaments to slide across each other, changing the length of the sarcomere and resulting in muscular contraction. The number of sites for crossbridges to form and the distance between these sites along the filamentous proteins govern the active force length relationship of the sarcomere. In humans, the active excursion of the sarcomere is about 2 μm.

For muscle fibers to contract forcefully and over significant lengths the sarcomeres have to be arranged in parallel and in series.

Both muscles A and B in Figure 2.5.2 are composed of 12 sarcomeres. Muscle B has a smaller number of sarcomeres in *parallel* than muscle A, and can produce only 75% of the active force of muscle A. Conversely, muscle A has a smaller number of sarcomeres in *series* and therefore has a smaller active range. As a result, muscle A produces a lower velocity of contraction than muscle B. Simply put, the arrangement of sarcomeres within

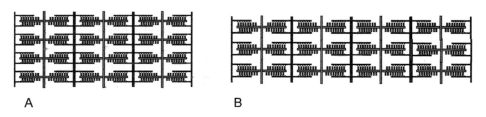

A   B

Fig. 2.5.2 Two muscles with an equal number but a different arrangement of sarcomeres.

a muscle has a powerful influence on the active and passive mechanical properties with the number of sarcomeres in series affecting the muscle's speed and active range, and the number of sarcomeres in parallel affecting the force-generating potential of the muscle.

For much larger muscles we can express the number of sarcomeres acting in parallel as the physiological cross sectional area (PCSA). The equation for PCSA is a rather simple one (Eq. 1) but the term can cause some confusion, since in muscles where the fibers are short compared to the belly there may be no simple anatomical plane from which this 'cross-sectional area' can be obtained directly by measurement.

$$PCSA = \frac{V \cdot cos\,(\theta),}{f_l} \qquad (1)$$

where V is the muscle volume, f_l is fiber length and θ is the pinnation angle.

However, we can construct a simple diagrammatic proof. Let us consider a pinnate muscle formed from three fibers, each consisting of three sarcomeres in parallel and four sarcomeres in series (Fig. 2.5.3).

The cross-sectional area of sarcomeres acting in the direction of the tendon = 3×3 cos θ (three sarcomeres in parallel in each of three fibers acting at an angle θ to the direction of the tendon). This is the volume of the muscle (36 sarcomeres) multiplied by the cosine of the pinnation angle (f_l) divided by length of the fibers (four sarcomeres per fiber). In the limiting case, where the pinnation angle is 0° (long-fiber muscle) the equation for physiological cross-sectional area reduces to V/f_l.

Powell and colleagues (1984) demonstrated that the product of PCSA and an estimate of specific active tension (the amount of force that can be produced actively by a muscle per unit area) could predict maximal force production in a number of muscles in the hind limbs of guinea pigs. Assuming the resting length of the sarcomere is nearly constant between muscles, the active range and velocity of contraction of muscle is determined by resting fiber length (essentially the number of sarcomeres $\times$ average resting length of the sarcomere). Muscles of reduced volume are able to produce lower levels of force; those with reduced fiber length have less active range and reduced velocity-generating capacity.

The specific tension of muscles may depend on a number of factors, including fiber type (slow or fast) and percentage of connective tissue. Slow fibers have greater oxidative capacity, have lower specific tensions and velocities than faster fibers, and are in greater proportion in postural muscles (e.g. soleus, vastus intermedius). In normally developing muscle the proportion of connective tissue is very small so its direct effect on specific tension is also small. However, under certain conditions the connective tissue fraction increases (see below).

Regulation of muscle force
The activity of alpha motor neurons (α-MNs) in the ventral portion of the spinal cord is regulated by signals descending from the motor cortex and the brainstem. The axon of the α-MN extends from the SC to a particular skeletal muscle and innervates a number

of muscle fibers distributed widely within the muscle. A single α-MN, and the fibers it innervates, is referred to as a motor unit (MU). In the extensors of the lower limb, an MU may incorporate more than 2000 fibers.

A single action potential formed by the α-MN causes a single mechanical twitch in the target muscle fibers. Repeated action potentials give rise to superposition of mechanical twitches and increased force. At higher frequencies a fused tetanus results and the MU is said to be maximally stimulated. This method of regulation of muscle force is called rate coding. There are limitations in the range of forces that can be supplied by this method since the twitch-tetanus ratio of forces is about 1:4.

A skeletal muscle and its nerve supply may consist of thousands of independent MUs. The force produced by a muscle is proportional to the number of MUs activated (or recruited). In voluntary contraction, the slower, smaller and lower threshold MUs tend to be recruited first followed by the larger, faster, higher-threshold units. This principle of action is called the Henneman principle (Henneman et al. 1965) and allows greater control over the force output of the skeletal muscle.

Normal muscle development

Before discussing the adaptation of muscle in SCP, it is instructive to consider the natural history of muscle development. In normal development the number of muscle fibers present is fixed by birth. Increases in muscle size after birth take place by hypertrophy, i.e. an increase in muscle fiber diameter. During the early years (0–5), separate populations of fast- and slow-twitch fibers emerge. Fibers continue to grow in area into adulthood. At around 25 years of age, the number of MUs (and muscle fibers) begins to decline and the fibers also begin to atrophy. There appears to be a preferential reduction in the cross-sectional area of type II (fast) fibers. By the time a person reaches his or her 8th decade they may have lost as much as 50% of their muscle mass because of fiber loss as well as fiber atrophy (Lexell et al. 1988). This has important implications for function. The elderly may lose so much strength that they cannot develop enough force in key muscles to complete everyday tasks such as the

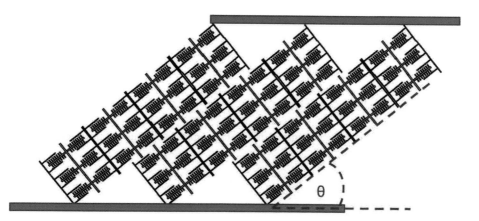

Fig. 2.5.3 Representation of sarcomere arrangement in a pinnate muscle.

133

sit-to-stand maneuver (Hughes et al. 1996). The natural history of sarcopenia in typically developing adults may have implications for mobility in those individuals where muscular strength is compromised by a pre-existing neurological condition.

Muscle adaptation in cerebral palsy

Muscles are organs capable of rapid adaptation to changes in the demands imposed on them whether these are in response to an altered neural drive or to an imposed external condition such as immobilization or disuse. Because of their plasticity they have often been called 'smart', but this is an unnecessary and inappropriate anthropomorphism. Rather, they are dumb animals in which complex molecular machinery transduces signals from the environment and regulates the activity of protein synthesis and degradation. The precise mechanism by which this is achieved is the subject of research in many laboratories, and is not completely elaborated. There have, however, been a number of factors identified that are central to muscle growth, muscle stiffness and muscle fiber length. It appears that an increase in the number of nuclei in the fibers, an increase in the number of satellite cells adjacent to muscle fibers, and hypertrophy of muscle fibers during infancy and childhood are affected by stress that is transduced by a number of signaling molecules including insulin-like growth factor (IGF) I and II.

At the time of writing, we know of no reports profiling the changes in protein regulation in SCP, but it is clear that a greater understanding of alterations of myogenic and atrogenic activity in the muscles may lead to the development of a whole generation of pharmaceutical interventions for children with neuromuscular disorders.

Molecular biology studies have the potential to show us much of the workings of the engine of adaptation but it is the physiological and histological studies that shed light on the accumulated physical changes in cell and organ structure and function which result.

The literature contains few histological studies on muscle from children or adults with SCP. The largest sample comes from the work of Castle et al. (1979). This group discovered a mixed picture of fiber atrophy and hypertrophy with type I (slow) and type II (fast) fiber predominance in different muscles with fatty infiltration a frequently observed feature. Unfortunately the motor function of the group was not detailed by the authors. The results from the work of Castle are in contrast to those of Rose et al. (1994) and Ito et al. (1996). Castle et al. (1979) reported mixed and mild changes to fiber-type distribution and size in their samples taken from 21 biopsies from the gastrocnemius, whereas the teams of Rose and Ito found type I predominance in most of their muscle samples. The histomorphometric picture is also dependent on the muscle from which samples are taken within the same individuals. Romanini and co-workers (1989) described type I dominance and increased size variation, type II atrophy and the presence of polygonal shaped fibers in the 'spastic' short adductors of a number of children but described only mild atrophy of type I and type II fibers of the semimembranosus. The results from gracilis were intermediate between the short adductors and the semimembranosus. In the affected upper limbs of tetraplegic individuals with cerebral palsy (CP), myosin heavy chain IIx (fast myosin found in type IIB fibers) has been found to be upregulated (Ponten et al. 2008). It appears that fiber type distribution and mean fiber diameter is an inconsistent feature in SCP varying according to the topography and severity of the condition in the individual person, as well as the individual muscle studied. This lack of consistency between studies suggests that alterations in structure and fiber type may be dependent on multiple influences (severity of upper motor lesion, disuse, altered pattern of use and musculoskeletal alignment).

One common feature of muscle in SCP is increased fiber-size variation. Rose et al. (1994) demonstrated that the variation in fiber diameter was associated with increased energy demands and prolongation of muscle activity during walking. The association between these variables indicates an explanatory relationship between the neuropathology of SCP, the secondary structural muscle impairments and functional deficits in this group. Romanini et al. (1989) suggested that the relative hypertrophy and atrophy of slow fibers within the same muscle indicates an overuse phenomenon with an initial increase in fiber size followed by exhaustion of these fibers and a gradual reduction in fiber size. Increased variation in fiber diameter may be indicative of a chronic denervation/reinnervation process. There is certainly evidence of abnormalities of the interaction of nerve and muscle in studies of the neuromuscular junction in children with SCP (Theroux et al. 2005).

Increases in connective tissue and fatty infiltration have been observed in some muscles showing extreme fiber size variation (Rose et al. 1994, Ito et al. 1996). Booth and colleagues (2001) used immunohistochemical techniques to show increased connective tissue in the vastus lateralis of children with SCP. They demonstrated relationships between total collagen content and the Modified Ashworth Score. In severe cases they reported very small diameter muscle fibers within an extensive extracellular matrix (ECM). This pattern is similar to that reported by Lieber and his colleagues (2003). In a study of the flexors of the upper limbs of children with SCP about to undergo muscle transfer surgery, they demonstrated the presence of small stiff fibers within an ECM of poor mechanical integrity. The proliferation of the ECM and the presence of very small fibers seems to be an end-stage phenomenon in muscle deformity affecting the active specific tension of muscle as well as reducing the lateral transmission of forces between neighboring fibers and fascicles (Huijing 1999). Lateral force transmission is an important method of distributing the tension generated by the activation of a single MU throughout a muscle. In the absence of these forces individual muscle fibers may be exposed to large and potentially damaging tensile forces.

Our understanding of muscle adaptation in SCP has been colored by groundbreaking studies (Tabary et al. 1972, Goldspink et al. 1974, Williams and Goldspink 1978) in which muscle-fiber length in animal models was studied under various conditions. Perhaps the most clinically influential finding was that fibers responded to imposed conditions of muscle stretch or muscle shortening. Clinicians have believed that muscle deformity (reduction in muscle length) is caused by a reduction in serial sarcomeres and a reduction in fiber length, but until recently there were no direct measurements of muscle-fiber length in SCP. Shortland et al. (2002), using ultrasonography, found that fascicles (groups of fibers visible with ultrasound imaging) in the medial gastrocnemius of childen with hemiplegia and diplegia were of similar length as in typically developing children. Lieber and Friden (2002) performed measurements of sarcomere length in the flexor carpi ulnaris of adults with spasticity and showed elongated sarcomeres and normal length fibers. However, recent results from ourselves and others suggest a differential effect of cerebral palsy on fiber length between different muscles (McNee and Shortland 2006, Mohagheghi et al. 2008). While the lengths of fibers in the medial gatrocnemius appear unaffected, there is a reduction in fascicle length in the lateral gastrocnemius of children with SCP, indicating that even neighboring muscles can be affected differentially. But what about the other muscles of the lower limb? Fascicle lengths taken using 2D and 3D ultrasound from selected muscles in typically developing children and adolescents and in independently ambulant children and adolescents with SCP positioned in the anatomical position reveal a compelling story (Fig. 2.5.4). A pattern emerges suggesting that the flexors of the limb (rectus femoris, tibialis anterior, and lateral gastrocnemius) have reduced fascicle (fiber) lengths while the extensors (vastus medialis, medial gastrocnemius) maintain or increase their fascicle length. It is difficult to explain these variations in fiber length in ambulant children with CP but it is possible that the large tensile forces to which the extensors of the limb are exposed result in sarcomere addition and maintenance of fiber length.

Our clinical impression is that muscle volumes and muscle belly lengths are reduced in SCP. It is only with the advent of magnetic resonance imaging (MRI) systems, and more recently freehand 3D ultrasound, that measurements of muscle volume and length have been made in individuals with SCP. Lampe and his co-workers (2006) measured muscle volumes and lengths throughout the lower limbs in a group of young adults with hemiplegia using MRI. They demonstrated reductions in muscle volume of up to 28% in the affected limb compared to the unaffected limb, with the distal muscles more involved. In individual

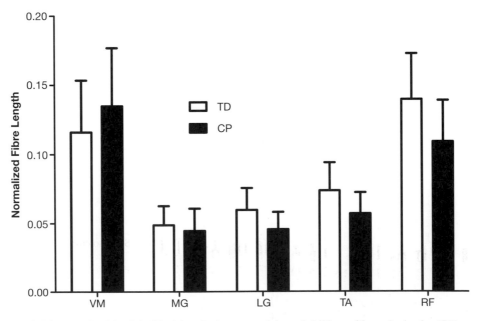

Fig. 2.5.4 Normalised fascicle (fibre) lengths in young adults and children with cerebral palsy (CP) and their typically developing peers (TD). VM, vastus medialis; MG, medial gastrocnemius; LG, lateral gastrocnemius; RF, rectus femoris; TA, tibialis anterior.

cases, they noted muscle volume reductions of 50%.Their results for muscle volume in hemiplegia in the distal musculature of the lower limb are similar to those reported by Elder et al. (2003) and Malaiya et al. (2007). Recently, we have completed a series of measurements of muscle belly volume and length in 24 ambulant children and adults (6–22 years) with bilateral CP and typically developing controls (Fig. 2.5.5). Muscle belly volumes and lengths normalized to body weight and lower limb length respectively, and data from a typically developing control group are also presented. We found significant hypotrophy for all 11 muscles in the individuals with SCP, and while there is no consistent pattern of deficit, we found distal muscles to be more affected than proximal ones and biarticular muscles more affected than monoarticular ones. Muscles in the group with SCP were significantly shorter in all muscles except one (vastus lateralis).

We have established that lower limb muscles are short in young people with SCP, but that muscle fibers are not always short! This seeming contradiction can be explained in terms of the pinnate muscle architecture of the lower limbs. Consider the idealized representation of the architecture of a pinnate muscle (Fig. 2.5.6). The contribution of fiber length to whole muscle length in muscles like these is relatively small. A pinnate muscle can become short by a reduction in the average diameter of the fibers or by a reduction in the number of fibers present. Our combined results for fiber length, muscle belly length and muscle volume suggest that muscle fiber atrophy or muscle fiber loss is responsible for much of the muscle belly shortness observed in SCP.

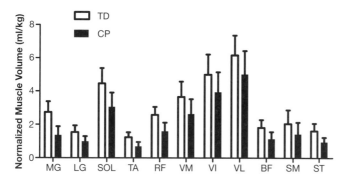

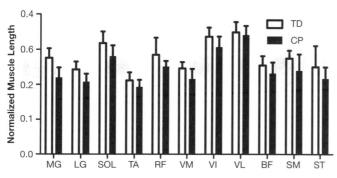

Fig. 2.5.5 Mean muscle belly volumes (a) and lengths (b) in ambulant children and young adults with cerebral palsy. MG, medial gastrocnemius; LG, lateral gastrocnemius; SOL, soleus; TA, tibialis anterior; RF, rectus femoris; VM, vastus medialis; VI, vastus intermedius; VL, vastus lateralis; BF, biceps femoris; SM, semimebranosus; ST, semitendinosus.

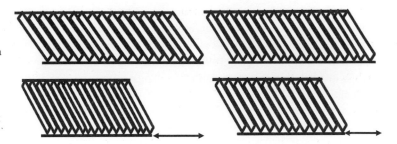

Fig. 2.5.6
A highly pinnate muscle may be short because of a reduction in fiber diameter or a reduction in fiber number (adapted from Shortland et al. 2002).

If muscle bellies are short it would seem likely that this shortness contributes, at least in part, to the limited passive range of motion we observe on clinical examination. However, there seems to be no relationship between the normalized resting length of the medial and lateral gastrocnemius bellies and passive dorsiflexion range at the ankle with the knee extended (Fig. 2.5.7). Our results from other range-of-motion measurements and muscle belly length measurements are similarly unrelated. The lack of relationship suggests the neurological and other factors that control muscle belly length are not the same as those controlling musculotendinous length. In other words, 'deformity', as we measure it in the clinic, does not inform us of muscle belly length or mechanical potential.

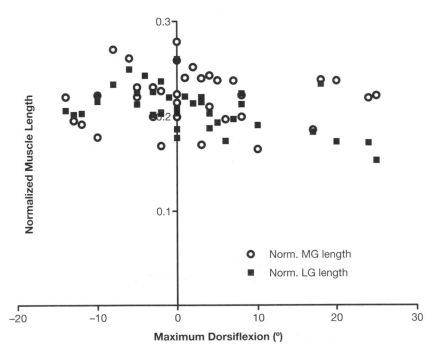

Fig. 2.5.7 The relationship between resting muscle belly length and maximum passive dorsiflexion (knee extended) for the medial (solid squares) and lateral (open squares) gastrocnemius in children and young adults with spastic cerebral palsy.

There are few data as yet relating muscle dimensions and functional capacity in individuals with SCP. Ohata and colleagues (2008) found a significant relationship between quadriceps femoris thickness and Gross Motor Function Classification System (GMFCS) level in ambulant and non-ambulant children with SCP. However, their population sample included a disproportionate number of children at GMFCS level V. It is possible that in non-ambulant children disuse is the dominant factor influencing muscle dimensions. Certainly, muscle atrophy is a product of disuse in typically developing individuals. Among the more physically able children and adults with SCP researchers are yet to determine if muscle belly dimensions are important predictors of function.

Muscle activation deficits in cerebral palsy

Although the mechanical potential of a muscle is governed largely by its physiological cross-sectional area, the capacity of an individual to generate force during a maximal voluntary contraction also depends on the percentage of motor units activated (recruitment) and the frequency of that activation (rate coding). Stackhouse and his co-workers (2005) tested the strength of the quadriceps and plantarflexors of typically developing children and ambulant children with SCP under different conditions. They asked children to voluntarily activate these muscle groups to a maximum, and they measured the force that the children could produce. They then augmented the voluntary contraction with supramaximal electrical stimulation (via electrodes placed on the skin surface). In this way they were able to distinguish the mechanical potential of the muscle group (under supramaximal stimulation) from the force that the child could produce voluntarily. They were able to demonstrate two interesting phenomena: (1) children with SCP could activate only half (plantarflexors) to two-thirds (quadriceps) of their available muscular resources; and (2) even when maximally stimulated, the muscles produced on average a quarter (plantarflexors) or half (quadriceps) of the force of the muscles of their typically developing peers. Their results demonstrate that weakness in SCP is both neurological and muscular in origin and these contribute in roughly equal measure. But are deficits in rate coding or recruitment or both responsible for 'neurological' weakness in SCP? Rose and McGill (2005) used fine-wire electrodes in the gastrocnemius and tibialis anterior of individuals with and without cerebral palsy to obtain instantaneous firing rates (IFRs) during graded submaximal contractions. At lower levels of neuromuscular activation, the IFRs of the two groups of children were similar. However, the children with SCP were unable to produce the higher firing rates necessary to reach the levels of neuromuscular activation produced by their typically developing peers obtained during maximum voluntary contractions. Their results may reflect either an inability to activate higher-threshold, higher-frequency motor units (a recruitment problem) or a failure to recruit lower-threshold motor units at higher frequencies (a rate-coding problem).

Clinical implications

The Relationship Between Neurological Deficit, Weakness and Muscle Deformity

SCP is a complex motor condition that produces significant secondary muscular impairments. Simple models of disuse or chronic stimulation do not explain the heterogeneity of our observations at the cellular level and, as yet, we do not have a complete understanding of the muscle pathologies observed in terms of altered neurological function. The number and variability of the muscular deficits between muscles and individuals may explain the variability of the response of our patients to intervention. However, certain features of the condition are consistent and serve as a starting point for building a speculative framework of understanding of muscular deformity and weakness.

Individuals with SCP have damage to the descending excitatory and inhibitory corticospinal tracts. Disruption of the excitatory tracts leads to the incomplete activation of the pool of α-MNs and possibly a reduced ability to recruit some of the high-threshold, higher-frequency units, while prolongation of motor unit firing due to lack of inhibition may encourage a fiber-type transformation from fast to slow. In muscles that are not subject to disuse, these factors in combination could account for the predominance of slow fiber type (possibly, the lack of development of a population of type II fibers) and increased variation in fiber size. It is possible that in more severe forms of SCP or in muscles that are more severely affected, motor unit firing may not be adequate to maintain the population of slower fibers, and a pattern of disuse emerges with a predominance of faster fibers. In both cases, the lack of activation of the smaller fibers may ultimately lead to the loss of motor units, fibrosis and fatty replacement, and the hypotrophy observed at the level of the muscle.

MUSCLE WEAKNESS AND LONG-TERM MOBILITY

Children with SCP are weak because of a combination of morphological and activation deficits but they are able to increase the strength of different muscle groups with progressive overload training (Damiano et al. 1995a, b). Our own results suggest that increases in strength may be due to an increase in muscle volume in part. We found increases in muscle volume after resistance training of the plantarflexors over a 10-week period (Fig. 2.5.8) that was maintained at a 12-week follow-up. However, strengthening programs seem to produce only moderate improvements in function (Damiano and Abel 1998). Perhaps the impact of strength training is compromised by the inability of individuals with SCP to select and coordinate muscle activation (Tedroff et al. 2006). In the elderly, muscular strength is an important determinant of function. Hughes and co-workers (1996) demonstrated that the elderly require near to the maximum strength of their quadriceps to complete a sit-to-stand task, and fail to complete the task as the height of the chair is lowered and the demands placed on their quadriceps increases. The loss of muscle strength in the elderly is due in the most part to sarcopenia (reductions in muscle size) which begins in the 3rd decade of life. The early loss of mobility in adults with CP is well documented. Probably the real value of intense muscular exercise is to increase the muscular reserve and extend mobility in SCP in the face of the natural history of muscular degeneration after maturity. Perhaps the effect of reduced muscle size is best explained by the conceptual graph showing the threshold in neuromuscular function necessary to perform a particular task (e.g. sit-to-stand) (Fig. 2.5.9).

Typically developing individuals reach this level of motor function early in their life (A) and are able to develop a substantial reserve in neuromuscular capacity above that required to perform the task (B). In old age, because of changes in muscle size and composition this reserve declines to a point (possibly in the individual's 8th or 9th decade) when

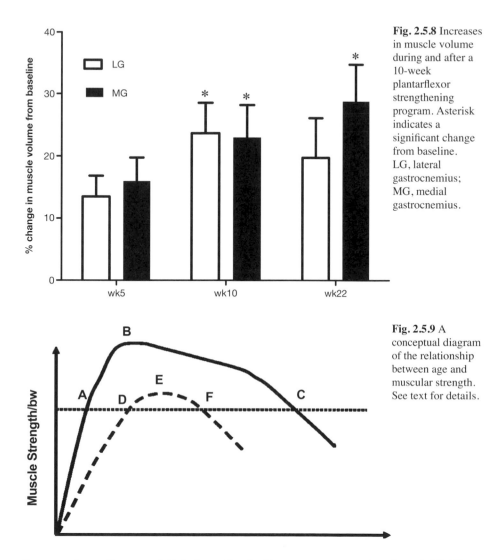

Fig. 2.5.8 Increases in muscle volume during and after a 10-week plantarflexor strengthening program. Asterisk indicates a significant change from baseline. LG, lateral gastrocnemius; MG, medial gastrocnemius.

Fig. 2.5.9 A conceptual diagram of the relationship between age and muscular strength. See text for details.

the muscular performance falls below a threshold necessary to complete the task (C). Those affected by SCP (dotted line) may develop the necessary neuromuscular performance to complete the task much later than their healthy peers (D) and at their peak motor function they may have less reserve (E). Because of this they fall below the threshold in muscular performance much earlier than typically developing individuals (F). In this context, we may need to reevaluate our treatment strategies and address the question: 'Are interventions that are designed to combat the positive features of the upper motor neuron lesion by weakening muscle to improve function in the short-term decreasing muscular reserve and restricting the long-term mobility of our patients in the long term?'

FUTURE WORK: CHARACTERIZING MUSCLE STRUCTURE AND FUNCTION BY
IMAGING

Muscle structure and function may be studied using standard and novel imaging modalities. At the cellular level, muscle physiologists use microscopes and staining techniques to illustrate the structure and content of the muscle cell (histology). These can be used to quantify cell density, cell shape, metabolic potential, accumulation of collagen and its direction, and levels of mRNA. These studies are restricted to static imaging of dead and fixed tissue but they have a very useful place in the study of cross-sectional data and provide valuable insight into the nature of pathological changes in neuromuscular disorders. Certainly, quantifying the genetic potential of muscle cells may grant us insights into the processes of adaption we would wish to direct and the syntheses of key proteins which we would look to control.

Ethical and practical considerations mean that harvesting and accessing of tissue samples in children is difficult. Studies in affected children are particularly rare and these studies tend to have small sample sizes and be inadequately controlled. Representative samples of the muscle may not be collected through a single biopsy and samples may suffer significant shrinkage, rendering the biopsies difficult to interpret. For these reasons, and because the individuals with SCP represent a heterogeneous group in which a variety of muscle abnormalities may be present, studies that rely on tissue samples may have limited scope.

At the level of the organ, we can quantify important structural and functional variables by different noninvasive imaging modalities. There are various techniques available and we will discuss a few of the more significant ones here. The gross morphology of muscle may be obtained by a number of techniques. MRI and peripheral computed tomography are established methods for estimating muscle volumes but require access to the radiology department and may be unsuitable for young children without sedation. Freehand 3D ultrasound represents a potential alternative. There are commercial and non-commercial organizations able to supply complete systems or software to generate complete 3D volumes by the attachment of a magnetic or other positional sensor to the ultrasound probe so that probe (and image) orientation and position can be calculated. A sequence of semi-structured ultrasound images are formed where any individual point within the image can be transformed to a 3D point in a global or local reference frame. An interpolation scheme is used to generate a volume-array consisting of regularly spaced voxels. In our laboratory, we use a cluster of markers attached to the ultrasound probe to provide positional and orientation information (Fig. 2.5.10).

Using MRI or ultrasound it is possible to make dynamic measurements of muscle movement. Delp and his co-workers (Asakawa et al. 2003) used a cine-contrast MRI technique to study the movement of the rectus femoris after transfer in subjects with cerebral palsy. They found that the movement of the rectus femoris during controlled motion of the lower limb was inconsistent with its proposed action as a knee flexor after surgical transfer. This is a good example of how imaging may reveal the dynamic action of muscles and help us to understand our interventions more clearly.

In our laboratory, we routinely observe increases in the echogenicity of ultrasound images taken from the muscles of children with SCP consistent with histological findings

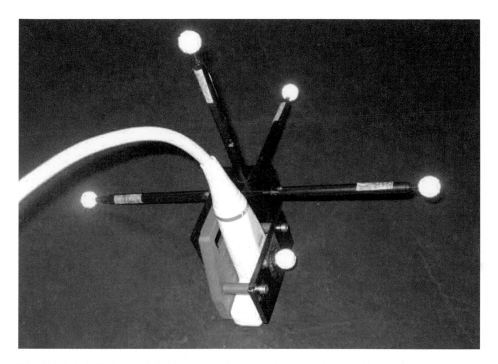

Fig. 2.5.10 A rigid cluster of markers attached to an ultrasound probe. The cluster provides 3D position and orientation data to inform the reconstruction of 3D ultrasound volumes.

already noted in this chapter (Fig. 2.5.11). The brightness of the image is related to the quantity of connective tissue within the image. It is possible to quantify the amount of echogenicity of an image and interpret the connective tissue content of the muscle if images are collected under similar conditions (probe frequency, gain etc). Using a simple measure of echo-intensity from 2D ultrasound images of the quadriceps, Pillen et al. (2007) could differentiate typically developing children and those with various neuromuscular conditions with a sensitivity of 90% and specificity of 92%. Kent-Braun and colleagues (2000) used standard MRI sequences and grayscale analysis to differentiate contractile and non-contractile components in skeletal muscle from young and old subjects. They demonstrated that older people have a significantly greater proportion of non-contractile tissue and that the proportion is inversely related to the level of activity in this group.

Diffusion-weighted MRI (DW-MRI) is a method that produces in vivo images of biological tissues weighted with the local microstructural characteristics of water diffusion. Because of this property, the technique has applications in quantifying the organization of highly orientated tissues. For example, Rose et al. (2007) used DW-MRI to quantify damage to the neural tracts in the internal capsule of preterm infants. A similar application in skeletal muscle might demonstrate lower anisotropy in muscle containing increased amounts of connective tissue or fat. Other microstructural features of muscle may also be quantified using DW-MRI. Karampinos and colleagues (2007) claimed that muscle fiber cross-sectional

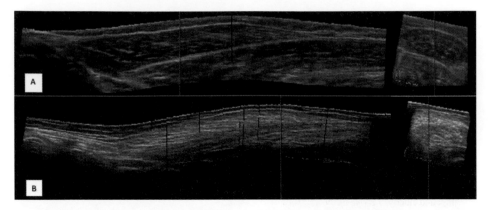

Fig. 2.5.11 Longitudinal and transverse sections through 3D ultrasound volumes from (a) a typically developing teenager and (b) a teenager with SCP. Note the larger degree of echogenic material in the image from the subject with SCP

asymmetry, a feature often found in histological studies of abnormal tissue, can be estimated using DW-MRI. Such techniques may be able to be used to gauge the level of involvement of individual muscles without recourse to invasive tissue sampling.

The combination of anatomical and dynamic imaging modalities, as well as imaging for tissue composition, is perhaps the most promising approach to understanding muscle pathology in SCP and its effect on human performance and long-term mobility. Noninvasive muscle investigations allow repeated measurements to be made with the potential of elucidating the natural history and the effects of intervention on muscle function.

Conclusions

- Histological data suggest complex and variable adaptations in the muscles of children with SCP.
- The muscles of the lower limb are small and short in children and young adults with SCP.
- There appears to be no relationship between muscle belly dimensions and passive range of movement indicating that the factors that control these variables are independent.
- We should use imaging techniques to better understand muscle structure and function.
- We should adopt novel approaches for improving muscle function in children and adolescents to preserve motor abilities in adulthood

REFERENCES

Asakawa DS, Pappas GP, Blemker SS, Drace JE, Delp SL (2003) Cine phase-contrast magnetic resonance imaging as a tool for quantification of skeletal muscle motion. *Semin Musculoskelet Radiol* **7**: 287–95.

Booth CM, Cortina-Borja MJ, Theologis TN (2001) Collagen accumulation in muscles of children with cerebral palsy and correlation with severity of spasticity. *Dev Med Child Neurol* **43**: 314–20.

Castle ME, Reyman TA, Schneider M (1979) Pathology of spastic muscle in cerebral palsy. *Clin Orthop Rel Res* **142**: 223–32.

Damiano DL, Abel MF (1998) Functional outcomes of strength training in spastic cerebral palsy. *Arch Phys Med Rehabil* **79**: 119–25.

Damiano DL, Kelly LE, Vaughn CL (1995a) Effects of quadriceps femoris muscle strengthening on crouch gait in children with spastic diplegia. *Phys Ther* **75**: 658–67.

Damiano DL, Vaughan CL, Abel MF (1995b) Muscle response to heavy resistance exercise in children with spastic cerebral palsy. *Dev Med Child Neurol* **37**: 731–9.

Elder GC, Kirk J, Stewart G, Cook K, Weir D, Marshall A, Leahey L (2003) Contributing factors to muscle weakness in children with cerebral palsy. *Dev Med Child Neurol* **45**: 542–50.

Goldspink G, Tabary C, Tabary JC, Tardieu C, Tardieu G (1974) Effect of denervation on the adaptation of sarcomere number and muscle extensibility to the functional length of the muscle. *J Physiol (Lond)* **236**: 733–42.

Henneman E, Somjen G, Carpenter DO (1965) Excitability and inhibitability of motoneurons of different sizes. *J Neurophysiol* **28**: 599–620.

Hughes MA, Myers BS, Schenkman ML (1996) The role of strength in rising from a chair in the functionally impaired elderly. *J Biomech* **29**: 1509–13.

Huijing PA (1999) Muscle as a collagen fiber reinforced composite: a review of force transmission in muscle and whole limb. *J Biomech* **32**: 329–45.

Ito J, Araki A, Tanaka H, Tasaki T, Cho K, Yamazaki R (1996) Muscle histopathology in spastic cerebral palsy. *Brain Dev* **18**: 299–303.

Karampinos DC, King KF, Sutton BP, Georgiadis JG (2007) In vivo study of cross-sectional skeletal muscle fiber asymmetry with diffusion-weighted MRI. *Conference Proceedings: Annual International Conference of the IEEE Engineering in Medicine & Biology Society 2007*, 327–30.

Kent-Braun JA, Ng AV, Young K (2000) Skeletal muscle contractile and noncontractile components in young and older women and men. *J Appl Physiol* **88**: 662–8.

Lampe R, Grassl S, Mitternacht J, Gerdesmeyer L, Gradinger R (2006) MRT-measurements of muscle volumes of the lower extremities of youths with spastic hemiplegia caused by cerebral palsy. *Brain Dev* **28**: 500–6.

Lexell J, Taylor CC, Sjöström M (1988) What is the cause of the ageing atrophy? total number, size and proportion of different fiber types studied in whole vastus lateralis muscle from 15- to 83-year-old men. *J Neurol Sci* **84**: 275–94.

Lieber RL, Friden J (2002) Spasticity causes a fundamental rearrangement of muscle-joint interaction. *Muscle Nerve* **25**: 265–70.

Lieber RL, Runesson E, Einarsson F, Friden J (2003) Inferior mechanical properties of spastic muscle bundles due to hypertrophic but compromised extracellular matrix material. *Muscle Nerve* **28**: 464–71.

Malaiya R, McNee AE, Fry NR, Eve LC, Gough M, Shortland AP (2007) The morphology of the medial gastrocnemius in typically developing children and children with spastic hemiplegic cerebral palsy. *J Electromyogr Kinesiol* **17**: 657–63.

McNee AE, Shortland AP (2006) The gross structure of myostatic contracture is different in the medial and lateral gastrocnemius in children with spastic cerebral palsy. *Abstracts of the American Academy for Cerebral Palsy and Developmental Medicine Annual Conference, Boston.*

McNee AE, Gough M, Morrissey MC, Shortland AP (2009) Increases in muscle volume after plantarflexor strength training in children with spastic cerebral palsy. *Dev Med Child Neurol* **51**: 429-35.

Mohagheghi AA, Khan T, Meadows TH, Giannikas K, Baltzopoulos V, Maganaris CN (2008) In vivo gastrocnemius muscle fascicle length in children with and without diplegic cerebral palsy. *Dev Med Child Neurol* **50**: 44–50.

Ohata K, Tsuboyama T, Haruta T, Ichihashi N, Kato T, Nakamura T (2008) Relation between muscle thickness, spasticity, and activity limitations in children and adolescents with cerebral palsy. *Dev Med Child Neurol* **50**: 152–6.

Pillen S, Verrips A, van Alfen N, Arts IM, Sie LT, Zwarts MJ (2007) Quantitative skeletal muscle ultrasound: Diagnostic value in childhood neuromuscular disease. *Neuromusc Dis* **17**: 509–16.

Ponten E, Lindstrom M, Kadi F (2008) Higher amount of MyHC IIX in a wrist flexor in tetraplegic compared to hemiplegic cerebral palsy. *J Neurol Sci* **266**: 51–6.

Powell PL, Roy RR, Kanim P, Bello MA, Edgerton VR (1984) Predictability of skeletal muscle tension from architectural determinations in guinea pig hindlimbs. *J Applied Physiol* **57**: 1715–21.

Romanini L, Villani C, Meloni C, Calvisi V (1989) Histological and morphological aspects of muscle in infantile cerebral palsy. *Ital J Orthop Traumatol* **15**: 87–93.

145

Rose J, Haskell WL, Gamble JG, Hamilton RL, Brown DA, Rinsky L (1994) Muscle pathology and clinical measures of disability in children with cerebral palsy. *J Orthop Res* **12**: 758–68.

Rose J, McGill KC (2005) Neuromuscular activation and motor-unit firing characteristics in cerebral palsy. *Dev Med Child Neurol* **47**: 329–36.

Rose J, Mirmiran M, Butler EE, Lin CY, Barnes PD, Kermoian R, et al. (2007) Neonatal microstructural development of the internal capsule on diffusion tensor imaging correlates with severity of gait and motor deficits. *Dev Med Child Neurol* **49**: 745–50.

Shortland AP, Harris CA, Gough M, Robinson RO (2002) Architecture of the medial gastrocnemius in children with spastic diplegia. *Dev Med Child Neurol* **44**: 158–63.

Stackhouse SK, Binder-Macleod SA, Lee SC (2005) Voluntary muscle activation, contractile properties, and fatigability in children with and without cerebral palsy. *Muscle Nerve* **31**: 594–601.

Tabary JC, Tabary C, Tardieu C, Tardieu G, Goldspink G (1972) Physiological and structural changes in the cat's soleus muscle due to immobilization at different lengths by plaster casts. *J Physiol (Lond)* **224**: 231–44.

Tedroff K, Knutson LM, Soderberg GL (2006) Synergistic muscle activation during maximum voluntary contractions in children with and without spastic cerebral palsy. *Dev Med Child Neurol* **48**: 789–96.

Theroux MC, Oberman KG, Lahaye J, Boyce BA, Duhadaway D, Miller F, Akins RE (2005) Dysmorphic neuromuscular junctions associated with motor ability in cerebral palsy. *Muscle Nerve* **32**: 626–32.

Williams PE, Goldspink G (1978) Changes in sarcomere length and physiological properties in immobilized muscle. *J Anat* **127**: 459–68.

2.6
CLASSIFICATION OF CEREBRAL PALSY AND PATTERNS OF GAIT PATHOLOGY

Sylvia Õunpuu, Pam Thomason, Adrienne Harvey and H. Kerr Graham

A classification is the grouping together of a number of individuals that share common attributes related to a specific disease process. Classification is necessary to define pathology at all levels from etiology, presentation, severity of involvement and functional abilities. With carefully defined classifications, we can better communicate among professionals about patients, estimate prognosis, make the most appropriate treatment decisions and realize the best outcomes. While there has been general consensus on the definition of cerebral palsy (CP) (Stanley et al. 2000, Rosenbaum et al. 2006), a wide variety of classifications have been put forward. Clover and Sethumadhavan (2003) have provided a very comprehensive history of how classification of CP has changed since the original description by Little in 1843 (Rang 1966) (Table 2.6.1). The following chapter will provide a brief description of a few classification systems used to define CP with a focus on functional classifications, which are the final stage at which treatment related to functional outcomes decisions must take place.

Why classification?
Before discussing a few of the many classification schemes of cerebral palsy (CP) that have been put forward, it seems necessary to review the reasons for classification. Bax et al. (2005) provided four primary reasons for the need to classify CP. These include the following: (1) to provide a description that provides a level of detail that can delineate the nature of the problem and its severity, (2) to provide prediction of both current and future service needs for an individual, (3) to provide comparison so that groups of patients with CP at one institution can be compared with those at another, and (4) to evaluate change so that one individual with CP can be evaluated at various times and change can be documented. These authors felt that further classification was needed, because the definition of CP was so broad. Classification systems have traditionally focused on the distribution of affected limbs, for example diplegia or hemiplegia, with an additional modifier to identify the type of muscle tone, for example spastic. Because of the complexity of presentation of individuals with CP a more in-depth classification system is needed to improve understanding and ultimately management of this disorder.

147

Reference	Year	Classification	
Little	1862	Hemiplegic rigidity Paraplegic rigidity Generalized rigidity Disordered movements without rigidity	
Sachs and Petersen	1890	Paralysis of intrauterine origin	Diplegia Paraplegia Hemiplegia
		Birth palsies	Diplegia Paraplegia Hemiplegia Diataxia (ataxia)
		Acute acquired palsies	Hemiplegia Paraplegia Diplegia Choreo-athetoid
Freud	1893	Unilateral disorders - hemiplegia Bilateral disorders - diplegia	Right or left Generalized rigidity Paraplegic rigidity Bilateral hemiplegia Choreo-athetosis Others
Wyllie	1951	Congenital symmetric diplegia Congenital paraplegia Quadriplegia or bilateral hemiplegia Hemiplegia with additional qualifications referring to all categories	Choreo-athetoid cerebral palsy Mixed forms of cerebral palsy Ataxic cerebral palsy Atonic diplegia
Minear	1956	A. Physiological	Spasticity, athetosis, rigidity, ataxia, tremor, atonia, mixed unclassified
		B. Topographical	Monoplegia, diplegia, paraplegia, hemiplegia, triplegia, quadriplegia
		C. Aetiological	Prenatal, natal anoxia, postnatal, cause described
		D. Trauma	Cause described
		E. Supplemental	Psychological evaluation Physical status, convulsive seizures, posture and locomotive behavior pattern, eye-hand behavior pattern, visual status, auditory status, speech disturbances
		F. Neuroanatomical	
		G. Functional capacity	Class I-IV
		H. Therapeutic	Class I-IV

Reference	Year	*Neurology*	*Extent*	*Severity*
Ingram	1955	Hemiplegia	Right or left	Mild Moderate Severe
		Double hemiplegia		Mild Moderate Severe

TABLE 2.6.1 (continued)
Comprehensive history of classification schemes for cerebral palsy since 1843

Reference	Year	Classification		
		Diplegia		
		Hypotonic	Paraplegia	Mild
		Dystonic	Triplegia	Moderate
		Rigid or spastic	Tetraplegia	Severe
		Ataxia		
		Cerebellar	Unitaleral	Mild
		Vestibular	Bilateral	Moderate
				Severe
		Ataxia diplegia		
		Hypotonic	Paraplegia	Mild
		Spastic	Triplegia	Moderate
			Tetraplegia	Severe
		Dyskinesia		
		Dystonic	Monoplegia	Mild
		Choreoid	Hemiplegia	Moderate
		Athetoid	Triplegia	Severe
		Tension	Tetraplegia	
		Tremor		
		Other		
Little Club	1959	Spastic cerebral palsy	Hemiplegia	
			Diplegia	
			Double hemiplegia	
		Dystonic cerebral palsy		
		Choreo-athetoid cerebral palsy		
		Mixed forms of cerebral palsy		
		Ataxic cerebral palsy		
		Atonic diplegia		

(From Clover and Sethumadhavan 2003, Table 1, p.287, by permission.)

Classifications of cerebral palsy

Minear (1956) has provided the most comprehensive classification system for CP which includes the following categories: (1) physiological (motor), (2) topographical (distribution of involvement), (3) etiological, (4) supplemental (patient capabilities from intellectual to visual), (5) neuroanatomical (brain lesion), (6) functional capacity (severity) and (7) therapeutic (level of treatment). The physiological classification refers to the motor aspects of impairment, which are categorized as follows: spastic, athetotic, rigid, ataxic, tremor, mixed and unclassified. The motor presentation of CP is defined in more detail in Chapters 2.3 and 2.4. The topographical classification refers to the anatomical location of involvement and is categorized as follows: monoplegia (one lower limb is principally involved); diplegia (both lower limbs are involved with minimal involvement of upper limbs); hemiplegia (ipsilateral involvement with the upper extremity more involved than the lower); triplegia (ipsilateral hemiplegia with contralateral monoplegia); quadriplegia (all four limbs involved – lower > upper); and double hemiplegia (all four limbs involved – upper > lower). The etiological classification represents several categories of cause: hereditary, acquired in utero, natal and postnatal. The etiology of CP was defined in more detail in Chapter 2.1. The supplemental categories include the other systems that can be involved in CP including: psychological, visual, auditory, posture, seizures and physical status. The neuroanatomical classification is dependent on comprehensive imaging capabilities, which will be discussed in Chapter 3.2. Even more than 50 years after Minear proposed the classification, the correlation of lesion presentation obtained by imaging and patient function is still not well understood. Finally Minear finishes with function and therapeutic classifications. The functional classifications defined the level of severity. Four levels were proposed: Class 1: patients with no practical limitation of activity; Class 2: patients with slight to moderate limitation of activity; Class 3: patients with great limitation of activity; and Class 4: patients who are unable to carry on any useful physical activity. These four levels, which were proposed in 1956, are similar to the newer five-level GMFCS Classification, which will be discussed later in this chapter. Minear further defined CP into therapeutic classifications: Class A: requiring no treatment; Class B: requiring minimal bracing and therapy; Class C: requiring bracing and treatment from a CP team; and Class D: requiring long-term institutionalization and treatment. In general, his classification has stood the test of time.

A simpler standardized classification scheme for CP was proposed more recently by Bax et al. (2005). This group proposed four major dimensions of classification: (1) motor abnormalities, (2) associated impairments, (3) anatomical and radiological findings, and (4) causation and timing (Table 2.6.2). The primary difference between the proposed classification and others is the proposal to eliminate the terms diplegia and hemiplegia due

TABLE 2.6.2
List of the major components of the classification of cerebral palsy as described by Bax et al. (2005)

Motor abnormalities
Nature and typology of the motor disorder: the observed tonal abnormalities assessed on examination (e.g. hypertonia or hypotonia) as well as the diagnosed movement disorders present, such as spasticity, ataxia, dystonia, or athetosis
Functional motor abilities: the extent to which the individual is limited in his or her motor function in all body areas, including oromotor and speech function

Associated impairments
The presence or absence of associate non-motor neurodevelopmental or sensory problem, such as seizures, hearing of vision impairments or attentional, behavioral, communicative and/or cognitive deficits, and the extent to which impairments interact in individuals with CP

Anatomic and radiological findings
Anatomic distribution: the parts of the body (such as limb, trunk or bulbar region) affected by motor impairments or limitations
Radiological findings: the neuroanatomic findings of computed tomography or magnetic resonance imaging, such as ventricular enlargement, white matter loss, or brain anomaly

Causation and timing
Whether there is a clearly identified cause, as is usually the case with postnatal CP (e.g. meningitis or head injury) or when brain malformations are present, and the presumed time frame during which the injury occurred, if known.

From Bax et al. 2005; reproduced by permission of Mac Keith Press.

to the substantial inconsistency in definition and imprecise use of these terms in both clinical practice and research. The authors recommend that the terms *unilateral* and *bilateral* be used in conjunction with a description of the motor disorder and functional motor classification in both the upper and lower extremities.

Classification of function using functional assessment scales

Since Minear's proposed classification in 1956 there have been a variety of efforts to improve the classification of function for persons with CP. The most commonly used classification of gross motor function in children with CP is the Gross Motor Function Classification System (GMFCS).

THE GROSS MOTOR FUNCTION MEASURE (GMFM)

Classification and measurement of gross motor function in CP are essential steps because they guide the family and the multidisciplinary management team to the natural history, and long-term prognosis of the condition. When planning treatment of gait problems, classification of gross motor function also guides decision-making towards appropriate management. The GMFM is the criterion for the measurement of gross motor function in children with CP, and has been shown to be valid, reliable and responsive to change (Russell and Rosenbaum 1989, Nordmark et al. 1997, 2000, Bjornson et al. 1998a, b, Russell et al. 2000, Russell and Leung 2003, Russell and Gorter 2005).

There are two versions of the GMFM. The original version consisted of 88 items, which were grouped into five dimensions of gross-motor function: lying and rolling, sitting, crawling and kneeling, standing and walking, and running and jumping (Russell and Rosenbaum 1989). A more recent version, which consists of 66 items, is computer scored, and features item maps. Because it has 22 fewer items, it is faster to administer. Since many of the 22 items that were removed from the GMFM-88 came from the lower end of the mobility scale, however, it is potentially limited for children who are very young or very severely involved (Russell and Leung 2003). In either case, measurement of GMFM requires specific training, an experienced physical therapist, and will take between 45 and 60 minutes on average to perform. Consequently, it should be considered to be an essential research tool: for example, in clinical outcome trials.

THE GROSS MOTOR FUNCTIONAL CLASSIFICATION SYSTEM (GMFCS)

The five gross motor curves (Fig. 2.6.1) which translate into the Gross Motor Functional Classification System (GMFCS) were introduced by Palisano and Rosenbaum (1997). This has now evolved into the GMFCS (Rosenbaum et al. 2002).

The gross motor curves are a useful matrix for identification of where a child is at a specific point in time in relation to their age and gross motor function. This is very useful in the prediction of future change. The vertical lines on the gross motor curves indicate the point at which 90% of final gross motor function is likely to be achieved and is much younger than often considered by clinicians. There are different descriptors for five different age bands and in general, the GMFCS becomes more reliable in older age groups at least up to the 6–12 age band (Nordmark et al. 1997). The child who is between 2 and 4 years old may

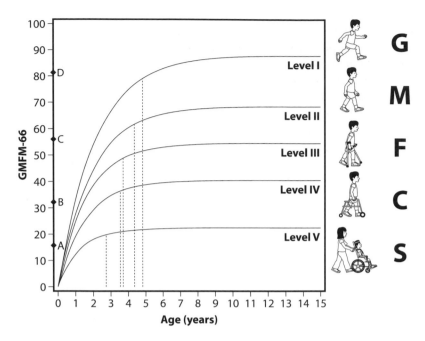

Fig. 2.6.1 Gross motor curves. Curves provide information about the predicted average development in groups defined by the Gross Motor Function Classification System levels. (Reproduced from Rosenbaum et al. 2002, Fig. 3, p 1361, by permission.)

be on the up swing of their gross motor curve, the child who is 6–12 years old may be on a stable plateau of gross motor function, and the youth between 12 and 18 years may be on a descending curve of gross motor function. These issues are highly relevant to management and clinical research. For example a child with spastic diplegia aged 2 years, GMFCS level II, who receives injections of botulinum toxin A (BoNT-A) for spastic equinus may make rapid gains in gross motor function and quickly move from walking only with assistance to walking independently. It is tempting for both the clinician and the parent to attribute the rapid gain in gross motor function solely to the effects of the injections of BoNT-A. Reference to the appropriate gross motor curve, however, indicates that such a child is following a curve with a rapid upward trajectory with or without intervention. For this reason, the reporting of clinical trials involving physiotherapy, the use of orthoses and injections of BoNT-A, in younger children with CP, must include an appropriate control group.

THE FUNCTIONAL MOBILITY SCALE (FMS) AND FUNCTIONAL ASSESSMENT QUESTIONNAIRE (FAQ)
Several groups have developed simple categorical scales for the assessment of functional ability and functional mobility in children with CP to be used as a longitudinal measure. These scales were designed to be responsive to change and can be used to document the

serial attainment of mobility scales and functional abilities, the deterioration or improvement in these skills after intervention, or other changes consequent on growth and development.

The FMS is a 6-level ordinal scale that rates the mobility of children with CP over three distances according to their need for assistive devices (Graham et al. 2004). The three distances of 5, 50 and 500 meters represent mobility in the home, school and wider community settings respectively. The scale is clinician administered through parent or child report and should reflect performance rather than capability, i.e. what the child actually does do rather than what they can do. For each of the three distances a rating of 1–6 is assigned. Figure 2.6.2 displays the FMS where 6 represents children who walk independently on all surfaces, 5 those who walk on level surfaces only, 4 those who use single point sticks, 3 the use of crutches, 2 the use of a walker and 1 represents wheelchair mobility. 'C' represents crawling and 'N' is for 'does not apply' and is assigned when children do not go anywhere for long distances using any of those mobility devices. The FMS is reliable and valid and has been shown to detect both deterioration and improvement in mobility that occurs in the rehabilitation period following single event multilevel surgery (Graham et al. 2004, Harvey et al. 2007).

The walking scale of the Gillette FAQ (Novacheck et al. 2000) is a 10-level parent-report walking scale encompassing a range of walking abilities from non-ambulatory to ambulatory in a variety of community settings and terrains (Fig. 2.6.3). It is a good measure of parental perspective and covers a wide variety of activities of daily living. Both the FMS and FAQ will be described in more detail in terms of case examples and treatment outcomes in Chapter 6.1.

Classification of function using motion measurement techniques

Optimum physical management of the child with CP requires comprehensive measurement of both function and gait. Three dimensional motion analysis techniques have facilitated the classification of gait function at both the joint level and in relation to patterns of movement across multiple joints. When proposed treatments impact the joint level, gait analysis provides the optimal information with which to make treatment decisions (such as orthopaedic surgery or bracing) and to evaluate treatment outcomes. Therefore any classification system being used to define treatment for the ambulatory person with CP, must consider measuring gait function at the individual joint level. Several strategies have been proposed for the classification of gait function based on joint kinematics in hemiplegia (Winters et al. 1987, Rodda and Graham 2001) and diplegia (Sutherland and Davids 1993, Rodda and Graham 2001, Rodda et al. 2004). Prior to this, gait patterns were described based on observational analysis alone (Rang 1990). Gait patterns have also been described using statistical techniques such as cluster analyses to describe gait patterns in CP (Wong et al. 1983, O'Malley et al. 1997, O'Byrne et al. 1998). However, the lack of direct correlation of these analyses to joint level understanding of function has limited their use as clinical tools.

Classification of unilateral involvement (hemiplegia)

The first attempt at classification of gait patterns with instrumented gait analysis in persons with hemiplegia was by Winters et al. (1987), who described a classification system using

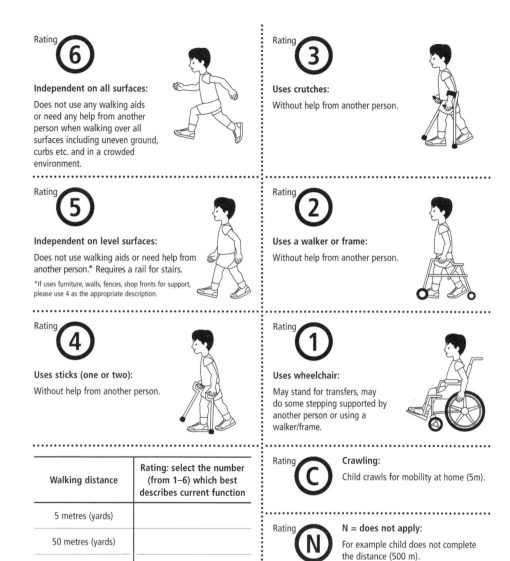

Rating **6**

Independent on all surfaces:

Does not use any walking aids or need any help from another person when walking over all surfaces including uneven ground, curbs etc. and in a crowded environment.

Rating **3**

Uses crutches:

Without help from another person.

Rating **5**

Independent on level surfaces:

Does not use walking aids or need help from another person.* Requires a rail for stairs.

*If uses furniture, walls, fences, shop fronts for support, please use 4 as the appropriate description.

Rating **2**

Uses a walker or frame:

Without help from another person.

Rating **4**

Uses sticks (one or two):

Without help from another person.

Rating **1**

Uses wheelchair:

May stand for transfers, may do some stepping supported by another person or using a walker/frame.

Walking distance	Rating: select the number (from 1–6) which best describes current function
5 metres (yards)	
50 metres (yards)	
500 metres (yards)	

Rating **C** **Crawling:**
Child crawls for mobility at home (5m).

Rating **N** **N = does not apply:**
For example child does not complete the distance (500 m).

Fig. 2.6.2 Functional Mobility Scale (FMS). The purpose of the FMS is to measure a child's current performance. Visual cues are provided along with descriptions to assist in defining current level of performance. (Reproduced from Harvey 2008, Fig. 4.1, p 112, by permission.)

Gillette Functional Assessment Questionnaire

Name:		UR:		Date:	

Please choose the answer below that best describes your child's usual or typical walking abilities Circle one number which best describes the highest level of walking ability.

1	Cannot take any steps at all
2	Can do some stepping on his/her own with the help of another person. Does not take full weight on feet; Does not walk on routine basis.
3	Walks for exercise in therapy and/or less than typical household distances.
4	Walks for household distances, but makes slow progress. Does not use walking at home as preferred mobility. (primarily walks in therapy or as exercise).
5	Walks for household distances routinely at home and/or school. Indoor walking only.
6	Walks more than 15-50 ft. outside the home but usually uses a wheelchair or stroller for community distances or in congested areas.
7	Walks outside for community distances, but only on level surfaces (cannot perform curbs, uneven terrain, or stairs without assistance of another person).
8	Walks outside the home for community distances, is able to get around on curbs and uneven terrain in addition to level surfaces, but usually requires minimal assistance or supervision for safety.
9	Walks outside the home for community distances, easily gets around on level ground, curbs, and uneven terrain, but has difficulty or requires minimal assistance or supervision with running, climbing and/or stairs.
10	Walks, runs, and climbs on level and uneven terrain and does stairs without difficulty or assistance.

Please tick all the things that your child is able to do, in addition to walking:

	Walk carrying an object		Jumps off a single step[3]
	Walk carrying a fragile object or glass of liquid		Hop on right foot[4]
	Walk up and down stairs using the railing		Hop on left foot[4]
	Walk up and down stairs without needing the railing		Step over an object, right foot first[4]
	Steps up and down curb independently		Step over an object, left foot first[4]
	Runs		Kick a ball with right foot[4]
	Runs well including around a corner with good control		Kick a ball with left foot[4]
	Can take steps backwards		Ride 2 wheel bike[5]
	Can manoeuvre in tight areas		Ride 3 wheel bike
	Get on and off a bus by him/herself[1]		Ice skate or roller skate[6]
	Skip rope[2]		Ride an escalator, can step on/off without help

[1] Including first step without crawling. Use of railing permitted.
[2] Consistently with successive jumps. Twirling rope by self or by other people
[3] Without falling upon landing
[4] Without holding on, without falling upon landing
[5] Without training wheels
[6] Without holding on to objects or another person

Fig. 2.6.3 Gillette Functional Assessment Questionnaire: Functional Walking Scales. The parent is expected to check one of the ten options that best reflects their child's typical ability to walk, and check boxes in list for other physical activities the child can do. (Reproduced by permission of the questionnaire's author, Dr Tom Novacheck.)

155

sagittal-plane kinematics for the ankle, knee, hip and pelvis. These patterns from type 1 through type 4 reflected increasing levels of involvement. Although the patterns present some overlap, they do provide a guide for surgical management. Type 1 represents a patient with an excessive equinus swing related to triceps surae over activity and/or anterior tibialis weakness (Fig. 2.6.4a). Since a true contracture is not present, the only management required is an orthosis to control the drop foot during swing phase. Type 2 represents an excessive equinus in swing as well as restricted ankle dorsiflexion in stance secondary to contracture of the plantarflexors. However, there is relative sparing of the knee and hip (Fig. 2.6.4b). Management of the patient with type 2 hemiplegia may require a procedure to obtain increased ankle dorsiflexion during stance, which might include a lengthening of the triceps surae and/or tibialis posterior. Type 3 represents a patient with the characteristics of types 1 and 2 as well as spasticity/contracture of the biarticular muscles crossing the knee. It usually features increased knee flexion at initial contact and stance as well as reduced and delayed peak knee flexion in swing (Fig. 2.6.4c). Appropriate management of a patient

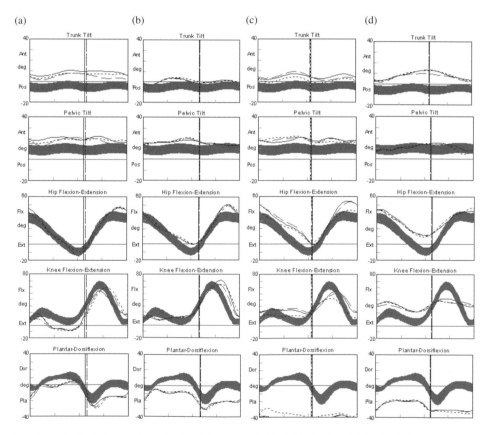

Fig. 2.6.4 Sagittal plane patterns for hemiplegia type 1 (a), 2 (b), 3 (c) and 4 (d) for the trunk, pelvis, hip, knee and ankle. Multiple gait cycles from an individual child for each type are plotted in relation to typical motion (grey band).

with type 3 hemiplegia requires similar management of the ankle (plantarflexors) as for type II as well as appropriate treatment of the muscle problems at the knee (hamstrings and rectus). Finally, type 4 represents a patient with the characteristics of types 1–3 as well as hip involvement with limited hip extension in terminal stance and increasing anterior pelvic tilt in stance (Fig. 2.6.4d). Management of the type 4 patient will require appropriate treatment of muscles crossing all three joints (ankle, knee and hip) (Stout et al. 2004).

A limitation of the Winters classification system is that no mention of common transverse-plane kinematic abnormalities was included and there was no inclusion of knee hyperextension which is a common pattern in hemiplegia. Rodda and Graham (2001) proposed a more comprehensive classification system. This included an additional sagittal-plane pattern of knee hyperextension in combination with excessive equinus in stance and swing, as well as transverse plane abnormalities of internal hip rotation (both of which are likely to occur in the more involved person with CP). Management of the type 4 pattern in the Rodda classification might include femoral derotation osteotomy and possible adductor lengthenings at the hip; hamstring lengthenings and rectus femoris transfer at the knee; and appropriate lengthening of the posterior calf to improve ankle motion. The Rodda classification is presented diagrammatically in Figure 2.6.5.

Classification of bilateral involvement (diplegia)

The classification systems for patients with diplegia are more complex, as bilateral involvement is present; and, in many cases, involvement is not symmetrical with different patterns on one side in comparison to the other. Rodda et al. (2004) recognized the issues related to asymmetry must be addressed in a classification system and included five sagittal-plane classifications, the final of which (type 5) recognizes the common presentation of asymmetrical involvement. A diagrammatic representation of this classification is presented in Figure 2.6.6. Group 1 represents patients with true equinus, Group 2 represents patients with jump gait with real equinus as well as knee and hip flexion, Group 3 represents apparent equinus with knee and hip flexion, Group 4 represents crouch with excessive ankle dorsiflexion and knee and hip flexion; and Group 5 represents asymmetric gait with a combination of issues, for example apparent equinus and jump gait. This classification system helps to define gait pathology, potential causes and ultimately a treatment strategy.

Classification by knee kinematic patterns

There are so many possible combinations of joint function in a patient with CP that some authors have chosen to study function at the joint level instead of across multiple joints. In a classic paper, Sutherland and Davids (1993) classified knee function in children with CP into four sagittal-plane patterns. Although they recognized the relationship between the function of one joint and its impact on adjacent joints, they felt that it was possible to define certain primary disorders at a single joint. The four primary patterns at the knee were titled jump knee, crouch knee, stiff knee and recurvatum knee. Each pattern was described by the sagittal-plane motion as defined by three-dimensional motion analysis (Fig. 2.6.7) as well as associated physical examination parameters and muscle activity. The identification of these patterns on an individual basis can lead to a more specific treatment plan as each

157

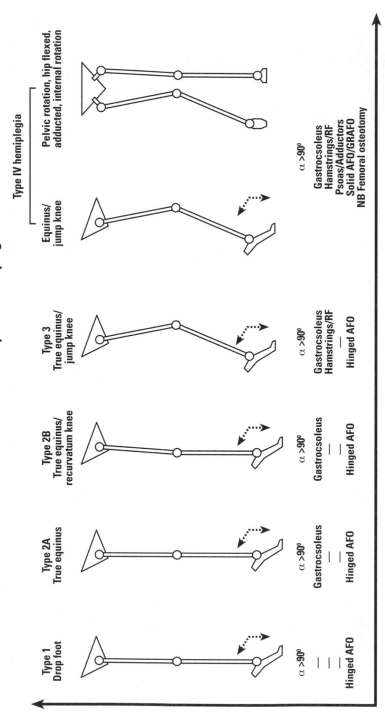

Fig. 2.6.5 Gait patterns: spastic hemiplegia. A visual representation of the gait patterns during mid-stance phase are illustrated for types 1 through 4. Suggested treatment options for the specific type are listed below. Additional patterns are identified which include subdividing type 2 into A typical and B recurvatum knee. A description of the transverse plane rotations of the pelvis and hip is acknowledged in type 4. AFO, ankle–foot orthosis; RF, rectus femoris; GRAFO, ground reaction ankle–foot orthosis. (Reproduced from Rodda and Graham 2001, Fig. 1, p 100, by permission.)

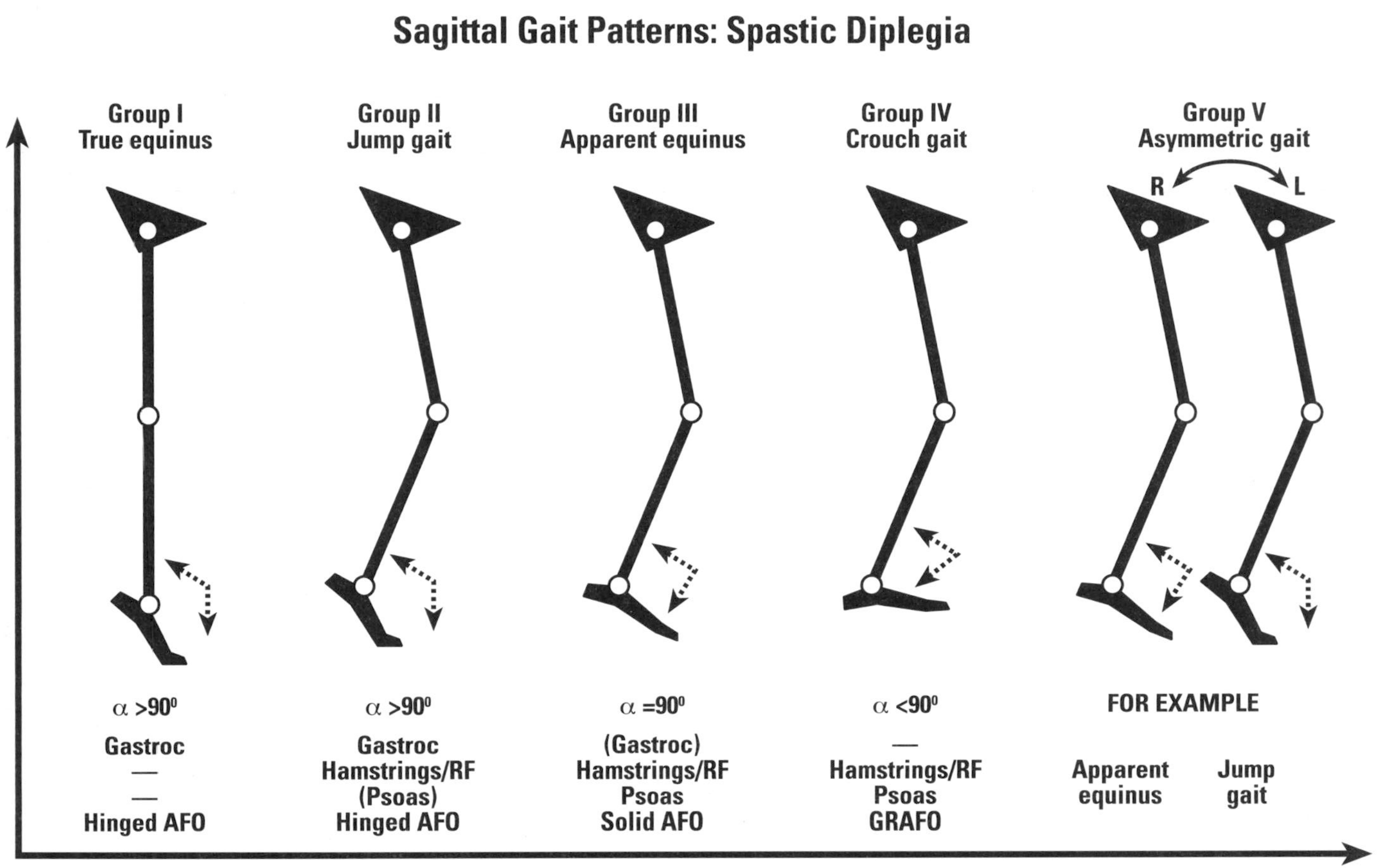

Sagittal Gait Patterns: Spastic Diplegia

Group I True equinus	Group II Jump gait	Group III Apparent equinus	Group IV Crouch gait	Group V Asymmetric gait
$\alpha > 90^0$	$\alpha > 90^0$	$\alpha = 90^0$	$\alpha < 90^0$	FOR EXAMPLE
Gastroc	Gastroc	(Gastroc)	—	Apparent equinus / Jump gait
—	Hamstrings/RF	Hamstrings/RF	Hamstrings/RF	
—	(Psoas)	Psoas	Psoas	
Hinged AFO	Hinged AFO	Solid AFO	GRAFO	

Fig. 2.6.6 Gait patterns: spastic diplegia. A visual representation of the gait patterns during mid-stance phase is illustrated for types I through V. The dominant problematic muscle groups and related treatment options are listed below each pattern. Asymmetrical gait patterns are also addressed as indicated in type V which is a combination of types I and IV. (Reproduced by permission and copyright (©) of the British Editorial Society of Bone and Joint Surgery; from Rodda et al. 2004, Sagittal gait patterns in spastic diplegia. *J Bone Joint Surg Br* **86**: 251–8.) AFO, ankle–foot orthosis; RF, rectus femoris; GRAFO, ground reaction force ankle–foot orthosis.

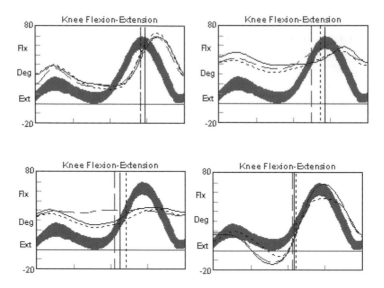

Fig. 2.6.7 Sagittal-plane knee patterns. The sagittal-plane knee kinematic patterns are plotted for the (a) jump, (b) crouch, (c) stiff and (d) recurvatum knees. These patterns are defined by stance or stance and swing phase characteristics. Multiple gait cycles from an individual patient for each type are plotted in relation to the typical motion (grey band).

pattern is consistent with a unique set of clinical and muscle function findings, as defined by dynamic electromyography, which can aid in guiding treatment.

Lin et al. (2000) described similar classifications for the knee with the inclusion of joint kinetic data. However, they described the 'stiff' knee classification as a 'mild' knee. Rodda and Graham (2001) took classification to the next step and described four sagittal-plane patterns which included the pelvis, hip, knee and ankle for patients with cerebral palsy.

Classification by joint kinetic patterns
Classification of gait in CP is now starting to go beyond kinematic patterns to focus on a combination of specific kinematic and kinetic patterns (Õunpuu 2002, Adolfsen et al. 2007). Joint kinetic patterns suggest a specific outcome of a combination of issues related to joint contracture, muscle strength, control and weakness. With these classifications, it is not so important whether the patient is defined as having hemiplegia or diplegia, since the classifications themselves provide one of the most important components for making treatment decisions that impact at joint level. This is because they represent the final outcome of all systems, which with the supporting information (passive range of motion, muscle strength and tone) allow treatment decisions to be made on the basis of function. The position of the trunk has substantial impact on lower extremity joint kinetics, however, and must always be taken into account when interpreting joint kinetic data. Joint kinetic patterns have been identified and discussed in the literature and in the previous edition of this book (Õunpuu 2004). A few sagittal-plane kinematic and kinetic patterns are described below to

further clarify their importance in defining function as it relates to level gait. It should be stressed that these represent an example of just a few of many possible combinations of joint kinematic and kinetic patterns, which in the future may lead to a more comprehensive and useful method of classifying gait problems in CP. Other joint kinetic patterns also have been identified and characterized. These include the hip-extensor moment pattern and the hip-adductor moment pattern (abductor avoidance) (Õunpuu 2004). Patterns such as these assist in the joint level classification of gait, which is ultimately needed for defining treatment and evaluating the outcomes of those treatments.

DOUBLE BUMP ANKLE MOMENT PATTERN
This ankle moment pattern is characterized by the shape of the internal ankle plantarflexor moment which is 'double bump' (Fig. 2.6.8). This is the one kinetic pattern that has been connected to a particular treatment protocol (Rose et al. 1993). The double bump ankle moment pattern is found in persons who have spasticity in their plantarflexors and who have a toe- or foot-flat initial contact during gait (for example, a child with 'jump gait'). Essentially, it represents a double firing of the triceps surae, usually as a result of gastrocnemius contracture and/or spasticity. The characteristics of the typically associated ankle joint kinematics and kinetics are described below.

Joint kinematic
• Neutral or excessive plantarflexion at initial contact
• Rapid dorsiflexion during loading response which results in a quick stretch of the spastic ankle plantarflexors that respond by contracting and producing premature plantarflexion
• Repeat dorsiflexion followed by plantarflexion in last half of stance (using a similar mechanism as above)
• Less than typical dorsiflexion from mid-stance through toe off.

Joint moment
• Plantarflexor moment 100% stance
• Absence of a dorsiflexor moment in loading response with development of a premature plantarflexor moment
• Followed by rapid decrease, increase and decrease in plantarflexor moment (double bump)
• Associated with dominant and continuous ankle plantarflexor contraction throughout stance.

Joint power
• Excessive power absorption in early stance (eccentric contraction of ankle plantar-flexors)
• Premature power generation in mid-stance (concentric contraction of ankle plantar-flexors)
• Inappropriate power generation in mid-stance drives body up, not forward

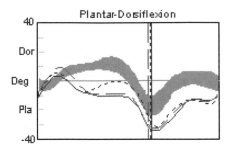

Plantar-Dorsiflexion

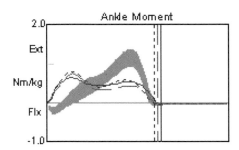

Ankle Moment

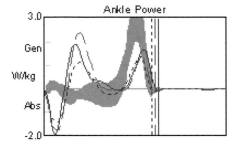

Ankle Power

Fig. 2.6.8 Double bump ankle pattern. The ankle kinematic, moment and power for the double bump ankle moment pattern is plotted for the sagittal plane. Multiple gait cycles from an individual patient are plotted in relation to the typical motion (grey band). The net internal ankle moment is plantarflexor throughout the stance phase indicating a toe initial contact and toe or forefoot contact through out stance. Increased ankle power absorption is noted in loading response and increased power generation is noted in mid-stance indicating an inefficient gait pattern.

- Second power absorption and generation in second half of stance
- Second power generation peak may be within or less than typical.

KNEE-EXTENSOR MOMENT PATTERN

The knee-extensor moment pattern is defined by the internal knee moment which is extensor through out the majority of stance phase (Fig. 2.6.9). For example in a child with crouch gait, inadequate hip-extensor and ankle-plantarflexor moments lead to excessive knee flexion or crouch and/or knee-flexion contractures, which in turn demand a compensatory knee-extensor moment pattern (Õunpuu 2002) (see Chapter 5.11). The knee-extensor moment pattern is characterized by continuous coactivity of the quadriceps and hamstrings. However, there is a net knee-extensor dominant moment, required to prevent collapse. The characteristics of the typically associated knee-joint kinematics and kinetics are described below.

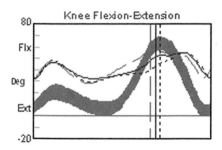

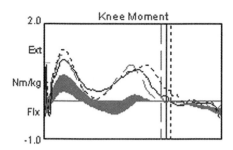

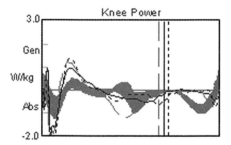

Fig. 2.6.9 Knee-extensor moment pattern. The knee kinematic, moment and power for the knee-extensor moment pattern are plotted for the sagittal plane. Multiple gait cycles from an individual patient are plotted in relation to the typical motion (grey band). The knee moment is extensor throughout the stance phase which is consistent with a crouch gait pattern and requires continuous quadriceps activity during stance to prevent collapse.

Joint kinematic
- Greater than normal knee flexion at initial contact
- Continued excessive knee flexion during 100% stance
- Minimal knee sagittal-plane range of motion in stance.

Joint moment
- Rapid development of extensor moment during loading response
- Knee-extensor moment 100% stance phase
- Associated with dominant and continuous quadriceps contraction throughout stance.

Joint power
- Typically minimal and varies depending on knee range of motion in stance.

163

KNEE-FLEXOR MOMENT PATTERN

The knee-flexor moment pattern is defined by an internal knee moment that is primarily flexor through out the stance phase (Fig. 2.6.10). This pattern is found in individuals with full knee extension or knee hyperextension on passive range of motion, plantarflexor spasticity contributing to an excessive plantarflexion/knee-extension couple and more often than not a forward trunk lean. The characteristics of the typically associated knee joint kinematics and kinetics are described below.

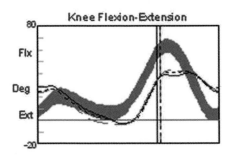

Fig. 2.6.10 Flexor moment pattern. The knee kinematic, moment and power for the knee-flexor moment pattern are plotted for the sagittal plane. Multiple gait cycles from an individual patient are plotted in relation to the typical motion (grey band). The knee moment pattern is primarily flexor throughout the stance phase, which is consistent with knee hyperextension or extension with a forward trunk position.

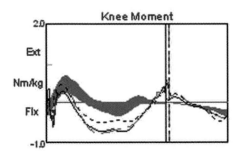

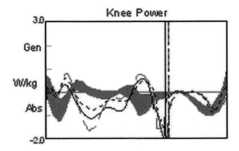

Joint kinematic
*   Greater than typical knee flexion to full knee extension at initial contact
*   Rapid knee extension after initial contact
*   Usually prolonged knee extension or hyperextension in mid to terminal stance.

164

Joint moment
- Rapid development of a knee-flexor moment during loading response
- Excessive knee-flexor moment during the majority of stance
- Associated with dominant and continuous knee-flexor activity; however, joint support may be provided by muscular contracture or ligamentous restrictions to further motion
- Variable knee moment in pre-swing.

Joint power
- Increased power absorption during period of rapid knee extension in stance
- Associated eccentric contraction of the knee flexors and/or stretching of the soft-tissue structures on the posterior aspect of the knee.

Summary

The classification of cerebral palsy is necessary for a variety of reasons. In the clinical setting, classification is needed to assist in optimal communication among medical professionals and between medical professionals and patients/families. It is needed to determine prognosis and define treatment options. In the research setting, classification is required to define homogeneous patient groups, to communicate effectively research results and to more clearly define and connect appropriate treatments with the 'right' patient. Standard and reproducible methods are needed in order for any classification system to be applicable in both the clinical and research environments. Moving forward, it will be important to establish consistency among medical professionals in both the definitions and classification systems used when treating persons with CP. In Chapter 6.1 the classification tools described above will be described in terms of their input for treatment decision-making and evaluation of persons with CP.

REFERENCES

Adolfsen SE, Õunpuu S, Bell KJ, DeLuca PA (2007) Kinematic and kinetic outcomes after identical multilevel soft tissue surgery in children with cerebral palsy. *J Pediatr Orthop* **27**: 658–67.

Bax M, Goldstein M, Rosenbaum P, Leviton A, Paneth N (2005) Proposed defintion and classification of cerebral palsy. *Dev Med Child Neurol* **47**: 571–6.

Bjornson KF, Graubert CS, Buford VL, McLaughlin J (1998a) Validity of the gross motor function measure. *Pediatr Phys Ther* **10**: 43–7.

Bjornson KF, Graubert CS, McLaughlin J, Kerfeld CI, Clark EM (1998b) Test retest reliability of the gross motor function measure in children with cerebral palsy. *Phys Occup Ther Pediatr* **18**: 51–61.

Clover AF, Sethumadhavan T (2003) The term diplegia should be abandoned. *Arch Dis Child* **88**: 286–90.

Graham HK, Harvey A, Rodda J, Nattrass GR, Pirpiris M (2004) The functional mobility scale (FMS). *J Pediatr Orthopaed* **24**: 514–20.

Harvey A, Graham HK, Morris ME, Baker RJ, Wolfe R (2007) The functional mobility scale: ability to detect change following single event multilevel surgery. *Dev Med Child Neurol* **49**: 603–7.

Harvey A (2008) *The Functional Mobility Scale for Children with Cerebral Palsy*. Gait CCRE Thesis Series, vol. 6. Melbourne, Austtralia: University of Melbourne. p 112.

Lin CJ, Guo LY, Su FC, Chou YL, Cherng RJ (2000) Common abnormal kinetic patterns of the knee in grait in spastic diplegia cerebral palsy. *Gait Posture* **11**: 224–32.

Minear WL (1956) A classification of cerebral palsy. *Pediatrics* **18**: 841–52.

Nordmark E, Hagglund G, Jarnlo GB (1997) Reliability of the gross motor function measure in cerebral palsy. *Scand J Rehabil Med* **29**: 25–8.

Nordmark E, Jarnlo GB, Hagglund G (2000) Comparison of the gross motor function measure and paediatric evaluation of disability inventory in assessing motor function in children undergoing selective dorsal rhizotomy. *Dev Med Child Neurol* **42**: 245–52.

Novacheck TF, Stout JL, Tervo R (2000) Reliability and validity of the functional assessment questionnaire as an outcome measure in children with cerebral palsy. *J Pediatr Orthop* **20**: 75–81.

O'Byrne JM, Jenkinson A, O'Brien TM (1998) Quantitative analysis and classification of gait patterns in cerebral palsy using a three-dimensional motion analyzer. *J Child Neurol* **13**: 101–8.

O'Malley MJ, Abel MF, Damiano DL, Vaughan CL (1997) Fuzzy clustering of children with cerbral palsy based on temporal-distance gait paramters. *IEEE Trans Rehabil Eng* **5**: 300–9.

Õunpuu S (2002) Gait analysis in orthopaedics. In: Fitzgerald R, Kaufer H, Malkani A, editors. *Orthopaedics*. St Louis: Mosby. p 86–107.

Õunpuu S (2004) Patterns of gait pathology. In: Gage JR, editor. *The Treatment of Gait Problems in Cerebral Palsy*. London: Mac Keith Press. p 231–5.

Palisano R, Rosenbaum P (1997) Development and reliability of a system to classify gross motor function in children with cerebral palsy. *Dev Med Child Neurol* **39**: 214–23.

Rang M (1966) *Anthology of Orthopaedics*. Edinburgh: E. & S. Livingstone. p 48–52.

Rang M (1990) Cerebral palsy. In: Morrissy R, editor. *Lovell and Winter's Pediatric Orthopedics*, vol. 1. Philadelphia, PA: J.B. Lippincott. p 465–506.

Rodda J, Graham HK (2001) Classification of gait patterns in spastic hemiplegia and spastic diplegia: a basis for a management algorithm. *Eur J Neurol* **8**: 98–108.

Rodda JM, Graham HK, Carson L, Galea MP, Wolfe R (2004) Sagittal gait patterns in spastic diplegia. *J Bone Joint Surg Br* **86**: 251–8.

Rose S, DeLuca P, Davis R, Õunpuu S, Gage J (1993) Kinematic and kinetic evaluation of the ankle after lengthening of the gastrocnemius fascia in children with cerebral palsy. *J Pediatr Orthop* **13**: 727–32.

Rosenbaum PL, Walter SD, Hanna SE, Palisano RJ, Russell DJ, Raina PS, Wood E, Bartlett DJ, Galuppi BE (2002) Prognosis for gross motor function in cerebral palsy: creation of motor development curves. *J Am Med Assoc* **288**: 1357–63.

Rosenbaum P, Paneth N, Leviton A, Goldstein M, Bax M, Damiano D, Dan B, Jacobsson B (2006) A report: the definition and classification of cerebral palsy. *Dev Med Child Neurol Suppl* **109**: 8–14.

Russell DJ, Rosenbaum PL (1989) The gross motor function measure: a means to evaluate the effects of physical therapy. *Dev Med Child Neurol* **31**: 341–52.

Russell DJ, Leung KM (2003) Accessibility and perceived clinical utility of the GMFM-66: evaluating therapists' judgements of a computer-based scoring program. *Phys Occup Ther Pediatr* **23**: 45–58.

Russell DJ, Gorter JW (2005) Assessing functional differences in gross motor skills in children with cerebral palsy who use an ambulatory aid or orthoses: can the GMFM-88 help? *Dev Med Child Neurol* **47**: 462–7.

Russell DJ, Avery LM, Rosenbaum PL, Raina PS, Walter SD, Palisano RJ (2000) Improved scaling of the gross motor function measure for children with cerebral palsy: evidence of reliability and validity. *Phys Ther* **80**: 873–85.

Stanley FJ, Blair E, Alberman E (2000) *Cerebral Palsies: Epidemiology and Causal Pathways*. London: Mac Keith Press. p 8–9.

Stout J, Gage JR, Van Heest AE (2004) Hemiplegia: pathology and treatment. In: Gage JR, editor. *The Treatment of Gait Problems in Cerebral Palsy*. London: Mac Keith Press. p 320–1.

Sutherland D, Davids J (1993) Common gait abnormalities of the knee in cerebral palsy. *Clin Orthop Relat Res* **288**: 139–47.

Winters TF, Gage JR, Hicks R (1987) Gait patterns in spastic hemiplegia in children and young adults. *J Bone Joint Surg Am* **69**: 437–41.

Wong MA, Simon S, Olshen RA (1983) Statistical analysis of gait patterns of persons with cerebral palsy. *Stat Med* **2**: 345–54.

2.7
THE NATURAL HISTORY OF AMBULATION IN CEREBRAL PALSY

Steven E. Koop

'What goes on four legs in the morning, on two legs at noon, and on three legs in the evening?'

'A man, who crawls on all fours as a baby, walks on two legs as an adult, and walks with a cane in old age.'

The riddle of the Theban Sphinx and the answer of Oedipus

The parents of a child with cerebral palsy have a question – just as the Sphinx did – but it is an even more challenging one: 'Will our child walk?' If only we could give a ready and confident answer! We want to be supportive and hopeful but we don't want to mislead. As trying as it might be, cerebral palsy is complex. Each child's circumstance poses many questions and each answer leads to more questions. Failure to recognize and grapple with the complexity of cerebral palsy can result in disappointment for children and parents. As the Sphinx suggested, human walking seems to have three phases: development of walking skills, mature walking function, and gradual decline with age. Individuals with cerebral palsy and sufficient motor control to walk seem to follow the same phases, with differences. The purpose of this chapter is to examine those differences and the questions that follow.

THE IMPORTANCE OF NATURAL HISTORY

A clear understanding of variations in development is required to justify intervention or 'treatment.' The outcome of an untreated health problem is known as the 'natural history' of the condition. It is reasonable for a physician to offer treatment if a person's health problem has unacceptable consequences now or if the problem, left alone, will have clear undesirable consequences in the future. If a child falls while running and sustains a badly displaced supracondylar humerus fracture, perhaps with bone protruding through the skin, the orthopedic surgeon moves quickly to thinking about treatment. The problem is clear and the need for intervention is plain: left untreated the fracture will become infected or heal in a position that will compromise function. The consequences of other health problems may be less clear. Two or three people in a hundred develop unexplained or 'idiopathic' scoliosis but only 10% of those individuals have a curve that exceeds 30°. Which person will it be? Does it matter? What can be done if the curve worsens?

The work of a physician who provides care for a child with cerebral palsy and altered walking skills is portrayed in Figure 2.7.1. At some point the consequences of one of a

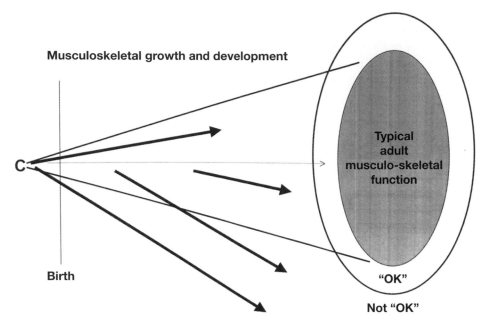

Musculoskeletal growth and development

Typical
adult
musculo-skeletal
function

Birth

"OK"

Not "OK"

Fig. 2.7.1 Natural history: the possible outcomes of a condition when left untreated.

group of disorders of the brain that originate between conception and infancy and alter movement and posture appear. Efforts are made to measure the impact of the disorder on current and future function. Will skills fall within the usual range of adult walking? Will skills be compromised but function 'acceptable?' or 'unacceptable?' How will the boundaries of 'acceptable' and unacceptable' be determined? Who will make that decision? If current or future function is not 'acceptable' what will be the goals of intervention? What interventions are possible? When should they be done? What must the child and family endure? How safe is the chosen intervention? What are the outcomes of intervention? Are the outcomes reliable? Will they last?

It may no longer be possible to know the true consequences of time and growth for children with cerebral palsy. Nearly every child receives some therapy. Many have worn braces. Others have received interventions for spasticity. Barnes and colleagues (2008), in a study of Pediatric Outcome Data Collection Instrument (PODCI) scores in children with cerebral palsy, found that 46% had undergone lower extremity musculoskeletal surgeries.

The typical development of human walking
Two forms of growth and development occur simultaneously in early childhood as walking function emerges: increase in physical size, and maturation of the neurological system. There are three distinct phases in physical growth. From birth to approximately 3 years of age the speed of growth is extraordinary but rapidly slowing. This is followed by several years of relatively constant juvenile growth. Adolescence is characterized by a phase of accelerated growth that ends with skeletal maturation. During the early years of rapid growth

there is substantial individual variation in motor task performance. It has been proposed that this variability is associated with a group of immature neural networks and that motor function is the result of experience-based selection of specific neural circuits that yield the most functional movement patterns (Forssberg 1985, 1999). Walking is one example of this process. Well known milestones mark neuromuscular maturation and walking. Infants acquire the ability to sit at approximately 6 months of age. They crawl near 9 months and walk with support at 10–15 months of age. Most are able to run at 18 months.

Sutherland and colleagues (1980) studied 186 children up to 7 years of age who were displaying typical development of walking skills. Their goals were to describe changes in gait in early childhood and define the parameters, or determinants, of mature walking. Reciprocal arm-swing and heel-strike were present in most of the children by 18 months and sagittal-plane angular rotations in their subjects were very similar to adult walking by 2 years of age. They found five important determinants of mature gait: single-limb stance, walking velocity, cadence, step length and the ratio of pelvic width to ankle spread. As maturation unfolds cadence decreases while walking velocity and step length increase. Key factors in the development of a mature pattern of the five determinants were increasing leg length and greater stability (which was manifested by increasing single-limb stance time). They found that a mature pattern of walking was established by three years of age. Beck and colleagues showed that walking patterns did not vary after four years of age when subjects were studied within 3 months (Beck et al. 1981). They found that an adult pattern of ground-reaction forces was present by 5 years. In a quantitative study of stride variability and dynamics Hausdorff and colleagues (1999) found that stride to stride control of walking is not fully mature until at least 7 years.

Rapid changes in physical size in early childhood present researchers with the problem of scaling data so that valid comparisons can be made between subjects of different stature and mass. Hof and Zijlstra (1997) suggested the problem could be solved by presenting the data in the form of nondimensional numbers and he proposed a group of dimensionless numbers related to gait mechanics. Following the observation that human walking can be likened to an inverted pendulum, Vaughan et al. (2003) used the nondimensional scaling method to examine the effects of growth and neuromaturation. They defined nondimensional step length (λ) and step frequency (ϕ) and examined them as children aged. Dimensionless velocity (β) was then calculated as $\beta = \lambda \cdot \phi$. The result was that dimensionless velocity β was found to be the square root of the Froude number (which relates the movements of animals of geometrically similar form but different size). When dimensionless velocity was calculated for a group of children of varying ages with normal walking it was found to increase until 70 months of age, after which it remained essentially unchanged into adulthood (Fig. 2.7.2).

Predictors of the ability to walk among children with cerebral palsy
The fourteen collaborating centers in the Surveillance of Cerebral Palsy in Europe (SCPE) found the prevalance of cerebral palsy to be 2.08/1000 live births (Surveillance of Cerebral Palsy in Europe 2002). In a subsequent study SCPE reported that by 5 years of age 54% of children walked without support, 16% walked with assistive devices, and 30% were unable

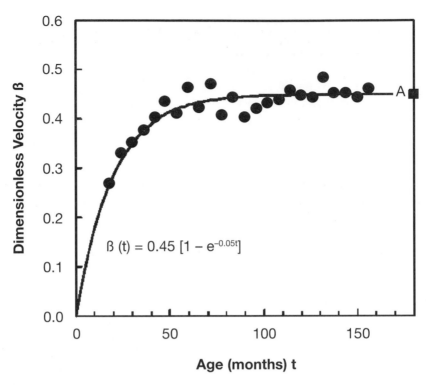

$$\beta (t) = 0.45 \, [1 - e^{-0.05t}]$$

Fig. 2.7.2 Dimensionless velocity (β) plotted as a function of a child's age. This parameter increases up to approximately 70 months of age and then remains unchanged, implying maturation of walking skills (Vaughan et al. 2003)

to walk. These are percentages consistent with a number of studies. Children with bilateral spasticity, dystonia, intelligence quotient less than 50, severe visual impairment or epilepsy are thought less likely to walk (Beckung et al. 2008). A retrospective analysis of 272 children in Brazil suggested the following gross motor milestones offered a good prognosis for walking: head control by 9 months of age, independent sitting by 24 months and crawling by 30 months (da Paz Junior et al. 1994). A prospective study of 31 children in Italy, observed over 30 months starting between nine and eighteen months of age showed two key predictors of walking ability. All children who walked were able to roll from supine to prone and raise their head by 18 months and all were able to sit without support by 24 months (with one exception) (Fedrizzi et al. 2000).

Wu et al. (2004) took a different approach in a retrospective review of 5366 children with cerebral palsy in California who did not walk at an age range of 24–42 months. They attempted to determine predictors of ambulation and then calculated univariate and multivariate odds ratios for achieving the ability to walk at least 20 feet without assistive devices by the age of 6 years (Table 2.7.1). Only 10% reached that level of walking ability. Demonstration of increased gross motor skills was associated with greater likelihood of being able to walk.

TABLE 2.7.1
Multivariate odds ratios for achieving full ambulation by 6 years of age among 2295 children with cerebral palsy who were nonambulatory at 2 years of age (from Wu et al. 2004)

Motor milestones	Odds ratio	p value
Does not roll	1	reference
Rolls, does not sit without support	4.6	0.0001
Sits without support, does not stand	12.5	0.0001
Pulls to stand	28.5	0.0001

These studies show an association between altered motor skills and delayed walking but offer no consistent or reliable method for answering the question every parent asks: 'Will my child be able to walk?'

Walking and the development of gross motor function in children with cerebral palsy

In response to the imprecise nature of descriptive terms used in cerebral palsy research and clinical work, Palisano and colleagues (1997) developed a 5-level classification system. The Gross Motor Function Classification System (GMFCS) is based on self-initiated movement with particular emphasis on trunk control (sitting) and walking. An effort was made to emphasize clinically meaningful function rather than limitations. The authors recognized that classification of motor function is dependent on age and they provided separate descriptions for four age groups: before the 2nd birthday, between the 2nd and 4th birthdays, between the 4th and 6th birthdays, and between the 6th and 12th birthdays. The expanded and revised GMFCS provided descriptions for a group between the 12th and 18th birthdays, provided operational definitions, and outlined distinctions between levels.

After their 6th birthday children in GMFCS level I walk without limitations. They are able to manage curbs and steps without assistance or the use of a handrail. They are able to run and jump but speed, balance and coordination may be limited. At level II individuals are able to walk in most settings. A challenging environment may prompt the use of a handheld mobility device for safety. Long distances or the need for rapid movement may result in the use of wheeled mobility. At level III household or indoor walking requires the use of handheld mobility devices. Movement from a floor or chair to standing requires physical assistance (another person or a firm support surface) and stairs mandate the use of a handrail. Movement in the broader community usually is accomplished with a manual or powered wheelchair. At level IV individuals use wheeled mobility in most settings. Standing for transfers or short distance walking requires the assistance of one or two persons. At level V ability to stand is extremely limited or absent. Equipment is needed to support sitting or standing and head alignment. All mobility is accomplished with a wheelchair.

In a subsequent study Rosenbaum and colleagues at CanChild Centre for Childhood Disability Research described patterns of gross motor development in children with cerebral palsy by severity using the Gross Motor Function Measure-66 (GMFM-66) and the GMFCS (Rosenbaum et al. 2002). A diverse population of 657 children with cerebral palsy (1–13 years of age) were assessed every 6–12 months over approximately 4 years (with an average of four assessments per child). Five distinct and significantly different motor growth curves that described patterns of gross motor development by GMFCS level were created.

The age by which children are expected to reach 90% of their motor development potential is termed Age-90. A clear trend existed in which children with greater cerebral palsy severity reached Age-90 at an earlier age. They also identified the GMFM-66 point limit and the range within which 50% of children reached their point limit (Table 2.7.2). A clear correlation was found between increased severity (GMFCS level) and limited motor development (GMFM-66 points).

The authors used four selected GMFM-66 items to illustrate the clinical interpretation of these curves. Item 21 (diamond A in Fig. 2.7.3) assesses whether a child can lift and

TABLE 2.7.2
Parameters of motor development for GMFCS

GMFCS		I	II	III	IV	V
GMFM-66	limit	87.7	68.4	54.3	40.4	22.3
	50% range	80.1–92.8	59.6–76.1	48.5–60	35.6–45.5	16.6–29.2
Age-90	years					
	50% range	4.8	4.4	3.7	3.5	2.7
	50% range	4.0–5.8	3.3–5.8	2.5–5.5	3.5	5.7

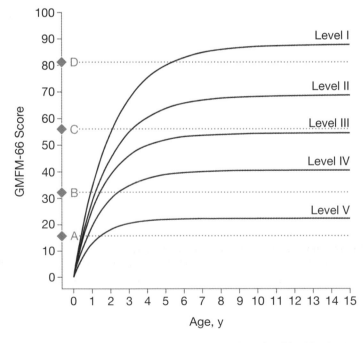

Fig. 2.7.3 Predicted average development by the Gross Motor Function Classification System levels (Rosenbaum et al. 2002)

maintain his/her head in a vertical position while sitting with trunk support from a therapist. A child with a GMFM-66 score of 16 would be expected to have a 50% chance of achieving this task. Item 24 (diamond B) assesses whether a child can sit unsupported by his/her arms for 3 seconds. Similar to item 21, children have a 50% chance of accomplishing this task at an average GMFM-66 score of 32 points. Item 69 (diamond C) measures a child's ability to walk forward ten steps without support (50% chance at GMFM-66 score of 56), and item 87 (diamond D) measures the task of walking down four steps with alternate feet and free arms (50% chance at GMFM-66 score of 81 points).

The authors felt their work would help parents understand their child's gross motor prognosis because a clear correlation was found between age, GMFCS level and the tasks included in the GMFM-66. They pointed out that none of the children had undergone selective dorsal lumbar rhizotomy or had received botulinum toxin or intrathecal lioresal (Baclofen) and no conclusions could be drawn about the effect of such interventions. While they demonstrated that children with cerebral palsy seem to reach a plateau in gross motor skills by 6–7 years of age they cautioned against assuming that interventions (therapy, medications or surgery) were of little value at that point. Beckung and colleagues (2007) confirmed the core findings of their work.

Walking function during adolescence

Many clinicians agree with the observation of Gannotti and her colleagues (2008): 'The natural history in children with cerebral palsy is a gradual decline in ambulatory function as children grow and age.' Day and colleagues (2007) performed a retrospective study of two groups of persons with cerebral who received services from the California Department of Developmental Disabilities, one group at 10 years of age (7550 individuals) and another at 25 years of age (5721 individuals). They created a scale of four levels of ambulatory ability. Group 1 walked well alone at least 6 m, balanced well, and moved up and downstairs without the need for a handrail. Group 2 walked well alone at least 6 m and balanced well but moved up and downstairs only with the use of a handrail. Group 3A walked unsteadily alone at least 3 m or walked only with assistive devices but did not use a wheel chair. Group 3B walked unsteadily alone at least 3 m or walked only with assistive devices and used a wheel chair. Group 4 did not walk. Among the children seen initially at age 10 years and then at 25 years of age, all of Group 1 maintained the ability to walk but 23% had lost skills. All of Group 2 remained ambulatory but 23% had improved their skills and 22% demonstrated loss of skills. In Group 3A 32% showed improvement in walking skills but 14% had lost the ability to walk. Loss of walking skills was more obvious in Group 3B: 5% improved but 34% no longer walked (and 6% had died).

Because this study was retrospective the GMFCS could not be used. The study did not take into account any past interventions and the authors acknowledged the possibility that receipt of services skewed the study group. Nonetheless Day and colleagues (2007) seemed to show that greater compromise in walking skills before adolescence predisposes a child to greater risk for deterioration or loss of walking function by early adulthood. They also demonstrated that some individuals may improve their walking skills, particularly those that do not use a wheelchair, but they offered no explanation.

173

McCormick and colleagues (2007) were able to use GMFCS as a measure of the stability of gross motor function changes from early adolescence into young adulthood. Although their study population included individuals as old as 38 years the mean age of the group was 22 years. Seventy of 103 individuals stayed at the GMFCS level they attained at age 12 years. Nine improved and 24 worsened in their GMFCS level with all changes being one level (with one exception, an individual who improved from GMFCS IV to II). Therefore none of the GMFCS I–III groups lost the ability to walk but seven of 35 (20%) at GMFCS IV became nonambulatory.

These studies suggest that some individuals are able to improve their walking skills during adolescence but others are losing function. Most clinicians believe that loss of function during adolescence is due to increased body mass, a relative loss of strength, and loss of flexibility leading to contractures. Gannotti and colleagues (2008) demonstrated a trend towards decreased walking velocity, increased mean knee flexion in stance and increased popliteal angle with age but could not demonstrate a link between these findings and age-related increases in body mass index. Well constructed longitudinal studies are needed to understand the effects of adolescent growth.

Walking function during adulthood

Day and colleagues (2007), cited earlier, followed a group of adults from age 25 to 40 years. The patterns noted in the group followed from 10 to 25 years of age were the same but the chances of improvement were much less. Only 5% demonstrated improved walking function while 30% lost function.

Andersson and Mattsson (2001) described the function of 221 adults at an average age of 38 years (range 20–58 years). In this group 162 (73%) had been able to walk at some point in their lives. Of those who were able to walk 17% reported improvement as an adult, 41% reported no change, 30% reported a loss of skills and 12% had stopped walking (nearly all by age 35 years). Bottos et al. (2001) described the function of 72 adults at an average age of 33 years (range 19–65 years). In their study population 76% had been able to walk (in some fashion) as an adolescent but only 43% had retained that ability. Of those who lost the ability to walk nearly all had stopped walking by age 40 years. Jahnsen and colleagues (2004b) described the function of 406 adults at an average age of 34 years (range 18–72 years). In a subgroup with spasticity who were ambulatory in early adulthood 26% reported improvement as an adult, 32% reported no change, 32% reported a loss of skills and 10% had stopped walking. Strauss and colleagues reported that 40% of individuals with cerebral palsy had lost the ability to walk by age 60 years (Strauss et al. 2004). Among those able to walk well alone at age 60 years, a 'marked decline' in ability was seen over the next 15 years.

Why is function lost? There are common themes. Nearly every study points out that adults with cerebral palsy are less active than their peers. Few adults with cerebral palsy participate in physical therapy or fitness programs. In Andersson and Mattsson's (2001) group only 36% participated in any therapy activities. Therefore deconditioning, coupled with increased body weight, may play a significant role. Jahnsen et al. (2003) administered the Fatigue Questionnaire (FQ) and the Life Satisfaction Scale (LSS) to 404 adults with cerebral palsy (mean age 34 years, range 18–72 years) and a normative population of individuals without cerebral palsy (mean age 45 years, range 19–80 years). The scores for total and physical fatigue were significantly higher in the adults with cerebral palsy. Factors cited by the respondents as causes of fatigue included limitations in physical and emotional function, deterioration in physical skills, pain, and low life satisfaction. Andersson et al. (2003) found evidence in a small study population that a 10-week program of progressive strength training improved strength and walking ability without increasing spasticity.

Pain is a problem for adults with cerebral palsy. In Jahnsen et al.'s (2004a) population, 72% reported pain. In 55% the pain was mild to moderate and in 17% the pain was severe. The pain had been present every day for at least one year in 28% of individuals with cerebral palsy. Only 15% of the normative population reported such pain. In Andersson and Mattsson's (2001) group 79% reported pain, with 22% stating that pain was present daily. Neck and back pain are the most common but pain is possible at every lower extremity joint from the hip to foot. Approximately two-thirds of adults with pain report pain present in two or more locations. Incomplete range of motion at one or more joints in the lower extremities (contracture) is present in 80% of adults with cerebral palsy. Increased tone or spasticity is a common report, coupled with decreased balance.

Fuzzy clustering: a new method for studying the natural history of walking in individuals with cerebral palsy and measuring the effects of intervention

Clustering is the work of partitioning of a data set into subsets so that (ideally) the data in each subset share some common trait. Fuzzy clustering is a technique for describing data that are not amenable to precise definition or measurement (Chau 2001). Methods exist to determine the number of clusters that might exist in a data set. Each point then has a degree of belonging to all of the identified clusters and a coefficient can be calculated to express the relative membership in a particular cluster. Fuzzy clustering has the potential to organize multidimensional gait data into approximate groupings for individuals with cerebral palsy which could, in turn, be compared to the characteristics of the cluster that represents normal walking. If relative membership in clusters shifts over time for a given individual then the effects of intervention (or lack of intervention) might be quantified (Vaughan and O'Malley 2005).

Summary of the natural history of walking skills for individuals with cerebral palsy

These observations fairly represent what we know about the walking skills of individuals with cerebral palsy:

1. 50%–80% of individuals with cerebral palsy will be able to walk in some manner.
2. While topographic classifications and types of motor control dysfunction offer insight about the probability of groups of individuals with cerebral palsy achieving the ability to walk they are imprecise and not useful for predicting an individual child's future walking ability.
3. Walking skills emerge and plateau later than in individuals without cerebral palsy
4. Instruments such as the Gross Motor Function Measure (GMFM), administered over time, are the most reliable method for predicting ultimate walking ability.

5. Five distinct levels of walking ability are described by the Gross Motor Function Classification System (GMFCS)
6. Deterioration in walking ability can be seen as early as adolescence.
7. Some individuals (10%–25%) are able to increase their walking ability in adolescence and young adulthood.
8. Deterioration is common in early adulthood (25–40 years of age) and as many as 10%–20% of individuals previously able to walk become nonambulatory by age 40 years. Improvement in walking skills is rarely seen in this period.
9. Individuals with greater walking ability (GMFCS I and II) experience less deterioration and are unlikely to become nonambulatory until late in life (over age 60 years).
10. Individuals with lesser walking ability (GMFCS III and IV) are at the greatest risk for early and substantial loss of walking skills and are at the greatest risk for becoming nonambulatory.
11. Decreased physical activity, decreased participation in physical therapy and fitness programs, loss of strength, contractures, and pain are the most common factors associated with deterioration in walking ability and overall physical function.

Questions
The natural arc of emerging skills, plateau in function, and decline in walking ability prompts many questions. For instance:

1. What is the role of physical therapy as gross motor skills emerge?
2. Is it possible to alter a child's apparent GMFCS level?
3. What is the role of tone-reducing interventions? How do we match them to the child?
4. What is the role of musculoskeletal surgery? What type, and when should they be performed?
5. How do some individuals improve their walking ability in adolescence and adulthood?
6. How do we detect and stop the deterioration in walking skills that starts in adolescence worsens in adulthood?

Of course, there are more questions and nuances in every question. We want to believe that we make a positive difference in the lives of the children we meet, and often we do, but there is much we do not understand about the effects of treatment. The section of the book dedicated to treatment methods and outcomes will serve as a start to our understanding.

REFERENCES

Andersson C, Mattsson E (2001) Adults with cerebral palsy: a survey describing problems, needs, and resources, with special emphasis on locomotion. *Dev Med Child Neurol* 43: 76–82.
Andersson C, Grooten W, Hellsten M, Kaping K, Mattsson E (2003) Adults with cerebral palsy: walking ability after progressive strength training. *Dev Med Child Neurol* **45**: 220–8.
Barnes D, Linton JL, Sullivan E, Bagley A, Oeffinger D, Abel M, Damiano D, Gorton G, Nicholson D, Romness M, Rogers S, Tylkowski C (2008) Pediatric outcomes data collection instrument scores in ambulatory children with cerebral palsy: an analysis by age groups and severity level. *J Pediatr Orthop* **28**: 97–102.

Beck RJ, Andriacchi TP, Kuo KN, Fermier RW, Galante JO (1981) Changes in the gait patterns of growing children. *J Bone Joint Surg Am* **63**: 1452–7.

Beckung E, Carlsson G, Carlsdotter S, Uvebrant P (2007) The natural history of gross motor development in children with cerebral palsy aged 1 to 15 years. *Dev Med Child Neurol* 49: 751–6.

Beckung E, Hagberg G, Uldall P, Cans C, Surveillance of Cerebral Palsy in Europe (2008) Probability of walking in children with cerebral palsy in Europe. *Pediatrics* **121**: 187–92.

Bottos M, Feliciangeli A, Sciuto L, Gericke C, Vianello A (2001) Functional status of adults with cerebral palsy and implications for treatment of children. *Dev Med Child Neurol* **43**: 516–28.

Chau T (2001) A review of analytical techniques for gait data. Part 1: Fuzzy, statistical and fractal methods. *Gait Posture* **13**: 49–66.

Da Paz Junior AC, Burnett SM, Braga LW (1994) Walking prognosis in cerebral palsy: a 22-year retrospective analysis. *Dev Med Child Neurol* **36**: 130–4.

Day SM, Wu YW, Strauss DJ, Shavelle RM, Reynolds RJ (2007) Change in ambulatory ability of adolescents and young adults with cerebral palsy. *Dev Med Child Neurol* **49**: 647–53.

Fedrizzi E, Facchin P, Marzaroli M, Pagliano E, Botteon G, Percivalle L, Fazzi E (2000) Predictors of independent walking in children with spastic diplegia. *J Child Neurol* **15**: 228–34.

Forssberg H (1985) Ontogeny of human locomotor control. I. Infant stepping, supported locomotion and transition to independent locomotion. *Exp Brain Res* **57**: 480–93.

Forssberg H (1999) Neural control of human motor development. *Curr Opin Neurobiol* **9**: 676–82.

Gannotti M, Gorton GE, Nahorniak MT, Gagnaire N, Fil A, Hogue J, Julewicz J, Hersh E, Marchion V, Masso PD (2008) Changes in gait velocity, mean knee flexion in stance, body mass index, and popliteal angle with age in ambulatory children with cerebral palsy. *J Pediatr Orthop* **28**: 103–11.

Hausdorff JM, Zemany L, Peng C, Goldberger AL (1999) Maturation of gait dynamics: stride-to-stride variability and its temporal organization in children. *J Appl Physiol* **86**: 1040–7.

Hof AL, Zijlstra W (1997) Comment on 'Normalization of temporal-distance parameters in pediatric gait'. *J Biomechan* **30**: 299–302.

Jahnsen R, Villien L, Stanghelle JK, Holm I (2003) Fatigue in adults with cerebral palsy in Norway compared with the general population. *Dev Med Child Neurol* **45**: 296–303.

Jahnsen R, Villien L, Aamodt G, Stanghelle JK, Holm I (2004a) Musculoskeletal pain in adults with cerebral palsy compared with the general population. *J Rehabil Med* **36**: 78–84.

Jahnsen R, Villien L, Egeland T, Stanghelle JK, Holm I (2004b) Locomotion skills in adults with cerebral palsy. *Clin Rehabil* **18**: 309–16.

McCormick A, Brien M, Plourde J, Wood E, Rosenbaum P, McLean J (2007) Stability of the Gross Motor Function Classification System in adults with cerebral palsy. *Dev Med Child Neurol* **49**: 265–9.

Palisano R, Rosenbaum P, Walter S, Russell D, Wood E, Galuppi B (1997) Development and reliability of a system to classify gross motor function in children with cerebral palsy. *Dev Med Child Neurol* **39**: 214–23.

Rosenbaum P, Walter S, Hanna SE, Palisano RJ, Russell DJ, Raina P, Wood E, Bartlett DJ, Galuppi BE (2002) Prognosis for gross motor function in cerebral palsy: creation of motor development curves. *J Am Med Assoc* **288**: 1357–63.

Strauss D, Ojdana K, Shavelle R, Rosenbloom L (2004) Decline in function and life expectancy of older persons with cerebral palsy. *NeuroRehabil* **19**: 69–78.

Surveillance of Cerebral Palsy in Europe (2002) Prevalence and characteristics of children with cerebral palsy in Europe. *Dev Med Child Neurol* **44**: 633–40.

Sutherland DH, Olshen R, Cooper L, Woo SL (1980) The development of mature gait. *J Bone Joint Surg Am* **62**: 336–53.

Vaughan CL, O'Malley MJ (2005) A gait nomogram used with fuzzy clustering to monitor functional status of children and young adults with cerebral palsy. *Dev Med Child Neurol* **47**: 377–83.

Vaughan CL, Langerak NG, O'Malley MJ (2003) Neuromaturation of human locomotion revealed by non-dimensional scaling. *Exp Brain Res* **153**: 123–7.

Wu YW, Day SM, Strauss DJ, Shavelle RM (2004) Prognosis for ambulation in cerebral palsy: a population-based study. *Pediatr* **114**: 1264–71.

177

Section 3

PATIENT ASSESSMENT

INTRODUCTION AND OVERVIEW

James R. Gage

This is an area that has changed enormously in my 30+ years of practice. When I took over the cerebral palsy service at Newington Children's Hospital in Connecticut in 1978, decisions were based almost entirely on clinical history and examination, which included visual observation of gait plus a few routine radiographs. At that time our knowledge of the cerebral control of locomotion was rudimentary, gait laboratories were not available for use in clinical practice, and sophisticated imaging techniques were non-existent. Surgical practice was largely based on empiricism and prior teaching, most of which was fallacious.

In those days, we started with a patient who walked badly and ended with a patient who walked differently, but not necessarily better. Furthermore, since we had no way to accurately assess our outcomes, there was no way that our future treatments could improve. The onset of the Motion Analysis Laboratory at Newington Children's Hospital, designed and built for us by United Technologies Research Corporation, changed all that. We suddenly had the capability to do accurate, preoperative and postoperative assessments of our patients even in cases in which single-event multiple lower-extremity procedures were carried out. As a result, ineffective procedures were rapidly discarded, and new and better ways of correcting or minimizing the pathology were gradually introduced with the long-term effect that cerebral palsy surgery has become much more predictable and reliable.

Since the Motion Analysis Laboratory opened at Newington Children's Hospital in 1981, computer technology has exploded in other areas as well. As an example, computer augmented tomography (CT) has revolutionized orthopaedic assessment and treatment of difficult spinal and hip deformities in cerebral palsy. It is now possible to obtain three-dimensional reconstructions, which allow the surgeon to visualize and plan specific treatment of these complex deformities. Similarly, MRI and PET scans have revolutionized brain imaging, and because of these tools treating physicians have a much better grasp of the nature of the cerebral pathology. This, in turn, allows a more accurate appraisal of potential response to various treatment modalities, as well as better ability to assess the patient's long-term functional prognosis.

179

Bioengineering also has come to the fore, such that computer simulation of various gait abnormalities is now possible. The long-term hope is that when we can model these deformities with sufficient accuracy, we may eventually be able to simulate proposed treatments as well. All of these developments will be discussed more completely in this section of the book.

3.1
CLINICAL ASSESSMENT

Joyce P. Trost

Clinical evaluation

In the assessment of ambulatory children with cerebral palsy (CP), many pieces are needed to create a comprehensive picture of the orthopaedic and neurological impairments confronting the patient. In order to prepare treatment plans and accurately assess outcomes of treatment, a balanced combination of medical history, detailed physical examination, functional assessment, imaging, observational gait analysis, computerized gait analysis, patient and family expectations or goals must be interpreted together.

The medical history

The medical history should include a collection of information regarding birth history, developmental milestones, medical problems, surgical history, current physical therapy treatment, and current medication. Parent report on current functional walking level at home, school, and in the community, as well as other functional skills such as stair-climbing, jumping and running will also have an effect on treatment plans and outcome analysis.

Birth history and other medical problems are important pieces of information for accurate diagnosis, future prognosis, treatment and goal-setting. Developmental milestones will give information regarding the maturity of a skill such as walking, and will often help in guiding families in setting appropriate goals for therapy or surgical intervention based on the natural history of the child's cerebral palsy. When considering surgical treatment, it is important to obtain the operative reports of previous surgeries to accurately assess current deformities, and necessary compensations. For example, iatrogenic weakness of the soleus muscle caused by heel-cord lengthening may require a different treatment plan from primary soleus weakness. Other surgical interventions to treat spasticity, such as selective dorsal rhizotomy, may be impacted by specifics of the etiology of the cerebral palsy. Rhizotomy is thought to be the most effective when done on children with primary spasticity associated with preterm birth, as discussed in Chapter 5.2. History is an important part of this decision.

Besides the medical history, it is helpful to know the reason for referral to the motion analysis laboratory, and current surgical or treatment considerations. Knowing about complaints of pain, and behavior or learning issues, will assist the clinician to perform a complete evaluation.

Functional outcome measures

Use of a parent report outcome evaluation tool such as the Functional Assessment Questionnaire (FAQ) (Novacheck et al. 2000), the POSNA (Pediatric) Outcomes Data Collection Instruments (PODCI) (Daltroy et al. 1998), or the evaluative Functional Mobility Scale (FMS) (Graham et al. 2004) to evaluate a child's skills may be beneficial. The FAQ is a validated 10-level parent-report functional measure of patient ambulation in the patient's own environmental context. A child who is typically able to keep up with peers achieves a score of 10. The scale decreases with decreasing ability for community ambulation. A companion FAQ-22, which has not been validated, can be used to report other functional skills related to ambulation such as running, jumping, and kicking (Table 3.1.1). The PODCI is also a validated parent report instrument designed to be used across ages and musculo-skeletal disorders to assess functional health outcomes. It measures outcomes that orthopaedic treatment can affect, and includes measures of upper- and lower-extremity motor skills, relief of pain and restoration of activity. Correlations have been found between the FAQ, PODCI, and gait measures in children, and when used in conjunction with gait data they provide a more complete survey of change (Tervo et al. 2002). The FMS is an evaluative measure of functional mobility in children with cerebral palsy and aged 4–18 years (Harvey et al. 2007). It quantifies functional mobility at both the activity level and

TABLE 3.1.1
Gillette Functional Assessment Questionnaire 22 skills

	Easy	A little hard	Very hard	Can't do at all	Too young for activity
Walk carrying an object	O	O	O	O	O
Walk carrying a fragile object or glass of liquid	O	O	O	O	O
Walk up and down stairs using the railing	O	O	O	O	O
Walk up and down stairs without using the railing	O	O	O	O	O
Steps up and down curb independently	O	O	O	O	O
Runs	O	O	O	O	O
Runs well including around a corner with good control	O	O	O	O	O
Can take steps backwards	O	O	O	O	O
Can maneuver in tight areas	O	O	O	O	O
Get on and off a bus by him/herself	O	O	O	O	O
Jump rope	O	O	O	O	O
Jumps off a single step independently	O	O	O	O	O
Hop on right foot *(without holding onto equipment or another person)*	O	O	O	O	O
Hop on left foot *(without holding onto equipment or another person)*	O	O	O	O	O
Step over an object, right foot first	O	O	O	O	O
Step over an object, left foot first	O	O	O	O	O
Kick a ball with right foot	O	O	O	O	O
Kick a ball with left foot	O	O	O	O	O
Ride 2 wheel bike *(without training wheels)*	O	O	O	O	O
Ride 3 wheel bike *(or 2 wheel bike with training wheels)*	O	O	O	O	O
Ice skate or roller skate *(without holding onto another person)*	O	O	O	O	O
Ride an escalator, can step on/off without help	O	O	O	O	O

participation domains of the International Classification of Functioning, Disability and Health (Rosenbaum and Stewart 2004). A unique feature of the FMS is its ability to distinguish between assistive device levels used by children, and the environmental setting that they are using them in. The FMS has shown sensitivity to quantify change after orthopaedic intervention in children with CP (Harvey et al. 2007).

Preliminary gait by observation

Prior to initiating the physical examination, it is helpful to collect a video in order to perform a gait by observation (GBO) analysis. This can focus the clinician during the physical examination. A complete discussion of the GBO comes later in this chapter.

Physical examination

An example of a standard physical assessment (PE) form used in the motion analysis laboratory at Gillette Children's Specialty Healthcare (Gillette) provides a useful reference to a comprehensive physical examination (Fig. 3.1.1). There are standardized definitions for the various elements of the assessment, which are intended to provide a more homogeneous evaluation.

The physical examination has six main goals: (1) to determine strength and selective motor control of isolated muscle groups, (2) to evaluate degree and type of muscle tone, (3) to estimate the degree of static deformity and/or muscle contracture at each joint, (4) to assess torsional and other deformities of the bone, (5) to describe fixed and mobile foot deformities, and (6) to assess balance, equilibrium responses, and standing posture

Physical examinations have limitations and benefits. The information collected during a physical examination is based on static responses, whereas functional activities, such as walking, are dynamic. Gait analysis data cannot be predicted by any combination of physical exam measurements either passive or active; however, there is a moderate correlation between time and distance parameters and strength and selectivity measures (Damiano and Abel 1998, Damiano et al. 2002a, Desloovere et al. 2006). The independence of gait analysis and PE measures supports the notion that each provides information that is important in the delineation of problems of children with cerebral palsy (Desloovere et al. 2006). The method of assessment, the skill of the examiner, and the participation of the child can all affect the usefulness of the examination. The degree of tone can change with the position of the child, whether s/he is moving or at rest, the level of excitement or irritability, or the time/day of the assessment. Objective evaluation of muscle strength is difficult in small children and children with neurological impairments (Bohannon 1989, Damiano et al. 2002a). In addition, motor control and the assessment of movement dysfunction are subjective and rely heavily on the experience and expertise of the examiner.

The area of foot and ankle evaluation in children and adults with CP has grown significantly over the past few years in the development of improved standardization of terminology, better standardized assessments, and computerized assessments of the foot (see Chapter 3.2 for the complete foot evaluation).

Gillette Children's Specialty Healthcare
Physical Assessment

Name:
MR#:
DOB:

	MOTION L	MOTION R	SELECTIVITY, STRENGTH L	SELECTIVITY, STRENGTH R
HIPS				
Flexion				
Extension				
Thomas test				
knee 0				
knee 90				
Abduction				
hips extended				
hips flexed				
Adduction				
Ober test				
Internal rotation				
External rotation				
Anteversion				
KNEE				
Extension				
Flexion				
prone				
supine				
Popliteal angle				
unilateral				
bilateral				
HS shift				
Extensor lag				
Patella alta				
TIBIA				
TF angle				
BM axis				
2nd toe test				
ANKLE SUBTALAR				
Dorsiflexion				
knee 90				
knee 0				
Confusion test				
Plantarflexion				
Anterior tibialis				
Posterior tibialis				
Peroneus longus				
Peroneus brevis				
Extensor hallucis longus				
Flexor hallucis longus				

STANDING POSTURE

BALANCE

COMMENTS

	FOOT POSITION L	FOOT POSITION R
FOOT NON-WEIGHTBEARING		
Subtalar neutral		
Hindfoot position		
Hindfoot motion		
eversion		
inversion		
Arch		
Midfoot motion		
Forefoot position 1		
Forefoot position 2		
Bunion def.		
1st MTP DF		
FOOT WEIGHTBEARING		
Hindfoot position		
Midfoot position		
Forefoot position 1		
Forefoot position 2		
SPASTICITY (Ashworth Scale)		
Hip flexors		
Adductors		
Hamstrings		
Rectus femoris		
Plantarflexors		
Posterior tibialis		
Ankle clonus		

Selectivity grade key
0 - Only patterned movement observed.
1 - Partially isolated movement observed.
2 - Completely isolated movement observed

Ashworth Scale
1 - No increase in tone
2 - Slight increase in tone
3 - More marked increase in tone
4 - Considerable increase in tone
5 - Affected part rigid

POSTURE / TRUNK
Abdominal Strength
Back Extensor Strength

LIG LAXITY

LEG LENGTH

Fig. 3.1.1 Physical examination is an important part of the problem solving process.

Muscle strength

Strength evaluation is necessary and is extremely important to ensure optimal clinical outcomes. It can be used to assess appropriateness for an intervention such as selective dorsal rhizotomy, or to assess the outcome of a multiple lower extremity procedure. There is increasing evidence that children with cerebral palsy are weak, and that motor function and strength are directly related (Kramer and MacPhail 1994, Damiano et al. 1995). There is an array of testing methods for the measurement of muscle strength in children with cerebral palsy depending on the type of equipment and time that you have available in the clinic. The most common in the clinical setting is manual muscle testing (MMT) using the Kendall scale (Kendall et al. 1971). Isometric assessment with a dynamometer is becoming more common in the clinic, and is often used in research and outcome studies. Isokinetic evaluations are used when evaluating strength throughout a range of motion. The individual characteristics of each testing situation must be considered in order to be able to interpret the results with any degree of validity.

The 5-point Kendall scale provides an easy and quick way to assess a child for significant weakness or muscle imbalance, and requires only a table and standardized positioning. It does, however, rely heavily on the examiner's judgement, experience, the amount of force generated by the examiner, and the accuracy of the positioning of the patient. Small yet clinically significant differences in strength may not be detected using this method. It is subjective and prone to examiner bias. However, under strict evaluation protocols, this method can still be useful (Wadsworth et al. 1987). For children who are under the age of 5, and who cannot follow complex directions for maximal force production, the manual muscle testing method, as well as any other method of strength assessment, is a vague screening tool at best.

Because of the wide variation that is seen with manual muscle assessment of isometric strength, the use of a hand-held dynamometer (HHD) has increased in the clinic and in research protocols to better quantify strength variation. The HHD approach has been shown to be a valid and reliable tool to measure isometric strength in patients with brain lesions (Bohannon and Smith 1987, Bohannon 1989) and in children with cerebral palsy (Berry et al. 2004). It does have an upper limit, however, and it will reach its maximum when used with stronger patients. Strength profiles for children with cerebral palsy are published (Wiley and Damiano 1998), as well as normative data for young children (Macfarlane et al. 2008). Validity of this examination still depends on appropriate positioning, whether stabilization is used, and the experience of the tester. Normalization is required for body weight and lever length for strength comparisons (Macfarlane et al. 2008).

Isokinetic strength assessment is used to measure torque generated continuously through an arc of movement. The length of time required for this assessment, the lack of portability of the equipment, and the difficulties young children have complying with this test modality precluded isokinetic strength testing from becoming standard in the pediatric clinical setting.

Selective motor control

Children with cerebral palsy have impaired ability to isolate and control movements, which contributes to their ambulatory and functional motor deficits. Selective motor control involves isolating movements upon request, appropriate timing, and maximal voluntary contraction without overflow movement. Therefore a muscle selectivity grading scale has been added to assessments. A typical scale includes three levels of control: 0, no ability to isolate movement; 1, partial ability to isolate movement; and 2, complete ability to isolate movement. The detailed definitions and descriptions for the lower extremity muscles groups assist in accurately describing a patient's motor control and are always reported together with strength ability (Table 3.1.2).

During a static examination, a child with hemiplegia may not be able to actively dorsiflex his foot on the involved side without a mass flexion pattern including hip and knee flexion. Consider a child who, on examination, demonstrates muscle strength of 3/5 (3 out of 5), with a selectivity grade of 0/2 (0 out of 2). During gait analysis this child may have difficulty with clearance of his foot in early swing phase due to the inability to perform dorsiflexion with his hip in extension. However, in midswing, dorsiflexion with inversion could occur because of the child's inability to regulate the pull of the anterior tibialis and the extensor digitorum longus. In this example, adequate dorsiflexion occurs, but the timing is late and the motion is not controlled as compared to a walk of a child with typical motor control. No surgical treatment would be able to address the problems of timing and balance; however, an orthosis may.

A frequent cause of crouch gait is soleus weakness secondary to tendo-Achilles lengthening (TAL) (Gage 1991). A TAL will lengthen both the gastrocnemius and soleus muscles, and allow excessive knee flexion in mid-stance. The inability of a patient to move the foot actively into plantarflexion, or a patient who exhibits knee flexion with toe-raising would suggest weakness of the soleus. This latter effect is a consequence of the gastrocnemius, which is both a knee-flexor and an ankle-plantarflexor, assisting the weakened soleus.

Hamstring weakness can also contribute to crouch gait since these muscles are biarticular and act as extensors of the hip (Delp et al. 1990, 1995). Strength and motor-control testing of the hip-extensors, abductors, and the abdominal muscles give information on whether weakness and impaired motor control contribute to the deviations observed at the trunk and pelvis (primary), or whether these deviations are due to pathology occurring in the limbs (secondary). Increased pelvic tilt and decreased hip extension in stance have many etiologies that include hip-extensor and abdominal weakness. This loss of proximal control allows the pelvis to rotate anteriorly during static standing and periods of the gait cycle when these muscle groups are unable to provide the needed eccentric control.

Muscle groups such as the quadriceps may become functionally long due to bio-mechanical malalignments that cause a stretch weakness at the end range of motion. Assessment of the active versus passive range of motion of a joint can give insight into true strength and control deficits. Knee-extensor lag as a measure of inadequate quadriceps strength is done with the hips in extension to eliminate the influence of hamstring tightness or shift. Assessment can be done supine with legs hanging over the edge of the table. The child is instructed to extend his knee fully without manual resistance, and the range of motion deficit is measured. Children who walk with a crouch-gait pattern may not have the ability to fully extend the knee at the end range of motion, but may have good isolation and strength at the end of the active range of motion.

TABLE 3.1.2
Selective motor control grading scale description

Hip flexion
Position: Patient seated supported or unsupported with hips at a 90° angle, legs over the side of the table. Arms folded across chest or resting in lap (not on the able or hanging on to the edge)

2 – hip flexion in a superior direction without evidence of adduction, medial or lateral rotation, or trunk extension
1 – hip flexion associated with adduction, medial or lateral rotation, or trunk extension that is not obligatory but occurs in conjunction with the desired motion through at least a portion of the range of motion
0 – hip flexion which only occurs with obligatory knee flexion, ankle dorsiflexion and adduction

Hip extension (hamstrings + gluteus maximus)
Position: Patient lying prone, head resting on pillow (prone on elbows not allowed). Knees in maximum possible extension. Pelvis stabilized as necessary

2 – hip extension in a superior direction without evidence of medial or lateral rotation, trunk extension, or abduction
1 – hip extension associated with medial or lateral rotation, trunk extension, or abduction that is not obligatory but occurs in conjunction with the desired motion through at least a. portion of the range of motion
0 – hip extension which only occurs with obligatory trunk extension, arm extension, or neck extension. May also include medial or lateral rotation, or abduction

Hip extension (gluteus maximus)
Position: Patient lying prone, head resting on pillow (prone on elbows not allowed). Knees in 90° or more flexion, hips in neutral extension, pelvis flat on table. Pelvis stabilized as necessary

2 – hip extension in a superior direction without evidence of medial or lateral rotation, knee extension, or hip abduction
1 – hip extension associated with knee extension, trunk extension, medial or lateral rotation, or abduction that is not obligatory but occurs in conjunction with the desired motion through at least a portion of the range of motion
0 – hip extension which occurs only with obligatory knee extension, trunk extension, medial or lateral rotation, or abduction

Hip abduction
Position: Side-lying, the hip in neutral or slight hip extension, neutral medial or lateral rotation, knee in maximum possible extension. Pelvis stabilized as necessary

2 – hip abduction in a superior direction without evidence of medial or lateral rotation or hip flexion
1 – hip abduction in a superior direction associated with hip flexion, or medial or lateral rotation that is not obligatory but occurs in conjunction with the desired motion through at least a portion of the range of motion
0 – hip abduction which occurs with obligatory hip flexion, or medial or lateral rotation

Hip adduction
Position: Side-lying body in straight line with legs, the hip in neutral or slight hip extension, neutral medial or lateral rotation, knee in maximum possible extension, opposite limb supported in alight abduction. Pelvis stabilized as necessary

2 – hip adduction in a superior direction without evidence of hip flexion, medial or lateral rotation, or tilting/rotation of the pelvis
1   hip adduction in a superior direction associated with hip flexion, or medial or lateral rotation, pelvis tilting/rotation that is not obligatory but occurs in conjunction with the desired motion through at least a portion of the range of motion
0 – hip adduction which occurs with obligatory hip flexion, or medial or lateral rotation

TABLE 3.1.2 continued
Selective motor control grading scale description

Knee extension
Position: Patient seated supported or unsupported with hips at a 90° angle, knees at 90° angle resting over the side of the table. Thigh stabilized as necessary
2 – knee extension in a superior direction, without evidence of hip or trunk extension, medial or lateral rotation of the thigh or hip flexion
1 – knee extension associated with hip or trunk extension, hip flexion, or medial or lateral rotation of the thigh that is not obligatory but occurs in conjunction with the desired motion through at least a portion of the range of motion
0 – knee extension which occurs with obligatory hip or trunk extension, hip flexion, or medial or lateral rotation of the thigh

Knee flexion
Position: Patient lying prone, head resting on pillow (prone on elbows not allowed). Knees in maximum possible extension. Pelvis and thigh stabilized as necessary
2 – knee flexion in a superior direction without evidence of hip flexion, medial or lateral thigh rotation, or tilting, rotation of the pelvis, or ankle plantarflexion
1 – knee flexion associated with a pelvic rise, hip flexion, medial or lateral rotation of the thigh, or ankle plantarflexion that is not obligatory but occurs in conjunction with the desired motion through at least a portion of the range of motion
0 – knee flexion which occurs with obligatory hip flexion, pelvic tilting or rotation, medial or lateral rotation of the thigh or ankle plantarflexion

Ankle dorsiflexion (anterior tibialis)
Position: Patient seated supported or unsupported with hips at a 90° angle, knees in extension (flexion may be allowed to achieve a range of dorsiflexion). Lower leg supported. Thigh stabilized as necessary
2 – ankle dorsiflexion and inversion without evidence of increased knee flexion, subtalar eversion, or extension of the great toe
1 – ankle dorsiflexion and inversion associated with increased knee flexion, subtalar eversion, or extension of the great toe that is not obligatory but occurs in conjunction with the desired motion through at least a portion of the range of motion
0 – ankle dorsiflexion and inversion which occurs with obligatory knee flexion, subtalar eversion, or extension of the great toe

Ankle plantarflexion (soleus)
Position: Patient lying prone, head resting on pillow (prone on elbows not allowed). Knees in 90° of flexion. Lower leg stabilized proximal to the ankle as necessary. Ankle in neutral plantarflexion/dorsiflexion position
2 – ankle plantarflexion in a superior direction without evidence of knee extension, subtalar inversion, eversion, or toe flexion
1 – ankle plantarflexion associated with knee extension, subtalar inversion, eversion, or toe flexion that is not obligatory but occurs in conjunction with the desired motion through at least a portion of the range of motion
0 – ankle plantarflexion which occurs with obligatory knee extension, subtalar inversion, eversion, or toe flexion

Ankle plantarflexion (gastrocnemius)
Position: Patient lying prone, head resting on pillow (prone on elbows not allowed). Knees in maximum extension, foot projecting over the end of the table. Lower leg stabilized proximal to the ankle as necessary. Ankle in neutral plantarflexion/dorsiflexion position
2 – ankle plantarflexion in a superior direction without evidence of subtalar inversion, eversion, or toe flexion
1 – ankle plantarflexion associated with subtalar inversion, eversion, or toe flexion that is not obligatory but occurs in conjunction with the desired motion through at least a portion of the range of motion
0 – ankle plantarflexion which occurs with obligatory subtalar inversion, eversion, or toe flexion

TABLE 3.1.2 continued
Selective motor control grading scale description

Ankle inversion (posterior tibialis)
Position: Patient seated supported or unsupported with hips at a 90° angle, thigh in lateral rotation, knees in flexion with lower leg stabilized proximal to the ankle. Ankle in neutral plantar/dorsiflexion
2 – inversion at the subtalar joint with plantarflexion of the ankle without evidence of toe flexion
1 – inversion at the subtalar joint with plantarflexion of the ankle associated with toe flexion that is not obligatory but occurs in conjunction with the desired motion through at least a portion of the range of motion
0 – inversion at the subtalar joint with plantarflexion of the ankle which occurs with obligatory and forceful toe flexion

Ankle eversion (peroneus brevis + peroneus longus)
Position: Patient seated supported or unsupported with hips at a 90° angle, thigh in medial rotation, knees in flexion with lower leg stabilized proximal to the ankle. Ankle in neutral plantar/dorsiflexion
2 – eversion at the subtalar joint with plantarflexion of the ankle without evidence of toe flexion. If head of 1st metatarsal is depressed, action of the peroneus longus is indicated
1 – eversion at the subtalar joint with plantarflexion of the ankle associated with toe flexion that is not obligatory but occurs in conjunction with the desired motion through at least a portion of the range of motion
0 – eversion at the subtalar joint with plantarflexion of the ankle which occurs with obligatory and forceful toe flexion

Ankle eversion (peroneus tertius)
Position: Patient seated supported or unsupported with hips at a 90° angle, knees in flexion with lower leg stabilized proximal to the ankle. Ankle in neutral plantar/dorsiflexion.
2 – eversion at the subtalar joint with dorsiflexion of the ankle and 2–5 toe extension.
1 – not applicable
0 – not applicable (peroneus tertius and extensor digitorum longus are anatomically combined. The two muscles always act together)

Great toe extension (extensor hallucis longus)
Position: Patient seated supported or unsupported with hips at a 90° angle, knees in flexion with lower leg supported. Ankle in neutral plantar/dorsiflexion
2 – extension of the metatarsophalangeal joint of the great toe without evidence of knee flexion or ankle dorsiflexion
1 – extension of the metatarsophalangeal joint of the great toe associated with knee flexion or ankle dorsiflexion that is not obligatory but occurs in conjunction with the desired motion through at least a portion of the range of motion
0 – extension of the metatarsophalangeal joint of the great toe with obligatory knee flexion, or ankle dorsiflexion

Great toe flexion (flexor hallucis longus)
Position: Patient seated supported or unsupported with hips at a 90° angle, knees in maximum extension with lower leg supported. Ankle in neutral plantar/dorsiflexion.
2 – flexion of the metatarsophalangeal joint of the great toe without evidence of knee extension or ankle plantarflexion
1 – flexion of the metatarsophalangeal joint of the great toe associated with knee extension or ankle plantarflexion that is not obligatory but occurs in conjunction with the desired motion through at least a portion of the range of motion
0 – flexion of the metatarsophalangeal joint of the great toe with obligatory knee extension, or ankle plantarflexion

Muscle tone assessment

When examining a child with cerebral palsy, it is important to determine the nature and extent of abnormal tone. Tone is the resistance to passive stretch while a person is attempting to maintain a relaxed state of muscle activity. Hypertonia has been defined as abnormally increased resistance to an externally imposed movement about a joint. It can be caused by spasticity, dystonia, rigidity, or a combination of these features (Sanger et al. 2003). Residual muscle tension assessments can be influenced by the degree of apprehension or excitement present in the patient as well as the position during the assessment. Time spent playing, talking with, or calming down the child/adult before and during the examination will often help with the accuracy of the examination. To improve the assessment of variations in muscle tone several different practitioners should do an assessment on different occasions. Standardization within a facility for testing positions and the use of a grading scale are imperative. Sanger et al. (2003) recommended the following process. Start by palpating the muscle in question to determine if there is a muscle contracture at rest. Next, move the limb slowly to assess the available passive range of motion. The limb can then be moved through the available range at different speeds to assess the presence or absence of a 'catch' and how this 'catch' varies with a variety of speeds. Next, change the joint's direction of motion at various speeds and assess how the resistance (including timing) varies. Lastly observe the limb/joint while asking the patient to move the same joint on the contralateral side. Observe and document any involuntary movement or a change in the resistance to movement on the side being assessed. By using a standard process for evaluation, the consistency and completeness of tone abnormality documentation will improve. Video analysis during portions of this assessment can have great clinical utility when the pattern of movement is reviewed later.

Spastic (as compared to dystonic) hypertonia causes an increase in the resistance felt at higher speeds of passive movement. Resistance to externally imposed movement rises rapidly above a speed threshold (spastic catch). The Ashworth scale (Lee et al. 1989), the Modified Ashworth scale (Bohannon and Smith 1987, Gregson et al. 1999, Clopton et al. 2005), Tardieu scale (Haugh et al. 2006) and an isokinetic dynamometer in conjunction with surface EMG (Engsberg et al. 1996, Damiano et al. 2002b) are methods used to assess severity of spastic hypertonia.

Dystonic hypertonia on the other hand shows an increase in muscle activity when at rest, has a tendency to return to a fixed posture, increases resistance with movement of the contralateral limb, and will change with a change in behavior or posture. There are also involuntary sustained or intermittent muscle contractions causing twisting and repetitive movements, abnormal postures, or both. We have used the the Hypertonia Assessment Tool-Discriminant (HAT-D) (Jethwa et al. 2007), a tool developed to distinguish between spasticity, dystonia and rigidity in the pediatric clinical setting. The reliability and validity for spasticity and rigidity is good, but only moderate for dystonia and mixed tone. The Barry–Albright Dystonia scale (BAD), a 5-point ordinal scale, is another measure of generalized dystonia (Barry et al. 1999). Mixed tone is often identified with a combination of both types of hypertonicity in the same patient. Mixed tone is more difficult to diagnose and quantify than pure spasticity. In children with cerebral palsy, however, it is important to assess the degree of mixed tone present, since the outcome of surgery may be less predictable. Fortunately, dynamic EMG and motion analysis are useful in determining when dystonia and mixed tone are present.

Range-of-motion and contracture

Differentiation between static and dynamic deformity may be difficult in the non-anesthetized patient (Perry et al. 1974). However, physical examination of muscle length will provide some insight into whether contractures are static or dynamic. Due to the velocity-dependent nature of spasticity, it is important that assessment of range-of-motion (ROM) is carried out slowly. Comparison of joint ROM with slow and rapid stretch, however, can be useful in the evaluation of spasticity (Boyd and Graham 1999). Physical examination can also help distinguish deviations caused by weakness rather than shortness of the antagonistic muscle group. Dynamic contracture will disappear under general anesthesia. Thus the ROM examination under general anesthesia will be more specific to musculotendinous contracture. Whether to perform muscle lengthening or use botulinum toxin injection can then be decided.

When assessing muscle contracture and muscle length either statically, or dynamically by gait analysis, awareness of the interaction of multiple muscle groups at a variety of levels is important. Differentiation between contracted biarticular and monoarticular muscles is important. The Silverskiöld test (Fig. 3.1.2) assesses the difference between gastrocnemius and soleus contracture. The Duncan–Ely test (Fig. 3.1.3) differentiates between contracture

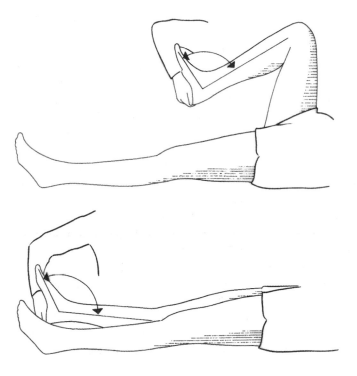

Fig. 3.1.2 (a) The Silverskiöld test differentiates tightness of the gastrocnemius and the soleus. In this test, the knee is flexed to 90°, the hindfoot is positioned in varus, and maximal dorsiflexion obtained. (b) As the knee is extended, if the ankle moves towards plantarflexion, contracture of the gastrocnemius is present.

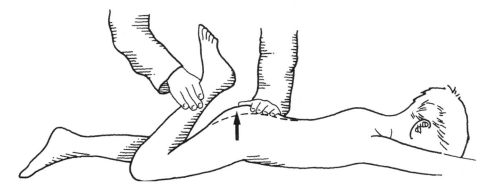

Fig. 3.1.3 The Duncan–Ely test exploits the fact that the rectus femoris is a hip-flexor and knee-extensor. The patient is positioned in prone. The knee is flexed. Flexion of the hip indicates the presence of rectus femoris contracture.

of the monoarticular vastii and the biarticular rectus femoris. However, Perry et al. (1976) showed that when these tests are performed in conjunction with fine-wire electromyography, both the monoarticular and the biarticular muscles crossing the joint will contract. For example, in the non-anesthetized patient, the Duncan–Ely test will induce contraction of not only the rectus femoris but also the iliopsoas, and the Silverskiöld test will induce contraction of both the gastrocnemius and the soleus. Under general anesthesia, however, these biarticular muscle tests will reliably demonstrate contracture of the biarticular muscle involved. Consequently, they should routinely be included as part of the presurgical examination under anesthesia.

HIP

The Thomas test is used to measure the degree of hip-flexor tightness. It is performed with the patient in a supine position and the pelvis held such that the anterior and posterior superior iliac spine (ASIS and the PSIS) are aligned vertically. Defining the pelvic position consistently rather than using the 'flatten the lordosis' method improves reliability. Hip-adductor tightness can be distinguished from gracilis, semimembranosus, and semitendinosus tightness by measuring hip abduction three ways with the patient supine: hip and knee both flexed (measures the length of adductors only), hip in neutral with the knee flexed off the side of the table (measures length of the adductors and gracilis), and hip in neutral and knee in full extension (measures the length of gracilis, medial hamstrings and adductors). Because of the origin and insertion points, the flexion and extension combinations of the hip and knee joint will help decipher which medial thigh muscles are tight. Stabilization of the pelvis is imperative for a correct measurement.

KNEE

A knee-flexion contracture can be caused by four components: (1) shortened hamstrings, (2) shifted hamstrings due to excessive anterior tilt, (3) shortened proximal gastrocnemius, and (4) capsular contracture. Measurements that reflect positional changes of the biarticular muscle groups are especially important at the knee since many biarticular muscles cross this joint. We routinely evaluate the degree of 'hamstring shift'. Hamstring shift is calculated by first measuring the unilateral popliteal angle, then the bilateral popliteal angle, and finding the difference between the two (Fig. 3.1.4a). 'Unilateral popliteal angle' is measured in the patient's normal resting supine position. The contralateral hip is in full extension, while the ipsilateral hip is flexed to 90°. The knee is then extended until the first endpoint of resistance is felt. The measurement of the degrees lacking from full extension will give the connective tissue and resting muscle extensibility. Cusick (1990) stated that the findings pertaining to the initial endpoint are more significant to functional ability than the stretched endpoint findings. The 'bilateral popliteal angle' measurement is done with the ipsilateral hip flexed to 90° and the contralateral hip flexed until the ASIS and PSIS are aligned vertically (comparable to the test for hip-flexion contracture described above) (Fig. 3.1.4b). If there is a significant 'hamstring shift', the popliteal angle, which is a measure of hamstring contracture, will significantly decrease as the pelvis is tipped posteriorly. The value of the popliteal angle with a neutral pelvis is a measure of the 'true hamstring contracture' and the value with the lordosis present is the 'functional hamstring contracture'. The difference between the two represents the degree of hamstring shift. Measurement of capsular tightness by fully extending the knee, with the hip in extension, completes the assessment of the knee.

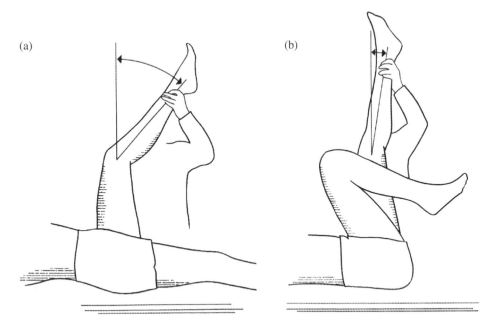

Fig. 3.1.4 Unilateral and bilateral popliteal angles are measured to calculate the hamstring shift. (a) The unilateral popliteal angle is measured with typical lordosis, contralateral hip extended, and the ipsilateral hip flexed to 90°. The number recorded is the degrees missing from full extension at the point of first resistance. (b) Bilateral popliteal angle is measured with the contralateral hip flexed until the ASIS and PSIS are vertical.

Excessive anterior pelvic tilt, which is common in diplegic and quadriplegic cerebral palsy, will produce a 'hamstring shift' in conjunction with an apparent knee flexion contracture (Hoffinger et al. 1993, Delp et al. 1996, Schutte et al. 1997). However, in children with crouch gait, hamstring length is frequently normal or even long. In this situation surgical lengthening of the hamstrings often serves to produce further weakening of hip extension, and exacerbates the excessive length of the hamstrings, with resultant additional hip flexion, anterior pelvic tilt and lumbar lordosis. Because of the relative length of the hamstring moment-arm at the hip and knee, Delp et al. (1996) estimated that for every 1° of excessive pelvic lordosis, there is a 2° increase in knee flexion. A hamstring shift > 20° is usually indicative of excessive anterior tilt either from tight hip flexor musculature, weak abdominals, or weak hip-extensors (Delp et al. 1996). Normal popliteal angle measurements of a 5- to 18-year-old should be 0°–49° for optimal functioning (mean 26°) (Katz et al. 1992). A 50° popliteal angle would be considered a mild deviation. Because of the difficulty in establishing dynamic hamstring length on physical exam and the danger of iatrogenic problems with excessive lengthening, dynamic hamstring length estimates should be obtained using gait analysis prior to consideration of any hamstring lengthening surgery.

Bone deformity

ANTEVERSION
Anteversion refers to the relationship between the axes of the femoral neck and the femoral condyles. This alignment is typically assessed as part of the static examination in the prone position (Fig 3.1.5).

Children with cerebral palsy commonly have excessive femoral anteversion, as do children with hypotonia and/or ligamentous laxity. Common compensations for excessive femoral anteversion to cover the femoral head include internal rotation of the femur and/or increase pelvic tilt. This, in turn, promotes the posture of internal limb rotation and excessive lumbar lordosis during gait that is common in children with cerebral palsy.

PATELLA ALTA
Patella alta is common in children who walk with excessive knee flexion. To screen for patella alta, the patient is positioned supine, knees extended. The top of the patella is then palpated. The superior edge of the patella is typically one finger width proximal to the adductor tubercle. Extensor lag is measured with the patient positioned supine, and the legs draped over the edge of the table. Extensor lag is defined as the difference between the active range and the passive range of motion during knee extension in this position (Fig. 3.1.6). Extensor lag is suggestive of patella alta and is indicative of quadriceps insufficiency. Patellar position can be measured with a lateral x-ray of the knee, taken in full extension (see Chapter 3.4).

TIBIAL TORSION
Tibial torsion can be measured three ways by physical examination: (1) measurement of a thigh–foot angle, (2) measurement of a bi-malleolar axis, or (3) the 2nd toe test. The

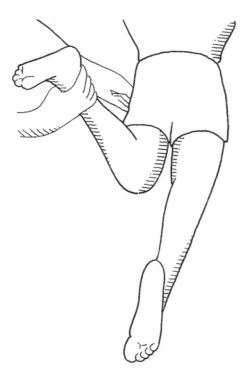

Fig. 3.1.5 Femoral anteversion. The clinician palpates the point of maximal trochanteric prominence. With the fulcrum of the goniometer at the midpoint of the knee, measurement of the angle of the tibia from the vertical is femoral anteversion.

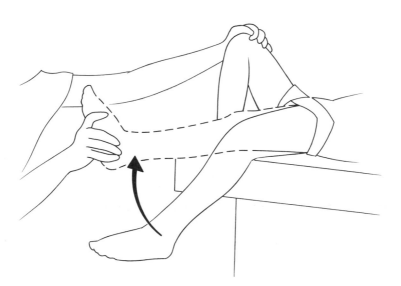

Fig. 3.1.6 Extensor lag. The patient is positioned supine. One knee is flexed and placed on the end of the mat to eliminate a total extension pattern. The patient is asked to straighten their free knee as far as possible. The difference between the active and passive knee extension is the extensor lag.

195

thigh–foot axis is measured with the patient prone. Hindfoot mobility is imperative for proper alignment (Fig. 3.1.7).

In a child with foot deformities, the bimalleolar axis may be more accurate than the thigh–foot angle. For the bimalleolar axis, the patient is positioned supine (Fig. 3.1.8). The benefit of the bimalleolar axis measurement is that the alignment and position of the foot does not impact the measurement. The 2nd-toe test allows visualization of the foot-progression angle with the knee extended. It eliminates the rotational component of knee movement, but requires that the foot be placed in subtalar neutral alignment (Fig. 3.1.9 a-c, Video 3.1.1 on Interactive Disc). In children with equinus contracture and/or severe varus or valgus foot deformities, therefore, this test cannot be performed accurately. Despite the absence of tibia torsion, the presence of a true knee valgus will increase the measurement of the 2nd toe test by the amount of true valgus that is present. Given the significant effect of even relatively minor degrees of tibial torsion on lever-arm dysfunction, none of these measures have been shown to be accurate enough to guide the amount of surgical correction. Therefore other methods of detection and measurement of tibial torsion are necessary. We have also been relying on the definition of tibial torsion using patient-specific data from motion analysis (the difference between the functional knee and bimalleolar axes) (Schwartz and Rozumalski 2005). Some centers may rely on computed tomography (CT) measurement of tibial torsion.

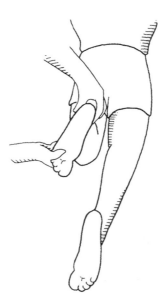

Fig. 3.1.7 Thigh–foot angle. The patient is positioned prone. Flex the knee to 90°, position hindfoot vertically, dorsiflex ankle to 90° taking care to avoid talonavicular subluxation. Place proximal arm of goniometer along posterior axis of femur, distal arm bisects the axis of the hindfoot with the point between the 2nd and 3rd metatarsals. The thigh–foot angle is the measurement of the angle.

Fig. 3.1.8 Mark the midpoints of the medial and lateral malleolus. With the knee fully extended in the supine position rotate the thigh segment until the medial and lateral femoral condyles are parallel in the frontal plane (a modified angle-finder can be used). Place the angle-finder on the malleoli. Using the angle-finder, document the angle between the malleolar axis and the condylar axis. This is the bimalleolar axis.

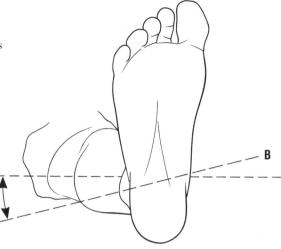

(a)

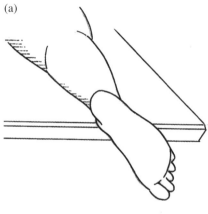

(b)

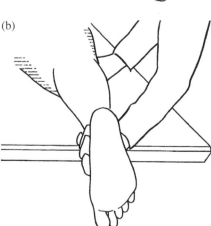

Fig. 3.1.9 The 2nd toe test (a) is a third method of measurement of tibial torsion. To perform this test, the foot must be flexible or well aligned. (b) Begin with the patient's knee fully extended, rotate the leg to position the 2nd toe pointing directly toward the floor. (c) Hold the thigh in this position while flexing the knee. Measure the angle from vertical. (See also Video 3.1.1 on the Interactive Disc.)

(c)

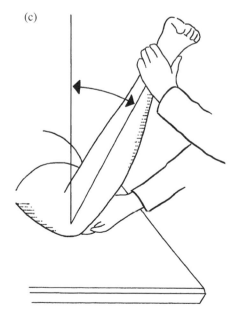

197

LEG LENGTH

Good assessment of limb-length inequality can be complicated by scoliosis, hip subluxation, pelvic obliquity, unilateral contracture of the hip-adductors, knee-flexion contracture, as well as other lower-extremity biomechanical abnormalities that would contribute to a functional limb length inequality. Clinical assessment requires good precision for repeatability and accuracy. Clinical limb length can be measured in supine using the inferior border of the ASIS and the distal aspect of the medial malleolus, or standing using blocks to equalize the ASIS or the iliac crest height. Radiographic assessment may be necessary if too many of these compounding factors are present on PE (see Chapter 3.4).

Posture and balance

Assessment of posterior, anterior, and mediolateral equilibrium responses should not be neglected when planning treatment. Many children with cerebral palsy will have delayed or deficient posterior equilibrium responses. Assessment of posture, including trunk, pelvis, and lower-extremity posture in static standing and during walking in the sagittal and coronal planes will often give insight to areas of weakness, poor motor control, and the compensation strategies that the child is using to circumvent them.

Gait by observation

Observational gait analysis consists of observing a subject without the use of formal gait analysis equipment. To improve the ability to make appropriate determinations and address all deviations, subtle and obvious, a systematic method should be used (Fig. 3.1.10). Various forms and scales have been developed to assist the observer in organizing the analysis as well as for reporting the observations (Perry 1992, Wren et al. 2007, Brown et al. 2008). The Observational Gait Scale (Mackey et al. 2003), and the Edinburgh Visual Gait Score (Wren et al. 2007) have been validated. However, they are scales for outcome measurement and may not fully describe what the clinician is seeing. Krebs et al. (1985) reported that observational gait analysis is more consistent with a single observer. They further observed that viewing a video of a patient walking is more consistent with both single and multiple observers than viewing the subject live with repeated walks. If slow-motion video is employed, they found that the consistency of observation improved markedly. The speed at which observers are able to process dynamic images of gait is much slower than the speed at which changes are taking place as someone walks. Many activities are occurring simultaneously at different joints, and in different planes. The brain can process only a few events at a time. Many gait abnormalities cannot be perceived without quantitative measurement of kinematics. In addition, the compensations that the patient employs may mask the primary gait deviations.

Currently, computerized gait analysis cannot provide much information about foot deformities. Consequently, careful clinical examination, weightbearing radiographs, and dynamic video in and out of current bracing or shoe wear is helpful. In addition, close-up video of the feet from all sides as well as video documentation of a Root sign (Fig. 3.1.11) (Root 1970). Forefoot wedging can also be done to assess the response of the foot to a variety of positions.

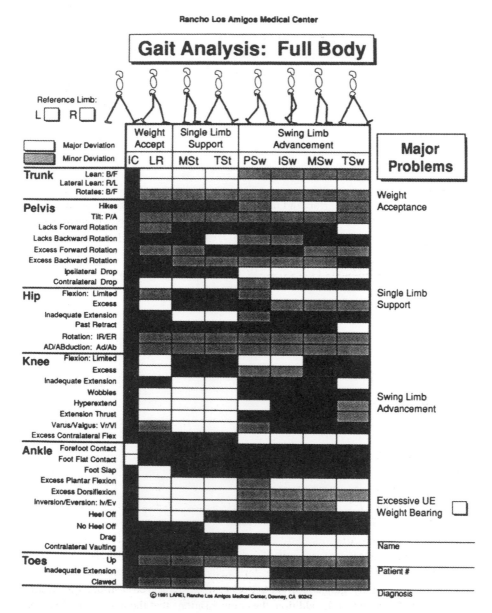

Fig. 3.1.10 Rancho gait by observation form (or Visual Gait Assessment) is an example of a gait-by-observation approach used to document deviations during ambulation. UE, upper extremity.

(a)

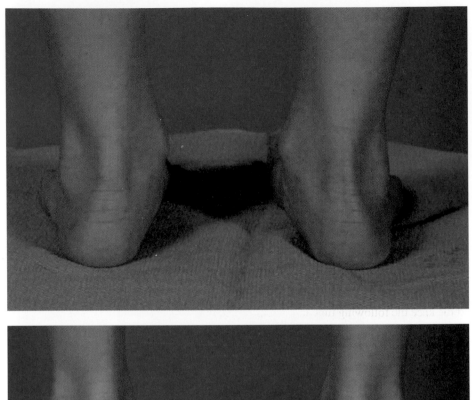

(b)

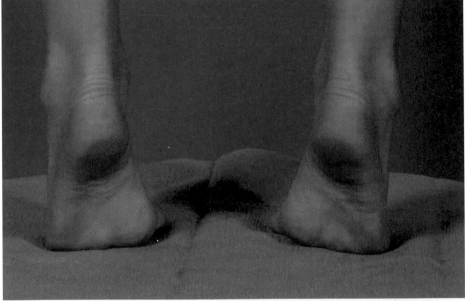

Fig. 3.1.11 (a) Flexible flat foot. (b) The Root test demonstrates a reconstitution of the medial longitudinal arch with inversion of the hindfoot during heel raises.

Finally, beginning with the feet during ambulation at initial contact, here are several questions which should be asked to complete GBO:

(1) What is the position of the foot at the end of terminal swing? Is the foot neutral or is it in a varus or valgus position?
(2) Is the ankle in a neutral position or equinus?
(3) Which portion of the foot contacts the floor first? Why?
(4) What is the foot-progression angle during stance and swing with respect to both the line of progression and the alignment of the knee?
(5) Is the foot plantigrade in stance?
(6) Does the foot maintain its appropriate contour throughout stance, for example, does the forefoot maintain its alignment with the hindfoot, and is the arch maintained?
(7) At which point in the cycle does any deviation in the foot occur?
(8) Does the foot go through the normal sequence of rockers, or is there premature plantarflexion in midstance, or delayed dorsiflexion in terminal stance?
(9) What are the positions of the toes in stance and swing? Is there toe clawing that is occurring in stance, or hyperextension of the first metatarsophalangeal joint in swing?

At the knee the following functions should be noted:

(1) What are the positions of the knee in terminal swing and at initial contact?
(2) Is there a loading response present?
(3) Does the knee come to full extension at any point in stance? If so, when?
(4) Does the knee hyperextend, or is the extension controlled?
(5) What is the maximum knee flexion in swing? When does it occur? Is it adequate for foot clearance?
(6) What is the knee position during stance and swing?
(7) Is the knee aligned with the foot?
(8) Is the shank aligned with the thigh?
(9) Is there a varus or valgus motion during loading?

Gait by observation is more difficult proximally. The mass of the trunk, and the soft tissue around the hips and pelvis, frequently obscure the motions that are occurring at these joints. Since selective motor control tends to be better in the proximal and worse in the distal joints, compensatory motions for distal gait problems often occur proximally *via* hip or trunk motion. However, without computerized gait analysis, it is difficult to determine whether the abnormal movements are compensations, or primary deviations. In looking at the trunk, pelvis, and hips it is necessary to note the following:

(1) Are the thigh and knee aligned to the plane of progression at initial contact? If not is the malrotation internal or external?
(2) Is there full hip extension in terminal stance?
(3) Is there excessive hip abduction in swing?

(4) What is the pelvic position? Is it excessively anterior or posterior?

(5) Are asymmetrical pelvic rotation and/or obliquity present?

(6) What are the trunk movements in each plane? Are these appropriate?

(7) Are the abnormal motions likely to be primary or compensatory?

(8) How are the arms moving during gait? Are they moving symmetrically and reciprocally or are they postured?

(9) Does the child elevate his/her arms to assist with balance?

And finally, some general questions to be considered in a GBO analysis:

(1) Is the stride length adequate and are the step lengths symmetrical?

(2) Does the walking pattern appear to be efficient or is there excessive body motion or other indications of excessive energy consumption?

(3) What influence do assistive devices or orthoses have on the child's walking pattern?

A comprehensive problem list can be derived by combining synthesizing the clinical examination, imaging data, GBO and 3-dimensional motion analysis information. Each piece of the examination process provides critical and unique information. It is necessary to fit this information together to get a complete picture of the child's gait problems and derive an appropriate treatment plan.

REFERENCES

Barry MJ, VanSwearingen JM, Albright, AL (1999) Reliability and responsiveness of the Barry–Albright Dystonia Scale. *Dev Med Child Neurol* **41**: 404–11.

Berry ET, Giuliani CA, Damiano DL (2004) Intrasession and intersession reliability of handheld dynamometry in children with cerebral palsy. *Pediatr Phys Ther* **16**: 191–8.

Bohannon RW (1989) Is the measurement of muscle strength appropriate in patients with brain lesions? A special communication. *Phys Ther* **69**: 225–36.

Bohannon RW, Smith MB (1987) Interrater reliability of a modified Ashworth scale of muscle spasticity. *Phys Ther* **67**: 206–7.

Boyd RN, Graham HK (1999) Objective measurement of clinical findings in the use of botulinum toxin type A for the management of children with cerebral palsy. *Eur J Neurol* **6**: s23.

Brown CR, Hillman SJ, Richardson AM, Herman JL, Robb JE (2008) Reliability and validity of the Visual Gait Assessment Scale for children with hemiplegic cerebral palsy when used by experienced and inexperienced observers. *Gait Posture* **27**: 648–52.

Clopton N, Dutton J, Featherston T, Grigsby A, Mobley J, Melvin J (2005) Interrater and intrarater reliability of the Modified Ashworth Scale in children with hypertonia. *Pediatr Phys Ther* **17**: 268–73.

Cusick BD, editor (1990) *Progressive Casting and Splinting*. Tucson, AZ: Therapy Skill Builders.

Daltroy LH, Liang MH, Fossel AH, Goldberg MJ (1998) The POSNA pediatric musculoskeletal functional health questionnaire: report on reliability, validity, and sensitivity to change. Pediatric Outcomes Instrument Development Group. Pediatric Orthopaedic Society of North America. *J Pediatr Orthop* **18**: 561–71.

Damiano DL, Abel MF (1998) Functional outcomes of strength training in spastic cerebral palsy. *Arch Phys Med Rehabil* **79**: 119–25.

Damiano DL, Vaughan CL, Abel MF (1995) Muscle response to heavy resistance exercise in children with spastic cerebral palsy. *Dev Med Child Neurol* **37**: 731–9.

Damiano DL, Dodd K, Taylor NF (2002a) Should we be testing and training muscle strength in cerebral palsy? *Dev Med Child Neurol* **44**: 68–72.

Damiano DL, Quinlivan JM, Owen BF, Payne P, Nelson KC, Abel MF (2002b) What does the Ashworth scale really measure and are instrumented measures more valid and precise? *Dev Med Child Neurol* **44**: 112–18.

Delp SL, Loan JP, Hoy MG, Zajac FE, Topp EL, Rosen JM (1990) An interactive graphics-based model of the lower extremity to study orthopaedic surgical procedures. *IEEE Trans Biomed Eng* **37**: 757–67.

Delp SL, Statler K, Carroll NC (1995) Preserving plantar flexion strength after surgical treatment for contracture of the triceps surae: a computer simulation study. *J Orthop Res* **13**: 96–104.

Delp SL, Arnold, AS, Speers RA, Moore CA (1996) Hamstrings and psoas lengths during normal and crouch gait: implications for muscle-tendon surgery. *J Orthop Res* **14**: 144–51.

Desloovere K, Molenaers G, Feys H, Huenaerts C, Callewaert B, Van de Walle P (2006) Do dynamic and static clinical measurements correlate with gait analysis parameters in children with cerebral palsy? *Gait Posture* **24**: 302–13.

Engsberg JR, Olree KS, Ross SA, Park TS (1996) Quantitative clinical measure of spasticity in children with cerebral palsy. *Arch Phys Med Rehabil* **77**: 594–9.

Gage JR (1991) *Gait Analysis in Cerebral Palsy*. London: Mac Keith Press.

Graham HK, Harvey A, Rodda J, Nattrass GR, Pirpiris M (2004) The Functional Mobility Scale (FMS). *J Pediatr Orthop* **24**: 514–20.

Gregson JM, Leathley M, Moore AP, Sharma AK, Smith TL, Watkins CL (1999) Reliability of the Tone Assessment Scale and the Modified Ashworth Scale as clinical tools for assessing poststroke spasticity. *Arch Phys Med Rehabil* **80**: 1013–16.

Harvey A, Graham HK, Morris ME, Baker R, Wolfe R (2007) The Functional Mobility Scale: ability to detect change following single event multilevel surgery. *Dev Med Child Neurol* **49**: 603–7.

Haugh AB, Pandyan AD, Johnson GR (2006) A systematic review of the Tardieu Scale for the measurement of spasticity. *Disabil Rehabil* **28**: 899–907.

Hoffinger SA, Rab GT, Abou-Ghaida H (1993) Hamstrings in cerebral palsy crouch gait. *J Pediatr Orthop* **13**: 722–6.

Jethwa A, Fehlings D, Macarthur C (2007) The development and evaluation of the Hypertonia Assessment Tool-Discriminant (HAT-D): a discriminative tool differentiating types of hypertonia in children. *Paediatr Child Health* **12** (Suppl A): 133–4.

Katz K, Rosenthal A, Yosipovitch Z (1992) Normal ranges of popliteal angle in children. *J Pediatr Orthop* **12**: 229–31.

Kendall HO, Kendall FP, Wadsworth GE, editors (1971) *Muscle Testing and Function*, 2nd edn. London: Williams and Wilkins.

Kramer JF, MacPhail HE (1994) Relationships among measures of walking effiency, gross mototr ability, and isokinetic stregth in adolescents with cerebral palsy. *Pediatr Phys Ther* **6**: 3–8.

Krebs DE, Edelstein JE, Fishman S (1985) Reliability of observational kinematic gait analysis. *Phys Ther* **65**: 1027–33.

Lee KC, Carson L, Kinnin E, Patterson V (1989) The Ashworth Scale: a reliable and reproducible method of measuring spasticity. *J Neurorehabil* **3**: 205–9.

Macfarlane TS, Larson CA, Stiller C (2008) Lower extremity muscle strength in 6- to 8-year-old children using hand-held dynamometry. *Pediatr Phys Ther* **20**: 128–36.

Mackey AH, Lobb GL, Walt SE, Stott NS (2003) Reliability and validity of the Observational Gait Scale in children with spastic diplegia. *Dev Med Child Neurol* **45**: 4–11.

Novacheck TF, Stout JL, Tervo R (2000) Reliability and validity of the Gillette Functional Assessment Questionnaire as an outcome measure in children with walking disabilities. *J Pediatr Orthop* **20**: 75–81.

Perry J (1992) *Gait Analysis: Normal and Pathological Function*. Thorofare, NJ: Slack.

Perry J, Hoffer MM, Giovan P, Antonelli D, Greenberg R (1974) Gait analysis of the triceps surae in cerebral palsy. A preoperative and postoperative clinical and electromyographic study. *J Bone Joint Surg Am* **56**: 511–20.

Perry J, Hoffer MM, Antonelli D, Plut J, Lewis G, Greenberg R (1976) Electromyography before and after surgery for hip deformity in children with cerebral palsy. A comparison of clinical and electromyographic findings. *J Bone Joint Surg Am* **58**: 201–8.

Root L (1970) Functional testing of the posterior tibial muscle in spastic paralysis. *Dev Med Child Neurol* **12**: 592–5.

Rosenbaum P, Stewart D (2004) The World Health Organization International Classification of Functioning, Disability, and Health: a model to guide clinical thinking, practice and research in the field of cerebral palsy. *Semin Pediatr Neurol* **11**: 5–10.

203

Sanger TD, Delgado MR, Gaebler-Spira D, Hallett M, Mink JW (2003) Classification and definition of disorders causing hypertonia in chilhood. *Pediatr* **111**: 89–97.

Schutte LM, Hayden SW, Gage JR (1997) Lengths of hamstrings and psoas muscles during crouch gait: effects of femoral anteversion. *J Orthop Res* **15**: 615–21.

Schwartz MH, Rozumalski A (2005) A new method for estimating joint parameters from motion data. *J Biomechan* **38**: 107–16.

Tervo RC, Azuma S, Stout J, Novacheck T (2002) Correlation between physical functioning and gait measures in children with cerebral palsy. *Dev Med Child Neurol* **44**: 185–90.

Wadsworth CT, Krishnan R, Sear M, Harrold J, Nielsen DH (1987) Intrarater reliability of manual muscle testing and hand-held dynametric muscle testing. *Phys Ther* **67**: 1342–7.

Wiley ME, Damiano DL (1998) Lower-extremity strength profiles in spastic cerebral palsy. *Dev Med Child Neurol* **40**: 100–7.

Wren TA, Do KP, Hara R, Dorey FJ, Kay RM, Otsuka NY (2007) Gillette Gait Index as a gait analysis summary measure: comparison with qualitative visual assessments of overall gait. *J Pediatr Orthop* **27**: 765–8.

3.2
FOOT BIOMECHANICS AND PATHOLOGY

Sue Sohrweide

Leonardo da Vinci stated that the human foot is both a masterpiece of engineering and a work of art. The healthy foot satisfies the seemingly paradoxical requirements of both shock absorption and thrust through an interaction of interrelated joints, connective tissue and muscles (Neumann 2002). This chapter provides a review of the bony anatomy of the foot and ankle complex, and the biomechanics of foot and ankle function, as well as giving a comprehensive evaluation of foot alignment in both the non-weightbearing and weightbearing positions.

Overview of bony anatomy

The foot and ankle complex consists of 28 individual bones (Fig. 3.2.1). The distal ends of the thin and long fibula laterally, and the thicker tibia medially, serve as a mortise for the second largest tarsal bone, the talus. The talus can be easily recognized by its large rounded head, broad articular facet on its upper surface, and by the two articular facets separated by a deep groove on its underside concave surface (Gray 1974). The plantar surface of the talus articulates with the calcaneus (os calcis), the largest of the tarsal bones and one that is well suited to accept the impact of the heel during walking (Neumann 2002). The head of the talus is quite prominent, and projects forward and medially to articulate with the navicular. The navicular, so named for its resemblance to a ship, has a concave proximal surface that articulates with the head of the talus. Distally, its surface articulates with the three cuneiform bones, so named for their wedge-like shape. The medial (1st), intermediate (2nd), and lateral (3rd) cuneiforms contribute to the creation of the transverse arch of the foot. The lateral cuneiform articulates with the cuboid, the most lateral of the tarsal bones, and so named for its six surfaces, three of which make articulation with adjacent bones (Neumann 2002). The five metatarsal bones articulate with the cuneiforms and cuboid proximally, and with the phalanges distally. The metatarsals are numbered from one through five, with the 1st metatarsal being the thickest, shortest, and most medial of the metatarsals. The 5th metatarsal is characterized by the tubercular eminence on the outer side of its base, serving as an attachment site for the peroneus brevis muscle. Each metatarsal has a slightly concave base (proximally), a shaft, and a rounded head (distal). The most distal bones comprising the foot are the phalanges, 14 in number, and referred to as proximal, middle, and distal. The 2nd–5th toes have a proximal, middle, and distal phalanx. The great toe has only a proximal and distal phalanx.

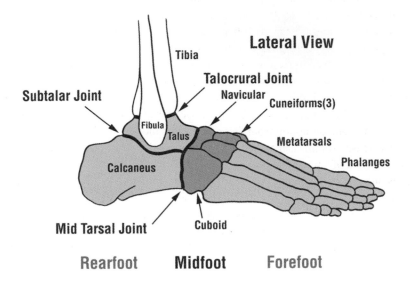

Fig. 3.2.1 Terminology to describe the bony anatomy and joints of the foot and ankle complex.

Articulations and functional divisions

Different terminology is often used by the various disciplines which deal with the foot and ankle, leading to possible misunderstanding and confusion. The following discussion regarding the articulations and functional divisions of the foot and ankle provides a uniform and consistent terminology for understanding both the simple and the complex aspects of the foot and ankle (Fig. 3.2.1).

The tibia, fibula and talus make up the ankle or talocrural joint. The articulation of the talus with the calcaneus is known as the subtalar or talocalcaneal joint. The calcaneus and cuboid laterally, along with the talus and navicular medially, create a complex joint commonly referred to as the midtarsal joint. This joint is also known as the transverse tarsal, or Chopart's, joint, and is S-shaped when viewed superiorly. The term '1st ray' refers to the 1st (medial) cuneiform and 1st metatarsal, '2nd ray' refers to the 2nd metatarsal and 2nd (intermediate) cuneiform, and '3rd ray' refers to the 3rd metatarsal and 3rd (lateral) cuneiform. The terms 4th and 5th ray refers to the 4th and 5th metatarsals only. The portion of the foot that lies behind the midtarsal joint (i.e. talus and calcaneus) is referred to as the rearfoot or hindfoot, with everything that lies in front of the midtarsal joint referred to as the forefoot. The forefoot can be further broken down into the division known as the midfoot, consisting of the five bones distal to the midtarsal joint, and proximal to the tarsometatarsal joint, i.e. the navicular, cuboid, and three cuneiforms.

Foot and ankle biomechanics

Perhaps the greatest source of confusion regarding the biomechanics of the foot and ankle arises from a lack of understanding of planes and axes of motion that occur within the foot and ankle. The sagittal, coronal (or frontal) and transverse planes are the three cardinal, or single, planes of motion that are most familiar to us (Fig. 3.2.2). The motion that occurs in these cardinal planes occurs through an axis that runs perpendicular to that cardinal plane. In other words, sagittal-plane foot motion (dorsiflexion and plantarflexion) occurs through a medial–lateral axis, coronal-plane foot motions (eversion/inversion) occur through an anterior–posterior axis, and transverse-plane foot motion (abduction/adduction) occurs through a superior–inferior axis. It should be noted that abduction and adduction of the foot occur in a different plane of motion from that of the same motions in the upper and lower extremities. The reason for this is that the foot does not continue in a straight line from the distal leg, but takes a 90° turn. Therefore ab/adduction of the foot occurs about an axis which is perpendicular to the plantar surface of the foot. If the foot were to continue on in a straight line from the leg, abduction and adduction would occur in the frontal plane. Interestingly, the foot has only a few joints whose axis of motion produces movement in only the cardinal planes, namely the 2nd, 3rd and 4th rays (dorsiflexion/plantarflexion), the IP joints (plantarflexion/dorsiflexion) and the MP joints (plantarflexion/dorsiflexion/

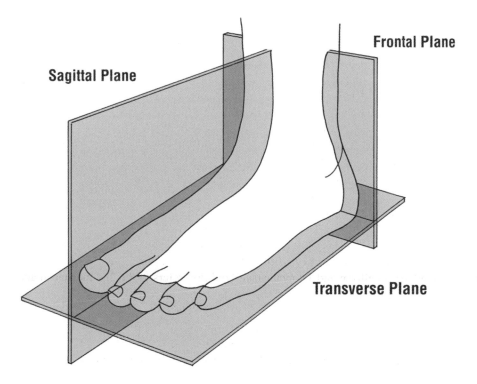

Fig. 3.2.2 The cardinal planes of the foot/ankle.

abduction/adduction). These are only a very small portion of the joints that are part of the foot and ankle complex. So what about the others?

Although the motions of the foot and ankle are defined in terms of these cardinal planes, the axes of motion are not perpendicular to these cardinal planes (Wright et al. 1964, Root et al. 1977). Because of the orientation of these joints, axes of motion pass through all three of the cardinal planes. Therefore motion which occurs at these joints occurs in all three planes, and is thus known as triplanar motion. Triplanar motion follows the all-or-nothing rule – meaning that if motion occurs in one plane, it is obligatory that motion also occurs in the other two. However, the amount of motion occurring in each plane depends entirely on the orientation of that axis and its proximity to the true, cardinal planes of motion. Triplane motion is often broken down into components of motion which are considered major, minor or clinically insignificant. The specific components of motion at each joint are discussed in detail in the sections below.

Pronation and supination are the terms that historically have been used to describe the triplanar motions in the foot and ankle. These two motions are pure rotations about an oblique axis resulting in the same end position as three separate rotations in the cardinal planes (Oatis 1988). Although these are the subject of debate, and are inconsistently used among disciplines, the terms 'pronation' and 'supination' should be used only with regard to the triplane motions of the foot and ankle, as they provide a consistent and logical description of the motion which is anatomically available. With that in mind, one must be aware that these motions of pronation and supination will be different in the foot and lower extremity when comparing the components of motion in an open chain (OC) versus a closed chain (CC) environment. An OC environment refers to a position where the distal segment is free, and therefore movement can only occur distal to the reference joint. OC pronation will produce elements of dorsiflexion, eversion and abduction. OC supination, on the other hand, produces elements of plantarflexion, inversion and adduction. A CC environment refers to a position where the distal body part is fixed, and therefore CC environments produce movement which occurs both proximal and distal to the reference joint (Fig. 3.2.3). CC pronation produces components of internal rotation of the tibia, adduction and plantarflexion of the talus, and eversion of the calcaneus. Because of this, CC pronation will cause a lowering of the medial longitudinal arch height. Pronation is a normal motion that facilitates the ability of the foot to adapt to uneven walking surfaces by unlocking the joints of the foot and creating a 'loose bag of bones'. It also facilitates flexion of the knee, allowing the lower extremity to function as a shock-absorber. In typical gait, pronation is a motion that begins at the time of initial contact, and continues until the time of foot flat in mid-stance. On the other hand, CC supination produces components of external rotation of the tibia, abduction and dorsiflexion of the talus, and inversion of the calcaneus. Because of this, CC supination will cause an increase in the height of the medial longitudinal arch. Supination is a normal motion creating a stable, rigid lever for push-off. This in turn will cause extension at the knee. During typical gait, supination of the foot begins in mid-stance, and peaks just prior to toe-off.

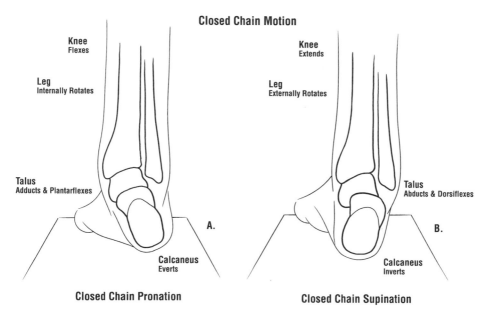

Fig. 3.2.3 Components of motion in closed chain (CC) pronation (A) and closed chain supination (B) of the foot/ankle.

Components of triplanar motion

ANKLE JOINT

The ankle, or talocrural joint, is most widely understood to be a joint which allows the motions of dorsiflexion and plantarflexion in the sagittal plane, with a medial–lateral axis of rotation which passes through the body of the talus and, on average, through the tips of both malleoli. It should be noted that variation in the orientation of this axis occurs within the typically developed population. However, the lateral malleolus is inferior and posterior to the medial malleolus, and therefore, the axis of rotation departs slightly from the pure medial–lateral axis (Fig. 3.2.4). The axis of rotation deviates from a pure medial–lateral axis about 10° in the frontal plane and 6° in the horizontal plane (Neumann 2002). Therefore the motion that does occur at the ankle joint is triplanar – pronation and supination – with the major component being that of dorsiflexion and plantarflexion. Minor components of motion at the ankle joint are ab/adduction, with clinically insignificant amounts of eversion/inversion.

SUBTALAR JOINT

The articulation between the talus and calcaneus is called the subtalar joint (STJ), and it is this joint which allows the foot to assume positions that are independent of the orientation of the ankle and leg above. Although much variation exists from one subject to another, the axis of rotation of the STJ is typically described as a line that pierces the lateral–posterior

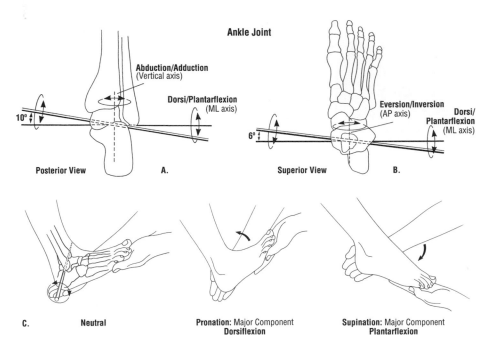

Ankle Joint

Abduction/Adduction
(Vertical axis)

Dorsi/Plantarflexion
(ML axis)

$10°$

Eversion/Inversion
(AP axis)

Dorsi/
Plantarflexion
(ML axis)

$6°$

Posterior View   **A.**   Superior View   **B.**

C.   **Neutral**   **Pronation:** Major Component
Dorsiflexion   **Supination:** Major Component
Plantarflexion

Fig. 3.2.4 The axis of rotation of the ankle joint as viewed posteriorly (A) and superiorly (B). The motion that occurs at the ankle joint is triplanar. Pronation and supination of the ankle joint will produce major components of dorsiflexion and plantarflexion, minor components of abduction and adduction, and clinically insignificant amounts of inversion and eversion (C). AP, anteroposterior; ML, medial–lateral.

heel and courses through the subtalar joint in an anterior, superior and medial direction (Neumann 2002). The typical axis of rotation of the STJ is positioned $42°$ from the horizontal plane and $16°$ from the sagittal plane (Fig. 3.2.5) (Manter 1941). Thus the motion which occurs at the STJ is also triplanar, providing for both pronation and supination. The major components of motion at the subtalar joint are eversion, inversion, abduction and adduction, with clinically insignificant amounts of dorsiflexion and plantarflexion.

MIDTARSAL JOINT

The midtarsal joint, often referred to as the transverse tarsal or Chopart's joint, is the functional articulation between the rearfoot (calcaneus and talus) and the midfoot (navicular and cuboid). Normal range of motion through the midtarsal joint varies dramatically in the literature, but it is generally agreed that motion at this joint rarely functions without an associated movement at nearby joints, especially the STJ (Neumann 2002). Two axes of rotation, the longitudinal axis and the oblique axis, at the midtarsal joint are described. The longitudinal axis runs in a nearly straight anterior–posterior direction (Fig. 3.2.6). Therefore the major component of motion for pronation is eversion, and for supination, inversion. In contrast, the oblique axis has a large vertical and medial–lateral pitch (similar to the ankle

210

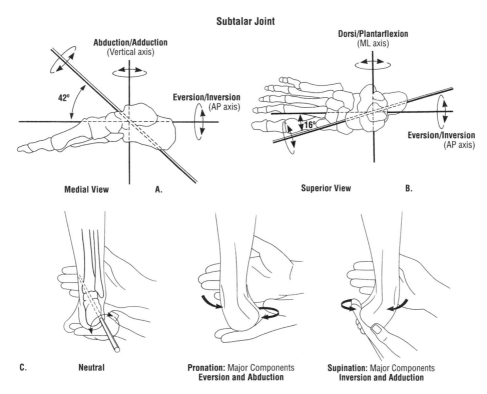

Subtalar Joint

Abduction/Adduction
(Vertical axis)

42°

Eversion/Inversion
(AP axis)

Medial View   A.

Dorsi/Plantarflexion
(ML axis)

16°

Eversion/Inversion
(AP axis)

Superior View   B.

C.   Neutral

Pronation: Major Components
Eversion and Abduction

Supination: Major Components
Inversion and Adduction

Fig. 3.2.5 The axis of rotation of the subtalar joint as viewed medially (A) and superiorly (B). The motion that occurs at the subtalar joint is triplanar. Pronation and supination of the subtalar joint will produce major components of eversion, inversion, abduction, and adduction, with clinically insignificant amounts of dorsiflexion and plantarflexion (C). AP, anteroposterior; ML, medial–lateral.

joint), and therefore the pronation that occurs about this axis has major components of dorsiflexion and abduction, and with supination, plantarflexion and adduction (Fig. 3.2.7). The midtarsal joint, and more specifically the oblique axis of the midtarsal joint, is often referred to as the 'little ankle' because, other than the ankle joint, it is the only place in the foot and ankle where dorsiflexion range of motion is available.

Evaluation of the foot

Despite the complexity of foot anatomy and biomechanics, evaluating the foot and understanding its function in both the non-weightbearing and weightbearing position is essential. As mentioned previously, the foot must function as both a mobile adaptor and a rigid lever at different points in the gait cycle. Correctly identifying structural abnormalities in the non-weightbearing position and the compensations that occur as a result of these abnormalities in weight bearing is essential to determining interventions to improve foot position and the function of the entire lower extremity.

Since every foot has its own neutral subtalar joint (STJ) position, the use of the non-weightbearing subtalar joint neutral position provides consistency in positioning the foot

211

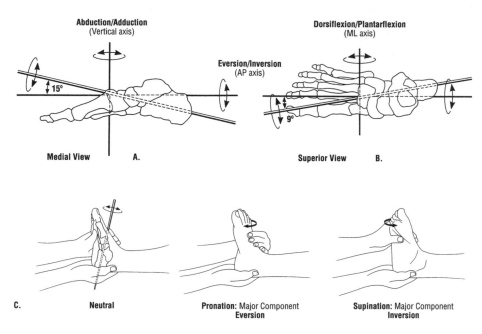

Midtarsal Joint: Longitudinal Axis

Abduction/Adduction
(Vertical axis)

Dorsiflexion/Plantarflexion
(ML axis)

Eversion/Inversion
(AP axis)

15°

9°

Medial View   **A.**

Superior View   **B.**

C.   **Neutral**

Pronation: Major Component
Eversion

Supination: Major Component
Inversion

Fig. 3.2.6 The axis of rotation of the midtarsal joint's longitudinal axis as viewed medially (A) and superiorly (B). Pronation and supination of the longitudinal axis of the midtarsal joint will produce major components of eversion and inversion, with clinically insignificant amounts of dorsiflexion, plantarflexion, abduction and adduction (C). AP, anteroposterior; ML, medial–lateral.

in order to assess and identify patient specific structural abnormalities and their resultant compensations in weightbearing. Root et al. (1977) originally defined subtalar joint neutral (STJN) as the position of the subtalar joint where it is neither pronated nor supinated. In addition, determining STJN and then naming positions of the rearfoot and forefoot in relation to the next most proximal segment is consistent with the orthopaedic naming of deformities in relation to the adjacent, proximal segment. This allows the evaluator a starting point from which to describe compensations/deviations in the foot that may (or may not) occur when going from the non-weightbearing to the weightbearing position.

This position is determined by palpation of the talonavicular joint. The importance of STJN position is controversial. Can the STJN position be reliably determined? Are the normalcy criteria proposed by Root et al. (1971) too restrictive and not clinically practical since few individuals have typical foot and lower-extremity structure? Normal gait may not even include a time when STJN should be obtained (Kirby 2002). However, with experience, rearfoot position in STJN can be identified with fair to good reliability (Pierrynowski et al. 1996, Elli et al. 2008).

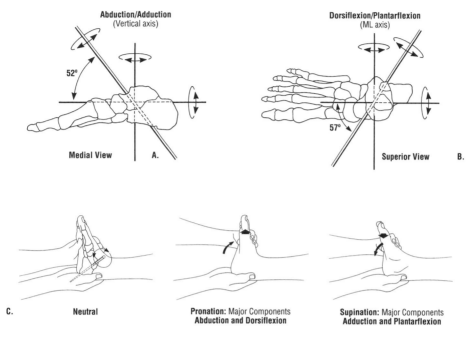

Midtarsal Joint: Oblique Axis

Abduction/Adduction (Vertical axis)

52°

Medial View   A.

Dorsiflexion/Plantarflexion (ML axis)

57°

Superior View   B.

C.   Neutral

Pronation: Major Components
Abduction and Dorsiflexion

Supination: Major Components
Adduction and Plantarflexion

Fig. 3.2.7 The axis of rotation of the midtarsal joint's oblique axis viewed medially (A) and superiorly (B). Pronation and supination of the oblique axis of the midtarsal joint will produce major components of dorsiflexion, abduction, plantarflexion and adduction. Inversion and eversion motion will be clinically insignificant (C). ML, medial–lateral.

Determining subtalar joint neutral (STJN)

Finding STJN is done through palpation at the articulation between the head of the talus and the navicular. Anatomical landmarks are used to assure accurate palpation of the head of the talus and the navicular. STJN is most easily found with the patient in the prone position with their feet hanging off the edge of the examination table. Palpation of the talus is performed with the thumb on the medial margin and the index finger on the lateral margin, while the opposite hand grasps the forefoot with the thumb placed over the 4th and 5th metatarsal heads, and the fingers gentle placed on the dorsum of the foot. Palpation of the head of the talus in non-weightbearing takes advantage of the fact that the foot dorsiflexes and abducts away from the head of the talus with pronation, and plantarflexes and adducts with supination. With pronation, the head of the talus will be felt medially behind the tuberosity of navicular. With supination, the head of the talus will disappear medially, and become prominent over the lateral side of the joint. Congruency of the talonavicular joint will be achieved when neither the medial nor lateral head of the talus protrudes and the examiner feels symmetry of the navicular on the head of the talus. In this position, the forefoot must be loaded against the neutral rearfoot. This is done by applying a gentle dorsiflexion force over metatarsal heads 4 and 5, until a soft end-point is encountered. This

213

force should not be so great as to cause dorsiflexion at the ankle joint. This position is known as the patient's STJN position. From this starting point, the patient's rearfoot and forefoot relationships are evaluated (Video 3.2.1 on Interactive Disc).

Evaluation of the rearfoot position in subtalar joint neutral

Once the foot has been placed in the STJN position, rearfoot position in relationship to the lower third of the leg is assessed (Fig. 3.2.8). By visualizing the relationship of the bisector of the calcaneus relative to the bisector of the lower third of the leg, the rearfoot alignment can be described. If this relationship is linear, the rearfoot position is said to be vertical. If the orientation of the rearfoot with respect to the lower third of the leg is inverted, this position is known as a varus position of the rearfoot. If the line bisecting the calcaneus is everted in relation to the lower third of the leg, this position is referred to as a valgus position of the rearfoot.

Evaluation of the forefoot position in subtalar joint neutral

Once the rearfoot position has been determined, forefoot to rearfoot relationship can be evaluated in each of the three cardinal planes. While maintaining STJN, forefoot position in the frontal plane can be described by assessing the angle between a line which is perpendicular to the bisection of the posterior calcaneus (replicating the plane of the calcaneal condyles) and the plane of the metatarsal heads. In this position, if the plane of the metatarsal heads is in the same plane as the line which is perpendicular to the bisection

Rearfoot Position (Frontal Plane)

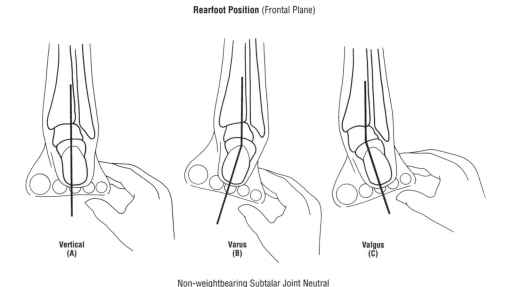

Vertical
(A)

Varus
(B)

Valgus
(C)

Non-weightbearing Subtalar Joint Neutral

Fig. 3.2.8 Evaluation of rearfoot position in relationship to the lower leg in the STJN position. If the relationship is linear, the rearfoot position is described as being vertical (A). If inverted, the rearfoot is said to be in a varus position (B), and if everted, the rearfoot is said to be in a valgus position (C).

214

of the calcaneus, the forefoot position is described as being neutral (Fig. 3.2.9). If the plane of the forefoot in relationship to the rearfoot shows the medial side of the foot to be higher than the lateral side (forefoot inverted) this position is described as a forefoot varus deformity (Fig. 3.2.10). If the opposite is seen, i.e. the lateral border of the foot is higher than the medial border (forefoot everted), this position is described as being a forefoot valgus deformity (Fig. 3.2.11). Typically, two types of forefoot valgus deformities exist. The first demonstrates that all of the metatarsal heads are everted, and this is referred to as a total forefoot valgus. The second is caused by plantarflexion of the 1st ray (1st cuneiform + 1st metatarsal), while the 2nd–5th metatarsal heads lie in the appropriate plane. The relationship of the forefoot to the rearfoot must also be assessed in the sagittal plane (Fig. 3.2.12). If the examiner visualizes a plane representing the ground surface applied to the plantar surface of the calcaneus, the plantar surface of the metatarsal heads should also lie on this plane. If the plane of the metatarsals sits below that of the calcaneus, the forefoot would be described as being plantarflexed in relation to the rearfoot, often referred to as a forefoot equinus deformity. In the transverse plane, the typical relationship between the forefoot and rearfoot requires the forefoot to have the same longitudinal direction as the rearfoot (Fig. 3.2.13). Deviations of the forefoot in the transverse plane toward the midline are referred to as adduction, and away from the midline as abduction.

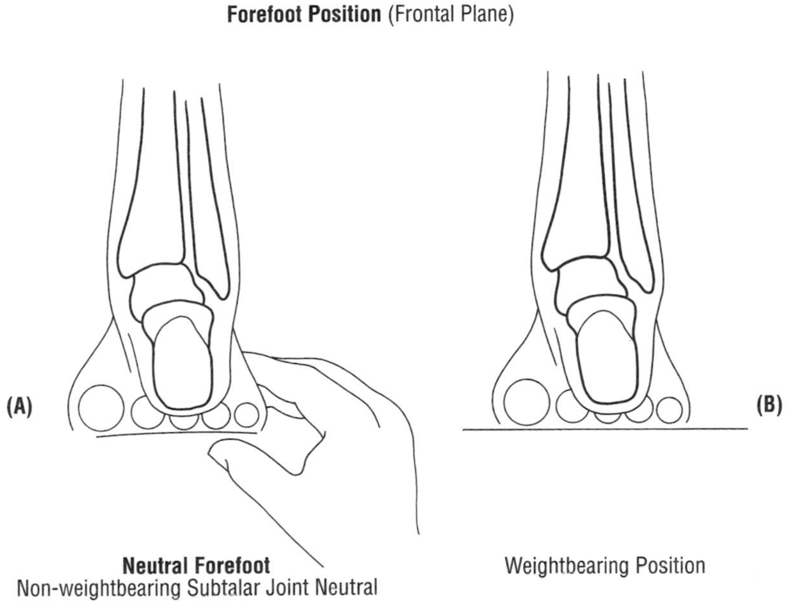

Forefoot Position (Frontal Plane)

(A)

(B)

Neutral Forefoot
Non-weightbearing Subtalar Joint Neutral

Weightbearing Position

Fig. 3.2.9 Evaluation of the STJN forefoot position in the frontal plane. If the plane of the metatarsal heads lies in the same plane as a line which is perpendicular to the bisection of the calcaneus, the forefoot position is described as neutral (A). No compensation is required in the weightbearing position (B).

215

Forefoot Position (Frontal Plane)

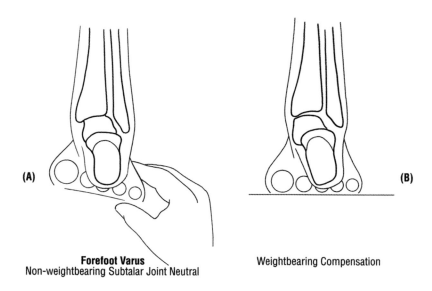

(A)

(B)

Forefoot Varus
Non-weightbearing Subtalar Joint Neutral

Weightbearing Compensation

Fig. 3.2.10 Evaluation of the STJN forefoot position in the frontal plane. If the plane of the metatarsal heads, in relationship to the rearfoot, shows the medial side to be higher than the lateral side (forefoot inverted), the forefoot is described as being in a varus position (A). A typical compensation for a forefoot varus deformity may be abnormal (increased amount) pronation (B).

Compensations

Compensation is defined as a change in the structural alignment or position of the foot to neutralize the effect of an abnormal force resulting in a deviation in structural alignment or position of another part (Gray et al. 1974). Compensations can be normal or abnormal. An athlete who is making a sharp cut to change direction while running requires compensation at the foot and ankle to accommodate the angle at which their foot approaches the ground in order to keep the foot firmly planted on the ground. This would be one example of a normal compensation through the foot and ankle. When structural deformities are present in the foot and ankle, as described in the section above, the foot has the ability to compensate for these deformities. Most often, these compensations occur through the motion of the subtalar and the midtarsal joint. Over time, abnormal compensations can lead to tissue stress and pain, as well as create lever-arm dysfunction which will negatively affect gait and posture.

Forefoot varus

The foot with a structural forefoot varus has an inverted orientation of the forefoot to the rearfoot when placed in the non-weightbearing STJN position. To compensate for this deformity during gait, this foot type typically demonstrates an abnormal amount of pronation

Forefoot Position (Frontal Plane)

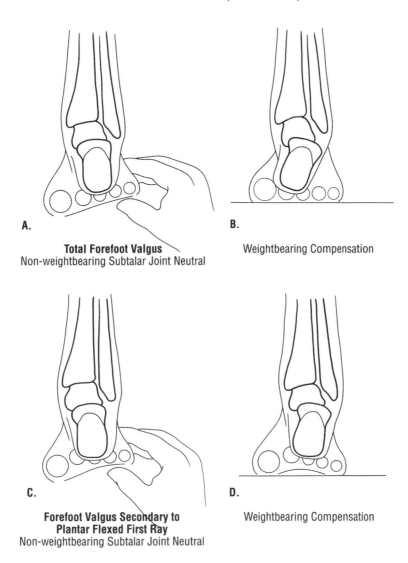

A.

Total Forefoot Valgus
Non-weightbearing Subtalar Joint Neutral

B.

Weightbearing Compensation

C.

**Forefoot Valgus Secondary to
Plantar Flexed First Ray**
Non-weightbearing Subtalar Joint Neutral

D.

Weightbearing Compensation

Fig. 3.2.11 Evaluation of the STJN forefoot position in the frontal plane. If the plane of the metatarsal heads, in relationship to the rearfoot, shows the lateral side to be higher than the medial (forefoot everted), the forefoot is described as being in a valgus position. This position may be secondary to a total forefoot valgus (A), or a plantarflexed 1st ray (C). A typical compensation for a forefoot valgus deformity may be abnormal (increased amount) supination (B and D).

Forefoot Position (Sagittal Plane)

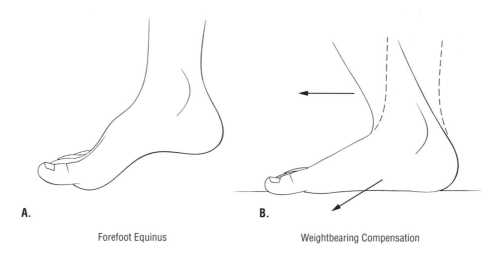

A.

Forefoot Equinus

B.

Weightbearing Compensation

Fig. 3.2.12 Evaluation of the STJN forefoot position in the sagittal plane. If the plane of the metatarsal heads sits below that of the calcaneus, the forefoot position would be described as a forefoot equinus deformity (A). Compensation may occur through the ankle joint or the oblique axis of the midtarsal joint (B).

during mid-stance. The reason for this is the fact that, when the medial calcaneal condyle has reached the ground in mid-stance, the forefoot, rather than being in contact with the floor, demonstrates an orientation where the medial border of the forefoot is elevated from the ground surface. To assist with the medial border reaching the ground, the STJ (if pain and motion allow) will continue pronating as the mid-stance phase of gait begins (Fig. 3.2.10). This excessive pronation is an abnormal compensation, and is manifested as eversion of the calcaneus, abduction of the forefoot, and lowering of the medial longitudinal arch. This compensated foot position leads to internal malrotation of the entire lower extremity as the talus plantarflexes and deviates medially. The clinician must appreciate the influence that the forefoot deformity has on the position of, not only the rearfoot, but the entire lower extremity, and address treatment accordingly. Placing a wedge under the medial forefoot may correct the compensated position of the rearfoot, confirming that the rearfoot position is flexible and being driven by the forefoot deformity. If correction of the rearfoot is not seen, a fixed rearfoot deformity may be present. However, hypermobility of the midfoot and diminished motor control and strength can limit the amount of correction seen with this maneuver.

Forefoot valgus
The foot with a structural forefoot valgus has an everted orientation of the forefoot in relation to the rearfoot when placed in the non-weightbearing STJN position. A typical compensation for this foot deformity may be abnormal supination during mid-stance. As

Forefoot Position (Transverse Plane)

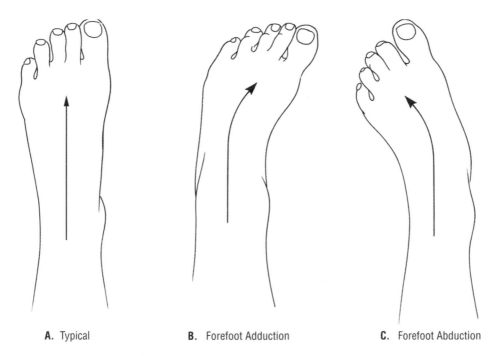

| **A.** Typical | **B.** Forefoot Adduction | **C.** Forefoot Abduction |

Fig. 3.2.13 Evaluation of the STJN forefoot position in the transverse plane. The relationship of the forefoot to the rearfoot should be linear (A). Deviations of the forefoot toward the midline are referred to as forefoot adduction (B) and away from the midline as forefoot abduction (C).

with the forefoot varus deformity, when the medial calcaneal condyle has reached the ground in mid-stance, the forefoot is not plantigrade. With this foot deformity, however, it is the lateral border of the foot which is elevated from the ground surface. In order to get the lateral border of the forefoot on the ground, the STJ (if pain and motion allow) will supinate (Fig. 3.2.11 B, D). This supination is occurring at a time in the gait cycle when the foot should be pronating, and is characterized by inversion of the calcaneus, adduction of the forefoot, and an increase in the height of the medial longitudinal arch. This abnormal compensation can be seen when a total forefoot valgus deformity is present, or with a rigid plantarflexed 1st ray. If a plantarflexed 1st ray is present, it is important to assess its mobility, as the ability or inability of the 1st ray to dorsiflex can greatly affect the way the foot will function in weightbearing. If the plantarflexed 1st ray is mobile, meaning that the 1st ray can be easily dorsiflexed to the level of the other metatarsal heads, this will most likely have little effect on overall foot position in weightbearing. If 1st ray mobility is limited, that is, it can not be dorsiflexed to the level of the other metatarsal heads, the weightbearing foot will function much differently than the foot with a mobile plantarflexed 1st ray. If, on the other hand, the plantarflexed 1st ray is rigid, assessment of rearfoot mobility is also necessary. If the hindfoot is flexible and the forefoot valgus deformity fixed, then correction of the forefoot will secondarily cause correction of the rearfoot. If the hindfoot is not flexible, then correction of the forefoot cannot produce rearfoot correction (Coleman and Chestnut 1977). The Coleman block test is a simple test to help determine the driving force behind the rearfoot position. To perform the test, the lateral border of the forefoot is placed on a block, varying anywhere from 0.5 to 2.5 cm, and the medial forefoot allowed to settle to the floor. If the rearfoot corrects with this test, then treatment should address only the forefoot. If the rearfoot does not correct, then treatment needs to address a combination of the forefoot and rearfoot. Similarly, use of lateral forefoot wedging can be used to assess the role the forefoot plays in the position of the rearfoot when a total forefoot valgus deformity is present.

Forefoot equinus

Forefoot equinus is a position of plantarflexion of the forefoot as compared to the rearfoot (Fig. 3.2.12). If adequate dorsiflexion range of motion is available at the ankle joint, no other compensation is required for this forefoot deformity. If ankle joint dorsiflexion is insufficient, compensation will have to occur through the oblique axis of the midtarsal joint, as that is the only other source of dorsiflexion range of motion in the foot and ankle complex. For this to occur, the STJ must be pronated in order to allow the needed mobility of the midtarsal joint. As with other abnormal compensations, this inappropriate timing and/or range of pronation may cause difficulty with pain and/or gait abnormalities.

Developmental trends

It is essential that those of us who deal with the pediatric patient appreciate normal and abnormal developmental parameters for the various stages of growth. In general, a newborn will demonstrate increased varus positioning of both the forefoot and rearfoot, metatarsus adductus, and excessive range of motion in the subtalar and ankle joints. There is little clinical evidence of a medial longitudinal arch until age 4–5. By 7–8 years of age, the child's foot should have developed the adult values of 0°–2° of rearfoot and forefoot varus, 5°–15° of metatarsus adductus, and significantly less range of motion through the ankle and subtalar joints (Gray et al. 1984). Clinical evaluation of the foot must be directly related to the child's age to determine if the deformity or problem is significant or not.

REFERENCES

Coleman SS, Chestnut WJ (1977) A simple test for hindfoot flexibility in the cavovarus foot. *Clin Orthop* **123**: 60–2.
Elli K, Schwartz M, Sohrweide S, Novacheck T (2008) Reliability of a subtalar joint neutral position. *GCMAS Annual Meeting* 208–9.
Gray G, Tiberio D, Witmer M, editors (1984) *When the Feet Hit the Ground Everything Changes. Neutral Subtalar Position*. Toledo, OH: The American Physical Rehabilitation Network.
Gray H (1974) The lower extremity. In: Pick T, Howden R, editors. *Gray's Anatomy*. Philadelphia, PA: Courage Books. p 203.
Kirby K (2002) Subtalar joint neutral versus tissue stress approach to mechanical foot therapy. In: Rasmussen J, editor. *Foot and Lower Extremity Biomechanics II: Precision Intricast Newsletters, 1997–2002*. Payson, AZ: Precision Intricast. p 9–13.
Manter JT (1941) Movements of the subtalar joint and transverse tarsal joint. *Anat Rec* **80**: 397–410.

Neumann DA (2002) Ankle and foot. In: Pfeiffer M, Weaver S, Folcher M, editors. *Kinesiology of the Musculoskeletal System – Foundations for Physical Rehabilitation*, 1st edn. St Louis, MO: Mosby. p 477–93.

Oatis C (1988) Biomechanics of the foot and ankle under static conditions. *Phys Ther* **68**: 1815.

Pierrynowski MR, Smith MB, Mlynarczyk JH (1996) Proficiency of the foot care specialist to place the rearfoot at subtalar neutral. *J Am Podiatr Med Assoc* **86**: 217–23.

Root, ML, Orien WP, Weed JH, Hughes RJ (1971) *Biomechanical Examination of the Foot*, vol. 1. Los Angeles, CA: Clinical Biomechanics Corp. p 34.

Root ML, Orien WP, Weed JH (1977) *Clinical Biomechanics: Normal and Abnormal Function of the Foot*. Los Angeles, CA: Clinical Biomechanics Corp. p 36.

Siegler S, Chen J, Schneck CD (1988) The three dimensional kinematics and flexibility characteristics of the human ankle and sub-talar joints. *J Biomechan Eng* **110**: 364–73.

Wright DG, Desai SM, Henderson WH (1964) Action of the subtalar joint and ankle joint complex during stance phase of walking. *J Bone Joint Surg Br* **46**: 361–82, 464.

3.3
NEUROIMAGING OF THE BRAIN

Beverly Wical

Neuroimaging adds significantly to our understanding of the pathogenesis and pathophysiology of the heterogeneous group of disorders responsible for cerebral palsy (Korzeniewski et al. 2008). In the newborn and postnatal period, imaging is directed towards identifying conditions or acute injury that may require treatment, as well as those that may be antecedents of cerebral palsy. In the older child, imaging often shows structural changes in the brain associated with motor impairment. Cranial ultrasonography, computed tomography (CT) and magnetic resonance imaging (MRI) are the main modalities utilized.

Cranial ultrasonography of the preterm and newborn brain is a clinical mainstay in identifying injury (Hintz and O'Shea 2008). It is safe, portable, and widely available. It is less sensitive than CT or MRI, however; abnormalities of the brainstem, cerebellum or cerebral convexities are not well visualized. Cranial ultrasound's predictive value may be hampered by interpreter reliability, particularly for less severe lesions (De Vries et al. 2004, Hintz et al. 2007).

CT is acutely sensitive for fresh hemorrhage, and is best for bone and scalp lesions. It is widely available, and the acquisition of images of newborn infants is not as dependent on the specialized skills of technologists as is cranial ultrasonography. Only axial images are typically acquired, limiting views of intracranial contents. Exposure to ionizing radiation occurs, causing concern regarding the amount received by young infants. As few as two or three CT procedures in infants may increase the risk of subsequent malignancy (Brenner and Hall 2007). Definitive long-term risks are still emerging, but we avoid CT in young infants whenever possible.

MRI provides the most detailed structural analysis of the developing brain. It adds to our understanding of the timing of injury, as well as the structural correlates of developmental and acquired disorders causing cerebral palsy. Additional techniques permit visualization of the venous structures and arterial tree. Diffusion weighted MRI, now in wide clinical use, allows the best timing of certain types of brain injury – particularly hypoxic–ischemic encephalopathy, and cerebral infarction. Emerging techniques such as diffusion tensor magnetic imaging allow exquisite delineation of white-matter tracts not previously possible. No ionizing radiation exposure occurs and no harm to humans has yet been identified from exposure to magnetic fields at the strengths used to produce medical images.

Neuroimaging of the fetus at risk for cerebral palsy
In utero ultrasonography is able to identify potential nervous system lesions associated with cerebral palsy. Ventriculomegaly on ultrasound is the most common cause for referral for

fetal MRI. From 18 weeks of gestation onward, MRI images can be obtained successfully from about 95% of fetuses (Zimmerman and Bilaniuk 2006). Despite this, early MRI may not correlate well with postnatal studies. The most common findings associated with fetal ventriculomegaly detected by ultrasonography are hydrocephalus, cortical malformations, or evidence of cerebral destruction due to infarction or hemorrhage. These are typically associated with cerebral palsy.

Neuroimaging of the preterm infant at risk for cerebral palsy

Routine screening cranial ultrasound is recommended between days 7 and 14 of life for infants born <30 weeks gestation; 65%–90% of intraventricular hemorrhage (IVH) occurs by the 7th day of life. Infants of 30–33 weeks gestation remain at risk for IVH, but at a substantially lower rate than children born earlier (Harris et al. 2007). Severe degrees of IVH (Fig. 3.3.1) are more reliably ascertained on ultrasound than mild IVH or white-matter lesions. Subtle abnormalities may be missed (Hintz et al. 2007).

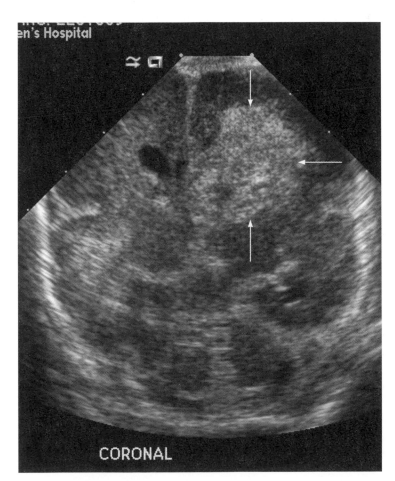

Fig. 3.3.1 Ultrasound of a child born at 24 weeks gestation; now 3 weeks of age (27 weeks). Head ultrasound shows parenchymal injury (arrows) consistent with grade IV IVH.

223

Identification of IVH is clinically important for assessing comorbidities and extent of injury (Hintz et al. 2005). Infants with documented IVH need serial ultrasonography because lesions may enlarge or new hemorrhage may occur. A repeat scan at conceptual age of 36–40 weeks may allow identification of infants with low-pressure ventriculomegaly (associated with white-matter injury) or lesions that increase risk for cerebral palsy but were not identifiable on early scans. Cystic lesions or ventriculomegaly may be found in infants near term with previously normal cranial ultrasounds (Goetz et al. 1995, Ito et al. 1997, Hayakawa et al. 1999).

Although most preterm infants with subsequent cerebral palsy have white-matter lesions on imaging, it is important to note that the majority of children with such abnormalities do not develop cerebral palsy. Of 344 children with ultrasounds documenting white-matter injury, only 24.4% were subsequently diagnosed with cerebral palsy. Of 76 with cystic periventricular leukomalacia, 57% had cerebral palsy. Of 164 children in the cohort diagnosed with cerebral palsy by the age of 2 years, over 30% had normal ultrasounds in the neonatal period (Ancel et al. 2006). Normal early and late cranial ultrasounds were found in 1473 infants with birthweights <1000 g and mean gestational ages of 26 weeks. Cerebral palsy occurred in 9.4% of the infants, and a Bayley Mental Development Index of <70 was found in 25.3% (Laptook et al. 2005).

The use of CT in those born preterm is limited. It may be used to verify findings identified on ultrasound, evaluate extent of hemorrhage, or assess position of intraventricular shunts or drains (Fig. 3.3.2).

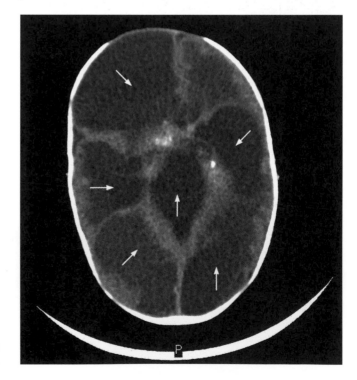

Fig. 3.3.2
CT demonstrating severe hydrocephalus due to meningitis in a child born at 34 weeks gestation. The child died. Arrows indicate fluid filled spaces replacing destroyed brain.

MRI best evaluates white-matter damage, hypoxic–ischemic encephalopathy, or other cerebral injury in the preterm infant. As in all other ages, MRI best delineates cerebral dysgenesis and other malformative processes. Atlases of the fetal and preterm infant brain are available and delineate the ontogenesis of development (Barkovitch 1990, Levine 2005). In early survivors of preterm birth with white-matter injury, MRI yields much more detailed information than screening ultrasounds. Abnormal signal change in the posterior limb of the internal capsule is a marker for significant risk of hemiplegia after grade III or IV IVH. In one study of preterm infants with such signal change on early MRI, all had hemiplegia by 12–24 months of age (De Vries et al. 1999). If the posterior limb of the internal capsule signal was symmetrical bilaterally, all had normal neuromotor outcome. If no abnormal signal is identified near the corona radiata white-matter tract on early MRI, essentially all infants will have a normal motor outcome. Similar findings occur in infants with periventricular leukomalacia. Lesions in the corona radiata above the posterior limb of the internal capsule are highly predictive of adverse motor outcome (Nanba et al. 2007). Early MRI assessment for white-matter injury correlates well with studies done at 18 months of age; this suggests that a second MRI may not be of much value in infants who had an early study (Sie et al. 2005). Moderate to severe white-matter injury on MRI in 167 preterm infants born at <30 weeks gestational age strongly correlated with a subsequent diagnosis of cerebral palsy (Woodward et al. 2006). Figures 3.3.3–6 demonstrate such injuries.

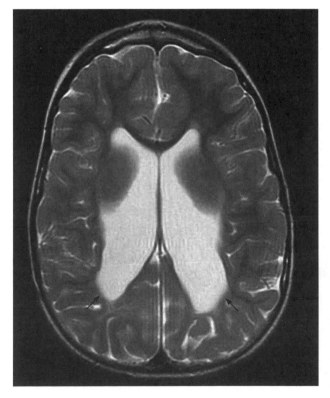

Fig. 3.3.3 MRI of a child with diplegia demonstrates the late sequelae of periventricular leukomalacia. Fluid in ventricles appears white. Ventricles are enlarged due to white-matter loss. Gray areas projecting into ventricles represent normal basal ganglia structure.

Moderate or severe injury was found in 21% of patients but nearly half of them did not have neurodevelopmental impairments when examined at 2 years of age.

Although strongly associated, abnormal imaging studies do not necessarily predict cerebral palsy. The degree and distribution of abnormalities must be must be considered (Dyet et al. 2006). A cohort of adolescents 15 years of age who had been very low-birthweight infants and survived without obvious neurologic impairment underwent MRI. Mild white-matter abnormalities were found in 13/56, yet there was no difference in the neurological examination between those with MRI changes and those without (Gaddlin et al. 2008).

Injury to the cerebellum in very preterm infants is now recognized as a cause of cerebral palsy, as well as ataxia or dystonia. It may be identified in up to a third of these infants. It is readily seen on MRI and images should be examined for this finding (Bodensteiner and Johnsen 2005, 2006, Limperopoulos et al. 2005, Kułak et al. 2007).

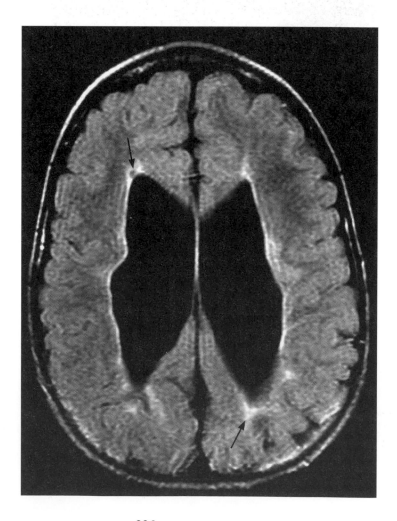

Fig. 3.3.4
MRI of a child with quadriplegia due to severe periventricular leukomalacia. Ventricles are enlarged. Arrows show areas of gliosis/scarring.

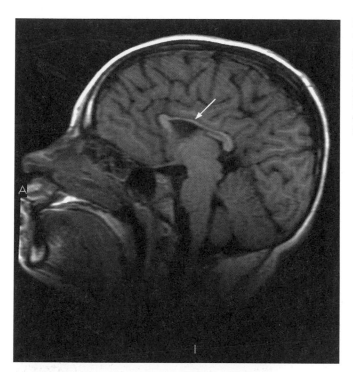

Fig. 3.3.5 MRI of a child with quadriplegia and greater involvement of legs demonstrates moderately severe periventricular leukomalacia and thinning of the corpus callosum as indicated by arrow.

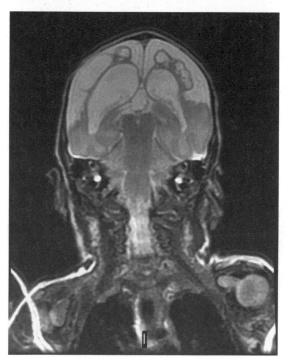

Fig. 3.3.6 MRI of a child with severe quadriplegia who experienced severe prenatal ischemia at 30 weeks gestation. Most of the brain has been destroyed and replaced with fluid-filled cysts (white areas).

227

Neuroimaging of the term newborn infant at risk for cerebral palsy

CT best identifies intraparenchymal, subdural, subarachnoid and intraventricular blood. It is indicated when an encephalopathic infant has a history of birth trauma, coagulopathy, or low hematocrit, as did the infant in Figure 3.3.7 – suggesting intracranial hemorrhage (Ment et al. 2002). If an infant is too unstable to undergo MRI, CT may be useful.

MRI is the study of choice for term newborn infants with encephalopathy, seizures, or features suggestive of cerebral malformation. Moderate to severe hypoxic–ischemic injury in the term infant (sustained either acutely or subacutely) is associated with the development of cerebral palsy. Early identification of those infants severely affected allows more accurate outcome predictions. Acute processes affecting blood flow or perfusion require diffusion-weighted imaging (DWI) and apparent diffusion coefficient (ADC) maps for optimal evaluation. Cytotoxic and vasogenic edema in areas most vulnerable to hypoxic injury cause signal change due to restricted diffusion of water (Zimmerman and Bilaniuk 2006). When hypoxic–ischemic injury is suspected, DWI should be performed between 48 and 120 hours of life. Images are likely to be most definitive at 72 hours post-injury, corresponding to the maximal edema and clinical encephalopathy. Newborn infants with significant asphyxia may have normal or near normal MRI/DWI in the first 24 hours post-injury, only to have significant signal change emerge after 48 hours. We have found the studies more reliable in the 48 hour–5 day window. Timing of scanning is crucial in obtaining accurate

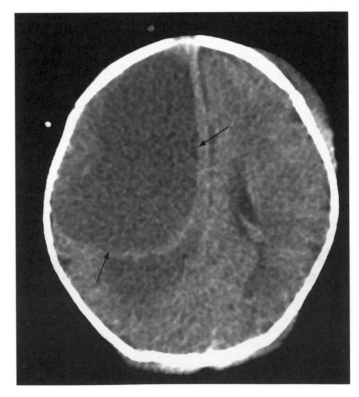

Fig. 3.3.7 CT from the first day after birth in a term infant demonstrates a large chronic hemorrhage that occurred in utero (see arrows).

228

information to aid in clinical decision-making and outcome predictions. If magnetic resonance spectroscopy is available in the same time frame, it may give additional information regarding extent of injury (Ment et al. 2002).

Certain MRI findings are associated with the most common patterns of asphyxia seen in the newborn (Zimmerman and Bilaniuk 2006, Okereafor et al. 2008). Findings reflect our knowledge of the pathophysiology of hypoxic brain injury in the full-term newborn infant. Profound acute asphyxia typically due to a catastrophic event just before delivery (uterine rupture, placenta abruptio) causes lesions in the putamen, ventrolateral thalamic nuclei, cortex and white matter along the central sulcus and the internal capsule (particularly the posterior limb). Findings on DWI imaging (such as in Fig. 3.3.8), although subtle in appearance, correlate strongly with this type of injury. A very young infant who suffers severe acute asphyxia from another cause (such as life-threatening apnea) may demonstrate a pattern of injury identical to the newborn infant. Infants with this constellation of imaging findings have a significant risk of death or disability (Fig. 3.3.9). Partial prolonged asphyxia (often occurring in utero, but also identified in the perinatal and postnatal periods) is associated with bilateral watershed infarctions both anteriorly and posteriorly as in Figure 3.3.10. Although the insult is global, the infarctions may be asymmetric. Severe partial prolonged asphyxia causes signal changes that are bihemispheric, large, and involve both gray and white matter. Diffusion imaging is most sensitive

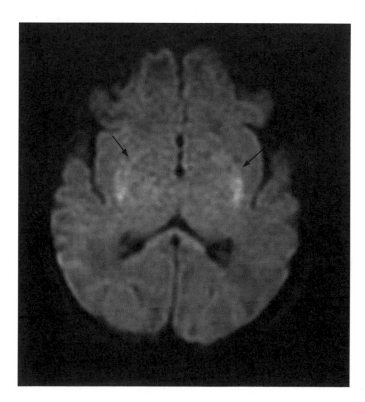

Fig. 3.3.8 MRI demonstrates late sequelae of severe acute hypoxic–ischemic encephalopathy. Faint signal changes (arrows) in the basal ganglia are the main abnormality. The child has severe spastic quadriplegia and microcephaly.

Fig. 3.3.9
MRI demonstrates late sequelae of severe acute hypoxic–ischemic encephalopathy. Faint signal changes (arrows) in the basal ganglia are the main abnormality; he also has microcephaly. The child has severe spastic quadriplegia.

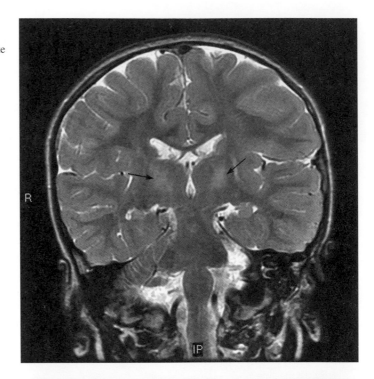

Fig. 3.3.10
Diffusion MRI demonstrates moderate to severe partial prolonged hypoxic–ischemic encephalopathy in a term infant. White areas indicated by arrows show a watershed pattern of injury.

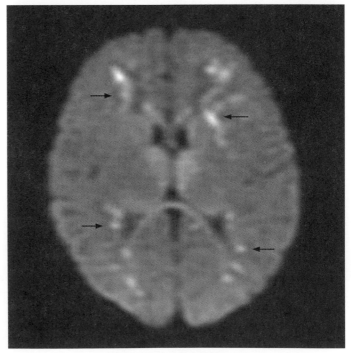

early on; imaging after resolution of acute injury reveals varying degrees of cortical necrosis, cystic encephalomalacia, or cerebral atrophy. These MRI findings are very highly correlated with significant cerebral palsy. If partial prolonged asphyxia is then combined with additional profound acute asphyxial injury, the imaging finding will show a combination of the deep gray matter and internal capsule lesions and extensive watershed infarctions. Cystic encephalomalacia, persistent deep gray-matter signal changes, and profound cerebral atrophy are sequelae found on follow-up MRI (Fig. 3.3.11). Outcomes associated with these findings include death or quadriparetic and dystonic cerebral palsy.

Other infants with less severe hypoxic–ischemic injury demonstrate moderate white-matter injury and diplegic cerebral palsy patterns predominate. Isolated thalamic injury and mild white-matter changes or normal patterns are not typically associated with cerebral palsy outcomes. The role of early MRI changes in those infants who have undergone hypothermic treatment for acute hypoxic–ischemic encephalopathy awaits further research for accurate outcome prediction.

Perinatal arterial ischemic stroke may occur in as many as 1:4000 term infants (Kirton and deVeber 2006). This was the single largest etiology (22%) in a series of 273 children born at term with a subsequent diagnosis of cerebral palsy (Wu et al. 2006a). Typically, no motor asymmetry is detected in the newborn infant but focal clonic seizures may occur. In the absence of a specific clinical presentation, diagnosis is dependent on neuroimaging. Cerebral infarction is easily identified by DWI within 24 hours or less of injury. The restricted diffusion is in an arterial distribution (Krishnamoorthy et al. 2000, Kuker et al.

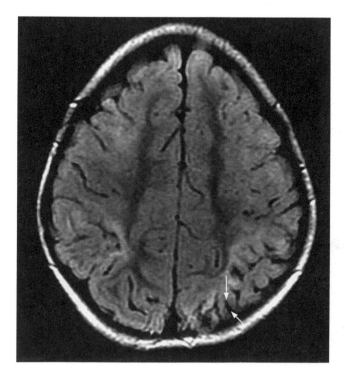

Fig. 3.3.11 MRI demonstrates late sequelae of severe acute and prolonged hypoxic–ischemic injury. Cortical atrophy is present (arrows).

2004). Figures 3.3.12–14 demonstrate the exquisite sensitivity of DWI and MR angiography techniques.

Approximately one-third of children with arterial stroke diagnosed in the newborn period will have cerebral palsy emerge later. Those with a later diagnosis have cerebral palsy 80% of the time. Most of these children have hemiplegia (Lee et al. 2005). In one study of 76 children with perinatal stroke, 68% developed cerebral palsy with 87% of those individuals manifesting a hemiplegic pattern (Golomb et al. 2008). Occlusion of the middle cerebral artery is the most common etiology, occurring two-thirds of the time on the left. Multiple infarctions can lead to triplegic or quadriplegic cerebral palsy. Cerebral venous infarctions, often associated with dural sinus venous thromboses, may be the cause of up to 30% of perinatal infarction. If located in a watershed distribution they may lead to diplegic cerebral palsy (Kirton and deVeber 2006). DWI is the best method to image ischemic white-matter change. Magnetic resonance venography (MRV) helps identify underlying venous sinus thrombosis.

If arteriovenous malformation, venous angioma, or tumor is suspected, additional studies with magnetic resonance angiography (MRA) or venography are indicated.

Cerebral dysgenesis is best identified by MRI. Severe malformative lesions such as lissencephaly, a form of severely abnormal cortical development (Fig. 3.3.15), or holoprosencephaly, the failure of the forebrain to divide (Fig. 3.3.16), occur in the first trimester of pregnancy. These are now frequently identified in the prenatal or newborn

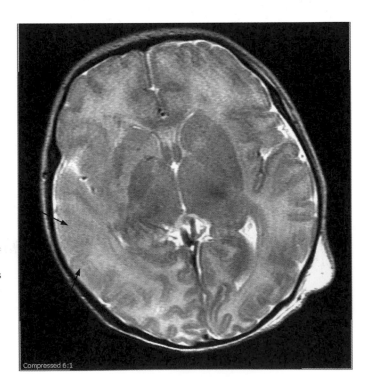

Fig. 3.3.12
MRI demonstrates acute infarction, focal edema, and gray-matter changes in the distribution of the right middle cerebral artery in a term infant 15 hours after birth. Arrows indicate blurring of gray- and white-matter junction.

232

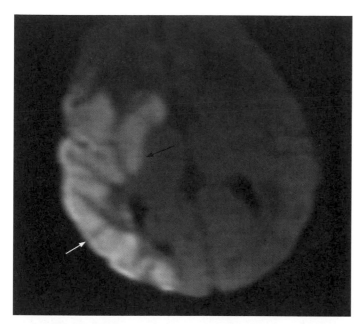

Fig. 3.3.13 Diffusion MRI of a term infant 15 hours after birth demonstrating acute infarction in the distribution of the middle cerebral artery. The infarcted area appears white in the illustration.

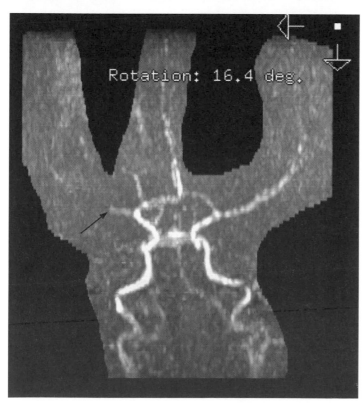

Rotation: 16.4 deg.

Fig. 3.3.14 MR angiogram of a term infant 15 hours after birth demonstrating complete occlusion of the right middle cerebral artery as indicated by arrow.

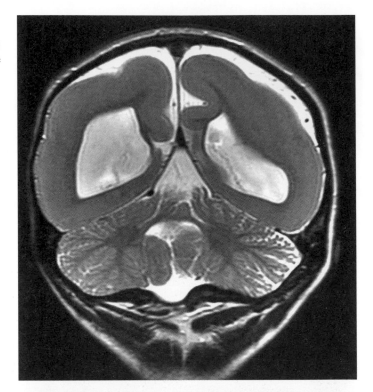

Fig. 3.3.15
MRI demonstrates
lissencephaly in a child
with quadriplegia. Note
absence of gyri and
resultant smooth
cortex.

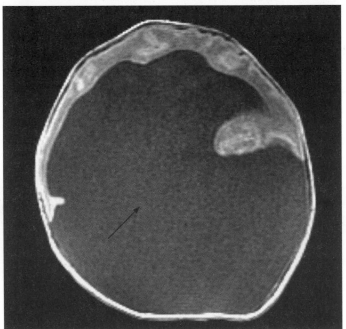

Fig. 3.3.16
MRI demonstrates
holoprosencephaly in a
child with quadriplegia.
Black area denotes
fluid-filled cyst behind
fused cortical remnant.

234

periods. Severe spastic quadriparesis is the outcome. More subtle malformations may be identified in infants with moderate encephalopathy without identifiable perinatal cause, those with multiple congenital anomalies, or those with seizures (Fig. 3.3.17). Along with infarction, cerebral malformations constitute a significant etiology for cerebral palsy in the term infant (Wu et al. 2006a, b).

Cerebral infection, particularly toxoplasmosis, rubella, cytomegalovirus, herpes simplex, syphilis, human immunodeficiency virus (HIV), varicella-zoster, and lymphocytic choriomeningitic viruses may account for 5%–10% of cases of cerebral palsy (Stanley et al. 2000). MRI is most useful to detect meningeal enhancement, cerebritis, abcess formation, focal ischemia and hemorrhage. Contrast enhancement after administration of gadolinium may provide increased sensitivity to cerebral and meningeal inflammation. CT is indicated to identify intracerebral calcifications; Figures 3.3.18 and 19 show classic imaging findings in a child affected by congenital cytomegalovirus.

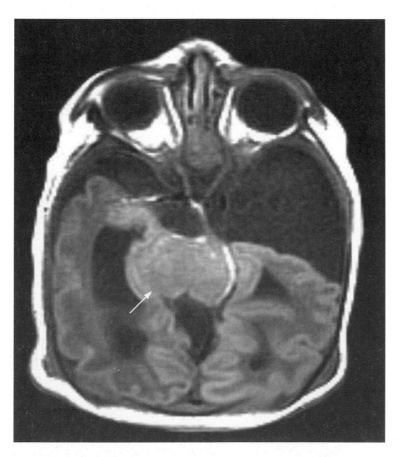

Fig. 3.3.17 MRI demonstrates fused diencephalon (arrow) in a child with quadriplegia. There is large a fluid-filled cyst in temporal area.

235

Fig. 3.3.18 CT of a child with congenital cytomegalovirus infection demonstrating periventricular calcifications (see arrows).

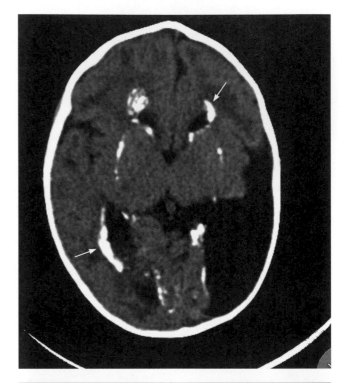

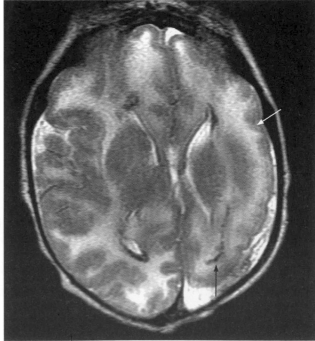

Fig. 3.3.19 MRI of a child with congenital cytomegalovirus infection demonstrating neuronal migration disorder. The arrows point to a dysplastic cortex.

Neuroimaging in the child diagnosed with cerebral palsy

Although cerebral palsy is a clinical diagnosis the location and type of structural brain injury correlates with cerebral palsy of differing types. CT scanning has demonstrated usefulness in identifying causation of cerebral palsy. Pooled studies of CT in 782 children with cerebral palsy showed abnormalities on 77% of scans (Ashwal et al. 2004). When just Class I studies were evaluated, 88% of children had abnormalities. The yield of abnormal studies varied with type of cerebral palsy: 89% in hemiplegic cerebral palsy and 36% in dyskinetic cerebral palsy. Despite these data, CT should not be a routine part of the evaluation of the child newly diagnosed with cerebral palsy.

MRI eclipses all other modalities in sensitivity and specificity for identifying associated conditions. Unless imaging results from the neonatal period are available for review and reveal clear structural changes consistent with the child's clinical condition, MRI is recommended for a child with the clinical signs of cerebral palsy. Lesions acquired in the prenatal or neonatal period may be clinically silent until later in the infancy or early childhood when motor impairment and spasticity emerge.

Data from 10 studies with a total of 644 children with cerebral palsy who underwent MRI scanning showed imaging abnormalities in 89% (range 68%–100%) (Ashwal et al. 2004). Injuries to white matter, basal ganglia, thalami or cerebellum were readily detected on MRI. Lesions were identified in 98% of children with quadriplegia, 96% with hemiplegia, and 70% with dyskinetic cerebral palsy. MRI is useful in determining when brain injury occurs. In studies of 345 children with various types of cerebral palsy, prenatal onset occurred in 37%, perinatal in 35%, and postnatal in 4%.

MRI gives neuroanatomic correlation with clinical types of cerebral palsy. Systematic review of studies utilizing MRI to evaluate 388 children with cerebral palsy found abnormal scans in 334 (86%) (Krägeloh-Mann and Horber 2007). Findings were related to the pattern of cerebral palsy in 83% of individuals. Periventricular white-matter lesions were the most common abnormalities found overall (56%). White-matter lesions were found in 90% of the preterm infants with cerebral palsy but only 20% of full-term infants with cerebral palsy showed similar pathology. As anticipated, spastic diplegic cerebral palsy occurred in 84% of the preterm infants. Gray-matter lesions (cortical or deep gray) were found in 18% (69/388) of infants. These affected term infants far more than pre-term infants (33% versus 3.5%), reflecting the pathophysiology of hypoxic–ischemic encephalopathy and white-matter injury in infants of different stages of maturation. Severe forms of quadriplegia and athetoid cerebral palsy were most common in children with gray-matter lesions. Again, this correlates with our understanding of the particular vulnerability of the deep gray-matter structures to hypoxic injury. Children with gray-matter lesions and unilateral MRI findings typically had hemiplegia most commonly associated with cerebral infarction; focal brain malformations were also frequently identified.

Identification of abnormalities on MRI is also related to preterm, term, or postnatally acquired injury (Figs 3.3.20, 21). Of 620 children with cerebral palsy, MRI showed abnormalities in 99% of preterm infants, 92% of term infants, and 79% of infants over 1 month of age (Ashwal et al. 2004).

Fig. 3.3.20
MRI demonstrating acute edema in a 4-month-old child who sustained non-accidental trauma. The arrows point to areas of cortical edema.

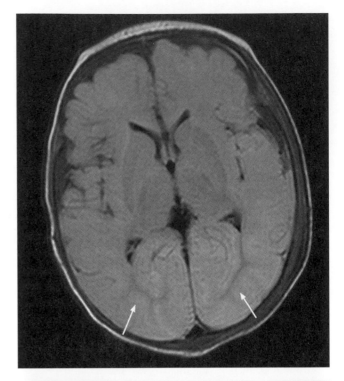

Fig. 3.3.21
MRI demonstrating late outcome of severe encephalomalacia and subdural hematomas (white areas). This MRI, taken 3 weeks later, is of the same child portrayed in Figure 3.3.20. Arrows point to areas of severe cortical injury, which will eventually be replaced by cysts.

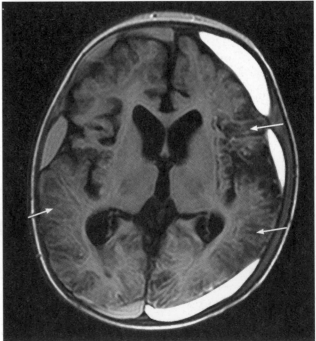

If children with brain malformations suffer motor symptoms that are consistent with the definition of cerebral palsy, they are now considered to have the disorder (Rosenbaum 2006). Data from scans of 1426 children with cerebral palsy identified major brain malformation on 12% of MRIs. Malformations of cortical development in the first trimester are typically most severe. If the lesion is unilateral (as a schizencephalic cleft or porencephalic cyst may be), hemiplegia is the usual result (Figs 3.3.22, 23).

MRI abnormalities thought to correlate with causation of cerebral palsy are very high in children with spastic types. In one study they were found in 123/129 (95%) children, including 45/45 with quadriplegia, 37/40 with diplegia, and 42/45 with hemiplegia (Kułak et al. 2007). However, depending on patient selection criteria and methodology, up to 15% of MRI studies are considered normal. Athetotic or dyskinetic cerebral palsy has a much lower incidence of MRI abnormality than the spastic subtypes; at least 30% of scans are unrevealing. A normal MRI of the brain does not preclude a diagnosis of cerebral palsy (Ashwal et al. 2004). In such children, careful re-evaluation of historical information and clinical monitoring over time for signs of slow neurologic deterioration are warranted. Imaging of the spinal cord should be considered in any child who has apparently normal bulbar function and intellect, yet has significant spastic quadriparesis.

Neuroimaging may need to be repeated in the child with cerebral palsy. New onset seizures with an abnormal EEG may be an indication for re-imaging. Alteration in a child's clinical history or examination suggestive of progressive symptoms, or new-onset neurological signs/symptoms superimposed on pre-existing cerebral palsy are indications for re-imaging, as well as diagnostic re-evaluation.

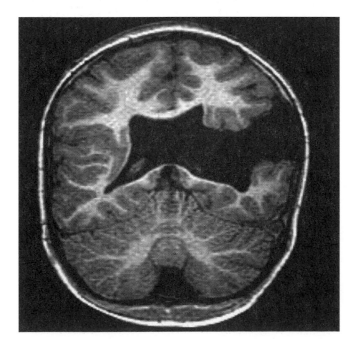

Fig. 3.3.22
MRI demonstrating a unilateral schizencephalic cleft in a child with hemiplegia.

Fig. 3.3.23 MRI demonstrating neuronal migration disorder in a child with hemiplegia. The arrows point to thickened cortex.

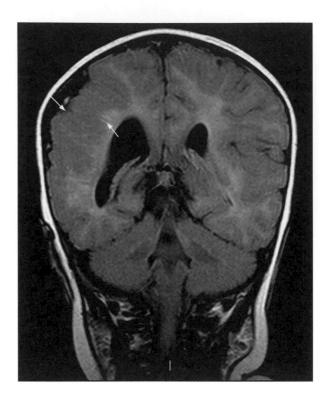

TABLE 3.3.1
Grades of intraventricular hemorrhage (from Papile et al. 1978, Dammann and Leviton 1997)

Grade I: Hemorrhage in the subependymal germinal matrix
Grade II: Hemorrhage into the ventricle, does not distend it
Grade III: Hemorrhage into ventricle with associated ventricular enlargement
Grade IV: Hemorrhage in the parenchyma; may not be expansion of IVH, but may be parenchymal
            hemorrhage due to venous infarction.

TABLE 3.3.2
MRI findings associated with certain patterns of cerebral palsy

Diplegia:
   Periventricular leukomalacia
Hemiplegia:
   Unilateral cortical encephalomalacia (cerebral infarction, trauma)
   Cystic encephalomalacia (intraparenchymal hemorrhage or venous infarction)
   Focal cerebral dysgenesis
   Unilateral schizencephaly
   Focal polymicrogyria/pachymicrogyria
Quadriplegia:
   Bilateral encephalomalacia (hypoxia–ischemia, bilateral trauma)
   Cerebral dysgenesis (lissencephaly, bilateral schizencephaly)
Athetoid:
   Abnormal signal change in basal ganglia, thalamus (hypoxia–ischemia in term infant, cerebellar infarction)

240

TABLE 3.3.3
Etiologies of cerebral palsy identified on MRI

Preterm brain injury
    Periventricular leukomalacia
    Ventriculomegaly (due to white-matter loss)
    Cystic lesions in white matter
Hypoxic–ischemic injury
    Basal ganglia and thalamic injury
    Encephalomalacia
    White-matter loss
    Cortical atrophy (elegyria)
    Cerebral atrophy
Cerebral infarction
    Prenatal: porencephalic cysts
    Perinatal: focal cortical encephalomalacia
Malformations
    Lissencephaly
    Schizencephaly
    Polymicrogyria/pachygyria
    Holoprosencephaly
    Cerebellar hypoplasia/malformation
Residuals of congenital infection
    Porencephalic cyst
    Schizencephaly
    Cystic encephalomalacia (focal/bilateral)
    Intracranial calcifications (best seen on CT)

REFERENCES

Ancel PY, Livinec F, Larroque B, Marret S, Arnaud C, Pierrat V, Dehan M, Nguyen S, Escande B, Burget A, Thiriez G, Picaud JC, Andre M, Breart G, Kaminski M (2006) Cerebral palsy among very preterm children in relation to gestational age and neonatal ultrasound abnormalities: the EPIPAGE cohort study. *Pediatrics* **117**: 828–35.

Ashwal S, Russman BS, Blasco PA, Miller G, Sandler A, Shevell M, Stevenson R, Quality Standards Subcommittee of the American Academy of Neurology and Practice Committee of the Child Neurology Society (2004) Practice parameter: diagnostic assessment of the child with cerebral palsy: report of the Quality Standards Subcommittee of the American Academy of Neurology and the Practice Committee of the Child Neurology Society. *Neurology* **62**: 851–63.

Barkovitch AJ (1990) *Practical Atlas of Neonatal Brain Development*. New York: Raven.

Bodensteiner JB, Johnsen SD (2005) Cerebellar injury in the extremely premature infant: newly recognized but relatively common outcome. *J Child Neurol* **20**: 139–42.

Bodensteiner JB, Johnsen SD (2006) Magnetic resonance imaging (MRI) findings in children surviving extremely premature delivery and extremely low birthweight with cerebral palsy. *J Child Neurol* **21**: 743–7.

Brenner DJ, Hall EJ (2007) Computed tomography – an increasing source of radiation exposure. *New Engl J Med* **357**: 2277–84.

Dammann O, Leviton A (1997) Duration of transient hyperechoic images of white matter in very-low-birthweight infants: a proposed classification. *Dev Med Child Neurol* **39**: 2–5.

De Vries LS, Groenendaal F, Van Haastert IC, Eken P, Rademaker KJ, Meiners LC (1999) Asymmetrical myelination of the posterior limb of the internal capsule in infants with periventricular haemorrhagic infarction: an early predictor of hemiplegia. *Neuropediatrics* **30**: 314–19.

De Vries LS, Van Haastert IC, Rademaker KJ, Koopman C, Groenendaal F (2004) Ultrasound abnormalities preceding cerebral palsy in high-risk preterm infants. *J Pediatr* **144**: 815–20.

241

Dyet LE, Kennea N, Counsell SJ, Maalouf EF, Ajayi-Obe M, Duggan PJ, Harrison M, Allsop JM, Hajnal J, Herlihy AH, Edwards B, Laroche S, Cowan FM, Rutherford MA, Edwards AD (2006) Natural history of brain lesions in extremely preterm infants studied with serial magnetic resonance imaging from birth and neurodevelopmental assessment. *Pediatrics* **118**: 536–48.

Gaddlin PO, Finnstrom O, Wang C, Leijon I (2008) A fifteen-year follow-up of neurological conditions in VLBW children without overt disability: relation to gender, neonatal risk factors, and end stage MRI findings. *Early Hum Dev* **84**: 343–9.

Goetz MC, Gretebeck RJ, Oh KS, Shaffer D, Hermansen MC (1995) Incidence, timing, and follow-up of periventricular leukomalacia. *Am J Perinatol* **12**: 325–7.

Golomb MR, Garg BP, Saha C, Azzouz F, Williams LS (2008) Cerebral palsy after perinatal arterial ischemic stroke. *J Child Neurol* 23: 279–86.

Harris NJ, Palacio D, Ginzel A, Richardson CJ, Swischuk L (2007) Are routine cranial ultrasounds necessary in premature infants greater than 30 weeks gestation? *Am J Perinatol* **24**: 17–21.

Hayakawa F, Okumura A, Kato T, Kuno K, Watanabe K (1999) Determination of timing of brain injury in preterm infants with periventricular leukomalacia with serial neonatal electroencephalography. *Pediatrics* **104**: 1077–81.

Hintz SR, O'Shea M (2008) Neuroimaging and neurodevelopmental outcomes in preterm infants. *Semin Perinatol* **32**: 11–19.

Hintz SR, Kendrick DE, Stoll BJ, Vohr BR, Fanaroff AA, Donovan EF, Poole WK, Blakely ML, Wright L, Higgins R, NICHD Neonatal Research Network (2005) Neurodevelopmental and growth outcomes of extremely low birth weight infants after necrotizing enterocolitis. *Pediatrics* **115**: 696–703.

Hintz SR, Slovis T, Bulas D, Van Meurs KP, Perritt R, Stevenson DK, Poole WK, Das A, Higgins RD, NICHD Neonatal Research Network (2007) Interobserver reliability and accuracy of cranial ultrasound scanning interpretation in premature infants. *J Pediatr* **150**: 592–6.

Ito T, Hashimoto K, Kadowaki K, Nagata N, Makio A, Takahashi H, Ikeno S, Terakawa N (1997) Ultrasonographic findings in the periventricular region in premature newborns with antenatal periventricular leukomalacia. *J Perinat Med* **25**: 180–3.

Kirton A, DeVeber G (2006) Cerebral palsy secondary to perinatal ischemic stroke. *Clin Perinatol* **33**: 367–386.

Korzeniewski SJ, Birbeck G, Delano MC, Potchen MJ, Paneth N (2008) A systematic review of neuroimaging for cerebral palsy. *J Child Neurol* **23**: 216–27.

Krägeloh-Mann I, Horber V (2007) The role of magnetic resonance imaging in furthering understanding of the pathogenesis of cerebral palsy. *Dev Med Child Neurol* **49**: 948.

Krishnamoorthy KS, Soman TB, Takeoka M, Schaefer PW (2000) Diffusion-weighted imaging in neonatal cerebral infarction: clinical utility and follow-up. *J Child Neurol* **15**: 592–602.

Kuker W, Mohrle S, Mader I, Schoning M, Nagele T (2004) MRI for the management of neonatal cerebral infarctions: importance of timing. *Child's Nerv Syst* **20**: 742–8.

Kułak W, Sobaniec W, Kubas B, Walecki J, Smigielska-Kuzia J, Bockowski L, Artemowicz B, Sendrowski K (2007) Spastic cerebral palsy: clinical magnetic resonance imaging correlation of 129 children. *J Child Neurol* **22**: 8–14.

Laptook AR, O'Shea TM, Shankaran S, Bhaskar B, NICHD Neonatal Network (2005) Adverse neurodevelopmental outcomes among extremely low birth weight infants with a normal head ultrasound: prevalence and antecedents. *Pediatrics* **115**: 673–80.

Lee J, Croen LA, Lindan C, Nash KB, Yoshida CK, Ferriero DM, Barkovitch AJ, Wu YW (2005) Predictors of outcome in perinatal arterial stroke: a population-based study. *Ann Neurol* **58**: 303–8.

Levine D (2005) *Atlas of Fetal MRI*. Boca Raton: Taylor and Francis.

Limperopoulos C, Benson CB, Bassan H, Disalvo DN, Kinnamon DD, Moore M, Ringer SA, Volpe JJ, Du Plessis AJ (2005) Cerebellar hemorrhage in the preterm infant: ultrasonographic findings and risk factors. *Pediatrics* **116**: 717–24.

Ment LR, Bada HS, Barnes P, Grant PE, Hirtz D, Papile LA, Pinto-Martin J, Rivkin M, Slovis TL (2002) Practice parameter: neuroimaging of the neonate: report of the Quality Standards Subcommittee of the American Academy of Neurology and the Practice Committee of the Child Neurology Society. *Neurology* **58**: 1726–38.

Nanba Y, Matsui K, Aida N, Sato Y, Toyoshima K, Kawataki M, Hoshino R, Ohyama M, Itani Y, Goto A, Oka A (2007) Magnetic resonance imaging regional T1 abnormalities at term accurately predict motor outcome in preterm infants. *Pediatrics* **120**: 10–9.

242

Okereafor A, Allsop J, Counsell SJ, Fitzpatrick J, Azzopardi D, Rutherford MA, Cowan FM (2008) Patterns of brain injury in neonates exposed to perinatal sentinel events. *Pediatrics* **121**: 906–914.

Papile LA, Burstein J, Burstein R, Koffler H (1978) Incidence and evolution of subependymal and intraventricular hemorrhage: a study of infants with birth weights less than 1,500 gm. *J Pediatr* **92**: 529–34.

Rosenbaum P (2006) Classification of abnormal neurological outcome. *Early Hum Dev* **82**: 167–71.

Sie LT, Hart AA, Van Hof J, De Groot L, Lems W, Lafeber HN, Valk J, Van der Knaap MS (2005) Predictive value of neonatal MRI with respect to late MRI findings and clinical outcome. A study in infants with periventricular densities on neonatal ultrasound. *Neuropediatrics* **36**: 78–89.

Stanley FJ, Blair E, Alberman E (2000) *Cerebral Palsies: Epidemiology and Causal Pathways.* London: Mac Keith Press.

Woodward LJ, Anderson PJ, Audtin NC, Howard K, Inder TE (2006) Neonatal MRI to predict neurodevelopmental outcomes in preterm infants. *New Engl J Med* **355**: 685–94.

Wu YW, Croen LA, Shah SJ, Newman TB, Najjar DV (2006a) Cerebral palsy in a term population: risk factors and neuroimaging findings. *Pediatrics* **118**: 690–7.

Wu YW, Lindan CE, Henning LH, Yoshida CK, Fullerton HJ, Perriero DM, Barkovitch AJ, Croen LA (2006b) Neuroimaging abnormalities in infants with congenital hemiparesis. *Pediatr Neurol* **35**: 191–196.

Zimmerman RA, Bilaniuk LT (2006) Neuroimaging evaluation of cerebral palsy. *Clin Perinatol* **33**: 517–544.

3.4
RADIOGRAPHIC EVALUATION OF THE PATIENT WITH CEREBRAL PALSY

Kevin Walker

Patients with cerebral palsy and other neuromuscular disorders are at an increased risk of developing musculoskeletal conditions ranging from hip subluxation to neuromuscular scoliosis. Therefore obtaining appropriate radiographic studies is an integral part of any clinical evaluation of a patient with cerebral palsy. Plain radiographs are appropriate for the initial evaluation of most patients in the outpatient clinic setting. Fundamentally, radiographs may serve one of three primary functions: (1) to evaluate a patient with a clinical deformity, (2) to screen for a disorder such as a hip subluxation, and (3) as a preoperative planning instrument. Further evaluation with other imaging modalities may also be indicated.

Pelvis radiographs

Patients with cerebral palsy are at risk of developing a subluxation of the hip (Lonstein and Beck 1986, Soo et al. 2006, Hagglund et al. 2007). The Gross Motor Function Classification System (GMFCS) is a validated instrument that characterizes the functional level of involvement of patients with cerebral palsy (Palisano et al. 1997). The rate of hip subluxation correlates with increasing GMFCS level from 0% for GMFCS I patients to 90% in GMFCS V patients (Soo et al. 2006). Indications for obtaining an anteroposterior (AP) pelvis radiograph include: (1) clinical signs of a hip subluxation including reduced hip abduction and/or femoral shortening, (2) patients with bilateral involvement age 18 months of age or older (Dobson et al. 2002), and (3) patients for whom lower-extremity surgery is anticipated. The following radiographic parameters can be assessed on the pelvis radiograph to identify a hip subluxation: the Reimers migration index, the integrity of Shenton's line, the acetabular index and the neck-shaft angle of the proximal femur (Fig. 3.4.1a). The Reimers migration index is calculated on the AP pelvis radiograph by measuring the percentage of the femoral head that is lateral to Perkin's line (Fig. 3.4.1b). A migration index greater than 30 % is considered abnormal (Reimers 1980). The migration index is particularly useful longitudinally over time such that on subsequent clinic visits any increase in the Reimers migration index will reflect a potential progression of the hip subluxation. Shenton's line is the line drawn on the AP pelvis radiograph from the inferior aspect of the femoral neck to the superior surface of the ipsilateral obturator foramen (Fig. 3.4.1b). In a radiograph of a reduced, normal hip, this line should be a continuous, uninterrupted arc. In a patient with a subluxation of the hip, this line is interrupted. The acetabular index (AI) is utilized to

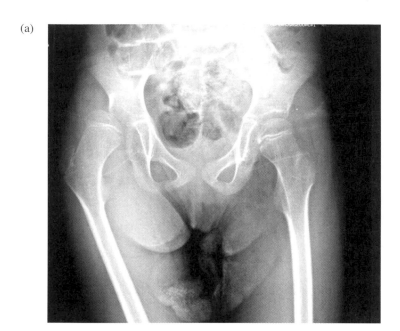

(a)

(b)

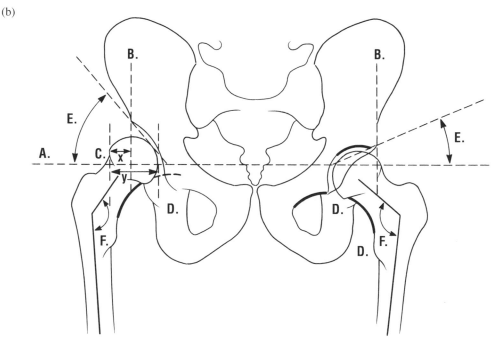

Fig. 3.4.1 (a) AP pelvis radiograph of patient with cerebral palsy with right hip subluxation. (b) Radiographic parameters of AP pelvis radiograph. (A) Hilgenreiner's line. (B) Perkin's line. (C) Reimers migration index (x/y). (D) Shenton's line. On the left side, Shenton's line is intact. On the right, Shenton's line is interrupted. (E) Acetabular Index. (F) Neck-shaft angle.

assess acetabular development in the skeletally immature patient. It is measured by determining the angle subtended by Hilgenreiner's line and a line drawn from the triradiate cartilage to the lateral border of the acetabulum (Fig. 3.4.1b). The AI normally decreases during the first 2 years of life and a normal value of 20° or less is present in children by age 2 years old. However, in a young child, an AI of up to 30° can be considered normal (Laurenson 1959, Tonnis 1976, Scoles et al. 1987). For a patient with cerebral palsy, an AI that is greater than 30° or that is significantly increased relative to the contralateral hip should be considered abnormal. Finally, the neck-shaft angle can be measured on the AP pelvis radiograph as well (Fig. 3.4.1b). The neck-shaft angle as measured on the radiograph can be affected by the rotational position of the femur. Obtaining the AP pelvis radiograph with the femur internally rotated will allow for accurate determination of the neck-shaft angle (Kay et al. 2000). The neck-shaft angle is increased in children with cerebral palsy (Bobroff et al. 1999). Femoral anteversion, neck-shaft angle and Reimer's migration percentage all correlate with GMFCS (Robin et al. 2008).

Hip surveillance
The risk of hip subluxation in patients with cerebral palsy varies with cerebral palsy subtype and GMFCS (Soo et al. 2006, Hagglund et al. 2007). The introduction of hip-surveillance protocols allows earlier detection of hip subluxation and has reduced the need for reconstructive surgery for subluxated or dislocated hips. Surveillance can identify children most at risk of hip subluxation, using radiological methods which are widely available (Gordon and Simkiss 2006). Implementation of hip surveillance programs has been advocated for patients with cerebral palsy with bilateral involvement as early as 18 months (Dobson et al. 2002) to 30 months of age (Scrutton et al. 2001) with radiographs repeated at 6- to 12-month intervals thereafter. Some authors recommend hip surveillance based on age and GMFCS level (Hagglund et al. 2007).

Knee radiographs

KNEE ALIGNMENT IN THE SAGITTAL PLANE
Patients with cerebral palsy are at risk for developing knee problems that include knee flexion contractures, anterior knee pain, patella inferior pole fractures, patella alta and crouched gait (Rosenthal and Levine 1977, Samilson and Gill 1984, Lloyd-Roberts et al. 1985, Topoleski et al. 2000, Senaran et al. 2007a). Radiographic evaluation of the patient who demonstrates knee flexion in gait should consist of an AP and lateral radiograph of the knee in maximum extension (Fig. 3.4.2). The lateral radiograph of the knee in maximum extension will enable the radiographic measurement of a knee flexion contracture if present. To assess patellar height, a lateral radiograph in 30° of flexion may also be obtained. A number of radiographic methods to measure patellar height have been described (Blumensaat 1938, Insall and Salvati 1971, Blackburne and Peel 1977, Caton et al. 1982, Norman et al. 1983, De Carvalho et al. 1985, Koshino and Sugimoto 1989, Grelsamer and Meadows 1992, Leung et al. 1996). By age 12 in boys, and by age 10 in girls, the patellar tendon length to patella height ratio of the Insall–Salvati method approximates that of the

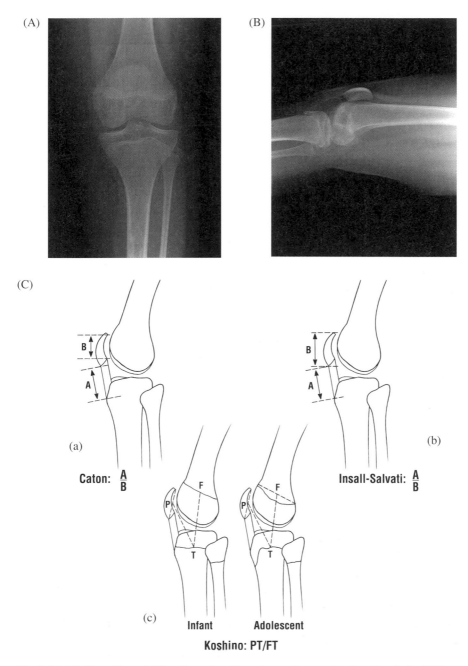

(A)

(B)

(C)

(a)

Caton: $\frac{A}{B}$

(b)

Insall-Salvati: $\frac{A}{B}$

(c)

Infant   Adolescent

Koshino: PT/FT

Fig. 3.4.2 AP (A) and lateral (B) radiographs of knee in maximum extension. Note lack of full extension on lateral radiograph. The knee-flexion contracture can be measured radiographically on the lateral x-ray by the angle formed by the long axis of the tibia and the long axis of the femur. (C) Radiographic methods of measuring patella height on lateral radiograph. (a) Caton–Deschampes ratio; (b) Insall–Salvati index (normal range is 1.0–1.2); (c) Koshino index (normal range is 0.9–1.3).

skeletally mature knee (Walker et al. 1998) (Fig. 3.4.2C). The Koshino index has been shown to be stable throughout a range of knee flexion from 30° to 90°. The normal range of the ratio is 0.9–1.3 (Koshino and Sugimoto 1989) (Fig. 3.4.2C). The Caton–Deschamps index also has been shown to be simple, reliable and reproducible during adolescence with low interobserver variation and without being affected by skeletal maturation (Aparicio et al. 1999) (Fig. 3.4.2C).

KNEE ALIGNMENT IN THE CORONAL PLANE

For patients with cerebral palsy, the primary deformities of their lower extremities most often are in the transverse plane, resulting in rotational deformities such as increased femoral anteversion. However, patients may also experience deformities in the coronal or frontal plane, resulting in genu varus ('bowed-leg') or genu valgus ('knock-kneed') deformities. For ambulatory patients, a standing 6-foot AP radiograph of both lower extremities from the hips (including the top of the pelvis when possible) to the ankles should be obtained (Fig. 3.4.3A). Careful attention must be paid to insure that the patella is positioned directly anteriorly over the distal femur in order to make certain that the limb is not rotated. Difficulty standing erect can also make these radiographs difficult to obtain and interpret. For issues of alignment in the coronal plane, the mechanical angles about the knee can be determined (Fig. 3.4.3B) (Paley et al. 1994).

Evaluation of limb-length difference

In patients for whom a limb-length difference is suspected based on a careful clinical examination, a block or lift of the amount corresponding to the estimated limb-length difference should be placed under the foot of the shorter limb for the radiograph. A standing 6-foot AP hip to ankle radiograph of both lower extremities should be obtained to measure the lengths of each leg and to calculate the difference. Care must be taken to ensure full knee extension to avoid misinterpretation. An alternative to a standing lower-extremity radiograph is a scanogram. A scanogram is a radiographic image in which the patient is supine and the radiographic tube and the radiographic film move together such that separate exposures are obtained at the level of each joint with a radiographic ruler incorporated into the image. The composite images of the joints can be used to measure the limb lengths and to calculate the difference. Asymmetric fixed knee flexion deformities make this method inaccurate in which case a CT scan for leg length should be considered. When evaluating a patient for a limb-length difference, it is also important to obtain an AP radiograph of the left hand in order to estimate the patient's 'bone age'.

Foot and ankle or distal tibia radiographs

Patients with cerebral palsy are at risk for developing equinovarus, equinovalgus or planovalgus foot deformities. Radiographic evaluation should consist of a standing AP and lateral radiograph of each foot. If a significant valgus deformity of the hindfoot is present clinically, an AP and a mortise radiograph of the ankle also may be helpful in order to evaluate the distal tibia for a valgus deformity.

(A)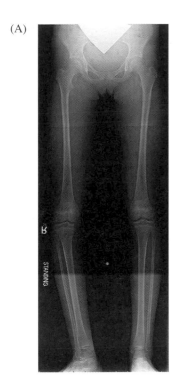

(B)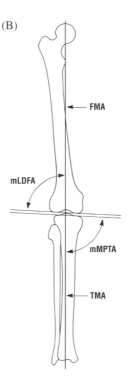

Fig. 3.4.3 (A) Standing anteroposterior hip to ankle radiograph of both lower extremities of a patient with spastic diplegia and right genu varum. (B) Diagram illustrating the mechanical alignment of the lower extremity in the coronal plane. The femoral mechanical axis (FMA) is determined by drawing a line from the center of the femoral head to the center of the distal femur in the middle of the intercondylar notch. The tibial mechanical axis (TMA) is determined by drawing a line from the middle of the proximal tibia between the spines of the tibial eminence to the middle of the distal tibial articular surface at the ankle. The mechanical angle of the knee is described by the angle formed by the FMA and TMA. In a knee without deformity, the mechanical angle is 0°. For patients with a deformity at the level of the knee, the true location of the deformity can be determined by establishing the mechanical angles of the distal femur and proximal tibia. mLDFA, mechanical lateral distal femoral angle (normal=88°–90°); mMPTA, mechanical medial proximal tibial angle (normal=88°–90°).

On the AP radiograph of the foot, the talocalcaneal angle and the talus–1st metatarsal angle can be measured (Fig. 3.4.4A). The AP talocalcaneal angle reflects the alignment of the hindfoot. The range of normal values is 10°–56°. A value greater than this range represents a valgus deformity of the hindfoot. A value less than the normal range is associated with a varus deformity of the hindfoot (Fig. 3.4.4B). The AP talus–1st metatarsal angle reflects the alignment of the forefoot. The normal range for this angle is 5°–15° (Vanderwilde 1988). The position of the navicular relative to the head of the talus can be assessed on the AP radiograph as well. Normally the navicular is positioned symmetrically on the head of the talus. Lateral subluxation of the navicular on the head of the talus is present in valgus foot deformities while medial subluxation is present in varus deformities (Fig. 3.4.4C).

249

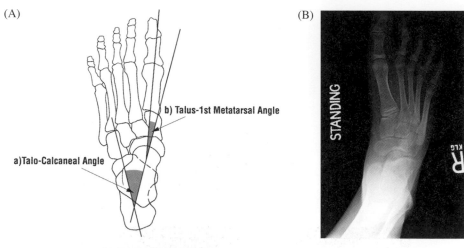

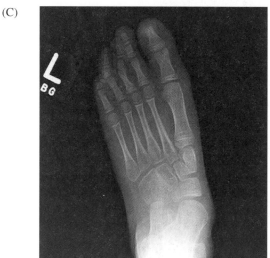

(A)

b) Talus-1st Metatarsal Angle

a)Talo-Calcaneal Angle

(B)

STANDING

(C)

Fig. 3.4.4 (A) Antereoposterior (AP) diagram of the foot. (B) Standing AP radiograph of foot with equinovarus foot deformity. The AP talocalcaneal angle is decreased and the navicular is displaced medially on the head of the talus. (C) Standing AP radiograph of foot with planovalgus foot deformity. The AP talocalcaneal angle is increased and the navicular is displaced laterally on the head of the talus.

On the lateral radiograph the talocalcaneal angle, the talus–1st metatarsal angle and the tibiocalcaneal angle (or 'calcaneal pitch' angle) can be assessed (Fig. 3.4.4D). The normal range of values for the lateral talocalcaneal angle is between 15° and 60°. A value lower than this range is associated with a varus deformity of the hindfoot. A value greater than this range is seen in valgus deformities (Fig. 3.4.4E). The tibiocalcaneal angle on the lateral radiograph ranges in value from 65° to 80°. This angle is increased in an equinus or plantarflexion deformity and it is decreased when there is a calcaneus or dorsiflexion deformity present.

(D)

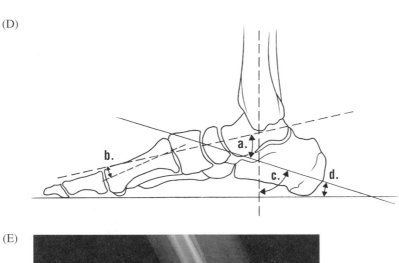

(E)

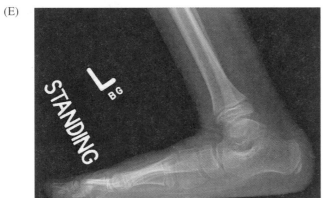

(F)

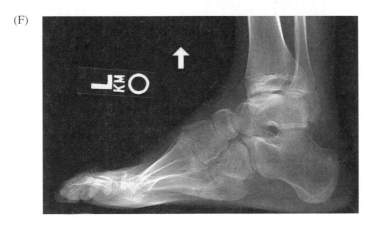

Fig. 3.4.4 continued (D) Lateral diagram of the foot. a, lateral talocalcaneal angle; b, talus–1st metatarsal angle; c, tibiocalcaneal angle; d, calcaneal pitch. (E) Standing lateral radiograph of foot with planovalgus foot deformity. The lateral talocalcaneal angle is increased. (F) Standing lateral radiograph of foot with cavovarus foot deformity. The 1st metatarsal is plantarflexed relative to the talus, resulting in a negative talus–1st metatarsal angle.

Calcaneal pitch is the angle of the calcaneus relative to the horizontal line of the ground. The lateral talus–1st metatarsal angle is a measure of the alignment of the forefoot relative to the hindfoot. A plantarflexed 1st metatarsal relative to the long axis of the talus is assigned a negative value. A normal range of values is from –5 to 20° (Vanderwilde et al. 1988). For patients with a cavus deformity of the foot, the angle will become increasingly negative (more plantarflexed) with progressively more severe deformities (Fig. 3.4.4F). For patients with a pes planus or planovalgus deformity, the angle will be progressively more positive. Assessing the alignment of the calcaneus relative to the tibia and the forefoot relative to the calcaneus on the standing lateral radiograph of the foot and ankle may be the only way to differentiate hindfoot equinus due to gastrocsoleus contracture from forefoot equinus due to pes cavus.

Spine radiographs
The incidence of neuromuscular scoliosis is not well defined in ambulatory patients with cerebral palsy. It is well understood that with increasing involvement and increasing GMFCS levels, the incidence of scoliosis increases significantly. It is also controversial what role tone-reduction procedures such as selective dorsal rhizotomy and intrathecal baclofen pumps play in the incidence of neuromuscular scoliosis (Johnson et al. 2004, Spiegel et al. 2004, Golan et al. 2007, Senaran et al. 2007b, Li et al. 2008, Shilt et al. 2008). For ambulatory patients with cerebral palsy, a careful evaluation of their spine for clinical signs of scoliosis should be part of their physical examination. Clinical signs of scoliosis include shoulder height inequality, trunk asymmetry or a thoracic rib hump deformity on Adams Forward Bend test. For patients in whom the physician is concerned that there is clinical evidence of scoliosis, for patients who have had a previous tone-reducing procedure and for more severely involved patients (GMFCS III, IV or V) standing, posterior–anterior (PA) and lateral full spine radiographs should be obtained (Fig. 3.4.5A). If a patient has difficulty standing, a limb-length difference or has significant joint contractures of their lower extremities, then sitting AP and lateral spine radiographs should be obtained instead. If an ambulatory patient with cerebral palsy has a curvature of their spine, they should be closely monitored with repeat spine radiographs obtained at routine intervals (approximately every 4–6 months) through the time period of their adolescence until they reach skeletal maturity. In more severely involved patients, spine radiographs may be obtained after skeletal maturity to monitor the spine for possible progression of the curvature. Neuromuscular spine deformities have a higher propensity for progression after skeletal maturity than idiopathic scoliosis (Thometz and Simon 1988). Sagittal deformities (hyper/hypolordosis and hyper/hypokyphosis) are more common in neuromuscular conditions. For both coronal- and sagittal-plane deformities, correlation with physical examination for flexibility or stress radiographs (flexion, extension, side-bending or traction) can be useful to differentiate fixed from postural deformities.

MEASUREMENT OF SPINAL CURVATURE ON RADIOGRAPHS
If the PA spine radiograph reveals a curvature of the spine, the magnitude of the curve is measured utilizing the Cobb method (Cobb 1948) (Fig. 3.4.5B). A spinal curve of 10° or

(A)

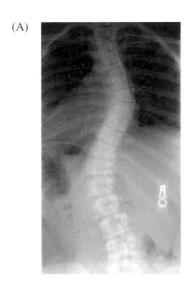

(B)

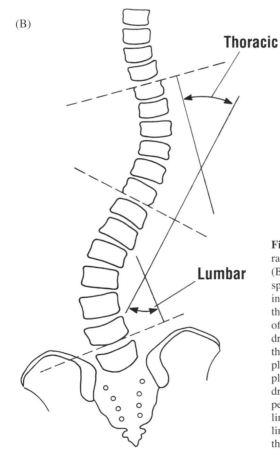

Thoracic

Lumbar

Fig. 3.4.5 (A) Posteroanterior whole spine radiograph of patient with scoliosis. (B) Cobb method of measuring magnitude of spinal curves. Step 1: identify end-vertebrae in the curve or curves. The end-vertebra is the last vertebra that tilts into the concavity of the curve and is the most tilted. Step 2: draw a line across the superior end-plate of the upper end-vertebra and the inferior end plate of the lower end-vertebra. (If the end-plate is difficult to visualize, the line can be drawn using the inferior aspect of both pedicles of the end-vertebra.) Step 3: draw a line perpendicular to each of the end-plate lines. The angle formed by these two lines is the Cobb angle.

less is considered normal. Scoliosis is defined as a curvature of the spine that results in a lateral deviation of the normal vertical line of the spine that is greater than 10°. On the lateral radiograph, a similar method can be used to measure relative kyphosis of the thoracic spine or lordosis of the lumbar spine in the sagittal plane. The thoracic spine should have 10°–40° of kyphosis and the lumbar spine should have 40°–60° of lordosis (O'Brien et al. 2005). Our understanding of the natural history of scoliosis for patients with cerebral palsy is based on previous studies that were historically done on institutionalized patients. General conclusions that can be drawn from these studies include the following: (1) patients with cerebral palsy are at an increased risk of developing scoliosis (Samilson and Bechard 1973), (2) the rate of scoliosis in institutionalized adult cerebral palsy patients varies from 25% to 64% and corresponds to severity of neurologic involvement (Samilson and Bechard 1973, Madigan and Wallace 1981), (3) patients who are nonambulatory and have total body involvement have an incidence of scoliosis of 62%, for bedridden patients the incidence approaches 100% (Saito et al. 1998), and (4) scoliosis may progress in severely involved patients with cerebral palsy after skeletal maturity (Thometz and Simon 1988).

Additional radiographic modalities

RADIOGRAPHIC EVALUATION OF FEMORAL ANTEVERSION
Children with cerebral palsy frequently have increased femoral anteversion. A number of different methods have been described to assess femoral anteversion radiographically (Weiner et al. 1978, Hernandez et al. 1981, Mahboudi and Horstmann 1986, Aamodt et al. 1995, Guenther et al. 1995, Miller et al. 1997, Sugano et al. 1998). For the radiographic evaluation of femoral anteversion for patients who do not have cerebral palsy, CT has been accepted as the criterion and has been proven to be more reliable and more accurate than biplanar radiographs (Kuo et al. 2003). However, in children with cerebral palsy, if optimal positioning of the femur is not possible, then neither 2D nor 3D CT is able to achieve clinically acceptable results (Davids et al. 2003). Ruwe et al. (1992) compared clinical examination of the patient in the prone position by palpation of the lateral trochanteric prominence with established techniques of radiographic evaluation in patients with cerebral palsy. The authors found that when clinical examination was compared with biplanar radiographs and CT scans, the clinical evaluation had the closest correlation to the actual femoral anteversion that was measured intraoperatively.

ADVANCED RADIOGRAPHIC EVALUATION OF ACETABULAR DYSPLASIA
Patients with cerebral palsy are at risk of developing a subluxation of the hip (Lonstein and Beck 1986, Soo et al. 2006, Hagglund et al. 2007). As mentioned previously, neuromuscular subluxation of the hip is often associated with acetabular dysplasia as well as an increased neck-shaft angle (Bobroff et al. 1999). CT imaging has been used to evaluate the location and extent of underlying acetabular deficiency and is a very important tool especially in the more severely involved children (GMFCS IV and V) (Fig. 3.4.6). These children often have hip-flexion contractures and pelvic obliquity making it difficult to interpret the plain radiographs. In able-bodied children with developmental hip dysplasia/dislocation,

254

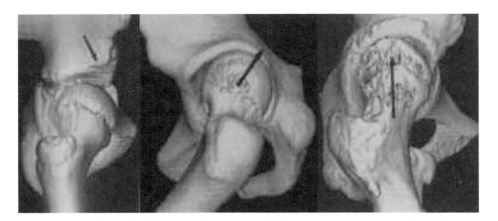

Fig. 3.4.6 Three-dimensional CT reconstruction of three children with cerebral palsy with acetabular dysplasia in different directions. (Reproduced from Kim et al, 1997, by permission)

acetabular deficiency is almost always anterior. Surgical procedures are recommended specific to this problem. For patients with cerebral palsy, the location of acetabular deficiency is variable, but is commonly posterior (Kim and Wenger 1997). However, in some patients the deficiency may actually be more global and may depend on the pattern of spasticity. In this setting, preoperative CT evaluation may provide information regarding the location and extent of underlying acetabular deficiency (Buckley et al. 1991, Chung et al. 2006). This knowledge is critical to perform the proper corrective surgery (see Chapter 5.7).

RADIOGRAPHIC IMAGING FOR SPONDYLOLYSIS
Spondylolysis is a frequent cause of low back pain in adolescent patients. The term spondylolysis refers to a defect of the pars interarticularis region of the posterior elements of the vertebra. It is often the result of repetitive extension or hyperextension-type activities and has been identified in 3%–5% of the population. It usually presents like other stress fractures with insidious onset not associated with an acute injury, but on occasion can be acute or can be found in the absence of clinical symptoms. Harada et al. (1993) identified spondylolysis in 21% of patients with spastic diplegia. Radiographic evaluation of the patient with cerebral palsy for possible spondylolysis should first consist of PA and lateral radiographs of the lumbar spine. If the area in question is limited to a specific level such as the L5–S1 level, a coned-down lateral radiograph at that level may more clearly visualize a defect. Oblique views of the lumbar spine may also help visualize a pars interarticularis defect. If plain radiographs are inconclusive, further imaging may be indicated. Options for additional imaging include a single photon emission computerized tomography (SPECT) scan, a reverse-gantry CT scan or MRI (Harvey et al. 1998). The SPECT scan will show increased scintigraphic uptake at a site of a pars fracture although this test can be negative if the defect is chronic. The SPECT scan may also be helpful to identify the prefracture stage as well to evaluate the healing potential of an established pars defect. The reverse-gantry

CT scan obtained using thin sections of the lumbar spine has been shown to have greater sensitivity and specificity than SPECT scans in identifying radiographically occult spondylolytic defects. Finally, MRI scans have been utilized as an imaging modality that can also be effective and reliable in the diagnosis of a pars defect. It may also be helpful when the CT scan does not show a defect in order to detect a prefracture stage similar to the SPECT scan. However, CT scans have the ability to evaluate healing on subsequent follow-up studies and are still considered the imaging method of choice by some authors in indeterminate cases (Harvey et al. 1998, Campbell et al. 2005, Hu et al. 2008).

EVALUATION OF BONE MINERAL DENSITY IN PATIENTS WITH CEREBRAL PALSY

Patients with cerebral palsy may be at risk of sustaining a fracture depending on a number of different risk factors. Some of these factors are GMFCS level/ambulatory status, anti-convulsant therapy, nutritional status and the need for immobilization (Presedo et al. 2007, Szalay et al. 2008). The risk of fracture also depends on bone strength. A number of variables affect bone strength as well, including bone mass, bone size and bone geometry. Bone mineral density (BMD) is the most widely measured property of bone. It correlates with bone strength and is an independent predictor of fracture risk. Bone mineral density is determined relative to a pre-established set of normative data and is reported as a Z-score. A Z-score of ±1.0 represents a finding 1 standard deviation from the norm. Each Z-score standard deviation decrease equals a 10%–20% decline in BMD. With each standard deviation decrease in BMD, the risk of fracture increases 1.5–2.5 times. The Dual Energy X-ray Absorptiometry (DEXA) Scan has been shown to be effective in assessing BMD in pediatric patients (Grissom and Harcke 2006). It is safe, affordable and precise, and it uses low doses of irradiation. For children with cerebral palsy, the DEXA scan of the lateral distal femur has been developed to overcome some of the limitations of classic DEXA scanning utilized for adults (Harcke et al. 1998, Henderson et al. 2002). However, it has not yet been correlated to predict fracture risk in this population. The DEXA scan also has limitations including the inability to distinguish features such as the structural shape of bone or the structural characteristics of the bone that affect strength (cortical versus cancellous bone, bone quality). Thus other means of assessing BMD have been developed: quantitative ultrasound (QUS) (Jekovcc-Vrhovsek et al. 2005), peripheral quantitative computed tomography (pQCT) (Binkley et al. 2005) and MRI (Modlesky et al. 2008). However, DEXA scans remain the most frequently utilized means of assessing BMD in this pediatric population.

Conclusion

In summary, a patient with cerebral palsy can develop a wide range of conditions affecting their lower extremities as well as their spine. They may also experience conditions that influence their bone mineral density which may put them at increased risk of sustaining a fracture. The radiographic evaluation is an integral part of the clinical evaluation of the patient with cerebral palsy and should provide the clinician with useful information to improve clinical decision-making.

REFERENCES

Aamodt A, Terjesen T, Eine J, Kvistad KA (1995) Femoral anteversion measured by ultrasound and CT: a comparative study. *Skelet Radiol* **24**: 105–9.

Aparicio G, Abril JC, Albinana J, Rodriguez-Salvanes F (1999) Patellar height ratios in children: an interobserver study of three methods. *J Pediatr Orthop B* **8**: 29–32.

Binkley T, Johnson J, Vogel L, Kecskemethy H, Henderson R, Specker B (2005) Bone measurements by peripheral quantitative computed tomography (pQCT) in children with cerebral palsy. *J Pediatr* **147**: 791–6.

Blackburne JS, Peel TE (1977) A new method of measuring patellar height. *J Bone Joint Surg Br* **59**: 241–2.

Blumensaat C (1938) Die Lageabweichumgen und Verrenkungen der Kniescheibe. *Ergebn Chir Orthop* **31**: 149–223.

Bobroff ED, Chambers HG, Sartoris DJ, Wyatt MP, Sutherland DH (1999) Femoral anteversion and neck shaft angle in patients with cerebral palsy. *Clin Orthop Relat Res* **364**: 194–204.

Buckley SL, Sponseller PD, Magid D (1991) The acetabulum in congenital and neuromuscular hip instability. *J Pediatr Orthop* **11**: 498–501.

Campbell RS, Gaines AJ, Hide IG, Papastefanou S, Greenough CG (2005) Juvenile spondylolysis: a comparative analysis of CT, SPECT and MRI. *Skelet Radiol* **34**: 63–73.

Caton J, Deschamps G, Chambat P, Lerat JL, Dejour H (1982) Les rotules basses: a propos de 128 observations. *Rev Chir Orthop* **68**: 317–25.

Chung CY, Park MS, Choi IH, Cho TJ, Yoo WJ, Lee KM (2006) Morphometric analysis of acetabular dysplasia in cerebral palsy. *J Bone Joint Surg Br* **88**: 243–7.

Cobb JR (1948) Outline for the study of scoliosis. In: Edwards JW, editor. *Instructional Course Lectures*, vol. 5. Ann Arbor, MI: American Academy of Orthopaedic Surgeons.

Cooke PH, Cole WG, Carey RP (1989) Dislocation of the hip in cerebral palsy. Natural history and predictability. *J Bone Joint Surg Br* **71**: 441–6.

Davids JR, Marshall AD, Blocker ER, Frick SL, Blackhurst DW, Skewes E (2003) Femoral anteversion in children with cerebral palsy: assessment with two and three dimensional computed tomography scans. *J Bone Joint Surg Am* **85**: 481–8.

De Carvalho A, Andersen AH, Topp S, Jurik AG (1985) A method for assessing the height of the patella. *Int Orthop* **9**: 195–7.

Dobson F, Boyd R, Parrott J, Nattrass G, Graham HK (2002) Hip surveillance in children with cerebral palsy: impact on the surgical management of spastic hip disease. *J Bone Joint Surg Br* **84**: 720–6.

Golan JD, Hall JA, O'Gorman G, Poulin C, Benaroch TE, Cantin MA, Farmer JP (2007) Spinal deformities following selective dorsal rhizotomy. *J Neurosurg* **106** (Suppl 6): 441–9.

Gordon GS, Simkiss DE (2006) A systematic review of the evidence for hip surveillance in children with cerebral palsy. *J Bone Joint Surg Br* **88**: 1492–6.

Grelsamer RP, Meadows S (1992) The modified Insall–Salvati ratio for assessment of patellar height. *Clin Orthop Relat Res* **282**: 170–6.

Grissom LE, Harcke HT (2006) Bone densitometry in pediatric patients. *Del Med J* **78**: 147–50.

Guenther KP, Tomczak R, Kessler S, Pfeiffer T, Puhl W (1995) Measurement of femoral anteversion by magnetic resonance imaging – evaluation of a new technique in children and adolescents. *Eur J Radiol* **21**: 47–52.

Hagglund G, Lauge-Pedersen H, Wagner P (2007) Characteristics of children with hip displacement in cerebral palsy. *BMC Musculoskelet Disord* **8**: 101.

Harada T, Ebara S, Anwar MM, Kajiura I, Oshita S, Hiroshima K, Ono K (1993) The lumbar spine in spastic diplegia. A radiographic study. *J Bone Joint Surg Br* **75**: 534–7.

Harcke HT, Taylor A, Bachrach S, Miller F, Henderson RC (1998) Lateral femoral scan: an alternative method of assessing bone mineral density in children with cerebral palsy. *Pediatr Radiol* **28**: 241–6.

Harvey CJ, Richenberg JL, Saifuddin A, Wolman RL (1998) The radiologic investigation of lumbar spondylolysis. *Clin Ragiol* **53**: 723–8.

Henderson RC, Lark RK, Newman JE, Kecskemthy H, Fung EB, Renner JB, Harcke HT (2002) Pediatric reference data for dual X-ray absorptiometric measures of normal bone density in the distal femur. *Am J Roentgenol* **178**: 439–43.

Hernandez RJ, Tachdjian MO, Poznanski AK, Dias LS (1981) CT determination of femoral torsion. *Am J Roentgenol* **137**: 91–101.

Hu SS, Tribus CB, Diab M, Ghanayem AJ (2008) Spondylolisthesis and spondylolysis. *J Bone Joint Surg Am* **90**: 656–71.

Insall J, Salvati E (1971) Patella position in the normal knee joint. *Radiol* **101**: 101–4.

Jekovec-Vrhovsek M, Kocijancic A, Prezelj J (2005) Quantitative ultrasound of the calcaneus in children and young adults with severe cerebral palsy. *Dev Med Child Neurol* **47**: 696–8.

Johnson MB, Goldstein L, Thomas SS, Piatt J, Aiona M, Sussman M (2004) Spinal deformity after selective dorsal rhizotomy in ambulatory patients with cerebral palsy. *J Pediatr Orthop* **24**: 529–36.

Kay RM, Jaki KA, Skaggs DL (2000) The effect of femoral rotation on the projected femoral neck-shaft angle. *J Pediatr Orthop* **20**: 736–9.

Kim HT, Wenger DR (1997) Location of acetabular deficiency and associated hip dislocation in neuromuscular hip dysplasia: three dimensional computed tomographic analysis. *J Pediatr Orthop* **17**: 143–51.

Koshino T, Sugimoto K (1989) New measurement of patellar height in the knees of children using the epiphyseal line midpoint. *J Pediatr Orthop* **9**: 216–81.

Kuo TY, Skedros JG, Bloebaum RD (2003) Measurement of Femoral Anteversion by biplane radiology and computed tomography imaging: comparison with an anatomic reference. *Invest Radiol* **38**: 221–9.

Laurenson R (1959) The acetabular index: a critical review. *J Bone Joint Surg Br* **41**: 702.

Leung YF, Wai YL, Leung YC (1996) Patella alta in southern China: a new method of measurement. *Int Orthop* **20**: 305–10.

Li Z, Zhu J, Liu X (2008) Deformity of lumbar spine after selective dorsal rhizotomy for spastic cerebral palsy. *Microsurgery* **1**: 10–2.

Lloyd-Roberts GC, Jackson AM, Albert JS (1985) Avulsion of the distal pole of the patella in cerebral palsy. A cause of deteriorating gate. *J Bone Joint Surg Br* **64**: 252–4.

Lonstein JE, Beck K (1986) Hip dislocation and subluxation in cerebral palsy. *J Pediatr Orthop* **6**: 521–6.

Mahboudi S, Horstmann H (1986) Femoral torsion: CT measurement. *Radiol* **160**: 843–4.

Madigan RR, Wallace SL (1981) Scoliosis in the institutionalized cerebral palsy population. *Spine* **6**: 583–90.

Miller F, Liang Y, Merlo M, Harcke HT (1997) Measuring anteversion and femoral neck shaft angle in cerebral palsy. *Dev Med Child Neurol* **39**: 113–18.

Modlesky CM, Subramanian P, Miller F (2008) Underdeveloped trabecular bone microarchitecture is detected in children with cerebral palsy using high-resolution magnetic resonance imaging. *Osteoporos Int* **19**: 169–76.

Norman O, Egund N, Ekelund L, Runow A (1983) The vertical position of the patella. *Acta Orthop Scand* **54**: 908–13.

O'Brien M, Kuklo T, Blanke K, Lenke L (2005) *Spinal Deformity Study Group Radiographic Measurement Manual*. Medtronic Sofamor Danek. p 4.

Paley D, Herzenberg JE, Tetsworth K, McKie J, Bhave A (1994) Deformity planning for frontal and sagittal plane corrective osteotomies. *Orthop Clin N Am* **25**: 425–65.

Palisano R, Rosenbaum P, Walter S, Russell D, Wood E, Galuppi B (1997) Development and reliability of a system to classify gross motor function in children with cerebral palsy. *Dev Med Child Neurol* **39**: 214–23.

Presedo A, Dabney K, Miller F (2007) Fractures in patients with cerebral palsy. *J Pediatr Orthop* **27**: 147–53.

Reimers J (1980) The stability of the hip in children. A radiological study of the results of muscle surgery in cerebral palsy. *Acta Orthop Scand Suppl* **184**: 1–100.

Robin J, Graham HK, Selber P, Dobson F, Smith K, Baker R (2008) Proximal femoral geometry in cerebral palsy. *J Bone Joint Surg Br* **90**: 1372–9.

Rosenthal RK, Levine DB (1977) Fragmentation of the distal pole of the patella in spastic cerebral palsy. *J Bone Joint Surg Am* **59**: 934–9.

Ruwe PA, Gage JR, Ozonoff MB, Deluca PA (1992) Clinical determination of femoral anteversion. A comparison of established techniques. *J Bone Joint Surg Am* **74**: 820–30.

Saito N, Ebara S, Ohotsuka K, Kumeta H, Takaoka K (1998) Natural history of scoliosis in spatstic cerebral palsy. *Lancet* **351**: 1687–92.

Samilson RL, Bechard R (1973) Scoliosis in cerebral palsy; incidence, distribution of curve pattterns, natural history and thoughts on etiology. *Curr Pract Orthop Surg* **5**: 183–205.

Samilson RL, Gill KW (1984) Patello–femoral problems in cerebral palsy. *Acta Orthop Belg* **50**: 191–7.

Scoles PV, Boyd A, Jones PK (1987) Roentgenographic parameters of the normal infant hip. *J Pediatr Orthop* **7**: 656–63.

Scrutton D, Baird G (1997) Surveillance measures of the hips of children with bilateral cerebral palsy. *Arch Dis Child* **76**: 381–4.

Scrutton D, Baird G, Smeeton N (2001) Hip dysplasia in bilateral cerebral palsy: incidence and natural history in children aged 18 months to 5 years. *Dev Med Child Neurol* **43**: 586–600.

Senaran H, Holden C, Dabney K, Miller F (2007a) Anterior knee pain in children with cerebral palsy. *J Pediatr Orthop* **27**: 12–16.

Senaran H, Shah SA, Presedo A, Dabney KW, Glutting JW, Miller F (2007b) The risk of progression of scoliosis in cerebral palsy patients after intrathecal baclofen therapy. *Spine* 32: 2348–54.

Shilt JS, Lai LP, Cabrera MN, Frino J, Smith BP (2008) The impact of intrathecal baclofen on the natural history of scoliosis in cerebral palsy. *J Pediatr Orthop* **28**: 684–7.

Soo B, Howard J, Boyd R, Reid S, Lanigan A, Wolfe R, Reddihough D, Graham HK (2006) Hip displacement in cerebral palsy. *J Bone Joint Surg Am* **88**: 121–9.

Spiegel DA, Loder RT, Alley KA, Rowley S, Gutknecht S, Smith-Wright DL, Dunn ME (2004) Spinal deformity following selective dorsal rhizotomy. *J Pediatr Orthop* **24**: 30–6.

Sugano N, Noble PC, Kamaric E (1998) A comparison of alternative methods of measuring femoral anteversion. *J Comput Assist Tomogr* **22**: 610–14.

Szalay EA, Harriman D, Eastlund B, Mercer D (2008) Quantifying postoperative bone loss in children. *J Pediatr Orthop* **28**: 320–3.

Thometz JG, Simon SR (1988) Progression of scoliosis after skeletal maturity in institutionalized adults who have cerebral palsy. *J Bone Joint Surg Am* **70**: 1290–6.

Tonnis D (1976) Normal values of the hip joint for the evaluation of X-rays in children and adults. *Clin Orthop Relat Res* **119**: 39–47.

Topoleski TA, Kurtz CA, Grogan DP (2000) Radiographic abnormalities and clinical symptoms associated with patella alta in ambulatory children with cerebral palsy. *J Pediatr Orthop* **20**: 636–9.

Vanderwilde R, Staheli L, Chew D, Malagon V (1988) Measurements on radiographs of the foot in normal infants and children. *J Bone Joint Surg Am* **70**: 407–15.

Walker P, Harris I, Leicester A (1998) Patellar tendon-to-patella ratio in children. *J Pediatr Orthop* **18**: 129–31.

Weiner DS, Cook AJ, Hoyt WA Jr, Oravec CE (1978) Computed tomography in the measurement of femoral anteversion. *Orthopedics* **1**: 299–306.

3.5

GAIT ANALYSIS: KINEMATICS, KINETICS, ELECTROMYOGRAPHY, OXYGEN CONSUMPTION AND PEDOBAROGRAPHY

James R. Gage and Jean L. Stout

Gait analysis as a measurement tool

Gait analysis should be thought about as a measurement tool. It provides useful information about the intricacies of the individual's gait, as well as about how far the individual's walking pattern deviates from normal. However, it does not provide a recipe for treatment as some seem to suggest (Watts 1994). That information lies solely within the knowledge base of the investigator who is using the data.

In a motion analysis laboratory, the elements of gait analysis usually include the following: (1) quantitative 3-dimensional measurement of motion (kinematics), (2) measurements of moments and power production occurring in the major articulations of the lower extremities (kinetics), (3) the on–off signals of individual muscles and/or muscle groups (dynamic electromyography), (4) metabolic energy assessment (oxygen consumption), and (5) dynamic foot pressure during gait (pedobarography). Thus gait analysis provides a precise 'snapshot in time' of an individual's pattern of walking or running. Comparison of that 'snapshot' to other databases can be extremely useful. For example, in a child with muscular dystrophy the progression of the condition can be assessed by comparing current data with that of the same individual at an earlier point in time; or in a child with spastic diplegic cerebral palsy, the results of a surgical intervention can be assessed by comparing the child's preoperative data to postoperative data taken a year or two post-surgery.

Comparison to an averaged database of individuals with normal gait also is useful, as it will tell the investigator not only how far the patient's gait is deviating from the typical standard, but also which joints are principally affected. With time an investigator may also learn to recognize patterns of gait deviations, which are characteristic of a particular disease or condition. For example, in children with spastic hemiplegic cerebral palsy there are four distinct patterns of involvement, which are difficult to separate without computerized gait analysis (Winters 1987). Furthermore, treatment protocols have been developed for each of these patterns such that, once the pattern is recognized, appropriate treatment for the individual can be determined (Stout et al. 2004). Motion analysis also provides useful information as to how difficulties with selective motor control, balance problems, and/or spasticity behave in motion. Computerized gait analysis is usually necessary as well to separate out 'coping responses' (see Chapter 2.4). Individuals with abnormal cerebral control, muscle contractures, and/or lever-arm dysfunction are forced to introduce other abnormalities into their gait to compensate or 'cope' with the problems imposed on them by their condition. In a child with spastic hemiplegia, this coping response may be something as simple as vaulting on the less involved side to compensate for a drop foot in swing. In severe hemiplegia (types III and IV), coping responses may alter gait to the extent that the child appears to have triplegic or quadriplegic involvement. Furthermore, coping responses frequently occur in different planes. A complex example of this might be a boy with spastic diplegia and right femoral anteversion who walks with his right hip internally rotated (transverse-plane deformity). He may compensate this with a combination of right pelvic retraction (transverse-plane compensation) plus persistent hip adduction on the right and hip abduction on the left (coronal-plane compensation). Sorting this out with gait analysis is difficult, but without gait analysis it is nearly impossible.

Interpretation of motion analysis can never be done in isolation. It always requires interpretation in conjunction with the patient's medical history as well as other measures of patient assessment. A careful history, which elucidates previous treatment such as orthopaedic surgery or focal spasticity management, may well provide the explanation for an otherwise puzzling gait deviation. Confounding factors such as pain, emotional stress, and/or medications also can impose significant changes on an individual's gait over a very short interval of time, which may lead to invalid interpretation of the gait data. Skilful interpretation of motion analysis data must incorporate information regarding the speed of walking, presence or absence of orthoses, and/or balance aids, all which may significantly alter gait (Schwartz et al. 2008).

The physical examination itself provides useful information about many things that gait analysis does not directly measure. These include information about lever-arm dysfunction (long bone torsions and/or foot deformities), muscle strength and/or contracture, degree of impairment of selective motor control, and body balance. With this additional knowledge, the examiner can start to distinguish between available joint motion (static contracture) versus the dynamic contracture imposed during gait by the particular pathology. Since abnormal muscle tone is absent under anesthesia, repeating the physical examination under general anesthesia just prior to surgical intervention will provide absolute knowledge as to the degree of static muscle contracture that is present, which may in turn result in modification of the surgical plan.

Appropriate imaging is also mandatory for accurate interpretation of motion analysis data. For example, by definition a child with coxa valga and anteversion (both of which are common in spastic diplegia) has lever-arm dysfunction, which will alter his/her gait pattern. The gait deviations produced by the deformity will be readily apparent without imaging, but the interpretation – the 'why' of what is occurring – will be more readily apparent with it. When an examiner is puzzled about abnormal kinematics or kinetics, it also is useful to augment the information with slow-motion video. At our laboratory, we have found that baffling kinematic or kinetic abnormalities of gait finally have found their explanation only after repeatedly viewing the individual's sagittal- and coronal-plane videos in slow motion. On the other hand, if one had only the video without the motion analysis, the gait abnormality might never have been fully appreciated.

Uses of gait analysis

Gait analysis has found many uses in the treatment of an individual with a neuromuscular disability. Because gait analysis can look at the specific deviations of individual lower-extremity joints, it has allowed us to be much more precise in our motor diagnoses. As a result it has allowed the formulation of a 'problem list' in which all gait deviations can be listed. This list then can be further categorized into primary (neurological), secondary (growth), and tertiary ('coping') deformities. Once this has been accomplished we can determine optimal treatment, which often includes interdisciplinary combinations such as spasticity reduction (neurosurgery) and correction of lever-arm dysfunction (orthopaedic surgery). These treatment programs have evolved over the years and will continue to evolve as we persist in critically assessing our outcomes. The current limitations in accurately modeling the foot make the use of gait analysis for decision-making around the foot and ankle a bit more limited. Consequently, in addition to motion analysis, we use close-up, slow-motion video, weightbearing radiographs, and pedobarography to augment our decision-making ability there.

Comparison of preoperative assessment to postoperative result has produced a learning curve (Schwartz et al. 2004, Paul et al. 2007). This has resulted in the replacement of some injurious procedures, such as tendo-Achilles lengthening in spastic diplegia, which lengthened both the relatively normal soleus and the abnormal gastrocnemius, with other procedures (Baumann, Strayer, etc.), which better address the specific problem (gastrocnemius spasticity/contracture) (Strayer 1958, Saraph et al. 2000). Motion analysis has demonstrated the role of lever-arm dysfunction in gait pathology and the benefits of correcting it, which were largely unappreciated prior to its advent (Gage 1991, Gage and Novacheck 2001, Erdemir and Piazza 2002, Gage and Schwartz 2002, 2004, Schwartz and Lakin 2003, Hicks et al. 2007). Preoperative versus postoperative analysis also has demonstrated the advantages of newer therapies such as spasticity reduction (selective dorsal rhizotomy or intrathecal baclofen pump) and single-event multilevel surgery, which allows simultaneous correction of all growth deformities (Gage and Novacheck 2001, Zwick et al. 2001, Schwartz et al. 2004, Rodda et al. 2006, Langerak et al. 2008).

Motion analysis has permitted us to evaluate the specific effect of orthoses (White et al. 2002, Bartonek et al. 2007). We routinely test children in and out of their orthoses both before and after planned interventions. This has allowed us not only to appraise the utility of the orthosis, i.e. whether or not it is improving function, but also to design more functional orthoses that are better suited to their specific tasks (Harrington et al. 1984, Van Gestel et al. 2008). Finally, gait analysis has proved to be very useful in prostheses, where successive designs of the device itself can be tested for functionality, but that discussion is beyond the scope of this text (Hicks et al. 1985).

Interpretation of gait analysis components

Each specific component of gait analysis contributes information that collectively focuses the interpreter to a problem list and ultimately to a treatment plan. The contribution of each component will now be discussed (Davids et al. 2003).

Kinematics

Normal kinematics are presented and defined in chapter 1.3 and in the DVD on Normal Gait, which is included with this book and will not be discussed further. Our purpose here is to discuss how these parameters are used in gait evaluation. Kinematics provide specific information as to 'what' is happening at the trunk, pelvis, and at each of the three major lower-extremity articulations (hip, knee, and ankle) bilaterally in all three planes (sagittal, coronal and transverse) throughout the gait cycle (Fig. 3.5.1). As such they are very useful

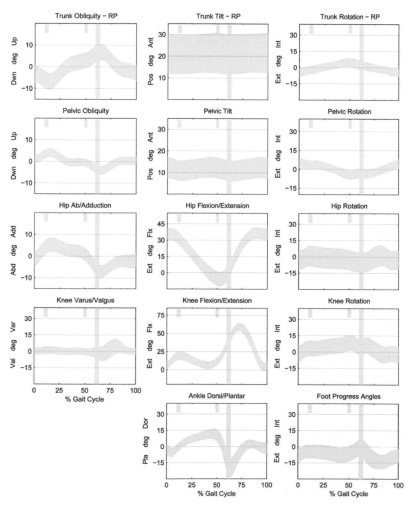

Center for Gait and Motion Analysis Gillette Children's Specialty Healthcare
Control Kinematics

Fig. 3.5.1 Normal kinematics of the coronal, sagittal and transverse planes including the trunk. Degrees of motion are on the ordinate and gait cycle percentage is on the abscissa. The vertical bar denotes toe-off and separates stance from swing.

263

for determining deviations of gait from that of a typical individual, looking at changes in a gait pattern over time and/or pre- and post-treatment. Linear measurements (velocity, step and stride length, stance time, etc.) are also kinematic variables.

When applying kinematics to the interpretation of a gait study, we look at things such as the timing of events within the gait cycle (stance and swing time, step and stride length, speed, etc.), the shape and magnitude of the graphs (modulation), range-of-motion, timing of specific events (toe-off, peak knee flexion in swing, etc.), and velocities (e.g. rate of knee flexion in initial-swing). We also observe things such as consistency from cycle to cycle and symmetry from side to side.

Presentation of Case MC (see Case 1 on Interactive Disc)

A case example may be the best way to demonstrate the application of gait analysis. This is a 14-year-old boy with right hemiplegic cerebral palsy, at Gross Motor Function Classification System (GMFCS) level II. He had had no previous orthopaedic intervention. In addition to his hemiplegia, he has learning, behavioral, and cognitive delays. He lives with a foster family, and as such no birth history or previous medical history is available. He was referred to our facility by a pediatric orthopaedist for recommendations to improve his walking (Fig. 3.5.2).

The kinematic findings of case MC are typical of a child with type IV hemiplegia using the classification scheme of Winters et al. (1987), and demonstrate nicely that kinematics

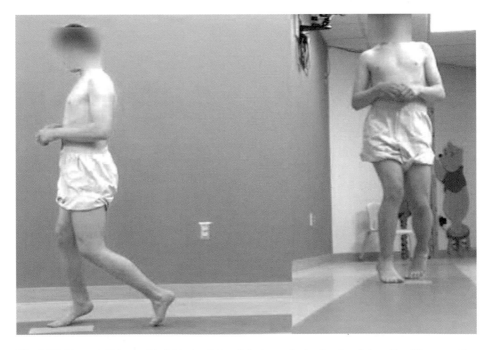

Fig. 3.5.2 14 year-old boy with right spastic hemiplegic cerebral palsy (see Interactive Disc, case 1).

264

often lend themselves to pattern recognition. The reason for this is that the pattern of abnormality of the sagittal-plane data of the ankle, knee, pelvis and hip (Fig. 3.5.3, center column) are typical of this particular hemiplegic pattern type. In the sagittal plane, we see the following abnormalities on the right (hemiplegic) side:

(1) continuous plantarflexion of the ankle throughout the gait cycle
(2) persistent knee flexion of 25° in stance phase with decreased and delayed timing of peak knee flexion in swing phase
(3) decreased total range of hip motion with incomplete hip extension in terminal stance phase
(4) a single bump pelvic tilt pattern consistent with poor pelvic–hip dissociation.

The transverse-plane graphs (Fig. 3.5.3, right column) demonstrate the following:

(1) persistent internal hip rotation throughout the gait cycle with mild pelvic retraction on the hemiplegic side.
(2) asymmetric pelvic rotation (pelvic retraction on the right side)
(3) left internal foot-progression angle (possible left internal tibial torsion).

Hemiplegia types III and IV are typically associated with excessive femoral anteversion. In this particular case, the measured internal hip rotation was consistent with excessive femoral anteversion. The relationship between anteversion and hip rotation was, however, inconsistent. Physical examination confirmed the fact that there was 60° of anteversion on the right side with relatively normal anteversion on the left. Even without anteversion, retraction of the pelvis on the involved side is typical in hemiplegia. In fact, when femoral anteversion and hemiplegia are present on the same side, it will often produce more pelvic retraction than we are seeing here. Since the foot progression angle is referenced to the coordinates of the laboratory, the 15° of internal foot rotation on the right was about what we would expect given that femoral torsion was internal by about 25° and there was a compensation of ~10° of pelvic retraction. On the left side, even after eliminating the internal bias of the pelvis, there was excessive internal foot progression suggesting a left internal tibial torsion, which was confirmed on clinical evaluation.

In general the coronal plane can be confusing because both primary and compensatory deviations can be present in this plane. There are also mathematical subtleties that render the coronal plane angles difficult to interpret. The coronal plane (Fig. 3.5.3, left column) demonstrates the following:

(1) pelvic obliquity (right side high, left side low)
(2) persistent adduction of the right hip and abduction of the left hip throughout the gait cycle.

In order to make sense of the gait pathology, one must remember that if balance and stability are to be maintained, abnormalities of gait require compensations. For example,

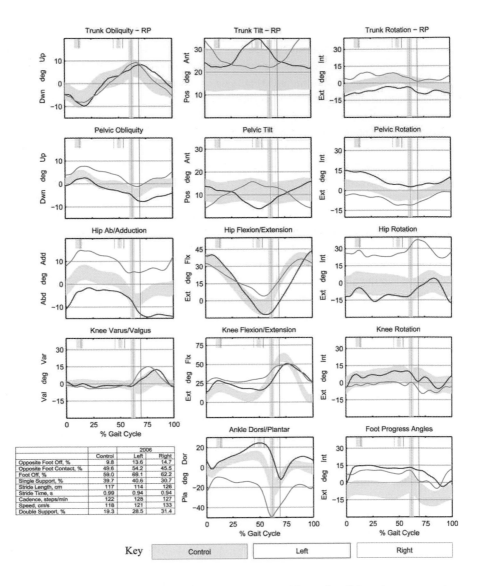

	2006		
	Control	Left	Right
Opposite Foot Off, %	9.8	13.6	14.7
Opposite Foot Contact, %	49.6	54.2	45.5
Foot Off, %	59.0	69.1	62.2
Single Support, %	39.7	40.6	30.7
Stride Length, cm	117	114	126
Stride Time, s	0.99	0.94	0.94
Cadence, steps/min	122	128	127
Speed, cm/s	118	121	133
Double Support, %	19.3	28.5	31.4

Fig. 3.5.3 The patient's sagittal-, transverse- and coronal-plane kinematics. Gait cycle percentage is on the abscissa and degrees of motion on the ordinate. The vertical bar at about 60% of the gait cycle delineates stance and swing. The gray band indicates the typical mean ± 1 standard deviation. The red line denotes the left side and the green line the right. The pathology is coming primarily from the right side. Both sides demonstrate deviations from normal, but the abnormalities on the left would be expected to normalize if the problems on the right were to be corrected. Sagittal-plane kinematics (center column) demonstrate the typical findings of a child with type IV hemiplegia (progressive anterior pelvic tilt from initial contact until pre-swing, incomplete hip and knee extension in stance, restricted knee flexion in swing, and ankle equinus). Transverse-plane kinematics (right column) demonstrate asymmetric pelvic rotation with retraction of the right hemipelvis, internal hip rotation throughout the gait cycle and internal foot progression. Coronal-plane kinematics (left column) demonstrate a pelvic obliquity (right side high, left side low). The right hip is continuously adducted and the left abducted throughout the gait cycle.

266

even though clinical measurement demonstrates that the right lower extremity is about 1 cm shorter than the left, the fact that he is walking in extreme equinus on the right and mild dorsiflexion on the left makes his right lower extremity functionally longer than the left. In addition, clinical examination suggests that his right hip-adductors are spastic, which would favor this pattern of pelvic obliquity. Finally, when one walks with pelvic retraction in the transverse plane, the hip-adductors on the retracted side and the hip-abductors on the protracted side are brought into the line of progression, which in typical gait is the flexion–extension plane (crab-walking is an extreme example of this). This probably accounts for the relative adduction on the right and abduction on the left throughout the gait cycle.

When one looks at the kinematics on the left side, it is readily apparent that they are also abnormal (that is, they fall out of the typical 2 standard deviation bandwidth). Again with some study and reflection, it will become apparent that most of the abnormalities on the left (with the exception of internal foot rotation, which is probably secondary to internal tibial torsion) are coming about because of gait compensations. As such if the abnormalities on the right side were to be corrected, most of the deviations on the left side could be expected to disappear.

MUSCLE LENGTHS

Muscle lengths are probably best thought of as a subset of kinematics. The methods by which they are derived have been discussed in the Normal Gait DVD. Our laboratory routinely outputs muscle-length graphs of hamstrings and psoas muscles (Fig. 3.5.4). It is difficult to assess the length and modulation of biarticular muscles during gait because affected individuals walk with abnormal limb positions/postures and biarticular muscles span more than one joint. Therefore these graphs have proven to be very useful in the assessment of biarticular muscle function in cerebral palsy and other neuromuscular gait disorders. Muscle-length graphs provide information on two aspects of a muscle's function: (1) its length throughout the gait cycle, and (2) its pattern of movement (modulation).

In our case example, it can be seen that the psoas and hamstring muscles on the left side are within the band of normal length and the curves have the appropriate shape, i.e. the muscles are modulating or moving normally. On the right side it can be seen that the psoas muscle begins and ends the gait cycle in the middle of the normal band, which implies that its functional length is normal. On the other hand, the medial and lateral hamstrings are functionally short at the beginning and end of the gait cycle. However, none of the three muscle groups on the right are modulating normally, which indicates that their range-of-motion is constricted.

It is important to realize that muscle-length graphs reflect only the functional length of the muscle during gait, and do not necessarily represent contracture. For example, if an individual without a disability chooses to walk with extended knees, an anterior pelvic tilt and excessive lumbar lordosis, his/her hamstrings will be functionally longer than the normal standard and the psoas muscles will be functionally shorter. Therefore, if the medial hamstrings are short referable to the standard in our example, it does not necessarily mean that the muscles are actually contracted or short. Rather, it means that in the postural pattern

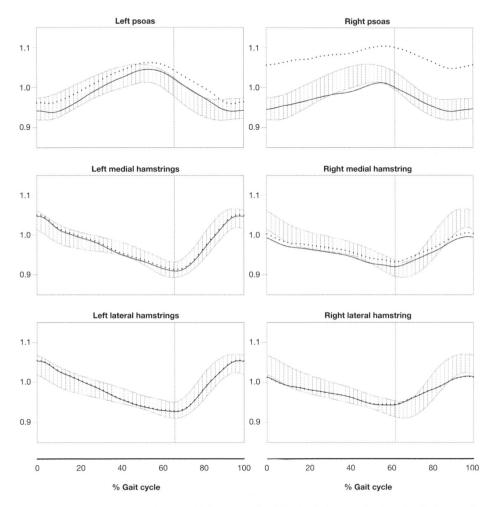

Fig. 3.5.4 Muscle-length graphs are useful when evaluating biarticular muscles. The hatched area of the graph indicates the typical mean ± 1 standard deviation. Percentage of gait cycle is on the abscissa and normalized origin to insertion length on the ordinate. The solid line depicts muscle length calculated with a generic model, dashed line depicts muscle length calculated with representation of the patient's anteversion (60° right, 25° left). The findings on the left are within normal limits. On the right, the resting length of the psoas is normal but its modulation (movement pattern) is restricted. The hamstrings are short in terminal swing at rest (medial > lateral) and modulation is markedly restricted. This finding is characteristic of muscle spasticity.

in which the patient is walking, muscles are *functionally* shorter than the normal standard. To best determine if his hamstrings were actually short, it would probably be necessary to assess his/her hips with the Thomas test under general anesthesia just prior to surgical intervention.

Abnormal muscle modulation (the pattern of muscle movement) often is an indication of inadequate muscle control and/or abnormal muscle tone. For example, many individuals with hamstring spasticity will demonstrate relatively normal hamstring length at rest with little or no modulation of the muscle during the gait cycle. In some of these individuals, surgical reduction of spasticity via selective dorsal rhizotomy will act to normalize the muscle's function (Fig. 3.5.5).

Biarticular muscle length will be discussed in more detail when we come to treatment. Muscle-length graphs have proven to be extremely useful in assessing biarticular muscle function in conditions such as crouch gait. For example, it has previously been assumed that the hamstrings always were short in crouch gait. However, muscle-length graphs demonstrate that the hamstrings are of normal length or long in about half of the cases. (Hoffinger et al. 1993, Delp et al. 1996, Schutte et al. 1997, Arnold et al. 2006, van der Krogt et al. 2008).

KINETICS

We learned earlier that *kinematics* were useful in describing 'what' specific gait anomalies were occurring. Furthermore, since they define the relationship between different body segments (links), they can be visualized. *Kinetics* find their best use in describing *why* a particular gait pathology is occurring. Kinetics involve the study of forces, moments, energy, and power associated with the kinematics. As with kinematics, normal kinetics were presented and defined earlier (Chapter 1.3 and DVD on Normal Gait). Kinetics are subdivided into *moments* and *powers*.

When applying kinetics to the interpretation of a gait study, on *moment graphs* we look at things such as the point of crossover from an extensor to flexor moment and whether it, in fact, occurs. We also look at the magnitude and shape of the moment in question, and if the moment appropriately corresponds to the timing of the dynamic electromyography (EMG). When interpreting *power graphs*, we again look at the timing, magnitude, and appropriateness of power compared to the typical standard. They tell us whether net power is being produced at the joint in question, and if so whether the muscle contraction is concentric (shortening) or eccentric (lengthening). Positive power indicates that power is being generated. Negative power indicates it is being absorbed.

In our case example (Fig. 3.5.6), the hip-moment graph of the hemiplegic right side is within normal limits, whereas the initial extension moment of the left hip is excessive. This probably reflects the excessive hip flexion on the left at the time of initial contact. At the knee, the initial extension moment of the vasti muscles is diminished on the right and there is a persistent knee-extension moment throughout the remainder of stance. This indicates that the ground reaction force is behind the knee and therefore continuous activity of the vasti is necessary to prevent the knee from buckling. The large extension moment in late stance and initial swing is probably secondary to spasticity of the rectus femoris. Remember

269

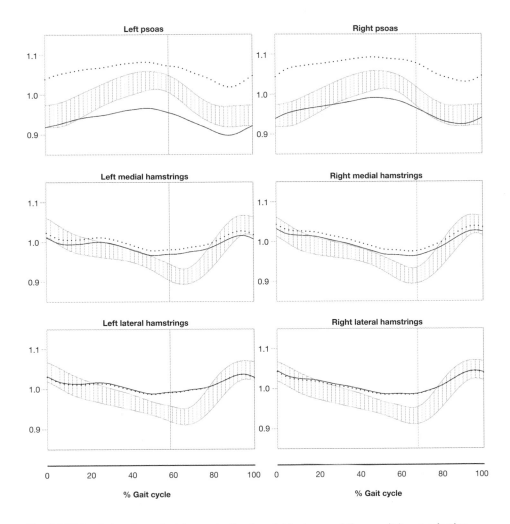

Fig. 3.5.5 Muscle-length graphs (a) pre-selective dorsal rhizotomy and (b, opposite) post-selective dorsal rhizotomy. Note that the restricted modulation of the psoas and hamstrings muscles, which was present prior to rhizotomy, has normalized following reduction of the child's spasticity.

that the three vasti and the rectus femoris act at different times in the gait cycle. The vasti support the knee during loading response whereas the rectus femoris controls the rate of knee flexion during pre-swing and initial swing. In this case, there is excessive damping of knee flexion such that we would expect that this young man might have problems with foot drag during the first half of swing phase. On the left side, the extension moment is also slightly

b)

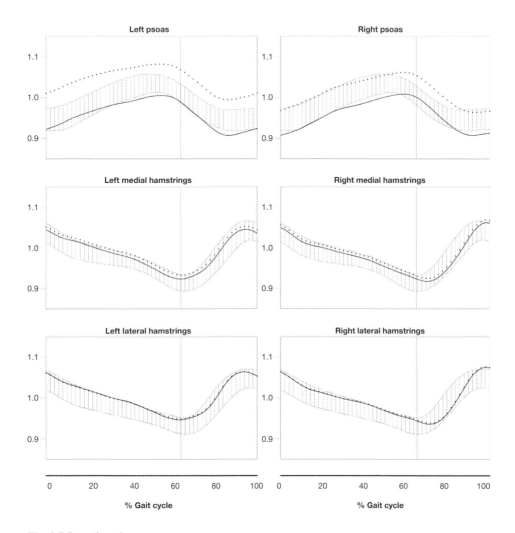

Fig. 3.5.5 continued

excessive throughout stance phase. This is probably secondary to the fact that the left knee is in mildly excessive flexion throughout stance phase as well. Note, however, that the magnitude of the extension moment produced by the rectus femoris during pre-swing on the left is normal as is the rate of knee flexion in pre-swing and initial swing. The left ankle-moment graph demonstrates a large plantarflexor moment that begins almost immediately

271

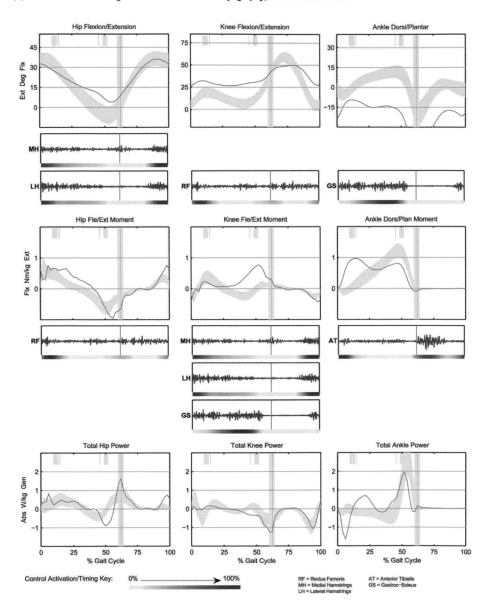

Fig. 3.5.6 and opposite Combination graphs of the right (a) and left (b) sides demonstrating sagittal plane kinetics and dynamic electromyography (EMG). The top row of graphs represent the kinematics of the sagittal plane, the bottom two rows the sagittal plane kinetics. Joint moments are illustrated in the middle row and joint powers in the bottom row. Graphs illustrating the dynamic EMG of muscles, which affect the joint, are pictured above and below the moment graphs. The findings derived from these graphs are discussed in the text that follows on page 274 in the case presentation.

(b)

Left Side Combined Electromyography, Kinematics & Kinetics

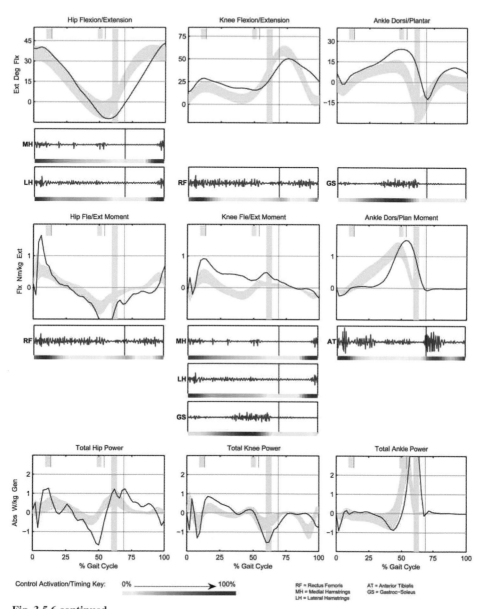

Fig. 3.5.6 continued

following toe contact. In this particular case, the abnormal moment is probably secondary to two factors: (1) the gastrocnemius is spastic, and (2) the abnormal landing position with the knee in 25° of flexion and the foot in 15° of equinus imparts an immediate stretch to the spastic muscle at initial contact, which in turn triggers a strong premature contraction. Close scrutiny of the plantarflexion moment reveals that it is biphasic. The reason for this will become apparent when we look at the ankle-power graph.

In our case example, the power graph of the hip extension (H1) power burst is somewhat diminished on the hemiplegic right side and mildly increased on the left. Again, this would be expected as several studies have shown that hemiplegic individuals derive the bulk of their power for propulsion from the less affected side (Olney et al. 1990, Fonseca et al. 2001, Detrembleur et al. 2003). The power graph of the knee is close to normal on the affected side. The right ankle demonstrates power absorption during loading response. This likely stimulates a central pattern generator (CPG) in the spinal cord, which results in a premature contraction of the triceps surae in mid-stance, as evidenced by the abnormal concentric power burst that follows. Following a short period of relaxation, there is a second firing of the triceps surae at the appropriate time in terminal stance, but of diminished magnitude compared to typical standard. Ankle power is normal on the left except that the magnitude of power at push-off is mildly increased.

ELECTROMYOGRAPHY

The role of EMG was discussed in Chapter 1.3. The challenges to EMG interpretation are multifactorial and include issues of detection techniques, signal recording and signal processing, as well as the challenges of understanding muscles that function isotonically (in both concentric and eccentric fashion) and isometrically within a given gait cycle (Yoon et al. 1981). As muscles change function, the relationships between the EMG signal and muscle force, muscle length, and endurance change as well. Speed of walking also plays an important role that must be kept in mind when interpreting EMG (den Otter et al. 2004, Schwartz et al. 2008). It is beyond the scope of this chapter to discuss all aspects of EMG instrumentation, electrodes, detection techniques, processing and normalization. The reader is referred to some excellent resources on these topics (Basmajian and DeLuca 1985, Perry 1992), and the DVD that accompanies this book. A short review of pertinent information follows.

The goal of EMG interpretation for an individual gait study in our laboratory is centered on three primary aspects related to timing: (1) identification of spasticity and other types of hypertonia, (2) evidence of selectivity, control, and muscular coordination, and (3) the contribution of individual muscles via fine wire techniques.

TIMING

Each muscle during the gait cycle has a characteristic pattern of activation and cessation of activity that is typically preserved with changes in speed in both children and adults (Perry 1992, Sutherland 2001, Hof et al. 2002, den Otter et al. 2004, Schwartz et al. 2008). With disability, timing can be disrupted for a number of reasons that may be related to the underlying neuromuscular deficit, but may be related to the mechanics or position of the joints and the demand for muscular activity at any given aspect of the walking cycle (Rose and McGill 2005). Timing of EMG signals, therefore, must not be interpreted in isolation. One choice is to interpret the EMG signals on a display that includes the corresponding kinematic and kinetic data (Fig. 3.5.6). By such a display we can determine whether muscle cessation is coordinated with a zero crossover point on the moment graph (when activity is no longer necessary), coordinated with decreased velocity of movement, or is independent of such factors. The display helps to determine whether the activity is a dynamic obstruction to function or appropriate support for a particular joint posture.

Perry (1992) described a series of EMG timing errors that are commonly seen at clinical gait laboratories. Each has significance to interpretation. For example, out of phase timing can be important in determining whether a muscle is appropriate for transfer (Fig. 3.5.7). This interpretation of timing has been used for both upper- and lower-extremity muscles (Gage et al. 1987, Van Heest et al. 2008). Premature timing, which begins before typical onset, may be a sign of spasticity. Each of the timing errors described by Perry is used to infer information about muscle function.

Timing of activity between muscles can be an important indicator of selective motor control and/or muscle coordination. If a group of muscles tested are simultaneously on, then simultaneously off, this is considered a sign of patterned movement or poor selective motor control (Fig. 3.5.8). Similarly, if all muscles tested demonstrate continuous activity, this would be another sign of limited control. Co-contraction of muscles is important and typical during some phases of the gait cycle, but not others. Obstructive co-contraction can be yet another sign of poor motor control.

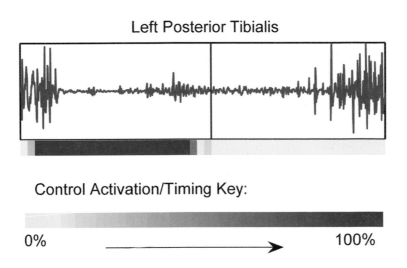

Fig. 3.5.7 Dynamic EMG of the tibialis posterior during a single gait cycle. The activity is out-of-phase. The muscle is quiet when activity is expected and active when none is expected. This muscle would be considered appropriate for transfer to make use of the out-of-phase timing. The colored bands indicate typical activity time.

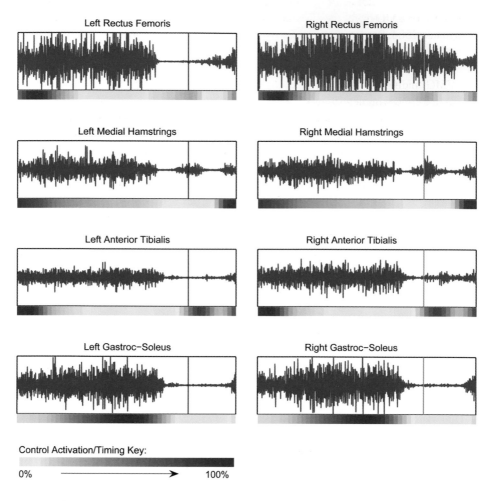

Fig. 3.5.8 EMG graphs of a patient who demonstrates a 'mass-flexion' pattern of activity. Notice that all muscles are all firing synchronously. This is noted bilaterally, but particularly on the left side. This pattern of activity is typical of an individual who has limited selective muscle control. Consequently locomotion is accomplished by reciprocating primitive patterns of mass flexion and mass extension of the hip, knee, and ankle.

DIFFERENTIATING TYPES OF HYPERTONIA

EMG can also be used to assist in the differentiation of types of hypertonia. Spasticity is evidenced in the EMG signal by premature firing, inappropriate bursts of activity associated with a particular motion, or clonus. It can also be noted by prolonged activity or continuous muscle activity. Differentiation of non-spastic types of hypertonia such as dystonia is more complicated. Characteristics of dystonia include repeated short bursts of activity

276

superimposed on more sustained tonic activity. Efforts are under way to separate the burst activity from the tonic activity, but in the clinical setting, the clinician often relies on experience or EMG data collection during non-gait type of activities (Grosse et al. 2004, Wang et al. 2004, Sanger 2008).

EMG FINDINGS IN CASE OF MC

The EMG findings of case MC (Fig. 3.5.6) demonstrate the asymmetry that one would expect in a child with hemiplegia. This is most clearly noted at the gastrocnemius. On the left side, a normal firing pattern is present. On the right, his hemiplegic side, he has premature firing of the muscle in terminal swing, and multiple bursts of activity in stance. The combination EMG, kinematic, kinetic plots demonstrate that he has a burst of activity coincident with the double bump moment pattern in stance and the inappropriate premature power generation in stance. Anterior tibialis activity on the right exhibits curtailed or early termination of EMG that does not return in terminal swing as is noted on the left. The amplitude of the rectus femoris is low, but inappropriate activity is present in swing phase during a time when knee flexion is blunted. Visually, hamstring activity does not appear to be different right to left. On each side, activity is prolonged into stance phase. Cessation of activity is noted at the timing of crossover of the hip-joint moment on the right side.

METABOLIC ENERGY ASSESSMENT (OXYGEN CONSUMPTION)

Metabolic expenditure measurement has long been used as a measure of gait efficiency, but is not a routine assessment in most clinical gait laboratories (Schwartz 2001). Despite limited clinical use, its relationship to overall gait pathology and a number of functional outcome tools has been demonstrated (Tervo et al. 2002). Evidence suggests that it can also be used as an indicator of the effect or magnitude of increased muscle tone, spasticity, or co-contraction (Unnithan et al. 1996). As a result, it has been useful in a number of intervention and outcome studies (Maltais et al. 2001, Schwartz et al. 2004, Thomas et al. 2004, Stout et al. 2008, Trost et al. 2008). While it is clear that the vast majority of children with cerebral palsy have increased energy expense for a variety of reasons previously described (Unnithan et al. 1996, 1999, Stout and Koop 2004, Potter and Unnithan 2005), the clinical utility for an individual child remains in the information it provides regarding the functional impact of the gait deviations that are unique to that child. Treatment decisions may be directed on the basis of the impact noted.

The rate of oxygen uptake (the amount of oxygen used per unit time) is the raw data collected. Just as with many other variables used in gait analysis interpretation, a normalization scheme is necessary to provide a common frame of reference between and across individuals of different ages and size etc. A non-dimensional normalization scheme allows comparisons across age, size, and sex (Schwartz et al. 2006). During any task (including walking), oxygen uptake comprises two components: a resting expenditure which consists of a basal metabolic rate and resting muscular consumption and a movement expenditure which consists of the antigravity and forward propulsion aspects of movement. The information can be expressed as gross expenditure (resting expenditure + movement expenditure) or net expenditure (gross expenditure − resting expenditure). Controversy exists over which has greater clinical utility (Baker et al. 2001, Schwartz et al. 2006, Brehm et al. 2007, 2008). Net expenditure provides the *energy of walking*, and is independent of the effects of growth (Baker et al. 2001, Schwartz et al. 2006). Independence from basal metabolic rate and biochemical differences, which vary with maturation, is also an important aspect (Potter et al. 1999, Potter and Unnithan 2005). All make it appropriate for long-term evaluation (Schwartz 2007). Gross expenditure, however, is more reproducible than net expenditure because it avoids the inherent increased error which results from the subtraction of values in the net protocol (Brehm et al. 2007, 2008). Evaluation of an individual child for clinically relevant changes may best be done by gross expenditure, particularly in the short term. A decision scheme has been suggested by Brehm and colleagues (2008) to determine when gross versus net energy reporting may be more appropriate in clinical planning.

Net non-dimensional energy expenditure for case MC is presented in Figure 3.5.9. He walks at a velocity within the typical range. His net energy expenditure is 1.78 times higher than typical for his given walking velocity. This falls just outside the 95% confidence interval of typical data. The average energy expenditure for children with type IV hemiplegia is 1.97, S.D. 0.35. This suggests the functional impact of the deviations identified for MC's gait is minimal.

DYNAMIC FOOT-PRESSURES DURING GAIT (PEDOBAROGRAPHY)

Dynamic pedobarography has been a continuously evolving technology ever since the first plantar pressures were captured in the early 20th century. Its use in pediatric gait analysis, in particular for children with cerebral palsy, continues to evolve as well. Today's systems typically measure pressure, vertical force, and foot contact area during the stance phase of the gait cycle. Both in-shoe systems and pressure-platform/mat systems have been used. There is a body of knowledge for both typically developing children (Bowen et al. 1998, Femery et al. 2002, Bertsch et al. 2004, Stebbins et al. 2005, Jameson et al. 2008, Linton et al. 2008), and in children with cerebral palsy (Oeffinger et al. 2000, Femery et al. 2002, Stebbins et al. 2005, 2006, Park et al. 2008, Westberry et al. 2008). System technology typically consists of calibrated force or capacitive sensors in which the electrical properties change under pressure creating a signal proportional to the pressure exerted. All systems use some method of normalization. Challenges to the interpretation of data include the fact that pressures increase with weight and speed of walking, and it is difficult without normative data for weight and speed to accurately assess the impact of any increased pressures present. Additionally, the influence of high pressures for a short duration of time versus lower pressures for longer duration is also important to consider. In our laboratory, we make use of the center of force progression to assess for areas where the pressure is maintained for a duration of time (Fig. 3.5.10). Methods to correlate to radiographic alignment show promise and potentially can be an important tool both preoperatively and postoperatively (Park et al. 2008, Westberry et al. 2008).

Plantar pressures (MatScan® by Tekscan Inc., Boston MA) for case MC demonstrate asymmetry right to left. Best viewed dynamically, the left side (his less involved side) demonstrates a forefoot heel-contact progression pattern. The right side clearly

Normalized O2 Consumption

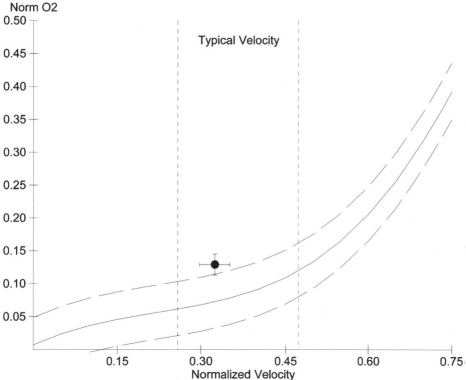

Fig. 3.5.9 A graph demonstrating energy expenditure. Non-dimensional normalized velocity is on the abscissa and net non-dimensional normalized rate of oxygen consumption on the ordinate. The two dashed vertical lines represent the 95% confidence interval of typical walking velocity. The solid line of the graph indicates typical net oxygen consumption at a particular velocity. The area between the two long-dashed lines represents the 95% confidence interval for net oxygen by velocity. Solid dot displays case data plus error bars. See text for a discussion of the findings.

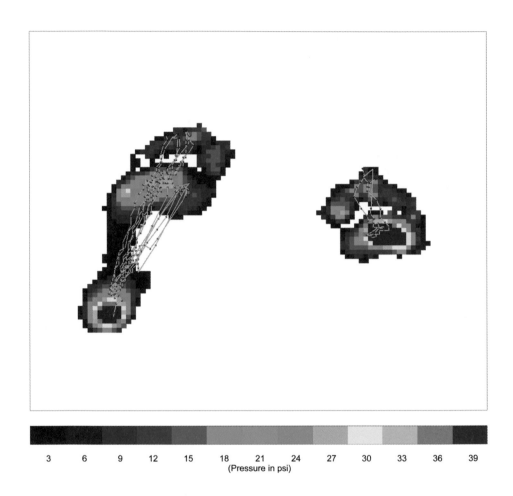

3   6   9   12   15   18   21   24   27   30   33   36   39

(Pressure in psi)

Fig. 3.5.10 Plantar pressure graphs of the patient's left and right sides. Colors indicate the magnitude of the pressure with red being the highest and blue the lowest. The red line on the foot indicates the progression of the center of pressure as the individual moves through the gait cycle. Notice that on the right side all of the patient's weight is borne on the forefoot and the pressure on the middle metatarsal heads is very high.

demonstrates weightbearing only across the metatarsal heads (see Video 3.5.1 on Interactive Disc for a presentation of pedobarography). The high-pressure areas indicated as red (greater than 36 pounds per square inch) measure 60–65 pounds per square inch at the left heel and 60–80 pounds per square inch at the right metatarsal heads (patient weight 136 lbs). The principal axis of each foot is internal bilaterally (Fig. 3.5.10).

Conclusions

In summary, we have attempted to point out how gait analysis can be used as a clinical tool to precisely document an individual's gait parameters at any point in time. In this particular chapter, we have demonstrated its value in detecting and/or localizing specific gait pathologies, which otherwise might not be apparent. This, in turn, enables the examiner to construct a problem list, which includes all major elements of the patient's pathology. Once we have this problem list in hand, we can go on to generate a specific plan of treatment. After that treatment is completed and the individual has fully recovered, a second gait analysis will allow the examiner to assess the results of the intervention. It is only with this kind of careful assessment that treatment errors can be determined and, in the future, avoided. In the case of cerebral palsy, prior to gait analysis we started with a patient with spasticity and gait pathologies who walked badly and ended with the same patient with spasticity and gait pathologies who walked differently. However, because we could not assess the specifics of the intervention, treatment protocols could never really improve.

Gait analysis is also useful for documenting the progression of a condition such as muscular dystrophy by comparing multiple analyses of the same individual over a period of time, and/or to evaluate the effect of the effect of an orthotic device or medication.

The analysis that was conducted on the patient presented in this chapter has allowed us to construct the following problem list:

(1) right femoral anteversion (about 60°)
(2) right knee-flexion contracture with associated patella alta and quadriceps insufficiency
(3) right psoas spasticity without contracture
(4) right hamstring spasticity and contracture
(5) right adductor spasticity and contracture
(6) right rectus femoris spasticity
(7) right triceps surae contracture (gastrocnemius > soleus)
(8) right dorsiflexor insufficiency with foot drop in swing
(9) left internal tibial torsion.

With this problem list in hand, we can now determine an appropriate program of treatment, which is discussed in the second section of this book.

REFERENCES

Arnold AS, Liu MQ, Schwartz MH, Õunpuu S, Delp SL (2006) The role of estimating muscle-tendon lengths and velocities of the hamstrings in the evaluation and treatment of crouch gait. *Gait Posture* **23**: 273–81.

Baker R, Hausch A, McDowell B (2001) Reducing the variability of oxygen consumption measurements. *Gait Posture* **13**: 202–9.

Bartonek A, Eriksson M, Gutierrez-Farewik EM (2007) A new carbon fibre spring orthosis for children with plantarflexor weakness. *Gait Posture* **25**: 652–6.

Basmajian JV, DeLuca CJ (1985) *Muscles Alive – Their Functions Revealed by Electromyography*, 5th edn. Baltimore: Williams and Wilkins.

Bertsch C, Unger H, Winkelmann W, Rosenbaum D (2004) Evaluation of early walking patterns from plantar pressure distribution measurements. First year results of 42 children. *Gait Posture* **19**: 235–42.

Bowen TR, Lennon N, Castagno P, Miller F, Richards J (1998) Variability of energy-consumption measures in children with cerebral palsy. *J Pediatr Orthop* **18**: 738–42.

Brehm MA, Becher J, Harlaar J (2007) Reproducibility evaluation of gross and net walking efficiency in children with cerebral palsy. *Dev Med Child Neurol* **49**: 45–8.

Brehm MA, Knol DL, Harlaar J (2008) Methodological considerations for improving the reproducibility of walking efficiency outcomes in clinical gait studies. *Gait Posture* **27**: 196–201.

Davids JR, Õunpuu S, DeLuca PA, Davis RB (2003) Optimization of walking ability of children with cerebral palsy. *J Bone Joint Surg Am* **85**: 2224–34.

Delp SL, Arnold AS, Speers RA, Moore CA (1996) Hamstrings and psoas lengths during normal and crouch gait: implications for muscle-tendon surgery. *J Orthop Res* **14**: 144–51.

den Otter AR, Geurts ACH, Mulder T, Duysens J (2004) Speed related changes in muscle activity from normal to very slow speeds. *Gait Posture* **19**: 270–8.

Detrembleur C, Dierick F, Stoquart G, Chantraine F, Lejeune T (2003) Energy cost, mechanical work, and efficiency of hemiparetic walking. *Gait Posture* **18**: 47–55.

Erdemir A, Piazza SJ (2002) Rotational foot placement specifies the lever arm of the ground reaction force during the push-off phase of walking. *Gait Posture* **15**: 212–19.

Femery V, Moretto P, Renaut H, Lensel G, Thevenon A (2002) Asymmetries in dynamic plantar pressure distribution measurement in able-bodied gait: application to the study of the gait asymmetries in children with hemiplegic cerebral palsy. *Ann de Readapt Med Phys* **45**: 114–22. (French.)

Fonseca ST, Holt KG, Saltzman E, Fetters L (2001) A dynamical model of locomotion in spastic hemiplegic cerebral palsy: influence of walking speed. Clin Biomech **16**: 793–805.

Gage JR (1991) *Gait Analysis in Cerebral Palsy*. London: Mac Keith Press. p 101–17.

Gage JR, Novacheck TF (2001) An update on the treatment of gait problems in cerebral palsy. *J Pediatr Orthop B* **10**: 265–74.

Gage JR, Schwartz MH (2002) Dynamic deformities and lever-arm considerations. In: Paley D, editor. *Principles of Deformity Correction*. Berlin, Heidelberg: Springer. p 761–75.

Gage JR, Schwartz M (2004) Pathological gait and lever-arm dysfunction. In: Gage JR, editor. *The Treatment of Gait Problems in Cerebral Palsy*. London: Mac Keith Press. p 180–204.

Gage JR, Perry J, Hicks RR, Koop S, Werntz JR (1987) Rectus femoris transfer to improve knee function of children with cerebral palsy. *Dev Med Child Neurol* **29**: 159–66.

Grosse P, Edwards M, Tijssen MA, Schrag A, Lees AJ, Bhatia KP, Brown P (2004) Patterns of EMG-EMG coherence in limb dystonia. *Mov Disord* **19**: 758–69.

Harrington ED, Lin RS, Gage JR (1984) Use of the anterior floor reaction orthosis in patients with cerebral palsy. *Bull Orthotet Prosth* **37**: 34–42.

Hicks J, Arnold A, Anderson F, Schwartz M, Delp S (2007) The effect of excessive tibial torsion on the capacity of muscles to extend the hip and knee during single-limb stance. *Gait Posture* **26**: 546–52.

Hicks R, Tashman S, Cary JM, Altman RF, Gage JR (1985) Swing phase control with knee friction in juvenile amputees. *J Orthop Res* **3**: 198–201.

Hof AL, Elzinga H, Grimmius W, Halbertsma J (2002) Speed dependence of averaged EMG profiles in walking. *Gait Posture* **16**: 78–86.

Hoffinger SA, Rab GT, Abou-Ghaida H (1993) Hamstrings in cerebral palsy crouch gait. *J Pediatr Orthop* **13**: 722–6.

Jameson EG, Davids JR, Anderson JP, Davis RB 3rd, Blackhurst DW, Christopher LM (2008) Dynamic pedobarography for children: use of the center of pressure progression. *J Pediatr Orthop* **28**: 254–8.

Langerak NG, Lamberts RP, Fieggen AG, Peter JC, van der Merwe L, Peacock WJ, Vaughan CL (2008) A prospective gait analysis study in patients with diplegic cerebral palsy 20 years after selective dorsal rhizotomy. *J Neurosurg Pediatr* **1**: 180–6.

Linton J, Barnes D, Johnson C, Lacy B, Hamilton ML (2008) Normative values for dynamic plantar pressures of typically developing children. *Dev Med Child Neurol* **50** (Suppl 4): 32–3.

Maltais D, Bar-Or O, Galea V, Pierrynowski M (2001) Use of orthoses lowers the O_2 cost of walking in children with spastic cerebral palsy. *Med Sci Sports Exerc* **33**: 320–5.

Oeffinger DJ, Pectol RW, Jr., Tylkowski CM (2000) Foot pressure and radiographic outcome measures of lateral column lengthening for pes planovalgus deformity. *Gait Posture* **12**: 189–95.

Olney SJ, MacPhail HE, Hedden DM, Boyce WF (1990) Work and power in hemiplegic cerebral palsy gait. *Phys Ther* **70**: 431–8.

282

Park KB, Park HW, Lee KS, Joo SY, Kim HW (2008) Changes in dynamic foot pressure after surgical treatment of valgus deformity of the hindfoot in cerebral palsy. *J Bone Joint Surg Am* **90**: 171–21.

Paul SM, Siegel KL, Malley J, Jaeger RJ (2007) Evaluating interventions to improve gait in cerebral palsy: a meta-analysis of spatiotemporal measures. *Dev Med Child Neurol* **49**: 542–9.

Perry J (1992) *Dynamic Electromyography. Gait Analysis: Normal and Pathological Function*. Thorofare, NJ: Slack. p 381–411.

Potter CR, Unnithan VB (2005) Interpretation and implementation of oxygen uptake kinetics studies in children with spastic cerebral palsy. *Dev Med Child Neurol* **47**: 353–7.

Potter CR, Childs DJ, Houghton W, Armstrong N (1999) Breath-to-breath noise in the ventilatory and gas exchange responses of children to exercise. *Eur J Appl Physiol Occup Physiol* **80**: 118–24.

Rodda JM, Graham HK, Nattrass GR, Galea MP, Baker R, Wolfe R (2006) Correction of severe crouch gait in patients with spastic diplegia with use of multilevel orthopaedic surgery. J Bone Joint Surg Am **88**: 2653–64.

Rose J, McGill KC (2005) Neuromuscular activation and motor-unit firing characteristics in cerebral palsy. *Dev Med Child Neurol* **47**: 329–36.

Sanger TD (2008) Use of surface electromyography (EMG) in the diagnosis of childhood hypertonia: a pilot study. *J Child Neurol* **23**: 644–8.

Saraph V, Zwick EB, Uitz C, Linhart W, Steinwender G (2000) The Baumann procedure for fixed contracture of the gastrosoleus in cerebral palsy. Evaluation of function of the ankle after multilevel surgery. *J Bone Joint Surg Br* **82**: 535–40.

Schutte LM, Hayden SW, Gage JR (1997) Lengths of hamstrings and psoas muscles during crouch gait: effects of femoral anteversion. *J Orthop Res* **15**: 615–21.

Schwartz M (2001) The effects of gait pathology on the energy cost of walking. *Gait Posture* **13**: 260. (Abstract.)

Schwartz MH (2007) Protocol changes can improve the reliability of net oxygen cost data. *Gait Posture* **26**: 494–500.

Schwartz M, Lakin G (2003) The effect of tibial torsion on the dynamic function of the soleus during gait. *Gait Posture* **17**: 113–18.

Schwartz MH, Viehweger E, Stout J, Novacheck TF, Gage JR (2004) Comprehensive treatment of ambulatory children with cerebral palsy: an outcome assessment. *J Pediatr Orthop* **24**: 45–53.

Schwartz MH, Koop SE, Bourke JL, Baker R (2006) A nondimensional normalization scheme for oxygen utilization data. *Gait Posture* **24**: 14–22.

Schwartz MH, Rozumalski A, Trost JP (2008) The effect of walking speed on the gait of typically developing children. *J Biomech* **41**: 1639–50.

Stebbins JA, Harrington ME, Giacomozzi C, Thompson N, Zavatsky A, Theologis TN (2005) Assessment of sub-division of plantar pressure measurement in children. *Gait Posture* **22**: 372–6.

Stebbins J, Harrington M, Thompson N, Zavatsky A, Theologis T (2006) Repeatability of a model for measuring multi-segment foot kinematics in children. *Gait Posture* **23**: 401–10.

Stout J, Koop S (2004) Energy expenditure in cerebral palsy. In: Gage JR, editor. *The Treatment of Gait Problems in Cerebral Palsy*. London: Mac Keith Press. p 46–7, 146–64.

Stout J, Gage JR, Van Heest AE (2004) Hemiplegia; pathology and treatment. In: Gage JR, editor. *The Treatment of Gait Problems in Cerebral Palsy*. London: Mac Keith Press. p. 314–44.

Stout JL, Gage JR, Schwartz MH, Novacheck TF (2008) Distal femoral extension osteotomy and patellar tendon advancement to treat persistent crouch gait in cerebral palsy. *J Bone Joint Surg Am* **90**: 2470–84.

Strayer LMJ (1958) Gastrocnemius recession; five-year report of cases. *J Bone Joint Surg Am* **40**: 1019–30.

Sutherland DH (2001) The evolution of clinical gait analysis part l: kinesiological EMG. *Gait Posture* **14**: 61–70.

Tervo RC, Azuma S, Stout J, Novacheck T (2002) Correlation between physical functioning and gait measures in children with cerebral palsy. *Dev Med Child Neurol* **44**: 185–90.

Thomas SS, Buckon CE, Piatt JH, Aiona MD, Sussman MD (2004) A 2-year follow-up of outcomes following orthopedic surgery or selective dorsal rhizotomy in children with spastic diplegia. *J Pediatr Orthop B* **13**: 358–66.

Trost J, Schwartz M, Novacheck T, Dunn M (2008) Selective dorsal rhizotomy. *Dev Med Child Neurol* **50**: 765–71.

Unnithan VB, Dowling JJ, Frost G, Bar-Or O (1996) Role of co-contraction in the O2 cost of walking in children with cerebral palsy. *Med Sci Sports Exerc* **28**: 1498–504.

283

Unnithan VB, Dowling JJ, Frost G, Bar-Or O (1999) Role of mechanical power estimates in the O2 cost of walking in children with cerebral palsy. *Med Sci Sports Exerc* **31**: 1703–8.

van der Krogt MM, Doorenbosch CA, Harlaar J (2008) Validation of hamstrings musculoskeletal modeling by calculating peak hamstrings length at different hip angles. *J Biomech* **41**: 1022–8.

Van Gestel L, Molenaers G, Huenaerts C, Seyler J, Desloovere K (2008) Effect of dynamic orthoses on gait: a retrospective control study in children with hemiplegia. *Dev Med Child Neurol* **50**: 63–7.

Van Heest AE, Ramachandran V, Stout J, Wervey R, Garcia L (2008) Quantitative and qualitative functional evaluation of tendon transfers in children with spastic hemiplegia. *J Pediatr Orthop* **28**: 679–83.

Wang SY, Liu X, Yianni J, Aziz TZ, Stein JF (2004) Extracting burst and tonic components from surface electromyograms in dystonia using adaptive wavelet shrinkage. *J Neurosci Methods* **139**: 177–84.

Watts HG (1994) Gait laboratory analysis for preoperative decision making in spastic cerebral palsy: is it all it's cracked up to be? *J Pediatr Orthop* **14**: 703–4.

Westberry D, Davids J, Jameson E, Pugh LI (2008) Comparative analysis of static foot alignment and dynamic loading patterns in ambulatory children with cerebral palsy. *Dev Med Child Neurol* **50** (Suppl 4): 62.

White H, Jenkins J, Neace WP, Tylkowski C, Walker J (2002) Clinically prescribed orthoses demonstrate an increase in velocity of gait in children with cerebral palsy: a retrospective study. *Dev Med Child Neurol* **44**: 227–32.

Winters TF Jr, Gage JR, Hicks R (1987) Gait patterns in spastic hemiplegia in children and young adults. *J Bone Joint Surg Am* **69**: 437–41.

Yoon Y, Mansour J, Simon SR (1981) Muscle activities during gait. *Orthop Trans* **5**: 229–31.

Zwick E, Saraph V, Strobl W, Steinwender G (2001) Single event multilevel surgery to improve gait in diplegic cerebral palsy – a prospective controlled trial. *Z Orthop* **139**: 485–9.

3.6
MODELING AND SIMULATION OF NORMAL AND PATHOLOGICAL GAIT

Jennifer L. Hicks, Michael H. Schwartz and Scott L. Delp

The diagnosis and treatment of gait abnormalities in children with cerebral palsy is challenging. A combination of several factors, including muscle spasticity, muscle weakness, bony malalignment, and neurological impairment may contribute to a patient's movement abnormality. In theory, correcting these factors with the appropriate treatment will improve the patient's gait pattern. Identifying the set of factors to target with treatment is difficult, however, since the abnormal gait pattern and set of contributing factors differ between patients. Further, the human body is a complex 3-dimensional linkage, and consequently muscles often have non-intuitive roles during locomotion that are difficult to discern from examining electromyographs (EMG) and joint motions (Fig. 3.6.1). Modeling and simulation of the musculoskeletal system is a powerful tool for quantifying muscle function during pathological gait, which can in turn help identify why a specific patient walks with an abnormal gait, and enable us to design an appropriate treatment plan.

'Modeling', in the context of gait, is a term that often conjures images of 3-dimensional musculoskeletal models and complex dynamic simulations. It is important to recognize that the term 'model' simply refers to a set of approximations used to represent a system of interest – in this case, the human body. For example, a model of the musculoskeletal system is needed to perform a conventional gait analysis. The process of inverse dynamics, which calculates joint angles and moments during gait (Davis et al. 1991), requires a model of the body that represents the rotational axes of the joints and the inertial properties of the body segments (i.e. masses and moments of inertia). Recent advances in the field of biomechanics allow us to extend this model in several ways to rigorously define the roles of skeletal alignment, muscle activations, muscle–tendon dynamics, and other factors in generating a normal gait pattern.

We can first extend the model used for inverse dynamics with a representation of 3-dimensional musculoskeletal geometry (Fig. 3.6.1, orange box). We represent each muscle as a path or set of paths between the muscle's origin and insertion, possibly with wrapping surfaces or via points to approximate the more complex geometries of tendon sheaths or overlapping muscles (Delp et al. 1990, Van der Helm et al. 1992). With this addition to the musculoskeletal model, we can calculate muscle moment arms, lengths, and velocities as a function of a subject's joint kinematics (Hoffinger et al. 1993, Delp et al. 1996, Schutte et al. 1997, Thompson et al. 1998). This type of model enables us to quantify, for example, the lengths and velocities of a patient's hamstrings muscles to determine if the muscles are slow or short during gait (Arnold et al. 2006a, b). We can also represent common bony deformities, like femoral anteversion, which alter muscle origins and insertions, and quantify the resulting changes in the moment arms or lengths of muscles (Schutte et al. 1997, Arnold et al. 2001, Arnold and Delp 2001).

As a next step, we can apply forces – along muscle paths, at the foot–ground interface, or from gravity – to the musculoskeletal model and observe the motions that result. In order to link forces to motions, we must formulate the model's equations of motion, which relate the accelerations of all the joints in the body to the forces applied to the body and the inertial parameters, position, and velocity of the body segments (Fig. 3.6.1, yellow box). By representing the action of forces on the body, we can gain valuable insight into the often non-intuitive role of muscles in supporting the body against gravity and propelling the body forward, as illustrated for several important lower-extremity muscles in Videos 3.6.1–6 on Interactive Disc. For example, as a consequence of dynamic coupling between joints in the body, muscles can accelerate joints they do not cross (Zajac and Gordon 1989, Riley and Kerrigan 1999, Arnold et al. 2005, Kimmel and Schwartz 2006). This phenomenon is well established for the soleus, often called the plantarflexion/knee-extension couple, as illustrated in Figure 3.6.2 and Video 3.6.6. The action of biarticular muscles also depends on dynamic coupling. For example, the hamstrings muscles may produce a knee-flexion acceleration through the muscles' knee-flexion moment and may generate a knee-extension acceleration through the muscles' hip-extension moment, via dynamic coupling (Arnold et al. 2005), as shown in Video 3.6.3. The net acceleration the hamstrings generate at the knee depends on the orientation of the body segments and the muscles' hip-to-knee moment arm ratio, an important consideration when examining the function of this muscle group often implicated in crouch gait. The musculoskeletal model's equations of motion capture the complexity of dynamic coupling and allow us to quantify muscle function in the presence of bony deformities, like excess tibial torsion or femoral anteversion, or in pathological locomotion patterns.

The next level of complexity in biomechanical modeling is forward-dynamic simulation of a subject's gait, driven by muscle-tendon actuators (see Fig. 3.6.1, red box and Video 3.6.7). Dynamic simulations represent muscle activation dynamics, linking muscle activations to forces as a function of a muscle's cross-sectional area, length, and velocity (Zajac 1989). We then use mathematical optimization to find a solution for the set of muscle activations that drives the model to follow a specified gait pattern and is consistent with experimentally measured EMG (Anderson and Pandy 2001, Thelen et al. 2003, Thelen and Anderson 2006). With a muscle-driven simulation of gait, we can assess how changes in a muscle's activation level or timing affect gait kinematics. For example, we can 'turn off' the rectus femoris muscle in the simulation of a child with stiff-knee gait to determine if this muscle inhibits knee flexion in swing phase (Reinbolt et al. 2008). Alternatively, we can increase the force applied by a muscle like the psoas or gastrocnemius in the simulation to determine if strengthening one of these muscles might similarly improve the patient's swing-phase knee flexion (Goldberg et al. 2004).

The musculoskeletal modeling tools described above have the potential to enhance our understanding of muscle function in normal and pathological gait and, in turn, improve the

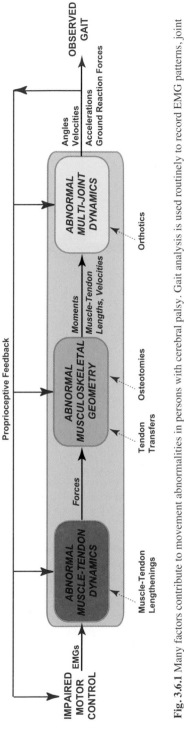

Fig. 3.6.1 Many factors contribute to movement abnormalities in persons with cerebral palsy. Gait analysis is used routinely to record EMG patterns, joint angles, and ground reaction forces during walking, but the transformation between EMG patterns and coordinated multi-joint movement is complex (gray-shaded region). Furthermore, to make treatment decisions clinicians must try to predict how the motions induced by muscles might change after treatment. Typically, treatments alter muscle-tendon dynamics or musculoskeletal geometry, which are difficult changes to measure. Computational models that characterize patients' muscle-tendon dynamics (red box), musculoskeletal geometry (orange box), and multi-joint dynamics of the body (yellow box) during walking may enhance the interpretation of motion analysis studies and improve the planning of treatments.

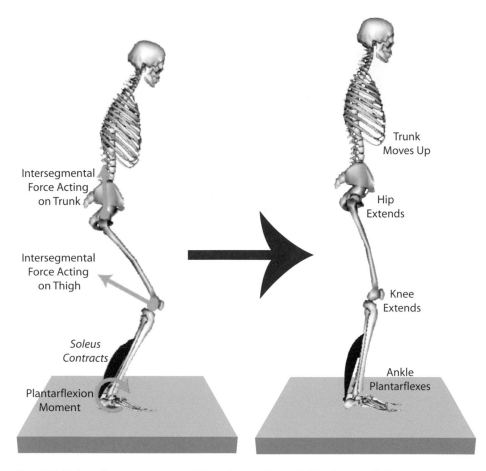

Fig. 3.6.2 Action of soleus as a result of dynamic coupling. *Left*: The force applied by soleus, a uniarticular muscle spanning the ankle, not only generates an ankle plantarflexion moment (bottom orange arrow), but also induces intersegmental forces throughout the body. The magnitudes and directions of these intersegmental forces depend on the force applied by the muscle, the moment arms of the muscle, the inertial properties of the segments, and the configuration of the body. In this example, the force applied by soleus produces a counter-clockwise angular acceleration of the shank. This acceleration requires the location of the knee joint to accelerate to the left and upward. The inertia of the thigh resists this acceleration, resulting in an intersegmental force at the knee (middle orange arrow). The intersegmental force at the knee accelerates the thigh, which in turn induces an intersegmental force at the hip (top orange arrow), and so on. *Right*: As a consequence of the intersegmental forces induced by soleus, the muscle accelerates not only the ankle, but all the joints of the body. At the body position shown, soleus accelerates the ankle toward plantarflexion, the knee toward extension, the hip toward extension, and the trunk upward. Over time, these accelerations give rise to changes in position. Thus, due to dynamic coupling, soleus does not function solely as an 'ankle plantarflexor' – in many situations, it does much more. In a similar fashion, other muscles induce intersegmental forces and accelerate joints that they do not span. (Figure adapted from Anderson et al. 2006.)

diagnosis and treatment of patients with gait disorders. Several challenges must be overcome to ensure these tools are useful in a clinical setting. First, although new freely available modeling tools (Delp et al. 2007) improve access to simulation, and increased computer processor speed reduces the time and cost required to generate muscle-driven dynamic simulations, creating a subject-specific simulation of each child who visits a gait analysis lab may not be practical. Second, expertise is required to interpret the results of any biomechanical analysis, since simulations cannot yet predict how a patient will walk after treatment. We can use several strategies to mitigate these concerns. First, we must use models of appropriate complexity to answer carefully posed questions about the cause of a particular gait abnormality or the consequence of a treatment. For example, we can determine if a muscle is slow or short during a patient's gait using a purely kinematic model – in this case we do not require a formulation of the model's equations of motion or a representation of muscle activation dynamics. Second, we must continue to validate our models and translate the insights gained from simulations into screening techniques that can be applied in a clinical setting. In the sections that follow, we discuss three clinical applications of modeling and simulation that utilize these principles. We conclude with a discussion of the remaining challenges for the modeling and simulation of pathological gait that will drive continued research.

Kinematic models to estimate hamstrings lengths and velocities in crouch gait

Many children with cerebral palsy walk with excessive knee flexion in terminal swing and stance, a movement pattern known as crouch gait. Spasticity or contracture of the hamstrings muscles is thought to restrict knee extension, thus contributing to the crouch gait of some patients (Baumann et al. 1980, Sutherland and Davids 1993, Crenna 1998, Tuzson et al. 2003). Hamstrings lengthening surgery is commonly prescribed to address a patient's diminished knee extension during gait. While some patients demonstrate improved knee kinematics, stride length, and locomotor efficiency after a hamstrings lengthening procedure (DeLuca et al. 1998, Abel et al. 1999), other patients fail to adopt a more erect gait posture after surgery or may experience negative complications, including the development of excessive anterior pelvic tilt or a stiff-knee gait pattern (Thometz et al. 1989, Hsu and Li 1990, DeLuca et al. 1998). The variable success of this procedure provides an impetus to better identify good candidates for hamstrings lengthening and understand the mechanisms of improvement after surgery. Common clinical indications for a hamstrings lengthening include excessive knee flexion during gait and/or a large popliteal angle; however, these measures do not directly assess whether a patient's hamstrings are short or slow during gait and are thus inhibiting the patient's knee extension. In a series of investigations, we examined whether analyses of the muscle-tendon lengths and lengthening velocities of patients' hamstrings during walking can help determine if a patient is likely to benefit from hamstrings surgery (Arnold et al. 2006a, b).

To address the utility of a musculoskeletal model in identifying good candidates for hamstrings lengthening surgery, we retrospectively analyzed the muscle-tendon lengths and velocities of 152 subjects treated at two different clinical centers for crouch gait (Arnold et al. 2006a). We estimated the subjects' preoperative and postoperative muscle-tendon lengths and velocities by combining kinematic data from a standard gait analysis with a 3-dimensional model of the lower extremity (Fig. 3.6.3). The lower-extremity model represented the geometry of the pelvis, femur, tibia, and the hip and knee joints, as well as the 3-dimensional paths of the hamstrings muscles (Arnold et al. 2001). We calculated the distance along the modeled path of the semimembranosus from origin to insertion at every 2% increment of the gait cycle for each subject to estimate the hamstrings' lengths and calculated the rate of change of this distance to estimate the hamstrings' lengthening velocities. We normalized the muscle-tendon lengths and velocities based on the average peak values measured in normal gait, which eliminated variations due to subject size (Arnold et al. 2001). To examine the relationship between hamstrings length and velocities and the outcome of surgery, we cross-classified subjects in a series of multi-way contingency tables based on the subjects' preoperative and postoperative gait kinematics, preoperative and

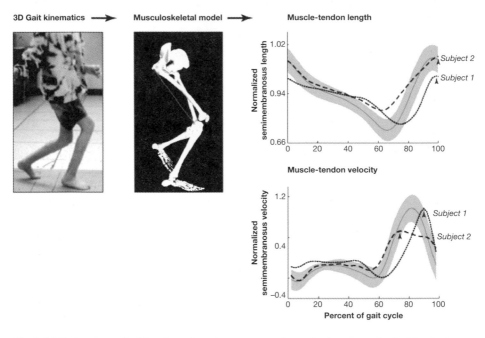

Fig. 3.6.3 Estimations of subjects' semimembranosus muscle-tendon lengths and velocities during walking. A computer model of the lower extremities (*center*) was used in combination with the subjects' joint angles and stride durations measured during gait analysis (*left*) to plot the muscle-tendon lengths and lengthening velocities of the semimembranosus vs gait cycle (*right*). The muscle-tendon lengths and velocities corresponding to each subjects' gait (e.g. Subjects 1 and 2, dashed lines) were normalized and were compared to the lengths and velocities averaged for unimpaired individuals (mean ± 2 S.D., shaded region) to determine if the subjects' hamstrings were operating at peak muscle-tendon lengths shorter than normal, or peak muscle-tendon velocities slower than normal (peak lengths and velocities indicated by arrows). Some of the subjects, such as Subject 2, walked with semimembranosus velocities that were substantially slower than normal. Such analyses may help to distinguish patients who have 'short' or 'spastic' hamstrings from those who do not, and thus may augment conventional methods used to describe patients' neuromusculoskeletal impairments and gait abnormalities. (Figure from Arnold et al. 2006.)

postoperative hamstrings lengths and velocities, and whether they received a hamstrings lengthening as part of their treatment. Using a log-linear analysis, we assessed whether subjects' outcomes were related to their length/velocity classifications (i.e. were the hamstrings short or slow before treatment and longer or faster after treatment?) and/or surgery classifications (i.e. did the subject receive a hamstrings lengthening?)

Our analysis of a diverse group of subjects treated for crouch gait at two leading clinical centers revealed that subjects with hamstrings that were neither short nor slow were less likely to exhibit improved knee kinematics after a hamstrings lengthening procedure (Arnold et al. 2006a). Further, the subjects who received an 'unnecessary' hamstrings surgery tended to have unimproved or worsened pelvic tilt. Within the subset of subjects who had improved knee extension after surgery, patients with short or slow hamstrings preoperatively tended to have longer or faster hamstrings after surgery (Arnold et al. 2006b). Evidence from prior experimental studies suggests that, in some instances, excessive passive forces generated by the hamstrings contribute to excessive knee flexion (Abel et al. 1999, Buczek 2002). Our examination of hamstrings lengths during gait, before and after surgery, corroborate these prior studies and suggest that surgically lengthening short hamstrings may improve knee extension by allowing these muscles to operate at increased lengths. Similarly, previous studies suggest that in some instances abnormal hamstrings excitation, triggered by spasticity, may limit the lengthening velocity of the hamstrings during gait (Perry and Newsam 1992, Crenna 1998, Granata et al. 2000, Tuzson et al. 2003). Our investigation of hamstrings velocities supports these findings and suggests that surgical lengthening of 'spastic' hamstrings may allow them to elongate with greater muscle-tendon velocities.

One argument against using an additional modeling step to calculate muscle-tendon lengths and velocities is that perhaps the same conclusions could be drawn from a subject's conventional gait analysis or clinical exam data. However, the presence of short or slow hamstrings was not evident from standard measures like hip or knee kinematics and popliteal angle (Arnold et al. 2006a). Since the estimates of muscle-tendon length used in our studies are based on a detailed model of musculoskeletal geometry and joint kinematics, they simultaneously account for muscle moment arms at the hip and knee, as well as the patient's 3-dimensional gait kinematics during walking.

In these studies, we demonstrated that a musculoskeletal model can help to identify subjects with abnormally short or slow hamstrings, and thus augment conventional gait analysis in identifying appropriate candidates for surgery. Estimating muscle-tendon lengths and velocities with a relatively simple modeling framework helped explain the functional consequences of surgery – we observed that in successful outcomes, the hamstrings operate at longer lengths or faster speeds, enabling more normal knee kinematics. A limitation of this type of analysis is that it does not allow us to estimate active or passive muscle-tendon forces. Further work, using muscle-driven dynamic simulations, is needed to quantify hamstrings activation and the joint accelerations this muscle group produces in both normal and pathological gait. We also recognize that multiple factors may contribute to the crouch gait of each subject. For example, muscle weakness or poor skeletal alignment may prevent improvement after a hamstrings surgery even if the length and velocity of the hamstrings are corrected to normal values. Thus the focus of the investigation in the next section is the contribution of bony deformities and crouched walking postures to the diminished knee extension observed in patients with crouch gait.

Induced acceleration analysis to quantify muscle function in subjects with crouch gait and tibial torsion

The excessive knee flexion exhibited by children with crouch gait tends to worsen over time if patients do not receive appropriate treatment (Sutherland and Cooper 1978, Bell et al. 2002). This chronic knee flexion increases the energy costs of walking (Campbell and Ball 1978, Waters and Lunsford 1985, Rose et al. 1990) and can lead to knee joint degeneration (Rosenthal and Levine 1977, Lloyd-Roberts et al. 1985, Bleck 1987). As discussed in the previous section, spasticity or contracture of the hamstrings may contribute to the excess knee flexion observed in some patients. Bony deformities like tibial torsion, which alter the dynamic coupling between joints (Fig. 3.6.2), may also contribute to crouch gait by reducing the capacity of muscles to accelerate the joints into extension, as suggested by several previous investigators (Stefko et al. 1998, Schwartz and Lakin 2003, Selber et al. 2004, Ryan et al. 2005). Correcting the deformity with a tibial derotation osteotomy is thought to improve bony alignment and help restore normal muscle function (see Chapter 5.2 for a clinical discussion of tibial torsion and derotation surgery), but this hypothesis has not been fully validated, nor is this surgery always successful. Simply walking in a crouched posture may also alter dynamic coupling and the joint angular accelerations generated by muscles during gait – changes that must be quantified to understand the implications of muscle weakness or abnormal activation. In the next set of investigations, we quantified the effect of crouched gait postures and the presence of a tibial deformity on the capacity of the lower-extremity muscles to extend the hip and knee joints (Hicks et al. 2007, 2008).

As in the previous section, we performed our analysis with a 3-dimensional model of the musculoskeletal system (Fig. 3.6.4) that represented the geometry of the joints and the paths of muscles in the lower extremity (Delp et al. 1990). The model in this study had 10 segments to represent the upper body and right and left legs, and 13 degrees of freedom to represent the articulations at the back, hip, knee and ankle joints. We included 92 muscle paths in the model, but focused our analysis on the major muscles capable of extending the hip or knee, including gluteus maximus, gluteus medius, vasti, hamstrings, and soleus (Arnold et al. 2005). Since we also sought to quantify the effect of tibial deformities on the joint accelerations induced by muscles, we developed a technique to simulate a torsional deformity of the tibia (Fig. 3.6.4, highlighted region), which modified muscle attachments sites and the relative orientation of the knee and ankle joints (Hicks et al. 2007). To calculate the joint accelerations that result from applying muscle forces or gravity to the body, we represented the inertial parameters of the body segments in the model (Delp et al. 1990) and the interaction between the foot and the ground (Anderson and Pandy 2003). By specifying these additional model properties, we were able to formulate the dynamic equations of motion which relate muscle forces to joint accelerations as a function of the body's position (Delp and Loan 2000).

To quantify the effect of tibial torsion and crouched postures on the capacity of muscles to extend the hip and knee, we used a technique commonly referred to as an induced

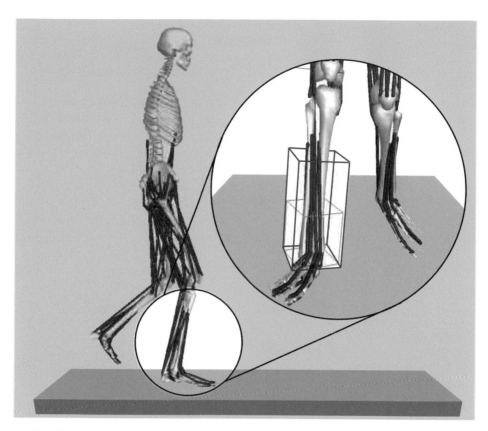

Fig. 3.6.4 Three-dimensional model of the musculoskeletal system used to determine the effect of tibial torsion deformities and crouched postures on muscle extension capacities. The model had 10 segments, 13 degrees of freedom, and 92 muscle paths. The model is shown with joint angles corresponding to the beginning of single limb support for a crouch gait. We added a deformable tibia to the model to simulate a range of torsional deformities (highlighted region). This deformity was implemented using two boxes (pink and blue): the inner box (pink), the ankle axis, and the foot were rotated by the torsion angle specified. There was a linear decrease in tibial torsion angle between the top of the inner box and the top of the outer box (blue). All bone deformation was distal to the proximal muscle attachments on the tibia.

acceleration analysis (Zajac and Gordon 1989). We positioned the musculoskeletal model with the joint angles from a normal or crouch gait pattern (Videos 3.6.8–10) and applied, in turn, a 1 Newton muscle force along the path of each of the lower-extremity muscles. Using the model's equations of motion, we then calculated the resulting accelerations of the knee and hip joint. These induced accelerations represent the *capacity* of each individual muscle to accelerate the joint towards extension, independent of the muscle's cross-sectional area, activation level, muscle-tendon length, or lengthening velocity. We similarly applied the force of gravity to each of the body segments and calculated the joint accelerations induced by gravity. To quantify the effect of tibial torsion on muscle extension capacities, we repeated this analysis for models with a range of excess, external torsion.

293

Analyzing the dynamics of the musculoskeletal model revealed that a crouched gait posture reduces the capacity of several major muscles to extend the knee (Hicks et al. 2008), including gluteus maximus, posterior gluteus medius, vasti, and soleus (Fig. 3.6.5, white bars). The exception was the hamstrings muscle group, whose extension capacity was

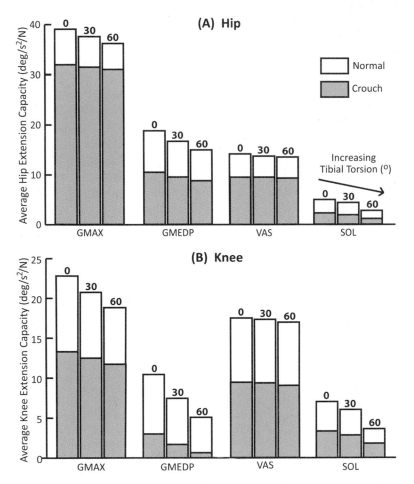

Fig. 3.6.5 The effect of external tibial torsion and crouched gait postures on the capacity of muscles to extend the hip (A) and knee (B) during single limb stance. The muscles shown, including gluteus maximus (GMAX), the posterior compartment of gluteus medius (GMEDP), vasti (VAS), and soleus (SOL), are the major muscles responsible for generating hip and knee extension accelerations in the single support phase of gait. The white bars show the average extension acceleration during normal single limb stance for each muscle in a model with 0°, 30° and 60° of excess, external tibial torsion. The gray bars show the average extension capacity during a representative moderate crouch gait for a model with 0°, 30° and 60° of excess tibial torsion. The capacity of all of these muscles to extend the hip and knee joint was substantially reduced when the model was positioned in a crouched gait posture. A torsional deformity of the tibia also reduced the capacity of several of these muscles, in particular the posterior gluteus medius and soleus, to extend the hip and knee joints. (Figure from Hicks et al. 2008.)

maintained in a crouched posture. Crouched gait postures also increased the flexion accelerations induced by gravity at the hip and knee. Several important muscles crossing the hip and knee were adversely affected by excessive external tibial torsion (Fig. 3.6.5, gray bars) when walking in either a normal or crouched gait posture (Hicks et al. 2007, 2008). For example, with an external tibial torsion deformity of 30°, the capacities of soleus, posterior gluteus medius, and gluteus maximus to extend both the hip and knee were all reduced by over 10% from the values calculated for an undeformed model.

The negative impact of both crouched postures and tibial deformities increased with the severity of the impairment, suggesting that crouch gait is a downward cycle. In a crouched posture, the joint-flexion accelerations induced by gravity increase and the capacity of muscles to generate joint-extension accelerations decrease, so an individual in a crouch gait must generate more muscle force to maintain a crouched posture. This increase in required muscle force is consistent with experimental studies that show greater muscle activity in flexed postures (Hsu et al. 1993) and reports of increased energy expenditure for crouch gait (Campbell and Ball 1978, Waters and Lunsford 1985, Rose et al. 1990). Larger muscle forces also increase joint loading, a likely contributor to knee abnormalities, like patella alta, observed in patients with crouch gait (Rosenthal and Levine 1977, Lloyd-Roberts et al. 1985). A tibial deformity tended to have the greatest impact on the soleus and gluteal muscles, which suggests that the deformity may be particularly deleterious in patients with pre-existing weakness of the gluteal or plantarflexor muscles. More optimistically, the findings of this study suggest that small improvements in gait posture, as a result of physical therapy or surgery, may help to reverse the natural progression of crouch gait. For example, our findings suggest that correcting a patient's tibial alignment may lead to small improvements in the capacity of the subject's muscles to extend the joints, which may lead to a more erect posture, and thus further improvement in muscle extension capacities.

The dynamic analysis used in these studies can be adapted to analyze the gait kinematics and bone geometry of individual patients to help estimate, for example, the contribution of a patient's tibial deformity to his or her crouch gait. This analysis requires a minor amount of additional computation beyond conventional inverse dynamics and may help to identify patients whose crouch gait would improve with targeted strength training or from surgery to correct bony malalignment. A notable restriction of this type of analysis is that it only allows us to calculate the capacity or potential of a muscle to accelerate the joints. The actual accelerations produced by a muscle also depend on its activation level, cross-sectional area, length, and velocity. The forces generated by muscles via activation during gait will be addressed in the next section on muscle-driven simulation.

Muscle-driven forward-dynamic simulations to understand stiff-knee gait
Many individuals with cerebral palsy walk with diminished knee flexion in the swing phase of gait, a movement abnormality known as stiff-knee gait. The insufficient knee flexion observed in these patients is often attributed to excessive swing-phase activation of the rectus femoris (Waters et al. 1979, Perry 1987, Sutherland et al. 1990), a biarticular muscle that generates a flexion moment at the hip and an extension moment at the knee. Stiff-knee gait is commonly treated with a rectus femoris transfer, a surgical procedure in which the

distal tendon of the muscle is detached from the patella and reattached to a site posterior to the knee (Gage et al. 1987, Perry 1987). The surgical transfer is thought to convert the rectus femoris to a knee-flexor (see Chapter 5.2 for a clinical discussion of the rectus femoris transfer), thereby eliminating the excessive swing-phase knee-extension moment produced by the muscle. The outcome of this procedure is sometimes unsuccessful and research by Asakawa and colleagues (2004) suggests that scarring after the transfer surgery may prevent the rectus femoris from acting as a knee-flexor. Analysis of the multi-joint motions produced by a muscle like rectus femoris is complex, but there is a strong clinical motivation to understand the possible contribution of abnormal rectus femoris activity to stiff-knee gait. We have developed forward dynamic simulations of able-bodied subjects and persons with stiff-knee gait to determine how the forces generated by rectus femoris and other muscles influence knee flexion during swing (Goldberg et al. 2003, 2004, Reinbolt et al. 2008). Quantifying the factors that influence knee flexion in swing can help us understand the biomechanical consequences of the rectus transfer procedure and identify appropriate candidates for surgery.

In this series of investigations, we generated muscle-actuated simulations of gait for both able-bodied individuals and children who walked with diminished swing-phase knee flexion. An example of a muscle-driven simulation of able-bodied gait is shown in Video 3.6.7. As in the previous section, we began with a computer model of the musculoskeletal system that represented the 3-dimensional geometry of the bones and joints and paths of the muscle-tendon units (Delp et al. 1990, Anderson and Pandy 1999). We then scaled the model to represent the experimentally measured size of the subject and generated the model's equations of motion, which relate applied forces to joint accelerations (Delp and Loan 2000). To create muscle-driven simulations, we represented the muscle-tendon units as actuators that generate forces as a function of the muscle's activation level, length, and velocity (Zajac 1989, Delp et al. 1990). We then solved for the muscle activations that enabled the model to follow the experimentally observed joint trajectories of the subject (Fig. 3.6.6). The muscle activations were determined using a mathematical optimization that minimized the difference between the measured gait kinematics and the motion of the model, while remaining consistent with experimentally-measured EMG (Anderson and Pandy 2001, Thelen et al. 2003, Thelen and Anderson 2006). Once this subject-specific simulation was generated, we made systematic changes to the simulation to address specific questions relevant to stiff-knee gait. For example, in one investigation, we altered the flexion velocity of the knee joint immediately prior to swing to quantify the effect of this parameter on peak knee flexion (Goldberg et al. 2003). We additionally examined the effect of perturbing the activation level or timing of the rectus femoris and other muscles to quantify the joint accelerations generated by the lower-extremity muscles during the double support and swing phases of gait (Goldberg et al. 2004, Reinbolt et al. 2008).

In our first simulation-based study of stiff-knee gait, we investigated the validity of one of the most common clinical indications for rectus transfer surgery: overactivation of the rectus femoris during early swing, which is thought to create excessive knee extension moments that restrict swing-phase knee flexion. Analysis of a large group of patients with stiff-knee gait demonstrated that these subjects do not exhibit larger than normal knee

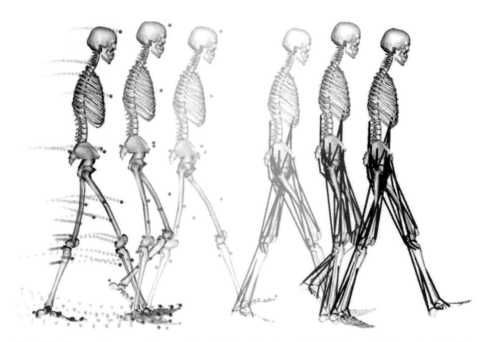

Fig. 3.6.6 Process for computing muscle activations in a dynamic simulation. A 3-dimensional, full-body musculoskeletal model with 21 degrees of freedom and 92 muscle-tendon actuators was used in conjunction with the subject's gait analysis data to create each subject-specific simulation. We scaled the body segment lengths and inertial properties for a generic model according to distances on the model and corresponding measures on the subject from experimental markers. We then used numerical optimization to solve for the set of muscle activations that drove the model to follow the subject's experimentally measured gait kinematics. The muscle excitations were constrained to be consistent with measured EMG patterns. The resulting simulations produced joint motions that were within a few degrees of measured joint motions.

extension moments in swing, but rather show reduced knee-flexion velocities at toe-off (Goldberg et al. 2003). This suggests that abnormal muscle activity prior to swing phase reduces the velocity of the knee going into swing, which results in the diminished and delayed knee flexion observed in these subjects. Our simulations of stiff-knee gait support this hypothesis. In particular, increasing subjects' knee flexion velocity at toe-off to normal values in the simulations increased the knee range of motion for all subjects by at least 7°. This first set of simulations indicated that the mechanism for improvement after rectus transfer surgery may be an alteration of rectus femoris function in pre-swing, which could improve knee flexion velocity at toe-off. Thus the focus of our next investigation was the influence of the rectus femoris and other lower-extremity muscles on knee flexion velocity at toe-off.

To establish a baseline for muscle function in pre-swing, we quantified the influence of each lower-extremity muscle on peak knee-flexion velocity in the double support phase of normal gait (Goldberg et al. 2004). Starting from a normal simulation of the double support phase, we systematically perturbed the force level in each muscle from its normal value.

We then stepped forward in time via numerical integration and observed the resulting peak knee-flexion velocity. We compared the perturbed and unperturbed simulations to determine the effect of increasing or decreasing a given muscle force on the peak knee-flexion velocity achieved. As expected, we found that increasing the force in the rectus femoris during double support decreased peak knee-flexion velocity (Fig. 3.6.7). Several other muscles had a significant impact on knee flexion as well. Increased force by the vasti or soleus had the effect of reducing peak knee-flexion velocity. In contrast, increased force by iliopsoas, gastrocnemius or hamstrings increased the peak knee-flexion velocity achieved.

This investigation of muscle function in normal gait has several clinical implications. First, the results of this analysis provide further evidence that diminished knee-flexion velocity at toe-off and abnormal pre-swing activation of rectus femoris may be an appropriate indication for surgery. These findings also shed light on why many patients treated for crouch or equinus gait subsequently develop a stiff-knee gait pattern (Thometz et al. 1989, Damron et al. 1993). Musculotendinous lengthening of the hamstrings or gastrocnemius muscles is commonly performed on these patients and may diminish the muscle's force-generating capacity, and thus its ability to create a knee-flexion moment during double support. Alternately, targeted strengthening of the iliopsoas, gastrocnemius, or hamstrings muscles may benefit many patients with stiff-knee gait.

To explore the contribution of abnormal pre-swing rectus femoris activation to diminished swing-phase knee flexion, we next examined a series of simulations of patients with stiff-knee gait (Reinbolt et al. 2008). In each subject-specific simulation, we eliminated the activation of the rectus femoris first during the pre-swing period, and then during the swing period, and observed the resulting peak knee-flexion angle in swing (see Fig. 3.6.8

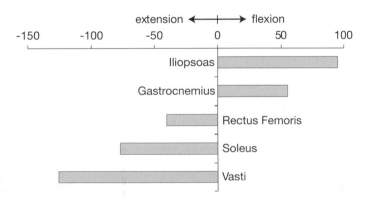

Fig. 3.6.7 The influence of selected muscles on peak knee-flexion velocity during double support. The influence of each muscle was calculated as the slope of the plot of change in peak knee-flexion velocity vs perturbation size in the simulation. The influence is a function of both the potential of each muscle to induce knee flexion velocity and the force exerted by the muscle during the simulation. Iliopsoas and gastrocnemius contributed the most to peak knee flexion during double support. Forces in vasti, rectus femoris and soleus decreased the knee-flexion velocity during double support. All other muscles had influences of less than 26°/s. (Figure from Goldberg et al. 2004.)

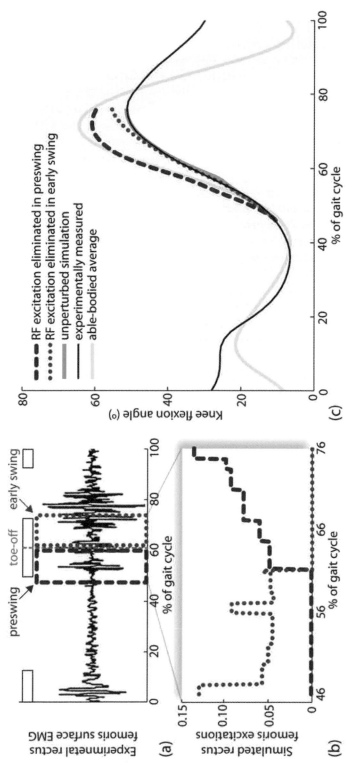

Fig. 3.6.8 Example of methods used to determine increase in peak knee-flexion angle in swing when rectus femoris activity was eliminated during pre-swing and separately during early swing. (a) Rectus femoris surface EMG of a subject with stiff-knee gait was recorded over an entire gait cycle. Normal rectus femoris EMG is indicated by horizontal white bars. Toe-off is indicated by a vertical dashed line at 61% of the gait cycle. Two time periods were selected for analysis: early swing (i.e. the period from toe-off to peak knee flexion) and pre-swing (i.e. the period before toe-off equal in duration to early swing). (b) Two simulation experiments were conducted by eliminating rectus femoris activity during pre-swing (dashed line) and separately during early swing (dotted line) to determine the muscle's effect on peak knee flexion. (c) Simulated changes in knee-flexion angles were different when rectus femoris activity was eliminated during pre-swing (dashed line) or early swing (dotted line). The unperturbed simulation (thick solid line) and experimentally measured (thin solid line) knee angles are shown for comparison. Normal knee flexion (shaded line) and 2 S.D. of the normal curve (shaded region) are shown as well. (Figure from Reinbolt et al. 2008.)

and Video 3.6.11 on Interactive Disc). We found that eliminating abnormal rectus activation in either pre-swing or early swing increased the peak knee flexion achieved during subjects' gait simulations. Improvements in peak knee flexion tended to be larger when subjects' pre-swing rectus activity was eliminated. These results confirm that pre-swing rectus femoris activity is at least as important as early swing activity and, for many subjects with stiff-knee gait, may limit knee flexion more than activity in early swing. Indeed, patients with a good surgical outcome tend to show an increased knee-flexion velocity at toe-off and a decrease in their knee-extension moment during double support (Goldberg et al. 2006). Our muscle-driven simulations have demonstrated that in evaluating rectus femoris activity for treatment of stiff-knee gait, both pre-swing and early swing EMG should be examined.

Although these studies provide valuable insight into the contribution of rectus femoris to stiff-knee gait, the mechanism by which patients improve after a rectus femoris transfer is still unclear. The transfer was originally intended to convert the rectus to a knee flexor, but several studies have shown that instead the muscle's knee extension capacity is merely reduced (Riewald and Delp 1997, Asakawa et al. 2002), possibly as a result of scarring between the rectus femoris and underlying vasti (Asakawa et al. 2004). An alternate mechanism of improvement is the reduction of the muscle's knee-extension moment, with preservation of its hip-flexion moment. We have begun a preliminary study to understand how surgical technique or scarring may influence outcome and to investigate the relative importance of the hip and knee moment arms of a transferred rectus (Fox et al. 2009). We created muscle-driven simulations of ten children with stiff-knee gait and altered the simulations to represent transfer of the rectus femoris to the sartorius or the iliotibial band, with and without scarring. Our preliminary results suggest that, while all surgical procedures improve the peak knee flexion observed in a simulation, scarring reduces the magnitude of improvement. For all procedures, the primary mechanism for improvement was the reduction of the knee-extension moment generated by rectus femoris, with a small additional benefit provided by maintenance of the muscle's hip flexion moment. While gait analysis tools alone are useful for characterizing stiff-knee gait, this series of modeling studies has demonstrated that dynamic simulation is an additional valuable tool to explore the underlying biomechanical causes of diminished knee flexion and the mechanisms leading to improvement after treatment.

Discussion and future directions

Modeling and simulation of the musculoskeletal system can provide insights into the pathomechanics of gait abnormalities and the functional consequences of treatments, as evidenced by the three examples presented in this chapter. The series of investigations we have described provide general guidelines, based on biomechanical principles, that can be used in combination with the data collected during a gait analysis to more rigorously identify the potential causes of an individual subject's movement disorder and more effectively plan treatment. For example, the methods used to estimate hamstrings lengths and velocities in the first investigation are currently used in several clinical centers to determine if a patient has short or slow hamstrings during gait, and thus may benefit from a lengthening procedure. Similarly, our analysis of models with tibial torsion deformities suggests that excess torsion may contribute to a patient's diminished knee extension when his or her external torsion is 30° or larger than normal. Our study of stiff-knee gait has also provided clinically useful guidelines. While one of the common clinical indications for a rectus transfer is over-activation in the swing phase, our simulations suggest that pre-swing rectus activity, which can reduce the flexion velocity of the knee joint at toe-off, may be a more important parameter in selecting appropriate candidates for surgery. In addition to these general guidelines, advances in technology and computational algorithms continue to decrease the time required to generate simulations of the pathological gait of individual subjects. Still, the limitations of current models must be reduced and the accuracy with which models represent individuals with neuromusculoskeletal impairments must be tested, before simulations can be widely used to guide treatment decisions for patients. Some of the important issues to be resolved in future studies are outlined below.

First, we must continue to refine and validate our models of the musculoskeletal geometry of children with cerebral palsy. The results of modeling and simulation studies, like the three examples presented in this chapter, are often sensitive to parameters like bony alignment, joint geometry, or muscle origin and insertion sites, which can alter muscle moment arms and muscle-tendon lengths and velocities during movement. Our analyses typically begin with a generic model of the musculoskeletal system that is scaled based on a subject's experimentally measured body size. We have developed techniques to model common bone deformities, like tibial torsion (Hicks et al. 2007) or femoral anteversion (Arnold et al. 2001), which deform the scaled musculoskeletal model based on clinically measured bony alignment. We can similarly modify generic models to simulate osteotomies (Free and Delp 1996, Schmidt et al. 1999) and tendon transfer surgeries (Delp et al. 1994). To validate our technique for modeling femoral anteversion, we compared the muscle-tendon lengths estimated by our deformable model to lengths determined from magnetic resonance images of four subjects with cerebral palsy (Arnold et al. 2001). We found very good agreement, with most length differences less than 5 mm in magnitude. Similar imaging studies are warranted to determine if the current modeling framework accurately represents variations due to other deformities, like tibial torsion or patella alta, or differences as a consequence of age, sex, or surgical treatment. In general, creating image-based models for all subjects is not likely to be practical, so we instead suggest a continued refinement of a hybrid approach. In particular, we recommend the use of subject-specific models that incorporate multi-dimensional scaling and algorithms for deforming bones, muscles, or joints based on a few patient-specific parameters from imaging or experimental measures (Chao et al. 1993, Arnold et al. 2001, Arnold and Delp 2001, Hicks et al. 2007).

The model of muscle-tendon mechanics used in simulations must also be further tested. While the current model captures many features of force generation in unimpaired subjects, it does not account for changes that may occur in neuromuscular disorders like cerebral palsy. For example, the model does not account for complexities associated with activation of spastic muscle, such as potential alterations in recruitment or rate modulation (Tang and Rymer 1981). In addition, our simulations have not considered the effects of muscle-tendon remodeling, such as alterations in the peak force of a muscle (Williams and Goldspink 1978) or changes in the elasticity of tendon (Woo et al. 1982) due to pathology or treatment.

Muscle-tendon models that characterize the effects of pathology, surgery, and other treatment modalities on muscle force-generating characteristics are needed to verify the accuracy of existing simulations and to enhance the value of new ones. A minimally invasive microendoscopy technique for imaging muscle (Llewellyn et al. 2008) may improve models of muscle-tendon mechanics in children with neuromuscular pathologies like cerebral palsy. This new imaging modality allows high-speed, real-time imaging of sarcomere dynamics in vivo, which will allow us to investigate how muscle architecture and dynamics change as consequence of pathology or treatment.

Perhaps the most profound limitation of the models described in this chapter is their exclusion of central nervous system control. For example, our analysis of the effect of tibial torsion on the capacity of muscles to extend the knee and hip joints did not consider how the nervous system may modulate muscle activation to compensate for this deformity. Additionally, the dynamic simulations of stiff-knee gait were performed open loop; that is, the synthesized motions had no ability to modulate the muscle excitation patterns through reflexes, as occurs in vivo. In general, the central nervous system may adapt to compensate for poor balance, muscle weakness, or in response to surgery or other treatment; however, our current modeling and simulation framework does not account for these adaptations. The incorporation of an accurate representation of sensorimotor control into dynamic simulations of abnormal movements is one of the critical challenges for developing models that can accurately simulate the outcome of treatment.

Continued work is also needed to ensure that the results generated by musculoskeletal simulations are accurate and clinically relevant. Sensitivity studies are valuable, allowing us to determine when the results of a particular analysis are strongly dependent on model parameters like joint geometry or muscle moment arms. Simulation results should be compared with experimental data to verify that a particular model is of sufficient complexity to answer the question posed. It is also important to examine whether the surgical recommendations provided by modeling and simulation studies lead to positive treatment outcomes in patients. To this end, we have begun a retrospective analysis of a large database of patients treated for crouch gait to determine if correcting the factors – like muscle spasticity, muscle weakness, or bony deformities – which contribute to a patient's excessive knee flexion, as determined by modeling and simulation, leads to good surgical outcomes. Since subject-specific modeling of each subject who visits a gait lab may not be practical, we have also begun to develop statistical models that use readily available preoperative variables from a subject's clinical exam or gait analysis to predict the likelihood that a particular treatment will be successful. The quantity of available preoperative data is prohibitively large, so we are using the knowledge gained in previous modeling and simulation studies to define a smaller subset of preoperative variables that enable robust predictions of surgical outcome and 'make sense' in terms of standard clinical and bio-mechanical knowledge. To ensure that computer modeling and simulation is accessible to researchers and clinicians, we have developed a freely available software package for musculoskeletal modeling and dynamic simulation, called OpenSim (Delp et al. 2007). This software is currently used by over 1000 researchers for a wide variety of applications, including the study of pathological gait.

302

We believe that computer models of the neuromusculoskeletal system play an important role in the assessment and treatment of gait abnormalities in persons with cerebral palsy, as illustrated by the examples presented in this chapter. Musculoskeletal simulations are necessary for explaining the biomechanical causes of movement abnormalities and the consequences of surgical procedures; this information is essential for developing improved treatment plans.

ACKNOWLEDGEMENTS

We are grateful to the members of the research team for each of the projects we describe in the chapter, including Allison Arnold, Jeffrey Reinbolt, Melanie Fox, Saryn Goldberg, Clay Anderson, May Liu, Sylvia Õunpuu, Marcus Pandy, James Gage, and Luciano Dias. We also acknowledge Roy Davis, Dennis Tyburski, Stephen Piazza, Silvia Blemker, Darryl Thelen, Katherine Bell, Melany Westwell, Jean Stout, Tom Novacheck, George Rab, Stephen Vankoski, Julie Witka, Kevin Granata, Chand John, and Joseph Teran for additional assistance with data collection, analysis, and interpretation. This work was funded by several grants from the NIH, including NIH R01-HD33929, NIH R01-HD046814, and the Roadmap for Medical Research U54 GM072970.

REFERENCES

Abel MF, Damiano DL, Pannunzio M, Bush J (1999) Muscle-tendon surgery in diplegic cerebral palsy: functional and mechanical changes. *J Pediatr Orthop* **19**: 366–75.

Anderson FC, Pandy MG (1999) A dynamic optimization solution for vertical jumping in three dimensions. *Comput Meth Biomech Biomed Eng* **2**: 201–31.

Anderson FC, Pandy MG (2001) Dynamic optimization of human walking. *J Biomech Eng* **123**: 381–90.

Anderson FC, Pandy MG (2003) Individual muscle contributions to support in normal walking. *Gait Posture* **17**: 159–69.

Anderson FC, Arnold AS, Pandy MG, Goldberg SR, Delp SL (2006) Simulation of walking. In: Rose J, Gamble JG, editors. *Human Walking*. Baltimore, MD: Williams and Wilkins.

Arnold AS, Delp SL (2001) Rotational moment arms of the medial hamstrings and adductors vary with femoral geometry and limb position: implications for the treatment of internally rotated gait. *J Biomech* **34**: 437–47.

Arnold AS, Blemker SS, Delp SL (2001) Evaluation of a deformable musculoskeletal model for estimating muscle-tendon lengths during crouch gait. *Ann Biomed Eng* **29**: 263–74.

Arnold AS, Anderson FC, Pandy MG, Delp SL (2005) Muscular contributions to hip and knee extension during the single limb stance phase of normal gait: a framework for investigating the causes of crouch gait. *J Biomech* **38**: 2181–9.

Arnold AS, Liu MQ, Schwartz MH, Õunpuu, S, Delp SL (2006a) The role of estimating muscle-tendon lengths and velocities of the hamstrings in the evaluation and treatment of crouch gait. *Gait Posture* **23**: 273–81.

Arnold AS, Liu MQ, Schwartz MH, Õunpuu, S, Dias LS, Delp SL (2006b) Do the hamstrings operate at increased muscle-tendon lengths and velocities after surgical lengthening? *J Biomech* **39**: 1498–506.

Asakawa DS, Blemker SS, Gold GE, Delp SL (2002) In vivo motion of the rectus femoris muscle after tendon transfer surgery. *J Biomech* **35**: 1029–37.

Asakawa DS, Blemker SS, Rab GT, Bagley, A, Delp SL (2004) Three-dimensional muscle-tendon geometry after rectus femoris tendon transfer. *J Bone Joint Surg Am* **86**: 348–54.

Baumann JU, Ruetsch, H, Schurmann K (1980) Distal hamstring lengthening in cerebral palsy: an evaluation by gait analysis. *Int Orthop* **3**: 305–9.

Bell KJ, Õunpuu S, DeLuca PA, Romness MJ (2002) Natural progression of gait in children with cerebral palsy. *J Pediatr Orthop* **22**: 677–82.

Bleck EE (1987) *Orthopaedic Management in Cerebral Palsy*. London: Mac Keith Press.

Buczek FL, Cooney KM, Concha MC, Sanders JO (2002) Novel biomechanics demonstrate gait dysfunction due to hamstring tightness. *Gait Posture* **16**: S57.

Campbell J, Ball J (1978) Energetics of walking in cerebral palsy. *Orthop Clin North Am* **9**: 374–7.

Chao EY, Lynch JD, Vanderploeg MJ (1993) Simulation and animation of musculoskeletal joint system. *J Biomech Eng* **115**: 562–8.

Crenna P (1998) Spasticity and 'spastic' gait in children with cerebral palsy. *Neurosci Biobehav Rev* **22**: 571–8.

Damron TA, Breed AL, Cook T (1993) Diminished knee flexion after hamstring surgery in cerebral palsy patients: prevalence and severity. *J Pediatr Orthop* **13**: 188–91.

Davis RB, Õunpuu S, Tyburski D, Gage JR (1991) A gait analysis data collection and reduction technique. *Hum Mov Sci* **10**: 575–87.

Delp SL, Loan JP (2000) A computational framework for simulating and analyzing human and animal movement. *Comput Sci Eng* **2**: 46–55.

Delp SL, Loan JP, Hoy MG, Zajac FE, Topp EL, Rosen JM (1990) An interactive graphics-based model of the lower extremity to study orthopaedic surgical procedures. *IEEE Trans Biomed Eng* **37**: 757–67.

Delp SL, Ringwelski DA, Carroll NC (1994) Transfer of the rectus femoris: effects of transfer site on moment arms about the knee and hip. *J Biomech* **27**: 1201–11.

Delp SL, Arnold AS, Speers RA, Moore CA (1996) Hamstrings and psoas lengths during normal and crouch gait: implications for muscle-tendon surgery. *J Orthop Res* **14**: 144–51.

Delp SL, Anderson FC, Arnold AS, Loan P, Habib A, John CT, Guendelman E, Thelen DG (2007) OpenSim: open-source software to create and analyze dynamic simulations of movement. IEEE *Trans Biomed Eng* **54**: 1940–50.

DeLuca PA, Õunpuu S, Davis RB, Walsh JH (1998) Effect of hamstring and psoas lengthening on pelvic tilt in patients with spastic diplegic cerebral palsy. *J Pediatr Orthop* **18**: 712–18.

Fox MD, Reinbolt JA, Õunpuu S, Delp SL (2009) Mechanisms of improved knee flexion after rectus femoris transfer surgery. *J Biomechan* **42**: 614–19.

Free SA, Delp SL (1996) Trochanteric transfer in total hip replacement: effects on the moment arms and force-generating capacities of the hip abductors. J *Orthop Res* **14**: 245–50.

Gage JR, Perry, J, Hicks RR, Koop S, Werntz JR (1987) Rectus femoris transfer to improve knee function of children with cerebral palsy. *Dev Med Child Neurol* **29**: 159–66.

Goldberg SR, Õunpuu S, Delp SL (2003) The importance of swing-phase initial conditions in stiff-knee gait. *J Biomech* **36**: 1111–16.

Goldberg SR, Anderson FC, Pandy MG, Delp SL (2004) Muscles that influence knee flexion velocity in double support: implications for stiff-knee gait. *J Biomech* **37**: 1189–96.

Goldberg SR, Õunpuu S, Arnold AS, Gage JR, Delp SL (2006) Kinematic and kinetic factors that correlate with improved knee flexion following treatment for stiff-knee gait. *J Biomech* **39**: 689–98.

Granata KP, Abel MF, Damiano DL (2000) Joint angular velocity in spastic gait and the influence of muscle-tendon lengthening. *J Bone Joint Surg Am* **82**: 174–86.

Hicks J, Arnold A, Anderson F, Schwartz M, Delp S (2007) The effect of excessive tibial torsion on the capacity of muscles to extend the hip and knee during single-limb stance. *Gait Posture* **26**: 546–52.

Hicks JL, Schwartz MH, Arnold AS, Delp SL (2008) Crouched postures reduce the capacity of muscles to extend the hip and knee during the single-limb stance phase of gait. *J Biomech* **41**: 960–7.

Hoffinger SA, Rab GT, Abou-Ghaida H (1993) Hamstrings in cerebral palsy crouch gait. *J Pediatr Orthop* **13**: 722–6.

Hsu LC, Li HS (1990) Distal hamstring elongation in the management of spastic cerebral palsy. *J Pediatr Orthop* **10**: 378–81.

Hsu AT, Perry J, Gronley JK, Hislop HJ (1993) Quadriceps force and myoelectric activity during flexed knee stance. *Clin Orthop Relat Res* **288**: 254–62.

Kimmel SA, Schwartz MH (2006) A baseline of dynamic muscle function during gait. *Gait Posture* **23**: 211–21.

Llewellyn ME, Barretto RP, Delp SL, Schnitzer MJ (2008) Minimally invasive high-speed imaging of sarcomere contractile dynamics in mice and humans. *Nature* **454**: 784–8.

Lloyd-Roberts GC, Jackson AM, Albert JS (1985) Avulsion of the distal pole of the patella in cerebral palsy. A cause of deteriorating gait. *J Bone Joint Surg Br* **67**: 252–4.

Perry J (1987) Distal rectus femoris transfer. *Dev Med Child Neurol* **29**: 153–8.

Perry J, Newsam C (1992) Function of the hamstrings in cerebral palsy. In: Sussman MD (Ed.) *The Diplegic Child: Evaluation and Management*. Rosemont, IL: American Academy of Orthopaedic Surgeons. p 299–307.

304

Reinbolt JA, Fox MD, Arnold AS, Õunpuu S, Delp SL (2008) Importance of preswing rectus femoris activity in stiff-knee gait. *J Biomech* **11**: 2362–9.

Riewald SA, Delp SL (1997) The action of the rectus femoris muscle following distal tendon transfer: does it generate knee flexion moment? *Dev Med Child Neurol* **39**: 99–105.

Riley PO, Kerrigan DC (1999) Kinetics of stiff-legged gait: induced acceleration analysis. *IEEE Trans Rehabil Eng* **7**: 420–6.

Rose J, Gamble JG, Burgos A, Medeiros J, Haskell WL (1990) Energy expenditure index of walking for normal children and for children with cerebral palsy. *Dev Med Child Neurol* **32**: 333–40.

Rosenthal RK, Levine DB (1977) Fragmentation of the distal pole of the patella in spastic cerebral palsy. *J Bone Joint Surg Am* **59**: 934–9.

Ryan DD, Rethlefsen SA, Skaggs DL, Kay RM (2005) Results of tibial rotational osteotomy without concomitant fibular osteotomy in children with cerebral palsy. *J Pediatr Orthop* **25**: 84–8.

Schmidt DJ, Arnold AS, Carroll NC, Delp SL (1999) Length changes of the hamstrings and adductors resulting from derotational osteotomies of the femur. *J Orthop Res* **17**: 279–85.

Schutte LM, Hayden SW, Gage JR (1997) Lengths of hamstrings and psoas muscles during crouch gait: effects of femoral anteversion. *J Orthop Res* **15**: 615–21.

Schwartz M, Lakin G (2003) The effect of tibial torsion on the dynamic function of the soleus during gait. *Gait Posture* **17**: 113–18.

Selber P, Filho ER, Dallalana R, Pirpiris M, Nattrass GR, Graham HK (2004) Supramalleolar derotation osteotomy of the tibia, with T plate fixation. Technique and results in patients with neuromuscular disease. *J Bone Joint Surg Br* **86**: 1170–5.

Stefko RM, de Swart RJ, Dodgin DA, Wyatt MP, Kaufman KR, Sutherland DH, Chambers HG (1998) Kinematic and kinetic analysis of distal derotational osteotomy of the leg in children with cerebral palsy. *J Pediatr Orthop* **18**: 81–7.

Sutherland DH, Cooper L (1978) The pathomechanics of progressive crouch gait in spastic diplegia. *Orthop Clin N Am* **9**: 143–54.

Sutherland DH, Davids JR (1993) Common gait abnormalities of the knee in cerebral palsy. *Clin Orthop Relat Res* **288**: 139–47.

Sutherland DH, Santi M, Abel MF (1990) Treatment of stiff-knee gait in cerebral palsy: a comparison by gait analysis of distal rectus femoris transfer versus proximal rectus release. *J Pediatr Orthop* **10**: 433–41.

Tang A, Rymer WZ (1981) Abnormal force–EMG relations in paretic limbs of hemiparetic human subjects. *J Neurol Neurosurg Psychiat* **44**: 690–8.

Thelen DG, Anderson FC (2006) Using computed muscle control to generate forward dynamic simulations of human walking from experimental data. *J Biomech* **39**: 1107–15.

Thelen DG, Anderson FC, Delp SL (2003) Generating dynamic simulations of movement using computed muscle control. *J Biomech* **36**: 321–8.

Thometz J, Simon S, Rosenthal R (1989) The effect on gait of lengthening of the medial hamstrings in cerebral palsy. *J Bone Joint Surg Am* **71**: 345–53.

Thompson NS, Baker RJ, Cosgrove AP, Corry IS, Graham HK (1998) Musculoskeletal modelling in determining the effect of botulinum toxin on the hamstrings of patients with crouch gait. *Dev Med Child Neurol* **40**: 622–5.

Tuzson AE, Granata KP, Abel MF (2003) Spastic velocity threshold constrains functional performance in cerebral palsy. *Arch Phys Med Rehabil* **84**: 1363–8.

Van der Helm FC, Veeger HE, Pronk GM, Van der Woude LH, Rozendal RH (1992) Geometry parameters for musculoskeletal modeling of the shoulder system. *J Biomech* **25**: 129–44.

Waters RL, Lunsford BR (1985) Energy cost of paraplegic locomotion. *J Bone Joint Surg Am* **67**: 1245–50.

Waters RL, Garland DE, Perry J, Habig T, Slabaugh P (1979) Stiff-legged gait in hemiplegia: surgical correction. *J Bone Joint Surg Am* **61**: 927–33.

Williams PE, Goldspink G (1978) Changes in sarcomere length and physiological properties in immobilized muscle. *J Anat* **127**: 459–68.

Woo SL, Gomez MA, Woo YK, Akeson WH (1982) Mechanical properties of tendons and ligaments. II. The relationships of immobilization and exercise on tissue remodeling. *Biorheology* **19**: 397–408.

Zajac FE (1989) Muscle and tendon: properties, models, scaling, and application to biomechanics and motor control. *Crit Rev Biomed Eng* **17**: 359–411.

Zajac FE, Gordon ME (1989) Determining muscle's force and action in multi-articular movement. *Exerc Sport Sci Rev* **17**: 187–230.

INTERLUDE
INTRODUCTION AND OVERVIEW
OF TREATMENT PHILOSOPHY

James R. Gage

Sometimes, when speaking to orthopaedic residents, I contrast the treatment of scoliosis with the treatment of cerebral palsy. In the former, the basic decision-making (whether to observe, brace, or operate) is fairly simple. Given some knowledge of the particular type of scoliosis and its natural history, the physician can comfortably decide upon a proper course of treatment. However, surgery is complex and difficult, and is only undertaken by a surgeon who is adequately trained to perform it.

With cerebral palsy, and particularly with children who have spastic diplegia, the converse is true. The procedures used to correct deformity and improve function are relatively easy to learn and perform. However, the decision-making (establishing treatment goals and identifying the surgical procedures necessary to reach those goals) is complex. The underlying neurological lesion and the problems it produces are multifaceted and difficult to fully understand. In addition, the gait deviations themselves are very difficult to sort out because they are a result of a mixture of neurological injury, abnormal growth and compensations. If these children are to be treated in a manner that will consistently optimize their function, the treating physician must thoroughly understand normal gait and the pathology which cerebral palsy imposes upon it.

However, if you have stayed with us to this point in the book, I think you now have a good base of knowledge and are ready to discuss treatment. When I came to Newington Children's Hospital in the late 1970s, I was already 5 years beyond my residency and thought I had a good knowledge of pediatric orthopaedics. I then met Dr Jim Cary, one of Newington's senior orthopaedists, who taught me a whole new approach to the treatment of a disabled child. At the beginning of each new resident rotation, Dr Cary would give the introductory lecture. In it, he laid down five principles for the treatment of a child with a disability (Cary 1976).

1. Define the end product in terms of long-range treatment objectives.
2. Identify the patient's problems, both immediate and future, with precision.
3. Analyze the effects of growth on the problems – with and without the proposed treatment.
4. Consider valid treatment alternatives, including non-treatment.
5. Treat the whole child, not just his motor–skeletal parts.

I have discovered over the years that those principles work well in addressing treatment of any child with a chronic disability. They are especially relevant in the treatment of cerebral palsy. We can only optimize the function of these children if we accurately evaluate them at the beginning of their treatment and set identifiable and realistic goals for function when treatment is complete and they are fully grown. We can make these children better, but unfortunately we can never fully restore normal function.

Nevertheless, families want (and often expect) their children to walk as near normally as possible. Consequently, at the beginning of a treatment program, the physician's first major task is to establish goals that the family understands and accepts. Adequate time should be set aside for the initial patient visit. Parents must understand that they are embarking on a multifaceted, multidisciplinary treatment program. For example, at our Center, after a careful history and initial evaluation to establish the diagnosis, we conduct a thorough discussion of the condition. This can easily consume more than an hour of time. Parents of a child with cerebral palsy usually come with anxiety about what's happened to their child, guilt that they are in some way responsible for their child's condition, and concern about the future. Support groups and brochures, which are written at a level that the parents can understand, are very useful when dealing with families who are unfamiliar with cerebral palsy. Because treatment involves a team, which includes therapists, orthotists, and physicians from various specialties, it is my personal feeling that these children are best treated in a center that can provide a full range of services.

This, then, is our task when faced with a child with cerebral palsy. We must do a thorough history and clinical examination, identify and categorize the problems, and then formulate valid treatment objectives. Since many body systems are involved and we wish to optimize the outcome in each area of involvement, evaluation is best done with a team of specialists.

The needs of a particular patient relate directly to the type of cerebral palsy and the degree of involvement. For example, because of their poor selective motor control, the major needs of a child with athetosis – which represents one of the abnormal tone patterns arising from injury to the basal ganglia – are usually communication and activities of daily living. Independent mobility may also be a goal, but this is usually accomplished with a power chair (often with a custom-built control system that has been specifically adapted for the child by an orthotist or engineer). In these children seizures and mental retardation (UK usage: learning disability) are uncommon. From an orthopaedic standpoint, fixed contractures are uncommon and, in general, surgery designed to improve ambulation is un-predictable and unlikely to succeed. As an example, if the hip-adductors are lengthened, these children may develop a fixed abduction deformity, something that is much less likely to occur in a child with pure spasticity. In addition to poor selective motor control, children with injury to the basal ganglia also have severe difficulties with balance and use of the upper extremities. Thus in this group of patients walking is rarely an achievable goal, and so the developmental pediatrician, therapists and orthotists are more likely to be the primary caregivers than the orthopaedic surgeon.

Children who are involved in all four limbs (quadriplegia) have a more extensive brain lesion than those with diplegia. Consequently they have more proprioception problems, poor selective motor control (only about 20% of them are able to ambulate as adults), and a higher incidence of mental retardation and seizures. From an orthopaedic standpoint, in children with total body involvement, ambulation is often not practical and/or possible. The goal is frequently independent or assisted transfers, with some limited household ambulation (if possible). The major orthopaedic problems of these children center on scoliosis, hip subluxation/dislocation and/or severe foot deformities. Consequently, the goal of the orthopaedist for these children is to prevent spinal deformity, maintain the hips located and mobile, prevent knee contractures, and keep the feet plantargrade and shoeable. Some type of residential care is necessary in the majority of these individuals as an adult.

Children with spastic diplegia and/or hemiplegia nearly always walk, and these children have the greatest potential for improvement. In general, however, orthopaedic treatment has not been problem-oriented and/or based on the pathophysiology of the condition. Consequently, many of the interventions done in the past were poorly conceived and often harmful. Muscle/tendon lengthening procedures were common (typically tendo-Achilles and/or hamstring lengthening), and bony deformities were generally ignored unless a hip subluxation or severe foot deformity was present. After each procedure children were immobilized in plaster for long periods followed by extensive therapy. The usual result was excessive morbidity and permanent weakness with little or no functional improvement. Furthermore, since the pathology was never addressed in a comprehensive manner, multiple surgical events were common. Consequently, these children spent most of their childhood either having or recovering from surgery. Mercer Rang (1990) referred to this as the 'Birthday Syndrome'; that is, 'the child had an operation every year and physical therapy all year long'.

Team treatment

Appropriate treatment of this complex condition demands not only a team, but also a team whose members communicate with each other. The team approach has become the cornerstone of our treatment program. That does not mean that the child needs to see each member of the team at each visit. For that matter, s/he may never need to see some members of the team at all. Rather, it means that each member of the team is familiar with all of the elements of the cerebral palsy problem and is also aware of the specific contributions that each member might offer to the solution of the problem. As such, each member of the team must be willing to refer the patient to the appropriate member of the team for treatment when s/he encounters a problem that is outside of her/his expertise. Because of the diverse nature of these children's problems, the team needs to be diverse as well. At Gillette, the cerebral palsy team includes specialists from developmental pediatrics, orthopaedic surgery, neurosurgery, ophthalmology, physical and occupational therapy, speech and hearing, orthotics, psychology, and social work. It is difficult to treat these children well without access to a specialized center that contains all of these disciplines. At the end of the clinic visit at our center, a clinical nurse reviews the problems with the patient and family to be sure all of the needs have been met.

In our program, the physician who first sees the child is generally a pediatric neurologist, a developmental pediatrician or a pediatric physiatrist. Each of these specialists is qualified to make the diagnosis of cerebral palsy, but the pediatric physiatrist usually does the initial treatment and follow-up. S/he supervises the child's physical/occupational therapy programs, orders appropriate orthoses, and monitors global development as well as the development of specific structures such as the hips and feet. In addition, the physiatrist has the training and expertise to apply stretching casts, administer oral drugs to control tone and/or use injectable drugs such as botulinum toxin and/or phenol to prevent the development of contractures. My personal feeling is that a pediatric orthopaedist should also see the child at about 1 year of age and then at appropriate intervals of 1 year or more depending upon the relationship between the physiatrist and orthopaedist and the physiatrist's comfort with orthopaedic problems.

Treatment protocols

The development of treatment protocols is an integral part of team treatment. These are needed to ensure that the diagnosis is correct, and that associated deformities are not missed. If this is not done, disasters are sure to arise. As an example, a 5-year-old child with the diagnosis of spastic diplegia was once referred to me by a qualified pediatric neurologist. Unfortunately, the correct diagnosis of medulloblastoma of the cerebellum was not made until after we started to notice progression of neurological involvement into her upper extremities and ordered an MRI study of her brain. The lesson is that the diagnosis is never certain until the specific, necessary, diagnostic studies have been done to rule out other treatable conditions. And even when the diagnosis of cerebral palsy is established, apparent neurological progression should trigger a referral back to the pediatric neurologist or neurosurgeon, as this may be indicative of a correctible problem (for example, hydro-cephalus secondary to shunt obstruction). On several occasions children have been referred to me with an undiagnosed subluxation of the hip simply because the treating physician did not suspect the condition and take a routine anteroposterior radiograph of the pelvis. We have found that without the benefit of treatment protocols, which are worked out and agreed upon by all members of the team, it is difficult to avoid such errors.

The treatment plan

At the appropriate time in the child's development, his/her tone should be assessed and a decision made as to whether or not surgical reduction of tone is warranted. For most children, the optimal window of time to consider spasticity reduction is between about 5 and 8 years of age. By this age the neurological and social development of the child is usually adequate to go through both the surgery and the rehabilitation that follows. In addition, if an intra-thecal baclofen pump is being considered, the child is usually not large enough to allow its implantation until at least 5 years of age. At our center we have put together a 'Spasticity Evaluation Team' to do this evaluation. This team consists of a pediatric orthopaedist, a physiatrist, and a neurosurgeon. Ideally it would be nice to have the luxury to refer most of the children in our clinic to the spasticity evaluation team, but this is not practical. Instead we rely on the expertise of the child's principle physician (physiatrist or orthopaedist) to determine whether or not referral to the spasticity evaluation team is warranted. If a child is ambulatory and is referred for spasticity evaluation, gait analysis will usually be done prior to that referral. In that way, the results will be available to the spasticity evaluation team at the time of the child's initial visit. Based on the evaluation by the spasticity evaluation team, one of four decisions is usually made:

1. Tone reduction is not indicated at this time.
2. Oral medications should be tried to control the abnormal tone.
3. The child is a good candidate for selective dorsal rhizotomy.
4. The child is a good candidate for the intrathecal baclofen pump.

If tone reduction is elected, the pediatric physiatrist monitors the post-operative rehabilitation.

Finally, once the child's gait has matured and is stable and issues relating to abnormal muscle tone have been addressed, consideration should be given to single-stage correction of his/her remaining growth deformities (muscle contractures and/or lever-arm dysfunction). Based on the pathophysiology of cerebral palsy, which we have discussed in previous chapters, we should now be well aware of the concept of 'balance between joints'. Many of the muscles in the lower extremities are biarticular so that if a surgeon performs a procedure at the ankle, it will also have an effect on the knee. Similarly, an isolated procedure at the knee will affect the ankle and the hip as well. We need to treat the child in a balanced and comprehensive way and so avoid Mercer Rang's 'Birthday Syndrome' (Rang 1990).

Therefore, at our Center, all of the child's orthopaedic deformities are corrected as part of a single surgical procedure. We refer to these multiple lower-extremity procedures as single-event multilevel surgeries (SEMLS). In the case of hemiplegia, one surgeon can do all the corrections. However, in children with diplegia, in order to allow correction of all of the bony and soft tissue deformities within a reasonable period of time, two teams of surgeons are used (one team operating on each side). The specifics of how this is accomplished will be discussed in more detail in subsequent chapters.

With this background in mind, we are now ready to discuss the various types of treatment that are available for cerebral palsy. We will begin with non-operative treatment. Following that we will discuss the surgical treatment of spasticity, and then go on to the correction of growth deformities (lever-arm dysfunction and muscle contractures). However, before we go on to treating this very complex and difficult condition, I'd like to leave you with the Serenity Prayer attributed to Reinhold Niebuhr: 'God, give us grace to accept with serenity the things that cannot be changed, courage to change the things which should be changed, and the wisdom to distinguish the one from the other.'

After more than 30 years of working in this field, I have come to believe that this simple prayer sums up the essence of caring for a child with cerebral palsy. To me, appropriate treatment of cerebral palsy is summed up adequately in those three lines.

REFERENCES

Cary JM (1976) *Principles for Caring for a Handicapped Child. Resident Lectures.* Newington Children's Hospital, Newington, Connecticut, USA.

Rang M (1990) Cerebral palsy. In: Morrissy R, editor. *Pediatric Orthopaedics.* Philadelphia, PA: J.B. Lippincott. p 465–506.

Section 4
NON-OPERATIVE TREATMENT

4.1
PHYSICAL THERAPY

Susan Murr and Kathryn J. Walt

Key points
- Maintaining range of motion, improving strength, and facilitating mobility are the three main components of physical intervention for children with cerebral palsy
- Goals for physical therapy should be functional and directed towards meaningful activity and participation in the child's environment
- Physical therapy episodes will occur across the lifetime and should be unique to the individual and may be dependent on the GMFCS level and age.

The motor impairments typically associated with cerebral palsy (CP) are such that physical therapy is often one of the first interventions recommended when a young child is diagnosed with cerebral palsy. In the past the goals of physical therapy were to normalize movement patterns, reduce neurological signs, and minimize the development of secondary impairments (Østensjø et al. 2003). The interventions were based upon the belief that activity limitations were directly influenced by motor impairments, but there were no empirical data to support that. Recently the idea of promoting function in children with neurological disorders in their natural environment has begun to be emphasized. In the words of Østensjø et al. (2003): 'From a functional perspective, therapy for children with CP should aim at enabling the children to master tasks and participate in activities that are important to the child and family.' Models of health status have also moved from the framework of disability to ability and from strictly individual to societal perspectives; the International Classification of Functioning, Disability and Health (ICF) has raised the awareness of physical therapists to focus on challenges to activity and participation.

Any discussion of the effect of CP on an individual and the possibilities for therapeutic intervention must consider that CP impacts many different body structures and functions with various levels of severity. The classification of severity that will be used throughout this chapter is the Gross Motor Function Classification System (GMFCS) (Palisano et al. 1997). Two specific age groups will be discussed: the young child from birth to 6 years, and the older child/adolescent, from age 12 and above. The in-between years often include other specific pharmacological and surgical interventions, and the therapy prescribed is related to rehabilitation after those interventions.

Considerations in working with the young child: birth to 6 years of age
From the perspective of the ICF, children with CP present with impairments in body function and structure such as abnormal muscle tone, strength, reflexes and range of motion (Law

315

et al. 2007). Children classified as GMFCS levels I–III have less impairment than children in levels IV and V. Significant activity limitations can also exist (i.e. dressing, feeding, functional mobility) as well as limitations in participation (i.e. playing alone or with friends, participating in school) in social and community roles for the child (Law et al. 2007). The environmental factors must also be considered and for the young child, the natural environment is typically home with loving adult caregivers. By the age of 3–5 years the child has often entered center-based education/school and is developing peer relationships. His/her environment is still limited because of overall development and the expectations for level of independence.

Previously held tenets related to treatment techniques, such as neurodevelopmental treatment, have been replaced by theories of motor control, motor learning, and dynamic systems theory. This philosophical and practical shift has been driven by factors such as current models of health status, family-centered principles, and improved theories of motor control and motor learning. From a dynamic systems perspective, adaptation of the environment and/or task is considered acceptable as a solution to a motor problem rather than focusing on changing the abilities of the child (Law et al. 2007). One randomized controlled trial that is in process is comparing a child-focused approach to intervention with a task/context-focused approach. In the child-focused approach, the therapist sets the goals, and the primary emphasis is on altering body functions and structures, with the assumption that changes at this level will bring about changes at the level of activity and participation. Change in the child's ability is sought first, and if there is not success at this level, environmental adaptations are then considered. Although there is greater emphasis on writing goals that are functional and measurable for the individual child, there is still evidence that typical movement patterns are considered the criterion (Law et al. 2007).

In the task/context-focused approach, the child's interest in motor-based tasks is identified as are the constraining factors either in the environment or the child himself, and treatment focuses on modifying the identified constraints. In this approach, the child will be encouraged to be successful using whatever compensations are determined by the child to be necessary to achieve the functional task, and the quality of the movement will not be the focus.

Infants and young children (birth to 3 years of age) are typically involved in an early intervention program, where a team performs the evaluation and determines the plan of care based upon the identified needs, the motivation and interest of the child and the family's goals. Treatment is often provided in the child's home, which is considered the most natural environment. Children aged 3–6 are transitioned to a center-based program and physical therapy may be provided, on a direct or consultative basis, to allow the child to participate more fully in his educational environment. Additional therapy may be provided in an outpatient setting during these years, with the various service providers collaborating so that functional activities are being practiced across a variety of settings.

Regardless of the framework, the goal of physical therapy is functional mobility and most therapists use a combination of interventions. There is limited evidence available to determine an optimal amount of intervention; studies comparing intensity yield little difference after a 6-month period (Bower et al. 2001). There may be support for a child and family's ability to complete a shorter-term intensive treatment regime. Episodic care, based upon a child's motivation to be learning a new motor skill, is indicated, especially in children at levels I–III of the GMFCS. More continuous care may be recommended for children at levels IV and V as the goal of therapy may be more directed at preventing secondary complications. These children are more dependent upon assistive technology for their functional mobility and evaluation of such equipment is a vital part of their intervention.

Treatment interventions include stretching and casting to maintain range of motion and alignment, strengthening to increase power and endurance, practice of functional activities, gait training with appropriate assistive device or treadmill, and potentially electrical stimulation, usually in combination with functional activities. Stretching, positioning and casting are often the first interventions recommended in a young child who has evidence of hypertonia, based upon the belief that soft tissue tightness or contracture responds to passive stretching. The stretch can be applied manually by the therapist or by external devices such as braces or equipment designed to provide elongation for a period of time. A review of literature was undertaken by Pin et al. (2006) in an attempt to answer the question, 'Does passive stretching improve passive joint range of movements and reduce spasticity more effectively in children with CP than no passive stretching?' They divided the stretching interventions into two categories: the first included manual stretching by holding a joint at the available end range of movement for seconds before releasing. The second involved sustained stretches achieved by holding a joint at end range by an external force such as a standing frame or other positioning equipment and the time frame was minutes to hours per day. They concluded that there was conflicting evidence on whether passive stretching can increase the passive range of motion in a joint, and the studies that showed improvements indicated a small effect size. There was some evidence suggesting that passive stretching may reduce spasticity in children with CP, but without carryover to functional activities such as walking. Statistically significant findings may or may not be clinically significant, but a minimal increase or even maintaining of joint range in a young, growing child, may be clinically significant and lead to increased function.

STRENGTHENING

Sufficient evidence exists that children with CP are weaker than their typically developing counterparts (Wiley and Damiano 1998). There is also excellent evidence that children with CP can enjoy and benefit from strengthening programs to increase balance and gait (Dodd et al. 2002), although such programs were originally avoided because of the fear of increasing spasticity. The young child, or the child with limited selective motor control, can work on strengthening during play and functional activities. If there is sufficient ability and understanding, strengthening can be accomplished by way of progressive resistive exercises. Resistance can be applied by resistance bands, free weights, or weight machines. Research supports two or three times per week for at least 6–10 weeks, working at 65% of maximum force generation as determined by dynamometry (Berry et al. 2004, Dodd and Foley 2007). Other strengthening activities may include aquatics, biking, participation in dance and other athletic activities, and hippotherapy (Fig 4.1.1). The child's interest and motivation, as well as family choice, can help direct the type of activity chosen.

Fig. 4.1.1 Biking is an excellent activity for strengthening and social participation. Noah enjoys riding as part of his therapy session, but also has a bike for use at home with his family and friends.

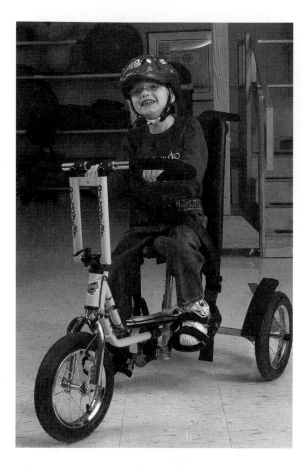

AMBULATION/LOCOMOTOR TRAINING

Children who are levels I–III on the GMFCS will generally choose walking as their primary form of locomotion at least in the household or other inside environments. Young children are encouraged to be upright and in weightbearing positions in either static or dynamic standing equipment or walkers, and then advance to less restrictive assistive devices as their strength, coordination and balance improve. Gait training is often a significant focus of physical therapy intervention, with increased attention to practice in the child's natural environment. Newer methods, which allow partial body weight support and treadmill training, provide an opportunity for increased practice and show promise for improving the gait and functional skills of young children with CP (Dodd and Foley 2007). Children at GMFCS levels IV and V will rely heavily on wheeled mobility for locomotion, and the perspective of introducing powered mobility for young children will enable them to participate more actively in their family and social environments. Parents who are initially hesitant to explore powered mobility as an option, thinking of it as a 'last resort', may indeed find that the benefits of increased independence and participation in activities of their child's choice affect their own attitudes and level of acceptance (Wiart et al. 2004).

FUNCTIONAL ACTIVITIES (FIG 4.1.2)

Young children learn about their environment and relationships with other people as their motor skills drive them. Children with CP often require additional support to facilitate their motor development and maximize their potential. This support typically comes in the form of hands-on treatment of the child or adaptation of the environment that enables the child to perform self-initiated activities. When a functional motor-therapy program was compared with a more traditional therapy program based on normalization of quality of movement, both groups of children were found to make gains in motor skills, but the former group improved more in using functional skills in daily-life situations (Ketelaar et al. 2001).

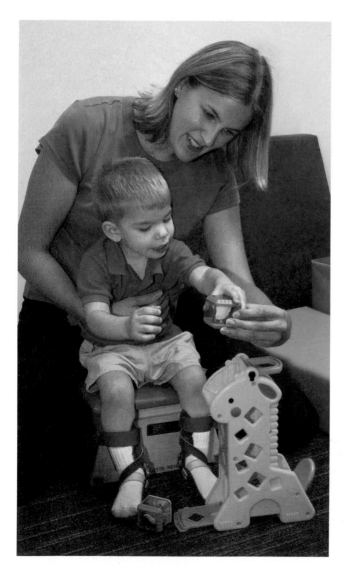

Fig. 4.1.2 Pierce is receiving external support for short sitting on the bench while he is encouraged to be reaching for blocks and dropping them into the shape-holder. He is having the experience of a functional activity even though he cannot complete it independently.

Considerations in working with adolescents

In the III Steps series, Palisano (2006) used the ICF to identify relationships of the components of care and clinical decision-making in pediatric physical therapy. He identified family centered care as a standard of pediatric practice. This includes sharing information, service coordination, and collaboration with caregivers and other providers. Other essential factors in pediatric practice include practice in daily activities and routines in a natural learning environment and also identifying outcomes that are meaningful to the child and family. With regard to adolescents, Palisano (2006) identified activity limitations due to secondary impairments related to alignment and limited range of motion. These limitations require increased demands on ambulation causing decreased functional walking. Physical therapy, therefore, should address balance impairments, ambulation and fitness relevant to joint protection and energy conservation.

Special considerations for adolescents with CP are also related to environmental factors and participation in life situations. This includes social interaction with peers and participation in school environment. The larger physical environment of middle schools and high schools typically places greater physical demands on the adolescent in negotiating through the hallways and across the campus. The main means of mobility should be reassessed, taking into consideration time constraints, energy, pain, and social attitudes. Increased demands on primary caregivers due to growth of the child may necessitate home environment and equipment changes. How the adolescent negotiates his or her environment, at home and in the community, may change because of age, size and independence issues. Functional capability and performance may also change during this time.

O'Neil et al. (2006) integrated the *The Guide to Physical Therapy* format with the ICF dimensions of body structure and function, activity, participation, and environmental factors. Functional outcomes, family-centered care, task-oriented approaches, and dynamic systems theory of motor learning are integral parts of physical therapy intervention. O'Neil et al. (2006) identified several areas to consider when making physical therapy recommendations for adolescents including functional mobility, past interventions, and secondary impairments.

Functional mobility skills that are required at home, at school and for community participation should be identified. This includes transfers, bed mobility, negotiating the bathroom, and moving from room to room. Floor mobility typically becomes emphasized less for adolescents than younger children who participate in age-appropriate floor activities with their peers. The school setting (where one must take into consideration such things as stairs, distance and time between classes, mobility within a classroom) should also be addressed for optimal participation. The individual education plan (IEP) and adaptive physical education should be utilized to enhance coordination of care (Fig. 4.1.3).

Past medical interventions such as spasticity management and orthopaedic interventions should be considered when making recommendations, developing the plan of care, and setting goals. In addition, secondary impairments, lower-extremity and postural alignment, and growth should be assessed on how these will also impact the plan of care and progress toward goals.

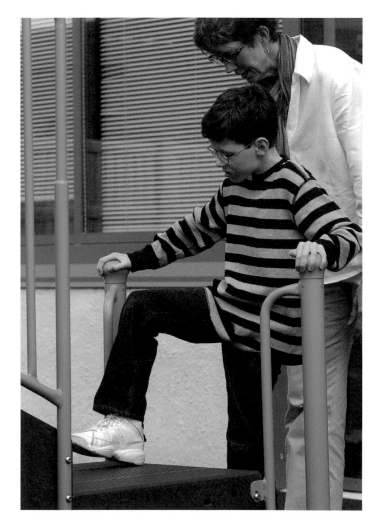

Fig. 4.1.3 Brandon is working on strengthening in the context of a functional activity. He requires sufficient lower-extremity strength to lift his body up onto a high step at a playground or on a school bus.

While the younger child may have been receiving direct physical therapy intervention through the school system based on individual educational needs, the adolescent may only have consultative services in middle school and high school. Therefore periodic physical therapy intervention is appropriate in an outpatient setting with increased frequency typically following medical interventions. The planned episode of physical therapy care should be framed by the primary movement problem that brought them in for evaluation. However, the goals and outcomes should address the movement problem in the context of a functional activity within the environment where the challenges exist. Physical therapy interventions used in the plan of care to achieve desired outcomes include stretching, strengthening, and cardiovascular endurance activities. In addition, functional activities and motor training, and facilitation of balance/postural control and coordination should also be emphasized.

Participation in fitness and recreation activities that provide ongoing strengthening and cardiovascular endurance, and which maintain flexibility for functional activities, should be implemented during and between the episodes of direct physical therapy intervention. Recently there has been more emphasis on lifetime fitness and recreation. Damiano (2006) emphasized the need for ongoing activity to promote physical conditioning especially during the aging process. Activities may include adaptive cycling (stationary and non-stationary), partial weightbearing gait training, aquatic programs, weight-lifting and other adaptive sports. However, there are barriers to participating in fitness and recreation activities for those with disabilities. Frequent reasons identified as barriers to participating in a wellness program include lack of interest by the child/family, lack of resources to implement a wellness program, economic limitations (including lack of reimbursement), lack of community programs, and competing priorities (Goodgold 2005). In addition, the frequency and intensity of exercise required to make physiological changes may be difficult to attain without guidance from a physical therapist.

Transition to adulthood and increasing independence should also be discussed and facilitated for adolescents in their high-school years. This includes self-advocacy, planning for transition, and preparation for independent living and/or transitioning to a college environment.

Clinical standardized tests and tools that may be helpful in goal-setting and measuring outcomes include the Functional Mobility Scale (FMS) (addresses mobility in home, school and community) and the Gross Motor Function Measure (if motor skills are assessed at less than 5 years of age). Cardiovascular endurance can be assessed using the Timed Up and Down Stairs (TUDS) test and the Energy Expenditure Index (EEI). Gait efficiency can be assessed using the Six-Minute Walk Test and the Timed Up and Go (TUG). Manual Muscle Testing and the Pediatric Berg Balance Test (14 items to assess balance) can also be useful assessment tools. In addition, the Canadian Occupational Performance Measure (child/parent perception of performance and participation) and the Child Health Questionnaire (QOL) are used to assess the adolescent's activity and participation and may be helpful in identifying meaningful goals for the adolescent (O'Neil 2006).

Recently, the Gross Motor Function Classification System (GMFCS) has been expanded to include 12- to 18-year-olds diagnosed with CP. Emphasis is on environmental factors and their potential impact on functional performance (Palisano et al. 2007). The FMS is another classification tool that compliments the GMFCS (Graham et al. 2004). The FMS scores functional mobility over three distances that would represent home (5 m), school (50 m), and the community (500 m). It also describes the assistive device used with each distance, with a score of 6 being the most mobile without an assistive device and a score of 1 describing wheelchair use for mobility. For example, a child who is at GMFCS level III, who ambulates in the home without an assistive device but uses the furniture for balance, uses a walker in his school and a wheelchair in the community, would have a score of 4–2–1. The FMS provides greater communication between health professionals in describing functional mobility and also has been shown to be sensitive to change following surgical intervention.

GMFCS levels I and II

Adolescents in level I and II GMFCS will be ambulatory in most environments, with the level II children possibly needing wheeled mobility for longer distances in the community due to environmental factors described above. Balance and coordination may also necessitate upper-extremity support for activities such as going up and down stairs (Palisano et al. 2007).

Adolescents who are in level I and level II on the GMFCS will benefit from physical therapy interventions that address stretching, cardiovascular endurance, strengthening, balance, and community ambulation. Stretching and strengthening continue to be essential to maintain postural and lower-extremity alignment so that functional ambulation can be optimized. Periodic strengthening programs continue to be recommended three times per week using 65% weight of a maximum voluntary contraction. Progressive strengthening programs are considered standard practice and are no longer thought to increase spasticity (Damiano et al. 1995a, b, Morton et al. 2005, O'Neil et al. 2006). Strengthening programs can be accomplished through free weights or weight-lifting machines. There are also programs utilizing motorized cycling (Fowler et al. 2007), bicycling, and swimming to facilitate strengthening and cardiovascular conditioning (Fig. 4.1.4). Partial weightbearing gait training can also be utilized to improve endurance and functional gait (Begnoche and Pitetti 2007, Provost et al. 2007). The latter group studied the effectiveness of using the partial weightbearing gait training in six children diagnosed with CP, aged 6–14 years. They were all in level 1 on GMFCS and able to participate using the Lite Gait, 30 minutes

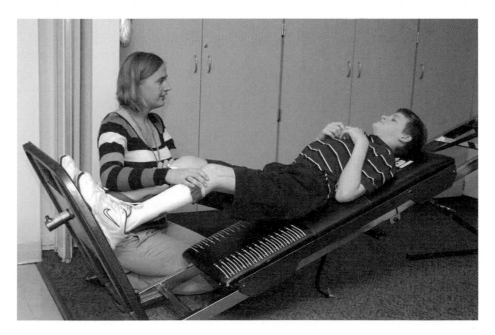

Fig. 4.1.4 Strengthening can be accomplished using body weight and gravity or with free weights or weight equipment.

323

twice a day, 6 days per week for 2 weeks. All children improved in endurance as measured on the EEI and also in functional gait with increased walking velocity and/or on the GMFM. Half of the children improved in balance as measured by single limb stance (Provost et al. 2007).

GMFCS level III

Adolescents in the level III category have more variability in their preference for mobility. Typically, they are capable of ambulating with an assistive device; however, in a school or community environment they may seek an alternative means of mobility because of time constraints, energy, and personal reasons. This could include self-propelling a manual wheelchair or use of powered mobility. Participation in sports will require adaptations because of mobility limitations (Palisano et al. 2007).

Adolescents in the level III category of the GMFCS will benefit from physical therapy interventions that address the most efficient means of mobility in each environment and supporting that mobility through strengthening and endurance activities. The effects of secondary impairments will also need to be addressed through daily stretching and range of motion. In a study by Bjornson et al. (2007), ambulatory activity level in youth diagnosed with cerebral palsy was compared to age matched typical peers. They used a Step Watch monitor to document average daily step counts and percentage of time the youth were active. They determined that the ambulatory activity level in youth with cerebral palsy is decreased overall in comparison with age matched typical peers. They also found that those in the GMFCS level III category have less activity compared to levels I and II. They concluded that the decreased activity level in the level III category was possibly due to having less variability in activity and less opportunity for activity (Bjornson et al. 2007). Due to limitations in ambulation, alternative means for improving cardiovascular endurance and strength are important (Fowler et al. 2007). This may include aquatic exercise, adaptive cycling and adaptive sports. Adolescents who are in level III can also participate in progressive strengthening programs within their abilities (Damiano et al. 1995a, b, Damiano 2006).

GMFCS levels IV and V

Adolescents in the level IV and V categories use wheeled mobility as their primary means of mobility and may also require positioning adaptations to their wheelchair for additional support. Operating a powered wheelchair may be the best option for independent mobility. Those in the level IV category may ambulate with assistance but usually not for functional purposes. They will require assistance from one or two people for transfers, but may be able to participate by supporting their weight through their lower extremities. In comparison, those in the level V category may require assistance via a mechanical lift because they are unable to support their own weight (Palisano et al. 2007).

Standing programs continue to be beneficial for maintaining bone integrity and also have positive effects on bowel programs, respiratory issues, and the digestive system (Stuberg 1992, Pin 2007). Daily standing programs are recommended 4–5 times per week for 60-minute sessions to minimize contractures, osteopenia, and other physiological benefits. Strengthening can be accomplished through other functional activities and positioning. This may include prone positioning, mat activities, aquatic therapy, and assisted ambulation. Gait trainers can be used to assist in ambulation and help to provide dynamic weightbearing through the lower extremities, provide opportunity for aerobic exercise, and also can facilitate positive social interaction.

Other essential aspects to consider in working with adolescents in the level IV and V categories include education in advocacy and self-directing cares and also providing resources for powered mobility, computer access, environmental controls, and community access. In addition, the family/caregiver may have concerns in regards to changing equipment needs. For example, a mechanical lift or ceiling lift may now be necessary for transfers because of the adolescent's size and limited functional mobility. Other intervention may involve training personal care attendants and/or group home staff in range of motion, positioning, transfers, and other home exercises.

REFERENCES

Begnoche DM, Pitetti KH (2007) Effects of traditional treatment and partial body weight treadmill training on the motor skills of children with spastic cerebral palsy: a pilot study. *Pediatr Phys Ther* **19**: 11–19.

Berry E, Giuliani CA, Damiano DL (2004) Intrasession and intersession reliability of handheld dynamometry in children with cerebral palsy. *Pediatr Phys Ther* **16**: 191–8.

Bjornson KF, Belza B, Kartin D, Logsdon R, McLaughlin JF (2007) Ambulatory physical activity performance in youth with cerebral palsy and youth who are developing typically. *Phys Ther* **87**: 248–57.

Bower E, Michell D, Burnett M, Campbell MJ, McLellan DL (2001) Randomized controlled trial of physiotherapy in 56 children with cerebral palsy followed for 18 months. *Dev Med Child Neurol* **43**: 4–15.

Damiano DL (2006) Activity, activity, activity: rethinking our physical therapy approach to cerebral palsy. *Phys Ther* **86**: 1534–40.

Damiano DL, Kelly LE, Vaughn CL (1995a) Effects of quadriceps femoris muscle strengthening on crouch gait in children with spastic diplegia. *Phys Ther* **75**: 658–67.

Damiano DL, Vaughan CL, Abel MF (1995b) Muscle response to heavy resistance exercise in children with spastic cerebral palsy. *Dev Med Child Neurol* **37**: 731–9.

Dodd KJ, Foley S (2007) Partial body-weight-supported treadmill training can improve walking in children with cerebral palsy: a clinical controlled trial. *Dev Med Child Neurol* **49**: 101–5.

Dodd KJ, Taylor NF, Damiano DL (2002) A systematic review of the effectiveness of strength-training programs for people with cerebral palsy. *Arch Phys Med Rehabil* **83**: 1157–64.

Fowler EG, Knutson LM, DeMuth SK, Sugi M, Siebert K, Simms V, Azen SP, Winstein CJ (2007) Pediatric endurance and limb strengthening for children with cerebral palsy (PEDALS) – a randomized controlled trial protocol for a stationary cycling intervention. *BMC Pediatr* **7**: 14.

Goodgold S (2005) Wellness promotion beliefs and practices of pediatric physical therapists. *Pediatr Phys Ther* **17**: 148–57.

Graham HK, Harvey A, Rodda J, Nattrass GR, Pirpiris M (2004) The Functional Mobility Scale (FMS). *J Pediatr Orthop* **24**: 514–20.

Ketelaar M, Vermeer A, Hart H, van Petegern-van Beek E, Helders PJ (2001) Effects of a functional therapy program on motor abilities of children with cerebral palsy. *Phys Ther* **81**: 1534–45.

Law M, Darrah J, Pollock N, Rosenbaum P, Russell D, Walter SD, Petrenchik T, Wilson B, Wright V (2007) Focus on function – a randomized controlled trial comparing two rehabilitation interventions for young children with cerebral palsy. *BMC Pediatr* **7**: 31. Available at http://biomedcentral.com/1471–2431/7/31, accessed May 28, 2008.

Morton JF, Brownlee M, McFadyen AK (2005) The effects of progressive resistance training for children with cerebral palsy. *Clin Rehabil* **19**: 283–9.

O'Neil ME, Fragala-Pinkham MA, Westcott SL, Martin K, Chiarello LA, Valvano J, Rose RU (2006) Physical therapy clinical management recommendations for children with cerebral palsy – spastic diplegia: achieving functional mobility outcomes. *Pediatr Phys Ther* **18**: 49–72.

Østenjsø S, Carlberg EB, Vøllestad NK (2003) Everyday functioning in young children with cerebral palsy: functional skills, caregiver assistance, and modifications of the environment. *Dev Med Child Neurol* **45**: 603–12.

Palisano RJ (2006) A collaborative model of service delivery for children with movement disorders: a framework for evidence-based decision making. *Phys Ther* **86**: 1295–305.

Palisano R, Rosenbaum P, Walter S, Russell D, Wood E, Galuppi B (1997) Development and reliability of a system to classify gross motor function in children with cerebral palsy. *Dev Med Child Neurol* **39**: 214–23.

Palisano RJ, Rosenbaum P, Bartlett D, Livingston M (2007) *GMFCS – E & R Gross Motor Function Classification System Expanded and Revised*. McMaster University: CanChild Centre for Childhood Disability Research.

Pin TW (2007) Effectiveness of static weight-bearing exercises in children with cerebral palsy. *Pediatr Phys Ther* **19**: 62–73.

Pin T, Dyke P, Chan M (2006) The effectiveness of passive stretching in children with cerebral palsy. *Dev Med Child Neurol* 48: 855–62.

Provost B, Dieruf K, Burtner PA, Phillips JP, Bernitsky-Beddingfield A, Sullivan KJ, Bowen CA, Toser L (2007) Endurance and gait in children with cerebral palsy after intensive body weight-supported treadmill training. *Pediatr Phys Ther* **19**: 2–10.

Stuberg WA (1992) Considerations related to weight-bearing programs in children with developmental disabilities. *Phys Ther* **72**: 35–40.

Wiart L, Darrah J, Hollis V, Cook A, May L (2004) Mothers' perceptions of their children's use of powered mobility. *Phys Occup Ther Pediatr* **24**: 3–21.

Wiley ME, Damiano DL (1998) Lower-extremity strength profiles in spastic cerebral palsy. *Dev Med Child Neurol* **40**: 100–7.

4.2
ORTHOSES

Tom F. Novacheck, Gary J. Kroll, George Gent, Adam Rozumalski,
Camilla Beattie and Michael H. Schwartz

Key points

- Prescription and fitting of orthoses can compensate for neuromotor deficiencies
- Orthoses are commonly prescribed to address deficiencies of both structure and function, though at times concerns in these areas are at odds and it may not be possible for any one orthosis design to be optimal in both of these areas
- Avoiding crouch and excessive knee stress is a central long-term goal of orthotic management
- Segmental analysis is necessary to assure proper alignment and function
- Proper lever-arm alignment should be restored to improve the plantarflexion/knee-extension couple
- A current focus is to improve testing and materials to optimize orthoses for stiffness and energy storage/return.

Review of relevant pathophysiology

In normal gait during the second half of stance phase, stability of the knee is maintained without quadriceps action through the plantarflexion/knee-extension couple (Chapter 1.3). That is, the action of the soleus at the ankle restrains forward motion of the tibia over the foot and in so doing maintains the ground reaction force in front of the knee (see Video 3.6.7 on Interactive Disc). The result is that the ground reaction force acting on the lever-arm of the forefoot produces an extension moment at the knee maintaining the knee in extension without the need for quadriceps activity. This dynamic action helps to prevent hyperflexion at the knee (also known as crouch gait).

Individuals with cerebral palsy often have (1) weak plantarflexors (gastrocnemius and soleus), (2) bony deformities of femoral anteversion in conjunction with external tibial torsion that misalign the foot relative to the knee axis, and (3) an unstable valgus foot that is not rigid enough to be an effective lever.

Each of these reduces the effectiveness of the plantarflexion/knee-extension couple for providing knee support in 2nd rocker and insufficient power for push-off in 3rd rocker (see Chapter 2.4). Therefore plantarflexor dysfunction can lead to both stance-phase (supportive) and swing-phase (propulsive) deficiencies. Fortunately, lever-arm dysfunction is usually correctable with appropriate orthopaedic surgery and/or bracing (Gage and Schwartz 2002). Provided there is satisfactory muscle function, upright posture can be restored and maintained.

Inadequate dorsiflexors or a dynamic imbalance in the relationship between the dorsiflexors and plantarflexors usually results in the inability to dorsiflex adequately in swing phase. This also causes problems with clearance. Midfoot deformity may result in a poor mechanical line of pull of the anterior tibialis decreasing its function for foot clearance.

Segmental evaluation of foot deformity is challenging (Chapter 3.2), but it is crucial to successful management with orthoses. Two common foot-deformity types exist in children with cerebral palsy. The rigid equinocavovarus foot is more difficult to manage with orthoses and is more common in hemiplegia. The equinovalgus foot deformity, predominantly seen in individuals with diplegic and quadriplegic cerebral palsy, is more supple and therefore more amenable to orthotic management. But, to be successful, the midfoot instability and forefoot varus deformity must be identified and managed. Treatment of these complex foot deformities may require surgical management (Chapter 5.8) in conjunction with orthotic prescription.

Historical perspective

While the history of orthotic management dates back to Hippocrates for the treatment of fractures with closed reduction and splinting, the recorded history for the treatment of neuromuscular conditions is shorter. Lewis A. Sayre, considered by many the 'father of orthopaedic surgery in North America', used a modified shoe device for maintaining congenital talipes equinovarus alignment in the mid-19th century (Wenger 1993). Winthrop Morgan Phelps, an American orthopaedic surgeon in the early 20th century, was primarily interested in the management of cerebral palsy. Although he was an orthopaedic surgeon, he advocated bracing rather than surgery as the primary method of controlling deformities in children with cerebral palsy (Phelps 1953). His braces, constructed primarily from leather and metal, were an offshoot from the knowledge gained during the era of polio epidemics. The introduction of plastics after World War II revolutionized the world of orthoses. Thermoplastics remain the mainstay for the fabrication of orthotics to this day. While plastics are certainly better than metal and leather, the search continues for strong, durable and lightweight materials that may have even better structural characteristics. Carbon fiber satisfies many of these goals. Its potential application is currently being investigated (Wolf et al. 2005, Desloovere et al. 2006, Novacheck et al. 2007).

Indications from patient assessment

HISTORY AND PHYSICAL
While a history of brace intolerance may indicate that the patient is not a brace candidate, it is not necessarily a contraindication as prior orthoses may have been improperly prescribed or fabricated. Adequate range of motion for typical alignment while walking is necessary to properly fit the orthosis and expect good function. This requires at least neutral ankle dorsiflexion with the knee in extension and no knee-flexion contracture. Foot alignment in non-weightbearing subtalar neutral indicates that the foot can be corrected and provides the specific indications for orthosis fabrication (see section on the total contact footplate, below). Weakness of the ankle-plantarflexors can be compensated for by an adequately supportive

orthosis of appropriate stiffness. Excessive plantarflexor spasticity may prevent orthosis wear and may need to be addressed. Femoral anteversion and tibial torsion diminish the effectiveness of a well made orthosis and should be identified and corrected to maximize effectiveness. Lever-arm malalignment can be assessed by examination in the orthosis to assure correct alignment of the foot relative to the knee, e.g. the 2nd toe test in the orthosis.

IMAGING

Weightbearing radiographs of the foot can facilitate assessment of foot deformity (Chapter 3.4). Radiographs in the orthosis can indicate whether the foot deformity is corrected and the foot is supported in functional alignment.

GAIT BY OBSERVATION

Gait by observation in and out of orthoses is one of the mainstays of assessment. Observational gait analysis qualitatively assesses the prerequisites of normal gait. Indications for a posterior leaf-spring (PLS) ankle–foot orthosis (AFO) include swing-phase clearance deficiency due to foot drop in swing or poor prepositioning of the foot for initial contact caused by equinus or coronal-plane muscle imbalance of the inverters/everters. Indications for a stiff PLS AFO or solid AFO include impaired stability in stance, identifiable by one or more of the following: slow walking speed, wide base of support, delayed toe-off, and short step length clearly identifiable visually. However, its numerous causes, described in the section above entitled 'Review of Relevant Pathophysiology', cannot be identified solely by observation. Improvements with an appropriate orthosis can facilitate understanding of its causes, e.g. improvement with an AFO of appropriate stiffness would suggest an unstable foot or weak ankle-plantarflexors as major contributors as opposed to hamstring contracture. Changes in foot-progression angle with the use of an orthosis suggest foot deformity as a cause.

QUANTITATIVE GAIT ANALYSIS

Each of these subjective evaluations for deficits can be objectively assessed with quantitative gait analysis (GA). Changes in each of these parameters with an orthosis can be assessed to identify effectiveness. If ineffective, is it due to pathology that cannot be treated orthotically? If so, the orthosis should be discarded. Or is the orthosis prescription incorrect? If so, can it be modified to improve its effect?

- Prolonged and excessive 2nd rocker
- Drop foot in swing
- Position of the ankle at initial contact
- Ankle-plantarflexor push-off power
- Foot-progression angle
- Prolonged stance phase with delayed toe-off
- Stance-phase sagittal-plane knee alignment relative to foot progression
- Sagittal-plane knee-extension moment.

As one of the prerequisites of normal gait, oxygen testing with and without the orthosis can be assessed to determine if the prescribed orthosis is improving efficiency.

Goals of treatment

Functional goals include improving the prerequisites of normal gait on level ground (stability, clearance, prepositioning, step length, efficiency). At younger ages, transitional activities – such as a child getting up to standing from the floor – may be more important. Sometimes goals conflict. One orthosis may not be optimal to address all of the goals. While a hinged AFO may help promote transitional activities from the floor to standing, it may also promote crouch gait while walking. Differences of opinion in goal setting can exist between physiatrists, physical therapists, and orthopaedists.

Some clinicians may want to minimize orthotic support in order to promote strengthening. Preventing joint motion and shielding the muscle from cyclical loading could promote atrophy. Evaluating the capacity that each child has for strengthening their ankle-plantarflexors will help determine how much ambulatory time should be spent in the orthosis. If the neurological impairment is too severe, motor control and strengthening capacity may be so limited that meaningful muscle strength may not be a reasonable goal. In this case, walking without AFO support leads to increased dependence on the hip-extensors and quadriceps which could have long-term adverse consequences for muscular strain and on the hip and knee joints.

Additional goals include protecting a body part during weightbearing activities, preventing contracture by immobilizing the musculotendinous unit in an elongated position with night splinting, and improving acceptance of the orthosis by ensuring optimal comfort and cosmesis through minimization of weight and bulk.

Treatment options

For practical purposes, hip–knee–ankle–foot orthoses (HKAFOs) are virtually never used to manage ambulatory problems in individuals with cerebral palsy. They are useful at rest to maintain proper alignment in children with total body involvement in an effort to prevent contracture and progressive hip subluxation.

Similarly, knee–ankle–foot orthoses (KAFOs) can be used at rest to maintain musculotendinous length of the hamstrings and gastrocnemius and prevent the development of knee flexion contracture. As a dynamic brace to assist with walking function, they are cumbersome and perhaps more applicable to paralytic than spastic conditions. Appropriate multidisciplinary management of hypertonia (see Chapters 4. 3–5.3) and correction of lever-arm dysfunction (see Chapters 5.5–5.8) can almost always simplify the problems adversely affecting walking function, and thereby eliminate consideration of a KAFO. Fixed joint contractures may prevent normal excursion of the joint while walking. They can cause many abnormalities including crouch gait and short step length. The orthotist should also recognize when an otherwise appropriate orthosis is not able to achieve its desired affect because of a hip or knee contracture. This is especially true when a floor reaction AFO has been prescribed and is being fitted.

For each of the AFO designs that are discussed here, the foot section of the orthosis should be considered separately. See Chapter 3.2 for information regarding foot deformity types and evaluation. If the goal of the orthosis is to assist with the dynamic function of walking, then the orthotist must first be able to assess alignment and fabricate an orthosis that will be well tolerated and restore alignment. The orthotist must recognize when this is not possible. Possible causes include rigid, uncorrectable foot deformity, tibial malrotation (external tibial torsion is the most common) and distal tibial valgus deformity. While the latter is a fairly common deformity in myelomeningocele, it can also occur in patients with cerebral palsy. It is more likely to be missed in cerebral palsy since it is less well documented.

SUPRAMALLEOLAR ORTHOSIS AND UNIVERSITY OF CALIFORNIA BIOMECHANICS LABORATORY ORTHOSIS

The supramalleolar orthosis (SMO) and the University of California Biomechanics Lab (UCBL) orthosis are commonly used for the treatment of cerebral palsy (Fig. 4.2.1). Both can control varus or valgus deformities of the hindfoot and compensate for forefoot deformities as described above. The SMO has greater leverage as it captures the distal tibia, ankle and hindfoot, allowing application of greater corrective forces to control varus and valgus, and resulting in greater control of more significant hindfoot and midfoot deformities. Careful identification of fixed forefoot deformities and incorporation of appropriate forefoot posting leads to an orthosis that is better able to achieve its functional goals of restoring proper lever arm alignment and can improve heel–toe gait by improving tibialis anterior alignment. The SMO on occasion will lessen foot drop in swing to some degree even though it does not passively control sagittal-plane ankle-joint alignment.

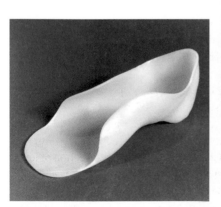
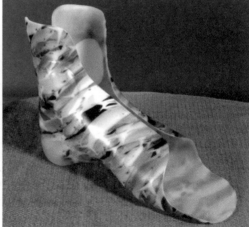

Fig. 4.2.1 UCBL (University of California Biomechanics Lab) orthosis (*left*), and supramalleolar orthosis (SMO) (*right*). Both orthoses provide hindfoot control, an arch mold, and medial/lateral borders for forefoot motion control. Length of the toe plate and medial/lateral borders vary depending on patient needs. The SMO captures the malleoli improving hindfoot varus/valgus control. Both can lead to improvements in foot-progression angle and stability in stance (shortening excessive stance-phase time).

ARTICULATED ANKLE–FOOT ORTHOSES

Articulated AFOs are commonly prescribed for children with cerebral palsy (Fig. 4.2.2). They have the advantage that they permit the ankle flexibility needed by small children to go from floor to stand and to climb stairs. They are frequently favored by physical therapists and physiatrists for young children. The flexibility of the ankle joint allows the ankle mobility required for the functional activities of getting up to a standing position, transitioning from one position to another, and stair-climbing. Many variations are possible. The hinge can be made from various materials with the theoretical advantage of providing a spring-like return to its resting, neutral position (although this remains clinically unproven). The joint range-of-motion can be unrestricted, or plantarflexion and/or dorsiflexion stops can be added to achieve different effects. The plantarflexion stop can prevent foot drop in swing.

Unfortunately, as children become older and larger, the articulated AFO with plantar-flexion stop may be inappropriate and can contribute to crouch. The articulated AFO design effectively treats the soleus and prevents contracture. The soleus is more commonly affected in children with hemiplegia than in children with diplegia (who generally only have gastrocnemius involvement). Articulated AFOs are therefore safer to use in hemiplegia, as children with hemiplegia are less likely to go into crouch. In children with diplegic involvement care must be taken that the soleus does not become overstretched.

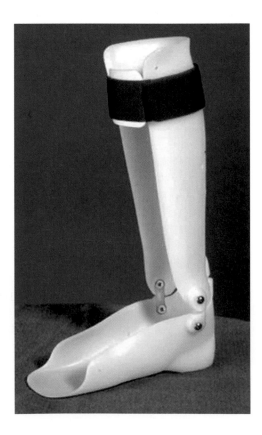

Fig. 4.2.2 Hinged AFO. The medial and lateral hinges allow free dorsiflexion and plantarflexion. In this case, however, plantarflexion is blocked by a posterior stop at 0°.

The overstretched soleus working in combination with a tight gastrocnemius which is held in neutral at the ankle may result in the knee being pulled into flexion. For these children an articulated AFO may, over time, create greater crouch (Fig. 4.2.3). In crouch, the one joint soleus muscle actually becomes excessively elongated. Care must be taken to avoid sacrificing long-term function for short-term goals in children with diplegia and quadriplegia by using this brace to maintain a plantigrade foot at the expense of increased knee flexion contributing to progressive crouch. If the gastrocnemius is contracted and this style of brace effectively prevents plantarflexion beyond neutral, the contracted gastrocnemius will pull the knee into flexion. Consequently, the action of the gastrocnemius is now restricted to knee flexion which becomes progressively easier to accomplish as the plantarflexion/ knee-extension couple becomes increasingly impaired. While the articulated AFO with plantarflexion stop may be a safe choice for young children, as children age, there are better ways to obtain functionally good results than by persisting with the articulated AFO.

POSTERIOR LEAF-SPRING ANKLE–FOOT ORTHOSES

The PLS AFO is a one-piece AFO consisting of a calf cuff that tapers to a band of various widths and pliability behind the ankle (the 'leaf') and widens back out to capture the heel and extend to the tip of the toes. The material used and the shape of the leaf affect the stiffness of the AFO (Fig. 4.2.4). The structural stiffness of the brace depends upon the thickness of the material, the radius of curvature of the leaf, and the stiffness characteristics of the material used (Sumiya et al. 1996, Nagaya 1997, Convery et al. 2004). Initially, the primary indication for the leaf-spring AFO was to prevent foot drop in swing phase and to ensure appropriate prepositioning of the foot for initial contact. The very lightweight dynamic AFO (DAFO) is appropriate in children for whom a foot drop in swing is still the primary indication (Fig. 4.2.5). The use of PLS AFOs has expanded to treat stance-phase 2nd rocker deficiencies as they can control dynamic equinus in stance. The elimination of premature heel rise avoids the inefficient mid-stance ankle power generation and improves stability in stance.

The 'appropriate' stiffness of the leaf remains an intriguing and challenging question. There has been little science to guide clinicians in this regard, but devices are being developed to test the stiffness characteristics of AFOs (Katdare 1999, Cappa et al. 2003). These devices can measure differences in stiffness between various leaf spring designs and materials (Novacheck et al. 2007). The augmentation of ankle-joint function between 2nd and 3rd rocker lies at the root of this challenge. Some materials and designs are intended to facilitate the storage of mechanical energy: that is, they have the ability to capture the mechanical energy that develops as the AFO bends into dorsiflexion, they store it until the limb is starting to unload in terminal stance, and then return that energy for push-off. Newer PLS designs (chevron, spiral, and carbon fiber) have been created to have a greater capacity for mechanical energy storage than the single-layer PLS AFO (Wolf et al. 2005).

In the future it may be possible to individualize the stiffness of the brace to meet the needs of the patient properly by resisting ankle dorsiflexion in 2nd rocker and returning the energy for push-off in 3rd rocker. Currently, the orthotist uses his/her expertise to adapt the stiffness of the AFO through design and material variables to comply with the physician's prescription. There are several studies which have addressed the contributions

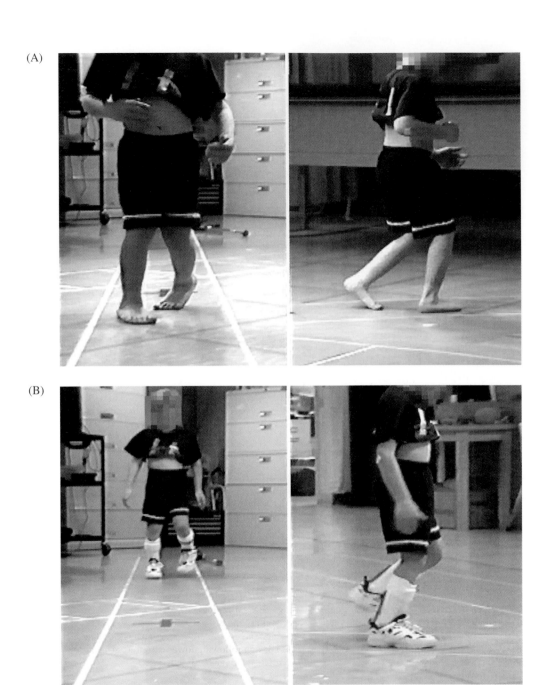

Fig. 4.2.3 Inappropriate hinged ankle–foot orthosis. Child with diplegic cerebral palsy with multilevel spasticity who has unfortunately undergone isolated heelcord lengthening. (A) Barefoot gait is in crouch with excessive ankle dorsiflexion. (B) The prescribed hinged AFO with free dorsiflexion is contraindicated: no improvements are seen with the orthosis. (See also Video 4.2.1 on Interactive Disc.)

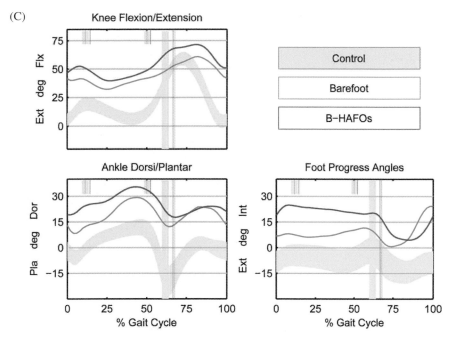

(C)

Knee Flexion/Extension

Ext ← deg → Flx

Control

Barefoot

B–HAFOs

Ankle Dorsi/Plantar

Pla ← deg → Dor

Foot Progress Angles

Ext ← deg → Int

0   25   50   75   100
% Gait Cycle

0   25   50   75   100
% Gait Cycle

Fig. 4.2.3 continued (C) Kinematic data show that crouch and excessive ankle dorsiflexion are both worse in the ankle–foot orthosis (AFO) (blue line) than barefoot (green line) compared to normal values (gray bands). Lever arm deformity and joint malposition result in intoeing gait which is also worse when tested with the orthoses. Surgical management will be required before this child can be an appropriate candidate for management with orthoses (likely a stiff PLS or floor reaction AFO).

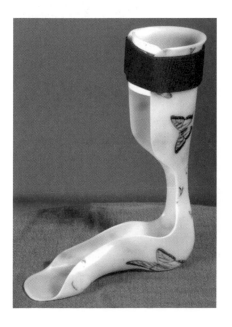

Fig. 4.2.4 Posterior leaf-spring (PLS) AFO. This PLS AFO is moderately stiff because of the thickness of the plastic as well as the radius of curvature and width of the leaf. This is a common AFO design following lower-extremity surgery to provide a relatively high level of stance phase support while strength is being regained postoperatively. As strength and motor control improve, the leaf can be trimmed to decrease stiffness. If muscle function is sufficient to avoid crouch, a University of California Biomechanics Laboratory orthosis or supramalleolar orthosis may be all that is required.

335

Fig. 4.2.5 Dynamic ankle–foot orthosis (DAFO). The DAFO is made out of very thin plastic, encapsulates the malleoli, and has dorsal wraps. Its primary indication is a dropfoot in swing.

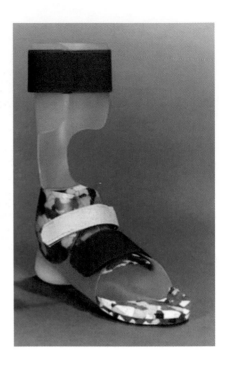

of stiff AFOs to the gait of patients who are plantarflexor deficient (Hullin et al. 1992, Thompson et al. 1999, Duffy et al. 2000). To date there is no practical way for the physician or orthotist to quantify the amount of stiffness required by a particular child to compensate for the abnormal 2nd and 3rd rockers in gait. Calculating the amount of energy storage that is appropriate to improve an individual's gait is even more challenging. Improvements in the design of orthotic testing devices will help answer these needs.

SOLID ANKLE–FOOT ORTHOSIS
Following the previous discussion of PLS designs, the reader will recognize that the solid AFO(SAFO) (Fig. 4.2.6) is simply a PLS design that is so stiff that the ankle joint does not move with use. Indications for SAFOs are increasingly severe spasticity and weakness, typically accompanied by poorer motor control. Controlling alignment and providing stability are the primary goals. Functional deficits are severe enough that ankle motion cannot be allowed as stability would be sacrificed.

FLOOR REACTION ANKLE–FOOT ORTHOSIS
The floor reaction AFO is a rear entry brace that has the maximal potential to restore the plantarflexion/knee-extension couple (Fig. 4.2.7) (Saltiel 1969). The floor reaction AFO is typically indicated for patients with severely compromised plantarflexor function, either as a primary pathology, or secondary to prior overlengthening of the heel cord. Prerequisites to the use of this style of AFO include full hip and knee extension and the absence of either tibial torsion or uncorrectable foot deformity that adversely affects the alignment of the

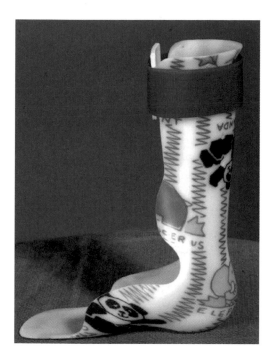

Fig. 4.2.6 Solid ankle–foot orthosis (SAFO). The SAFO eliminates ankle motion and is indicated if impairments of distal strength and motor control do not allow a less restrictive orthosis. Appropriate goals could include improvements in foot-progression angle, equinus in stance, dropfoot in swing, and protection of the knee from hyperextension or crouch in stance.

foot relative to the knee (Harrington et al. 1984). If present, surgical correction is required to establish the prerequisites before using the orthosis. If knee-extensor function is deficient (typically associated with patella alta), the floor reaction AFO can be used to minimize or eliminate crouch and relieve stress on the knee.

TOTAL CONTACT FOOTPLATE

An unrecognized coronal plane forefoot (varus or valgus) deformity is a frequent cause of inability for the patient to tolerate the orthosis or failure to provide adequate function. As a result of improved recognition and understanding of these deformities, both orthotic and surgical treatments have led to restoration of foot function as an effective lever arm for the ankle plantarflexors. Surgical correction is addressed in Chapter 5.8. A foot plate can be incorporated to compensate for the forefoot deformity using internal forefoot posting to bring the floor up to meet the foot (Fig. 4.2.8). This foot plate can be used as a foot orthosis alone or incorporated into UCBL orthoses, SMOs and AFOs.

One of the primary objectives of nearly any lower-extremity orthosis is to maintain neutral calcaneal alignment. This is effective when the pathology of the foot is identified exclusively as a rearfoot deformity. Conversely, when the pathology of the foot is identified exclusively as a forefoot deformity the treatment modality must focus on the forefoot to maintain neutral calcaneal alignment. When a forefoot deformity is not properly supported, it will cause significant rotation within an orthosis. For example, insufficient support of forefoot varus will most often present as redness or blistering at the 5th metatarsal, navicular, talus, and lateral calcaneus.

Fig. 4.2.7 Floor reaction ankle–foot orthosis (AFO). The floor reaction AFO can be either solid or hinged with a dorsiflexion stop set between 0° and 10° (A). Note the hinge depicted here is reversed.
(B) 15-year-old boy with diplegic cerebral palsy developed slight worsening of crouch during adolescence and anterior knee pain due to excessive patellofemoral stress. He has an insufficient plantarflexion/knee-extension couple due to ankle-plantarflexor weakness (2+/5). As a result, ankle dorsiflexion in midstance is excessive. Prior treatment includes selective dorsal rhizotomy and correction of lever-arm dysfunction. He is a good candidate for this orthosis (C) as he has good bone alignment (out of brace foot-progression angle is normal) and spasticity is minimal (normal range of knee motion in swing phase). (D) Ankle dorsiflexion is blocked at 10° (normal functional range) preventing excessive forward movement of the tibia over the plantigrade foot. He is no longer in crouch in mid-stance due to the effect of the orthosis. Knee pain resolved as a result of the 2nd rocker ankle restraint provided by the orthosis. At skeletal maturity, management was simplified to UCBL orthosis without recurrence of knee pain or crouch. B, bilateral; GRAFO, ground reaction ankle–foot orthosis. (See also Videos 4.2.2a and b on Interactive Disc.)

(A)

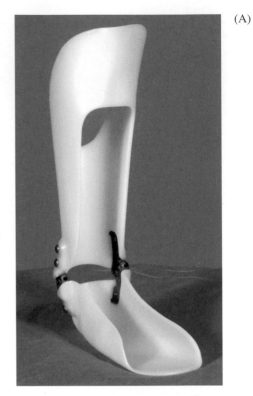

(B)

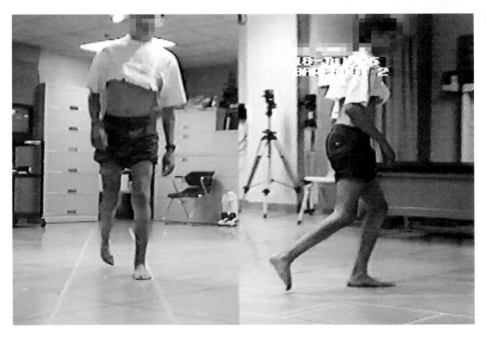

(C)

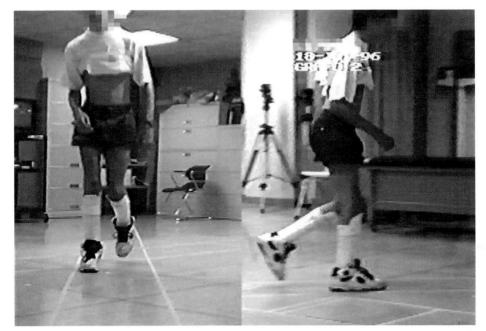

(D)

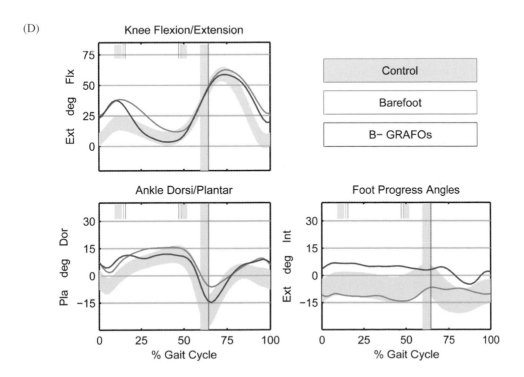

Knee Flexion/Extension

Control

Barefoot

B- GRAFOs

Ankle Dorsi/Plantar

Foot Progress Angles

% Gait Cycle

% Gait Cycle

339

The 'total contact footplate' design utilizes a modifiable forefoot post inside the orthosis aimed at treating forefoot deformities (Fig. 4.2.8a). When fabricated properly, the total contact footplate essentially brings the floor up to meet the foot (Fig. 4.2.8b) and prevents rotation within the orthosis. This design requires unique casting, modification, fabrication, and fitting techniques.

The first step in treatment is a thorough foot evaluation to identify the specific type and degree of forefoot deformity (see Chapter 3.2 for details). If a forefoot deformity is identified, there are several critical factors which must be considered to determine if a total contact footplate is an appropriate treatment option.

Indications for total contact footplate
- Joint flexibility sufficient to attain subtalar neutral
- Presence of a forefoot varus or valgus
- Rigid plantarflexed 1st ray.

Contraindications for total contact footplate
- Rigid midfoot deformities
- Marked in-toeing prior to orthotic intervention (when treating forefoot varus).

It is imperative that the alignment of the foot is maintained in subtalar neutral during the casting process (including the forefoot in the frontal plane). This is also true for the cast modification process. Reducing the angle of the deformity promotes pronation of the forefoot in seeking to find the floor through 2nd rocker. This excessive motion results in rearfoot eversion and loss of subtalar neutral. It is this motion/rotation that causes redness or blistering within an orthosis.

Upon weightbearing, there should be a significant improvement in the alignment of the knee and the foot-progression angle. With this design it is worthy to note that forefoot abduction with pronation can mask the appearance of internal femoral and/or tibial torsion related in-toe gait. Total contact correction of forefoot varus will reveal these proximal torsions with noticeably increased in-toeing during ambulation. The ankle should be well maintained in subtalar neutral and the 1st metatarsal head should not make contact with the plantar surface of the AFO. The plantar surface support of the midfoot should terminate just proximal to the 1st metatarsal head. There is an aggressive drop-off at the end of the midfoot support, mimicking the contour of the plantar surface of the 1st metatarsal shaft and head (Fig. 4.2.8c). It is this aggressive support of the forefoot and midfoot which helps to maintain subtalar neutral and prevents the 1st metatarsal head from dropping. The greater the forefoot deformity, the more elevated the 1st metatarsal head will be.

When fitting the total contact footplate, it is essential to pre-position the foot to don the orthosis. It is this 'pre-positioning' of the foot which makes an orthotic design that utilizes dorsal wraps difficult to don correctly. This requires holding the rearfoot in subtalar neutral to reveal the forefoot deformity. Once this position is achieved, release the rearfoot but continue to hold onto the forefoot. Slide the foot into the orthosis until the calcaneus is well situated in the heel of the orthosis. There should be no medial or lateral migration of the

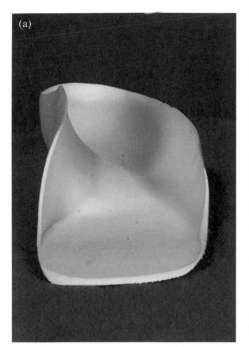

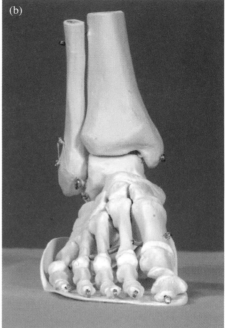

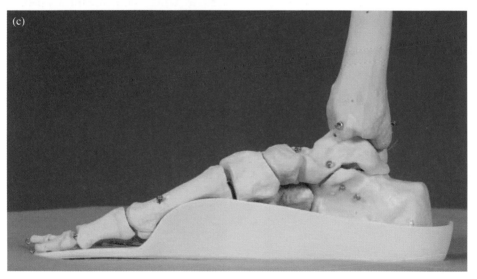

Fig. 4.2.8 The 'total contact footplate' (TCF). (a) The most common design incorporates an arch mold that extends distally on the medial side of the forefoot under the metatarsals to compensate for a forefoot varus deformity and avoid the midfoot collapse and hindfoot valgus that would result when weightbearing. An extended lateral border is necessary to contain the foot and control abduction. (b) The 1st metatarsal is supported in an elevated position to maintain alignment of the hindfoot and midfoot. (c) Note the aggressive drop-off at the end of the midfoot support, mimicking the contour of the plantar surface of the 1st metatarsal shaft and head.

forefoot once located into the orthosis. Secure the instep strap ensuring that the heel remains well seated in the orthosis. To maintain optimal positioning of the foot into the orthosis, a dynamic instep strap design is recommended. A dynamic instep strap provides medially or laterally directed corrective forces at the ankle. Secure calf strap and any other straps needed to maintain proper foot and ankle alignment.

Trimlines are critical to the success and function of the orthosis. The lateral forefoot trimline must extend sufficiently to encompass the 5th metatarsal head to prevent forefoot abduction. The medial forefoot border can be trimmed proximal to the metatarsal head, with the exception of a skew foot diagnosis.

Once the patient has ambulated with the orthosis for 20 minutes, remove the orthosis and the patient's sock. Inspect the limb for pressure areas. Insufficient midfoot support can result in increased redness and pressure at the 5th metatarsal, lateral calcaneus, navicular, and head of the talus. Excessive midfoot support can result in redness and pressure at the base of the 5th metatarsal, 5th metatarsal shaft, and lateral malleolus. Heat relief of these reddened areas rarely solves the problem. Reddened areas are generally the result of insufficient or excessive midfoot support. Therefore reduction of pressure is accomplished through modification of the midfoot support.

Consistently following these techniques can result in improved bony alignment of the foot as confirmed radiographically (Fig. 4.2.9). The focus of this discussion has been on compensating for a forefoot varus, but the total contact footplate can also be used for a forefoot valgus by incorporating the appropriate forefoot lateral posting (as determined in subtalar neutral) to maintain correct hindfoot and midfoot alignment.

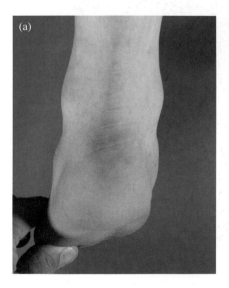 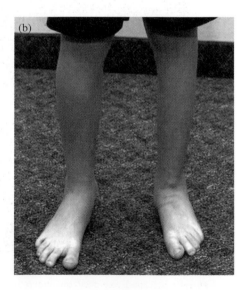

Fig. 4.2.9 Case study using posterior leaf-spring ankle–foot orthosis with total contact footplate. 12-year-old boy with cerebral palsy. (a) The left foot in non-weightbearing has a neutral hindfoot, midfoot instability, and forefoot varus. (b) In weightbearing, the foot is in planovalgus (note inward rotation of the tibia and knee).

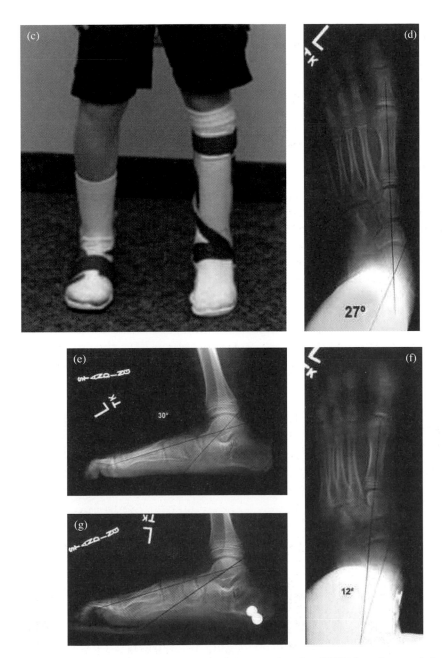

Fig. 4.2.9 continued (c) In an AFO with a total contact footplate (TCF), foot alignment is improved (note also the improved knee and tibial alignment relative to the foot). Barefoot standing AP (d) and lateral (e) radiographs document dorsal and lateral talonavicular subluxation, abduction of the forefoot, and plantarflexed talus. Standing anteroposterior (AP) (f) and lateral (g) radiographs in posterior leaf-spring ankle–foot orthosis with TCF show improved alignment. (See also Video 4.2.1 on Interactive Disc.)

343

Supporting evidence

Motion analysis laboratories have been used over the past 15–20 years to objectively evaluate the effects of AFOs on gait function in children with cerebral palsy. Numerous studies have reported significant improvements in linear parameters of velocity, step and stride length, and single limb stance support time when children with cerebral palsy are tested while wearing their AFOs (Dursun et al. 2002, Romkes and Brunner 2002, White et al. 2002, Buckon et al. 2004, Lam et al. 2005, Radtka et al. 2005). These improvements indicate substantial functional improvement. In addition, net oxygen can be reduced 6%–9% when children with cerebral palsy are tested while wearing their AFOs (Maltais et al. 2001). Hainsworth et al. (1997) reported that ROM and gait deteriorated when AFOs were not worn in 12 children between 3 and 7 years of age with cerebral palsy.

In addition to global functional improvements, AFOs have been shown to improve abnormal gait parameters specific to ankle joint function (Abel et al. 1998, Rethlefsen et al. 1999). Abel saw a reduction of abnormal power burst in mid-stance and an increase in the late stance ankle moment indicating improved ability to support body weight in a more appropriate alignment at the ankle in patients with either equinus or pes planovalgus.

Consistent and substantial changes in kinematics or kinetics at the pelvis, hip or knee have not been identified. Despite improvements in parameters of both global and ankle function, little effect of AFOs on proximal joints of the lower limb have been noted (Õunpuu et al. 1996, Abel et al. 1998, Rethlefsen et al. 1999, Crenshaw et al. 2000, Buckon et al. 2004, Radtka et al. 2005). On the other hand, improvements in the proximal joints are seen in paralytic conditions such as myelomeningocele and poliomyelitis (Hullin 1992, Thompson 1999, Duffy 2000).

The primary effect of an orthosis is a correction of positional and movement pathology at the foot and ankle. This has secondary effects on all joints in all planes through the coupled dynamics of the lower extremity. By shifting gait to a more normal pattern, and positioning joints more functionally, orthoses can change overall gait efficiency, in addition to correcting ankle and foot kinematics. Several studies have shown improvements in gait efficiency with use of orthoses (Mossberg et al. 1990, Waters and Mulroy 1999, Maltais et al. 2001, Smiley et al. 2002). More recently, Brehm and colleagues (2008) examined the interaction between changes in gait pattern induced by orthoses, and changes in energy observed in children with cerebral palsy. Their study revealed that while part of the efficiency improvements could be attributed to improvements in gait pattern, a significant portion was due to an increase in walking speed. The portion of efficiency increase arising from gait pattern changes was attributable in part to an improvement in terminal-swing and mid-stance knee extension, the latter improvement probably secondary to an enhanced plantarflexion/knee-extension couple. While overall positive changes for gait efficiency were found, the response was highly variable. Some children benefitted from the orthoses, while others did not – or even worsened. This finding suggests the need for further analysis to understand how to develop optimized orthoses.

The question of whether specific AFO designs lead to identifiable differences has received some attention. In a retrospective review of 115 patients with cerebral palsy, White et al. (2002) found that gait improvements were independent of specific AFO design.

A variety of styles provided similar results. Buckon et al. (2004) showed that various configurations of AFOs (solid, articulated and PLS) all normalized ankle kinematics in stance, increased step/stride length, decreased cadence, and decreased energy cost of walking. As would be expected, articulated AFOs result in greater ankle dorsiflexion in terminal stance than solid AFOs and pre-swing plantarflexion power is preserved (Rethlefsen et al. 1999). There is no evidence that tone reducing features incorporated in the footplate of a standard AFO provide additional benefit in gait parameters (Crenshaw et al. 2000). Articulated AFOs were shown to be superior to dynamic AFOs (supramalleolar) in improving gait parameters in children with hemiplegic CP (Romkes and Brunner 2002). Further, the dynamic AFO did not reduce muscle overactivity as well as the solid AFO (Lam et al. 2005). Despite this finding, the dynamic AFO was equally effective at correcting equinus in stance and swing and less restrictive of ankle movement. The authors noted that since they are lighter and less bulky, compliance was improved. It is well known that children in general will choose the lightest, smallest, and least restrictive style brace, even in the absence of significant differences in gait parameters or energy expenditure (Smiley et al. 2002).

An articulated AFO with free dorsiflexion could have adverse effects on crouch. The articulated AFO controls the spastic and/or contracted gastrocnemius at the ankle, but the abnormal two-joint muscle pulls the knee into flexion. In other words, the articulated AFO allows crouch. As mentioned above, despite the beneficial effect that the articulated AFO has on maintaining ankle power generation (Rethlefsen et al. 1999), the authors were concerned that there is excessive ankle dorsiflexion in terminal stance with articulated as compared to solid AFOs . They warned that articulated AFOs should only be considered for 'children who do not have a preexisting tendency to crouch'. Buckon et al. (2004) did note that some children with greater involvement did have a worsening of knee extensor moment, excessive ankle dorsiflexion and greater energy cost with an articulated AFO. Radtka et al. (2005), on the other hand, did not see the same adverse effects at the knee with the articulated AFO. The patients in this study may have had lesser involvement.

Many children with neurologic dysfunction have deficits of ankle plantarflexion function both for stance phase stability and for propulsion of the limb into swing. It would be desirable to use an AFO which is properly tuned to provide support in mid-stance and energy return in 3rd rocker, or push-off. Theoretically, that is the goal of the PLS AFO. It is often prescribed for this purpose and can be fabricated in a variety of designs. Current designs seem to succeed in achieving the first goal, but not the second. While the PLS AFO did improve foot drop in swing and increased power absorption in midstance, it did not augment push off power in terminal stance (Õunpuu et al. 1996). It is flexible enough to allow dorsiflexion, but had no effect on knee kinematics. These authors conclude that 'the name "posterior leaf spring" is misleading in terms of the function of this AFO during gait in persons with CP, as this brace does not augment power-generating capabilities at the ankle'. There is evidence to support the idea that there exists an optimal AFO for any one patient. A small group of children with hemiplegia were given two different custom-fit AFOs, one plastic and one carbon fiber. Motion analysis data were collected barefoot, with only shoes, and with each of the AFOs. The results indicate that many aspects of gait improve when using the AFOs, such as pre-positioning of the limb and walking velocity.

However, not all of the changes were significant when compared to the shoe-only condition. The authors conclude that, although the use of AFOs in this group of children improved their gait, it is important to remember that it is the combination of shoes and orthoses that affects the wearer (Desloovere et al. 2006).

Technical evaluation of orthosis stiffness is an area of increasing interest. Several devices that measure the mechanical characteristics of AFOs in 2nd and 3rd rocker have been developed and tested. These devices can be quite simple, such as a static, manual device used to test PLS AFO stiffness in dorsiflexion (Sumiya et al. 1996). There are also dynamic stiffness testers, which have shown the ability to detect the difference between AFOs built to be stiff, moderately stiff, and flexible, and to differentiate between orthoses made of different materials (carbon fiber, copolymer, and polypropylene) (Katdare 1999, Novacheck 2007). More sophisticated test mechanisms allow for two degrees of freedom, flexion/extension and ab/adduction (Cappa et al. 2003). There have also been devices built to interface with motion capture systems (Katdare 1999, Nelson et al. 2003). These devices are mechanically much simpler and can measure the stiffness dynamically thus providing a direct measurement of mechanical energy storage. However, the need for a motion-capture system limits the practicality of these devices.

One of the more comprehensive devices includes an adjustable mechanical analog of the full leg and foot which is manually driven to simulate both dorsiflexion and toe flexion (Fig. 4.2.10) (Bregman et al. 2008). This allows dynamic stiffness to be measured at both the ankle and metatarsal joints without the need of a motion capture system.

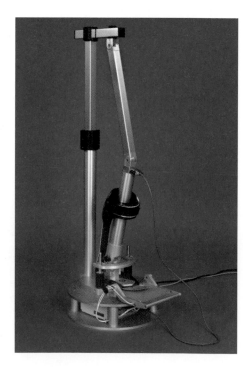

Fig. 4.2.10 Biarticular Reciprocating Universal Compliance Estimator (BRUCE). This comprehensive device includes an adjustable mechanical analog of the full leg and foot. It is manually driven to simulate both dorsiflexion and toe flexion. In this figure a carbon fiber ankle–foot orthosis (AFO) is mounted for testing. A wide range of AFO and footplate sizes can be accommodated. The orthosis can be secured with or without shoes. Forces and moments are monitored continuously to determine the dynamic material and structural properties.

All of the devices have been validated and can measure the mechanical characteristics of AFOs with good repeatability. However, the functional relationship between patient characteristics, AFO characteristics and AFO performance has yet to be determined.

Due to the variability in AFO design, material and manufacturing as well as patient diagnosis, ability and activity level, determining the optimal AFO stiffness is a challenging problem. Basic questions still need to be answered: (1) is a specific AFO effective for a given set of patient characteristics? (2) Is there such a thing as an optimal AFO stiffness? (3) If there is an optimal AFO stiffness, does it provide better function than the current best practice? (4) Finally, assuming that there is an optimal AFO, is there a relationship between the optimality criteria, the mechanical characteristics of the AFOs and patient characteristics such as weight, walking speed, and strength?

REFERENCES

Abel M, Juhl GA, Vaughan CL, Damiano DL (1998) Gait assessment of fixed ankle-foot orthoses in children with spastic diplegia. *Arch Phys Med Rehabil* **79**: 126–33.

Bregman D, Rozumalski A, Koops D, De Groot V, Schwartz MS, Harlaar J (2008) A new method for evaluating ankle foot orthosis stiffness: BRUCE. Abstracts of the 17th Annual Meeting of ESMAC, Antalya, Turkey, 28 (Suppl 2) S45.

Brehm MA, Harlaar J, Schwartz MH (2008) Effect of ankle-foot orthoses on walking efficiency and gait in children with cerebral palsy. *J Rehabil Med* **40**: 529–34.

Buckon C, Thomas SS, Jakobson-Huston S, Moor M, Sussman M, Aiona M (2004) Comparison of three ankle-foot orthosis configurations for children with spastic diplegia. *Dev Med Child Neurol* **46**: 590–8.

Cappa P, Patane F, Pierro MM (2003) A novel device to evaluate the stiffness of ankle foot orthosis devices. *J Biomech Eng* **125**: 913–17.

Convery P, Grieg RJ, Ross RS, Sockalingham S (2004) A three center study of the variability of ankle foot orthoses due to the fabrication and grade of polypropylene. *Prosthet Orthot Int* **28**: 175–82.

Crenshaw S, Herzog R, Castagno P, Richards J, Miller F, Michaloski G, Moran E (2000) The efficacy of tone-reducing features in orthotics on the gait of children with spastic diplegic cerebral palsy. *J Pediatr Orthop* **20**: 210–16.

Desloovere K, Molenaers G, Van Gestel L, Huenaerts C, Van Campenhout A, Callewaert B, Van de Walle P, Seyler J (2006) How can push-off be preserved during use of an ankle foot orthosis in children with hemiplegia? A prospective controlled study. *Gait Posture* **24**: 142–51.

Duffy CM, Graham HK, Cosgrove AP (2000) The influence of ankle foot orthoses on gait and energy expenditure in spina bifida. *J Pediatr Orthop* **20**: 356–61.

Dursun E, Dursun N, Alican D (2002) Ankle-foot orthoses: Effect on gait in children with cerebral palsy. *Disabil Rehabil* **24**: 345–7.

Gage JR, Schwartz MH (2002) Dynamic deformities and lever-arm considerations. In: Paley D, editor. *Principles of Deformity Correction*. Berlin: Springer. p 761–75.

Hainsworth F, Harrison MJ, Sheldon TA, Roussounis SH (1997) A preliminary evaluation of ankle orthoses in the management of children with cerebral palsy. *Dev Med Child Neurol* **39**: 243–7.

Harrington E, Lin RS, Gage JR (1984) Use of the anterior floor reaction orthosis in patients with cerebral palsy. *Orthot Prosthet* **37**: 34–42.

Hullin M, Robb LE, Loudon IR (1992) Ankle–foot orthosis function in low-level myelomeningocele. *J Pediatr Orthop* **12**: 518–21.

Katdare K (1999) *The non-linear stiffness of ankle-foot orthoses: measurement and prediction*. University of Minnesota, Minneapolis: Biomedical Engineering Graduate Program. (Dissertation.)

Lam W, Leong JCY, Li YH, Hu Y, Lu WW (2005) Biomechanical and electromyographic evaluation of ankle foot orthosis and dynamic ankle foot orthosis in spastic cerebral palsy. *Gait Posture* **22**: 189–97.

Maltais D, Bar-Or O, Galea V, Pierrynowski M (2001) Use of orthoses lowers the O_2 cost of walking in children with spastic cerebral palsy. *Med Sci Sports Exerc* **33**: 320–5.

Mossberg KA, Linton KA, Friske KF (1990) Ankle–foot orthoses: effect on energy expenditure of gait in spastic diplegic children. *Arch Phys Med Rehabil* **71**: 490–4.

Nagaya M (1997) Shoehorn-type ankle–foot orthoses: prediction of flexibility. *Arch Phys Med Rehabil* **78**: 82–4.

Nelson K, Kepple T, Lohmann Siegel K, Halstead L, Stanhope S (2003) Ankle foot orthosis contribution to net ankle moments in gait. Abstracts of the 27th Annual Meeting of ASB, Toledo, OH.

Novacheck TF, Beattie C, Rozumalski A, Gent G, Kroll G (2007) Quantifying the spring-like properties of ankle–foot orthoses (AFOs). *J Pediatr Orthop* **19**: 98–103.

Õunpuu S, Bell KJ, Davis RB, DeLuca PA (1996) An evaluation of the posterior leaf spring orthosis using joint kinematics and kinetics. *J Pediatr Orthop* **16**: 378–84.

Phelps W (1953) Braces – lower extremity – cerebral palsies. *Am Acad Orthopaed Surg Instruct Course Lect* **10**: 303–6.

Radtka S, Skinner SR, Johanson ME (2005) A comparison of gait with solid and hinged ankle–foot orthoses in children with spastic diplegic cerebral palsy. *Gait Posture* **21**: 303–10.

Rethlefsen S, Kay R, Dennis S, Forsten M, Tolo V (1999) The effects of fixed and articulated ankle–foot orthoses on gait patterns in subjects with cerebral palsy. *J Pediatr Orthop* **19**: 470–4.

Romkes J, Brunner R (2002) Comparison of a dynamic and a hinged ankle-foot orthosis by gait analysis in patients with hemiplegic cerebral palsy. *Gait Posture* **15**: 18–24.

Saltiel J (1969) A one-piece, laminated, knee locking, short leg brace. *Orthot Prosthet* **23**: 68–75.

Smiley S, Jacobsen FS, Mielke C, Johnston R, Park C, Ovaska GJ (2002) A comparison of the effects of solid, articulated, and posterior leaf-spring ankle–foot orthoses and shoes alone on gait and energy expenditure in children with spastic diplegic cerebral palsy. *Orthopedics* **25**: 411–15.

Sumiya T, Suzuki Y, Kasahara T (1996) Stiffness control in posterior-type plastic ankle–foot orthoses: affect of trimline. Part 1; a device for measuring ankle moment. *Prosthet Orthot Int* **20**: 129–31.

Thompson J, Õunpuu S, Davis RB, DeLuca PA (1999) The effects of ankle–foot orthoses on the ankle and knee in persons with myelomeningocele: an evaluation using three-dimensional gait analysis. *J Pediatr Orthop* **19**: 27–33.

Waters R, Mulroy S (1999) The energy expenditure of normal and pathologic gait. *Gait Posture* **9**: 207–31.

Wenger DR (1993) Clubfoot. In: Wenger DR, Rang M, editors. *The Art and Practice of Children's Orthopaedics*. New York: Raven. pp. 138–67.

White H, Jenkins J, Neace WP, Tylkowski C, Walker J (2002) Clinically prescribed orthoses demonstrate an increase in velocity of gait in children with cerebral palsy: a retrospective study. *Dev Med Child Neurol* **44**: 227–32.

Wolf S, Knie I, Rettig O, Fuchs A, Doderlein L (2005) Carbon fiber spring AFOs for active push-off. *Paper presented at the Annual Gait and Clinical Motion Analysis Society Meeting, Portland, Oregon, 6–9 April.*

4.3
PHARMACOLOGIC TREATMENT WITH ORAL MEDICATIONS

Marcie Ward

Key points

The goals for the use of oral medications should be clearly delineated prior to starting treatment.

- Side effects and risks of the oral medications limit their utility. The physician must evaluate the patient's response to these medications to determine whether or not the benefits outweigh any risks or side effects
- The trial and error process to determine the utility of these oral medications requires that the treating physician and the family communicate regularly
- Because these oral medications act at different sites, their use in combination may produce a greater clinical effect
- Blood work may be necessary to follow for the potential adverse event of hepatotoxicity.

Review of relevant pathophysiology

The oral medications for spasticity work at various points along the tonic stretch–spinal reflex arc, or at the level of the muscle itself (Fig. 4.3.1). Many of these medications work either to increase GABAergic inhibition, or to inhibit excitatory neurotransmitters. Dantrolene sodium, however, works by inhibiting the release of calcium ions from the sarcoplasmic reticulum thereby diminishing the force of the contraction of the muscles (Pinder et al. 1977). Some medications are used for their anticholinergic effects on the central nervous system that reduce extrapyramidal movements. The multiple sites of action of these commonly used spasticity drugs make it possible to use the medications in conjunction with one another to potentially produce an adjunctive effect on the patient's tone and spasticity.

Historical perspective

Historically, spasticity management options in children were limited to oral medications, phenol neurolytic blocks, range of motion exercises, casting, bracing, and orthopaedic surgical lengthening of muscles and tendons. Now, with other treatments available, which are often more effective at reducing tone globally such as intrathecal baclofen (ITB) and selective dorsal rhizotomy (see Chapters 5.1 and 5.2) or more selectively, such as botulinum toxin injections (see Chapter 4.4), the use of oral medications is less common. There are

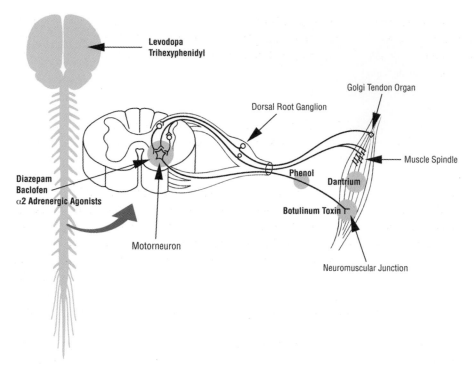

Fig. 4.3.1 The tonic stretch–spinal reflex arc and sites of action of medications for spasticity and dystonia.

still many instances where the use of the oral medications is warranted and necessary. For instance, not all communities can support the maintenance of an ITB pump and families may lack resources to travel for those needs. Also, in the young child, it may not be possible to fit an ITB pump in the abdominal space because of their small size. Furthermore, some families are reluctant to pursue ITB therapy due to fears of placing a 'foreign object' in their child, or fears of surgery. In such a child, realizing the maximal utility of the oral medications may be the best way to globally reduce tone, improve comfort and ease the caregiver burden. Still other children who are treated with focal spasticity medications (botulinum toxin and phenol) may have trouble with night-time spasms and discomfort, and may benefit from bedtime dosing of oral medications to improve sleep and comfort. Certainly, the child with dystonic tone may benefit from ITB therapy, but if their tone is not significant enough to warrant a pump, they may benefit from a trial of the anticholinergics or the dopaminergic agonists to improve function and reduce unwanted movements.

Indications from patient assessment
History and physical examination reveal indications for the use of oral medications in the management of tone or movement disorders for patients with cerebral palsy. Currently, laboratory tests and imaging do not have a direct role for evaluating a child in this situation. Movement analysis testing may have a limited role in helping to identify dystonic tone that

may be more amenable to treatment with anticholinergics and dopamine agonists. For the most part, however, oral medications should be considered if spasticity and abnormal tone are found on physical exam, and noted in the history to be interfering with movement, comfort and care.

HISTORY

Diagnosis of the cause of abnormal tone begins with the patient's history. The child whose birth history is consistent with an event known to potentially produce an injury to the brain, may be presumed to have cerebral palsy secondary to that event. Full investigation of cerebral palsy is guided by the practice parameters outlined by the American Academy of Neurology (Ashwal et al. 2004). It is imperative that the practitioner confirms that the antecedent event fits with the tone pattern noted on physical exam, lest the true etiology of the abnormal tone be overlooked. The majority of children with cerebral palsy experience some degree of spastic tone. Many of these children also display some aspect of dystonic tone to varying degrees. Pure athetoid tone is rarely seen, but is expected in patients with lesions isolated to the basal ganglia, from kernicterus, for example. Depending on the expertise of the treating physician, consultation with a pediatric physiatrist, or a pediatric neurologist may be considered to confirm the diagnosis and offer opinions regarding treatment options.

Discussion of how the abnormal tone is impacting the child's daily life is paramount. Is the child in pain? Is his care or positioning challenging due to high tone? Is she sleeping through the night comfortably? Other associated medical problems can exacerbate movement disorders and hypertonia, so a careful global assessment is also necessary to assess for noxious stimuli including pain generators, infection, skin ulceration, gastric reflux, anxiety and sleep disorders. Some of these factors can contribute to a 'vicious cycle' of tone, which can be averted by eliminating the noxious stimuli.

PHYSICAL EXAMINATION

Examination of the patient with abnormal tone involves evaluating range of motion, resting tone, tone with rapid stretch of the muscles, tone that is produced by active movement, motor control, and strength. Identification by physical exam of the types of tone involved in the patient's movement disorder can be helpful in choosing an oral medication. The practitioner may choose to treat dystonic tone differently than spastic tone. Tone that is only seen during active movement may represent dystonia that could respond more favorably to the anticholinergics and dopaminergic medications. Furthermore, on physical exam the practitioner can often identify how abnormal tone may interfere with positioning or cares, and may also reveal how painful spasms or pain with range of motion impacts comfort.

Goals of treatment

Oral medications are typically considered to treat tone that is interfering with daily care, and comfort of the child. They globally reduce abnormal tone, so they are more commonly used

351

for children with more severe impairments of function (levels IV or V on the Gross Motor Function Classification System). They are less often used in the child with hemiplegia or diplegia, unless it is severe. Oral medications are less often used to treat hypertonia that results solely in gait impairment. The history and physical examination in combination provide insight for the practitioner regarding how the abnormal tone is affecting the patient's quality of life, and guides the practitioner toward appropriate goals of treatment with oral medications.

Treatment options

Treating spasticity in the child with cerebral palsy may call for oral medications as the primary treatment or as an adjuvant in the patient-care plan. Consideration must be given to the goals of treatment and to the potential side effects and risks of the oral medications.

Unfortunately the majority of oral medications are not likely to 'cure' high tone and rarely do they eliminate spasticity or movement disorders entirely. The goals for treatment with oral medications need to be explained to the family so that their expectations remain realistic. Often oral medications can reduce spasticity and the frequency of uncomfortable muscle spasms; they can decrease opisthotonic posturing, undesirable movements, and pain. If so, comfort and ease of care improve. Goals such as these are reasonable and warrant consideration of oral medication use.

Oral medications are not necessarily the end point of the child's spasticity treatment plan. Sometimes they are used as a temporary intervention until other more definitive options (ITB, selective dorsal rhizotomy or orthopaedic surgery) are considered by the team of care-providers or the child's family.

Nearly all of these medications, however, have the possible side effect of sedation and therefore cognitive impairment. Many of them are metabolized in the liver and have the potential for hepatotoxicity. Still others may produce physical dependence on the medication, requiring a slow taper if the medication be discontinued. To avoid the consequences of withdrawal, the care-provider must deliver regular and ongoing doses. This is particularly challenging as these medications typically work best on a schedule of about three times a day dosing.

The trial-and-error process to determine the utility of these oral medications requires that the treating physician and the family communicate regularly. As each medication is tried, it is increased slowly to a maximum allowable dose followed by an assessment of the patient's tone, goals, comfort and ease of care, to identify whether or not the medication is effective. If the medication is not effective at the maximum dose or if side effects preclude the physician from continuing to increase the dose, the medication may need to be discontinued and deemed ineffective for the goals that were set. If there is some improvement in the tone, but further tone control is desired, a second medication can be added. As with the first medication, the dose is titrated up slowly, monitoring the patient's response for efficacy and side effects.

A discussion of many of the agents commonly used for spasticity and movement disorder in cerebral palsy follows. It cannot be overemphasized that if these medications are to be tried, the physician must evaluate the patient's response to determine whether or not the benefits outweigh any risks or side effects of the medications.

Pain and anxiety disorders are not uncommon in children with cerebral palsy and can interfere with function. Treatment of these concerns can be useful for improving the function of children with neurological impairments. Though worth mentioning here, a complete discussion of anxiolytics and analgesics lies outside the scope of this chapter.

BENZODIAZEPINES

Spasticity has been treated with benzodiazepines for many years. Diazepam has been used over the greatest number of years (Whyte and Robinson 1990). Like many of the oral medications for spasticity management, benzodiazepines do not have labeling for this indication despite their long-standing use, and safety and efficacy have not been studied in children under 6 months of age.

Schmidt et al. (1967) studied the effect of diazepam on cats and identified that the mechanism of action is increasing presynaptic inhibition at the spinal-cord level. Subsequent to that study, those findings were confirmed in two human studies (Verrier et al. 1975, Kaieda et al. 1981). Diazepam is thought to directly augment GABA postsynaptic action, creating an inhibitory effect at the spinal reflex arc, as well as at the supraspinal level and the reticular formation. It reduces monosynaptic and polysynaptic reflexes (Schlosser 1971) and is particularly useful in reducing painful spasms that may produce insomnia (Mathew and Mathew 2005).

Diazepam is metabolized in the liver along a complex pathway that is more efficient in children, but less efficient in neonates and adults. Its metabolites are protein-bound. In the patient with malnutrition or a low serum albumin, free metabolites may increase the risk of side effects. Peak levels typically occur about one hour after administration of diazepam so more frequent dosing allows more consistent relief of symptoms. The half-life is variable at 15–95 hours (depending on the patient's age and metabolism); for clonazepam the half-life is about 30–40 hours (Drugdex System 2008).

Side effects of the benzodiazepines typically include somnolence, ataxia, inco-ordination, respiratory depression, fatigue, euphoria, hypotension, diarrhea, and rash. Physiologic dependence does occur and, therefore, if the medication is to be discontinued it needs to be weaned in order to avoid symptoms of withdrawal (Drugdex System 2008). If withdrawal does occur it will typically be manifested by agitation, irritability, tremor, twitching, nausea, insomnia, fever, and perhaps seizures. Since the half-life is quite long, symptoms of withdrawal may not occur until 2–4 days after the medication is acutely discontinued (Gracies et al. 1997).

Pediatric dosage for diazepam starts at 0.12 mg/kg/day divided into three or four daily doses, to a maximum of 0.8 mg/kg/day or 60 mg (Gracies et al. 1997). Certainly if sedation occurs, the dosage needs to be decreased. For clonazepam, the dosage begins at 0.01mg/kg/day divided into two or three daily doses. This may be increased to 0.3 mg/kg/day, up to a maximum of 20 mg/day. Diazepam is available in tablet form as well as in a liquid form, and clonazepam is available in tablet form and in an oral dissolvable tablet (Drugdex System 2008).

BACLOFEN

Baclofen is labeled for the treatment of spasticity and is often used to treat spasticity associated with cerebral palsy. It acts at the level of the spinal cord binding to GABA-B receptor sites, agonizing the site and suppressing the release of excitatory neurotransmitters. Augmenting GABAergic activity reduces spasticity. Monosynaptic responses are more affected than polysynaptic responses (Curtis et al. 1981, Hill and Bowery 1981). Baclofen is completely absorbed orally and metabolized partly by the liver and otherwise nearly fully secreted by the kidneys. The half-life of baclofen is 2–4 hours.

Side effects of oral baclofen therapy may include somnolence, hypotonia, weakness, nausea, vomiting, and dizziness (Drugdex System 2008). Oral baclofen may lower the seizure threshold (Young 1997, Krach 2001). Physiologic dependence can develop, such that sudden withdrawal may result in rebound spasticity, muscle spasms, hallucinations, confusion, seizures, and temperature elevations (Krach 2001, Patel and Soyode 2005). Therefore weaning of baclofen is recommended if the medication is to be discontinued. As a precaution, if a patient is undergoing surgical intervention with the possibility of postoperative ileus, the dose should be tapered down as low as possible prior to surgery (Krach 2001). This prevents the critical situation of managing baclofen withdrawal in a patient who cannot tolerate oral baclofen or absorb oral baclofen. Tone and spasms during the postoperative period can be managed with intravenous diazepam.

Dosage recommendations in children include initial dosing of 5–15mg daily divided twice daily and increasing the dose and frequency to a maximum of 40 mg/day in children less than 8 years old, and 60 mg in children older than 8, divided three times a day. The dose should be increased approximately every 3 days while observing for symptoms of sedation (Drugdex System 2008). Maximum dosage is often quoted at 60 mg per day but some practitioners have prescribed as much as 160 mg per day to control tone adequately as long as unacceptable side effects are not encountered (Young 1997). Baclofen is available in tablet form or intrathecal preparation (see Chapter 5.1). Many pharmacies will compound an oral suspension form of baclofen, but the medication settles out of solution rapidly. Therefore the actual dispensed dosages may not be uniform (Krach 2001). Families must be reminded to shake the liquid well before every use.

DANTROLENE SODIUM

Dantrolene sodium is a unique medication for the treatment of spasticity. It is labeled for such and its action is at the level of the muscle itself. It works by inhibiting the release of calcium ions from the sarcoplasmic reticulum and thus diminishing the force of the muscle's contractions. Dantrolene sodium has its greatest effect on the fast contracting muscles and has no effect on cardiac muscle (Young and Delwaide 1981). It does, however, cause weakness in non-spastic muscles as well, as it is not selective for spastic muscles alone. This factor makes it a less appealing medication for the treatment of spasticity in the ambulatory patient with cerebral palsy (Young 1997). Caution should be taken in prescribing dantrolene sodium for the patient who has severe myocardial disease, has borderline pulmonary function or who is ambulatory (Young and Delwaide 1981).

Dantrolene sodium is metabolized by the liver and excreted in the urine. This medication does carry a black box warning for hepatoxicity (Drugdex System 2008), which is seen in about 1.8% of patients treated. For this reason monitoring liver enzymes is recommended. If elevated transaminases are identified, the medication should be tapered and discontinued. Fatal hepatitis is thought to occur in about 0.3% of patients treated. This has typically occurred in women over the age of 30 who have received doses greater than or equal to 300 mg per day for more than 2 months (Ward et al. 1986). Because of the concomitant affects that valproate may have on the liver, combining these medications is not recommended. Dantrolene sodium's active metabolite reaches peak levels within 4–8 hours with a half-life of about 8.7 hours (Drugdex System 2008).

The most common side effects of dantrolene sodium are weakness and fatigue. It may also lead to malaise, dizziness, diarrhea, and visual disturbances (Drugdex System 2008).

In prescribing dantrolene sodium, pediatric dosages begin at 0.5–1.0 mg/kg once daily. This dose may be increased by 1.5 mg/kg every 7 days to a maximum dose of 12 mg/kg/day or 400mg/day. Dantrolene sodium is available in tablets or in intravenous preparation (Whyte and Robinson 1990, Drugdex System 2008).

ALPHA-2 ADRENERGIC AGONISTS

The alpha-2 adrenergic agonists have been found in some studies to benefit spasticity of multiple origins including multiple sclerosis, spinal cord injury and stroke (Nance 1997, Young 1997). For this reason they have been used for the treatment of spasticity including that which results from cerebral palsy.

Alpha-2 adrenergic agonists act at the level of the brain and the spinal cord, likely presynaptically hyperpolarizing the motoneurons and perhaps decreasing the release of excitatory neurotransmitters, thus decreasing the spastic response (Young 1997, Krach 2001, Patel and Soyode 2005). Alpha-2 adrenergic agonists have also been identified as having antinociceptive effects (Nance 1997), a property shared with baclofen.

Tizanidine is the most commonly used alpha-2 adrenergic agonist in the treatment of spasticity. It is metabolized in the liver with a half-life of about 2½ hours. Hepatotoxicity can occur with tizanidine with an incidence of 2–5%. For this reason it is highly recommended that the practitioner monitor liver enzymes throughout the treatment course (Krach 2001, Edgar 2003). Clonidine has also been used for the treatment of spasticity, but is metabolized in part through the renal system, peaking in its function at 1.5–5 hours with a half-life of 12–16 hours (Drugdex System 2008).

Side effects in using alpha-2 adrenergic agonists include sedation, hypotension, and dry mouth (Drugdex System 2008). Weingarden and Belen (1992) identified that the side effects of hypotension can be minimized using a transdermal preparation of clonidine rather than an oral form. Although lowering the seizure threshold is not a typical concern in starting an alpha-2 adrenergic agonist, Feron et al. (2008) published one case report of new onset seizures after starting clonidine in a child with cerebral palsy for the treatment of attention deficit disorder.

In prescribing oral tizanidine it is recommended that the practitioner start with 1 mg (for those younger than 10 years of age) or 2 mg (over 10 years of age). The practitioner may choose to begin dosing at bedtime to avert problems associated with the side effect of drowsiness. Peak plasma levels are found 1–2 hours post-ingestion. Maintenance dosing for tizanidine typically is 0.3–0.5 mg/kg/day divided four times a day (Edgar 2003, Patel and Soyode 2005). Clonidine is started at 0.05 mg by mouth at bedtime and increased by 0.05 mg every 7 days to a maximum of 0.3 mg per day divided three times a day. A transdermal form of clonidine is available as well (Patel and Soyode 2005).

LEVODOPA

Levodopa has been suggested as a possible treatment for management of movement disorders in children with cerebral palsy. Its primary indication is for the treatment of Parkinson disease. It relieves the symptoms of Parkinson disease including resting tremor, rigidity and dyskinetic movements. Levodopa is thought to primarily help with hypertonia resulting from extrapyramidal injury (dystonia). It has been investigated for its utility in adults after stroke and demonstrated significantly improved recovery of motor function (Scheidtmann et al. 2001). It may improve the dystonic or extrapyramidal movements in some cases of cerebral palsy (Brunstrom et al. 2000). It should be noted that levodopa is the treatment of choice for dopamine-responsive dystonias. As dopamine-responsive dystonias can be misdiagnosed as cerebral palsy, a dramatic response to the drug may suggest a misdiagnosis (Fink et al. 1988, Nygaard et al. 1994). If marked improvement in the movement disorder occurs with levodopa, the practitioner may need to consider workup for dopamine responsive dystonia, especially in the patient with an unclear etiology for cerebral palsy.

Levodopa is a dopamine precursor. Levodopa's mechanism of action is as a dopamine receptor agonist. It is known to cross the blood brain barrier where it is presumably converted to dopamine in the central nervous system (Drugdex System 2008). Levodopa's half-life is substantially increased when combined with carbidopa and therefore, lower dosages of levodopa are needed to obtain therapeutic results.

Side effects of levodopa treatment include dyskinesias, and nausea (Drugdex System 2008). Lowering the dose may improve the nausea, but the adverse side effects may limit the ability to reach an optimal therapeutic effect.

Estimating the dosage of levodopa is challenging in the pediatric patient, as there are no guidelines for its use in children. The author's experience is that it is generally safe to begin with 50 mg twice daily in small children and 100 mg twice daily for older children and teenagers. Ultimately levodopa should be given three times a day by gradually increasing the patient's dose by 50 mg per day as they demonstrate freedom from side effects. Maximum dosing of levodopa in children usually does not exceed 600–800 mg per day (Edgar 2003). The medication should be given with meals to avoid nausea.

TRIHEXYPHENIDYL

Trihexyphenidyl is only approved for the treatment of Parkinson disease and for extrapyramidal reactions, but it has been studied in the treatment of dystonia associated with cerebral palsy (Hoon et al. 2001, Sanger et al. 2007).

Trihexyphenidyl is an anticholinergic that works centrally. It is believed that trihexyphenidyl blocks the action of acetylcholine on the central muscarinic receptors. In animal models of asphyxia a relative preservation of cholinergic interneurons in the striatum has been identified, compared with the degree of preservation of their postsynaptic targets and the degree of injury to the dopaminergic neurons. It is believed that this results in a relative increase in cholinergic activity (Burke and Karanas 1990). By reducing cholinergic transmission with trihexyphenidyl, the balance between the dopaminergic and cholinergic drive is reestablished resulting in decreased dystonia (Sanger et al. 2007).

The metabolism of trihexyphenidyl is unknown. It is excreted in the urine with a half-life of 3.7 hours (Drugdex System 2008). Side effects are relatively minimal but may include dry mouth, constipation, blurred vision, dizziness, nausea, confusion and psychosis (Drugdex System 2008). Most side effects appear to be well tolerated. Dosing recommendations are to begin trihexyphenidyl at 2–2.5 mg per day and increase by 2–2.5 mg every other week to a maximum dose of 60 mg per day. Trihexyphenidyl comes in tablets or in a liquid (Edgar 2003).

Supporting evidence/outcome data

Benzodiazepines
Research into the effects of diazepam on spasticity in children began over 40 years ago with the work of Engle (1966). Using a double-blind crossover study, diazepam yielded greater subjective clinical improvement in 12 of 16 children compared to placebo. The subjective findings of clinical improvement were not specific to spasticity. For instance, behavioral improvements were noted in those children as well. Behavioral improvements may be attributed to the general relaxation of the child (Whyte and Robinson 1990). A more recent study found that diazepam was superior to placebo in a double-blind randomized placebo-controlled study, in which 180 children were given a bedtime dose of either diazepam or placebo. Caregivers reported that children who received diazepam slept better. Feeding, bathing, play, and exercise times were less stressful for the children, with less crying and less irritability (Mathew and Mathew 2005). When prescribing benzodiazepines, however, it should be noted that behavioral side effects occur in about 9% of children with cerebral palsy (Kalachnik et al. 2002).

Baclofen
Milla and Jackson (1977) reported a double blind, placebo-controlled crossover study of baclofen for the treatment of spasticity on 20 children with cerebral palsy. Dosages began at 10 mg per day in divided doses and were gradually increased, in three increments over 9 days. For children aged 2–7 years, maximum daily dose was 40 mg, and for children older than 7 years old maximum daily dose was 60 mg. Oral baclofen was found to be superior to placebo in decreasing tone and allowing active and passive range of motion (Milla and Jackson 1977). A double-blind study demonstrated reduced tone in children with cerebral palsy in dosages of up to 30 mg per day for children age 6 and under, and 70 mg per day in children over the age of 6 (Schwartzman et al. 1976). Baclofen has been reported to

357

decrease the response to pain and noxious stimuli in adult patients with spasticity, a potential added benefit with this medication (Pinto et al. 1972).

DANTROLENE SODIUM

The efficacy of dantrolene sodium in the treatment of spasticity has been studied extensively. In 18 patients (only some of whom were children), dantrolene sodium resulted in a 50% moderate to marked improvement in spasms and unwanted movements compared to placebo (Chyatte and Basmajian 1973). Subsequently dantrolene sodium was found to be superior to placebo in improving physiologic measurements in children with cerebral palsy (Joynt and Leonard 1980). Some of the most convincing research comes from Haslam and colleagues in 1974. Twenty-three children in a double-blind placebo-controlled crossover study were overall found to have improvement in reflexes and scissoring with dantrolene sodium at dosages of 1–3mg/kg four times a day. In contrast, two studies reported little improvement or equivocal results. Fifteen children treated with dantrolene sodium for 8 weeks were felt to have little improvement (Ford et al. 1976). Similarly, 28 children in a double-blind placebo controlled crossover study were reported to have experienced equivocal effects with dantrolene sodium (Denhoff et al. 1975).

ALPHA-2 ADRENERGIC AGONISTS

The majority of the research conducted involving alpha-2 adrenergic agonists and their effect on spasticity has been done in adult patients with spinal-cord injury, multiple sclerosis and cerebral vascular accidents (Young 1997, Krach 2001, Montane et al. 2004). Tizanidine has been found to be effective in treating spasticity in patients with multiple sclerosis and spinal-cord injury (Nance 1997), but no pediatric studies have been published. Similar research has been done supporting the use of clonidine in treating spasticity associated with adult spinal cord injury, but only one case report (that of a 17-year-old patient with cerebral palsy who failed treatment with diazepam and baclofen) supports the use of clonidine in treating spasticity due to cerebral palsy (Dall et al. 1996). In this report, transdermal clonidine 0.1mg was used with subjective improvement in tone.

LEVODOPA

The only literature documenting the benefits of levodopa on spasticity in cerebral palsy is a case report in which a 16-year-old patient with spastic quadriplegic cerebral palsy and truncal dystonia was given a trial of 100 mg of levodopa daily. After 2 weeks a decrease in unwanted movements was noted and, at 200 mg daily, further functional improvement was identified. With further increases in the dose, benefits decreased, leading the author to conclude that the ideal dose for this patient was 200 mg daily. The authors documented the decreased unwanted upper extremity movements with a motion measurement system as well as decreased dynamic electromyographic activity after treatment (Brunstrom et al. 2000).

TRIHEXYPHENIDYL

Fahn (1979) reported that children had better relief of dystonia with trihexyphenidyl than adults did. Children tended to respond favorably with fewer adverse events (Fahn 1983). In a double-blind, randomized, placebo-controlled trial, Burke et al. (1986) identified a positive effect from trihexyphenidyl in younger dystonic patients (mean age 18.9 years). Upper-extremity function and verbal expression were found by parental report to improve in some children with extrapyramidal cerebral palsy after trihexyphenidyl was initiated (Hoon et al. 2001). In the most recent study of the use of trihexyphenidyl in dystonic cerebral palsy, 23 children aged 4–15 years of age with secondary dystonia were started on trihexyphenidyl 0.1 mg/kg/day which was increased over a 9-week period, up to a maximum of 0.75mg/kg/day. After the 9-week period trihexyphenidyl was tapered off over the following 5 weeks. Objective motor assessments were performed at base line, 9 weeks, and 15 weeks. Upper-limb function was significantly improved by 15 weeks in some of the subjects, but this was not seen at the 9-week evaluation. The authors concluded that there may be value in continuing trihexyphenidyl for a sufficient period of time to determine whether or not benefit may be realized. However, the overall results were equivocal for the use of trihexyphenidyl in treating children with secondary dystonia from cerebral palsy (Sanger et al. 2007).

Case example 1

A 3-year-old child with quadriplegic cerebral palsy demonstrated muscle tone that was mostly spastic in nature. The child had some difficulty with sleeping through the night and cares were challenging for the family because of spasticity. A trial of oral baclofen was started at 2.5 mg at bedtime in an effort to improve his sleep by gaining control over his overall tone. The dose was increased every 3 days by 2.5–5 mg three times a day. His tone improved, but spasms continued to interfere with sleep. A nightly dose of diazepam was added. Because tone was satisfactorily reduced during the day, daytime diazepam was not started. If sedation had been problematic with this regimen, a trial of an alpha-2 adrenergic agonist or dantrolene sodium was the next consideration.

Case example 2

A 9-year-old child with dystonic cerebral palsy secondary to anoxic injury at birth was troubled by poor control of her right upper extremity which compromised the completion of many of her activities of daily living. In the past oral baclofen did not improve her upper-extremity function, and it caused cognitive clouding limiting the ability to increase the dose. A trial of levodopa was started at a dose of 100 mg twice daily which was increased by 50 mg a week, to a steady state of 100 mg three times per day with improvement in symptoms. In an effort to obtain further improvements in symptoms, the dose was increased further to a maximum of 600 mg per day with further benefit noted. If benefits from levodopa had not been noted, this medication would have been tapered and discontinued. A trial of trihexyphenidyl would then be considered.

Summary

Many oral medications are available that may be used to treat abnormal muscle tone and movement disorders in the child with cerebral palsy. The practitioner should choose medications, weighing the efficacy of the oral medications against the side effects and risks. Avoiding sedation in a child with functional cognitive skills is imperative. Goals of the treatment should be discussed with the patient and the family so that realistic expectations about the benefits of the medication are understood prior to initiating treatment. Potential side effects and precautions must be made clear to the patient and their family so that the impact of the side effects can be evaluated as dosing is optimized. Since there are different sites of action for these oral medications, the practitioner may choose to use the medications in combination in an effort to produce a potentially greater clinical effect.

REFERENCES

Ashwal S, Russman BS, Blasco PA, Miller G, Sandler A, Shevell M, Stevenson R (2004) Practice parameter: diagnostic assessment of the child with cerebral palsy: report of the Quality Standards Subcommittee of the American Academy of Neurology and the Practice Committee of the Child Neurology Society. *Neurology* **62**: 851–63.

Brunstrom JE, Bastian, AJ, Wong M, Mink JW (2000) Motor benefit from levodopa in spastic quadriplegic cerebral palsy. *Ann Neurol* **47**: 662–5.

Burke RE, Karanas AL (1990) Quantitative morphological analysis of striatal cholinergic neurons in perinatal asphyxia. *Ann Neurol* **27**: 81–8.

Burke RE, Fahn S, Marsden CD (1986) Torsion dystonia: a double-blind, prospective trial of high-dosage trihexyphenidyl. *Neurology* **36**: 160–4.

Chyatte SB, Basmajian JV (1973) Dantrolene sodium: long-term effects in severe spasticity. *Arch Phys Med Rehabil* **54**: 311–15.

Curtis DR, Lodge D, Bornstein JC, Peet MJ (1981) Selective effects of baclofen on spinal synaptic transmission in the cat. *Exp Brain Res* **42**: 158–70.

Dall JT, Harmon RL, Quinn CM (1996) Use of clonidine for treatment of spasticity arising from various forms of brain injury: a case series. *Brain Inj* **10**: 453–8.

Denhoff E, Feldman S, Smith MG, Litchman H, Holden W (1975) Treatment of spastic cerebral-palsied children with sodium dantrolene. *Dev Med Child Neurol* **17**: 736–42.

DRUGDEX(r) System (retrieved 20 Dec 2008) http://www.thomsonhc.com. Greenwood Village, CO: Thomson Healthcare.

Edgar TS (2003) Oral pharmacotherapy of childhood movement disorders. *J Child Neurol* **18**: S40–9.

Engle HA (1966) The effect of diazepam (valium) in children with cerebral palsy: a double-blind study. *Dev Med Child Neurol* **8**: 661–7.

Fahn S (1979) Treatment of dystonia with high-dosage anti-cholinergic medicine. *Neurology* **29**: 605.

Fahn S (1983) High dosage anticholinergic therapy in dystonia. *Neurology* **33**: 1255–61.

Feron FJ, Hendriksen JG, Nicolai J, Vles JS (2008) New-onset seizures: a possible association with clonidine? *Ped Neurol* **38**: 147–9.

Fink JK, Filling-Katz MR, Barton NW, Macrae PR, Hallett M, Cohen WE (1988) Treatable dystonia presenting as spastic cerebral palsy. *Pediatrics* **82**: 137–8.

Ford F, Bleck EE, Aptekar RG, Collins FJ, Stevick D (1976) Efficacy of dantrolene sodium in the treatment of spastic cerebral palsy. *Dev Med Child Neurol* **18**: 770–83.

Gracies JM, Elovic E, McGuire J, Simpson DM (1997) Traditional pharmacological treatments for spasticity. part I: Local treatments. *Muscle Nerve Suppl* **6**: S61–91.

Haslam RH, Walcher JR, Lietman PS, Kallman CH, Mellits ED (1974) Dantrolene sodium in children with spasticity. *Arch Phys Med Rehabil* **55**: 384–8.

Hill DR, Bowery NG (1981) 3H-baclofen and 3H-GABA bind to bicuculline-insensitive GABA B sites in rat brain. *Nature* **290**: 149–52.

Hoon AH Jr, Freese PO, Reinhardt EM, Wilson MA, Lawrie WT Jr, Harryman SE, Pidcock FS, Johnston MV (2001) Age-dependent effects of trihexyphenidyl in extrapyramidal cerebral palsy. *Ped Neurol* **25**: 55–8.

Joynt RL, Leonard JA Jr (1980) Dantrolene sodium suspension in treatment of spastic cerebral palsy. *Dev Med Child Neurol* **22**: 755–67.

Kaieda R, Maekawa T, Takeshita H, Maruyama Y, Shimizu H, Shimoji K (1981) Effects of diazepam on evoked electrospinogram and evoked electromyogram in man. *Anesth Analg* **60**: 197–200.

Kalachnik JE, Hanzel TE, Sevenich R, Harder SR (2002) Benzodiazepine behavioral side effects: review and implications for individuals with mental retardation. *Am J Ment Retard* **107**: 376–410.

Krach LE (2001) Pharmacotherapy of spasticity: oral medications and intrathecal baclofen. *J Child Neurol* **16**: 31–6.

Mathew A, Mathew MC (2005) Bedtime diazepam enhances well-being in children with spastic cerebral palsy. *Pediatr Rehabil* **8**: 63–6.

Milla PJ, Jackson AD (1977) A controlled trial of baclofen in children with cerebral palsy. *J Int Med Res* **5**: 398–404.

Montane E, Vallano A, Laporte JR (2004) Oral antispastic drugs in nonprogressive neurologic diseases: a systematic review. *Neurology* **63**: 1357–63.

Nance PW (1997) Tizanidine: an alpha2-agonist imidazoline with antispasticity effects. *Todays Ther Trends* **15**: 11–25.

Nygaard TG, Waran SP, Levine RA, Naini AB, Chutorian AM (1994) Dopa-responsive dystonia simulating cerebral palsy. *Pediat Neurol* **11**: 236–40.

Patel DR, Soyode O (2005) Pharmacologic interventions for reducing spasticity in cerebral palsy. *Ind J Pediatr* **72**: 869–72.

Pinder RM, Brogden RN, Speight TM, Avery GS (1977) Dantrolene sodium: A review of its pharmacological properties and therapeutic efficacy in spasticity. *Drugs* 13: 3–23.

Pinto Ode S, Polikar M, Debono G (1972) Results of international clinical trials with lioresal. *Postgrad Med J* **48** (Suppl 5): 18–25.

Sanger TD, Bastian A, Brunstrom J, Damiano D, Delgado M, Dure L, Gaebler-Spira D, Hoon A, Mink JW, Sherman-Levine S, Welty LJ (2007) Prospective open-label clinical trial of trihexyphenidyl in children with secondary dystonia due to cerebral palsy. *J Child Neurol* **22**: 530–7.

Scheidtmann K, Fries W, Muller F, Koenig E (2001) Effect of levodopa in combination with physiotherapy on functional motor recovery after stroke: a prospective, randomised, double-blind study. *Lancet* **358**: 787–90.

Schlosser W (1971) Action of diazepam on the spinal cord. *Arch Int Pharmacodyn Ther* **194**: 93–102.

Schmidt RF, Vogel ME, Zimmermann M (1967) Effect of diazepam on presynaptic inhibition and other spinal reflexes. *Naunyn-Schmiedebergs Archiv Exp Path Pharmakol* **258**: 69–82. (German.)

Schwartzman JS, Tilbery CP, Kogler E, Gusman S (1976) Effects of lioresal in cerebral palsy. *Folia Med* **72**: 297–302.

Verrier M, MacLeod S, Ashby P (1975) The effect of diazepam on presynaptic inhibition in patients with complete and incomplete spinal cord lesions. *Can J Neurol Sci* **2**: 179–84.

Ward A, Chaffman MO, Sorkin EM (1986) Dantrolene. A review of its pharmacodynamic and pharmacokinetic properties and therapeutic use in malignant hyperthermia, the neuroleptic malignant syndrome and an update of its use in muscle spasticity. *Drugs* **32**: 130–68.

Weingarden SI, Belen JG (1992) Clonidine transdermal system for treatment of spasticity in spinal cord injury. *Arch Phys Med Rehabil* **73**: 876–7.

Whyte J, Robinson K (1990) *Pharmacologic Management*. Philadelphia, PA: Lea and Febiger. p 201–26.

Young R (1997) Current issues in spasticity management. *Neurology* **3**: 261–75.

Young RR, Delwaide PJ (1981) Drug therapy: spasticity. *N Engl J Med* **304**: 96–9.

4.4
PHARMACOLOGIC TREATMENT WITH BOTULINUM TOXIN

Guy Molenaers and Kaat Desloovere

Review of relevant pathophysiology

Treatment of spasticity is central in clinical management of children with cerebral palsy (CP) (Graham et al. 2000, Papavasiliou 2009). A variety of anti-spasticity interventions are available to treat these patients, such as oral medication, selective dorsal rhizotomy, and intrathecal baclofen. Botulinum toxin type A (BoNT-A) is a relatively new treatment available for children with CP. This neurotoxin is injected intramuscularly and is selectively taken up at the cholinergic nerve terminal, where it blocks the release of acetylcholine, causing selective, temporary muscular denervation. Although BoNT-A has a high potential therapeutic value as tone reducer, it should be noted that botulinum toxin, secreted by the bacterium Clostridium botulinum, can also be considered as one of the strongest poisons of the world, and is potentially lethal if not used in a safe way.

Seven immunologically distinct forms of botulinum neurotoxin exist, designated as serotypes A, B, C1, D, E, F and G (Aoki 2001). The serotypes differ in neurotoxin complex size, activation level, intracellular site of action, acceptor/receptor sites, muscle weakening efficacy, duration of action and target affinity (Aoki 2002). BoNT-A has been commercially available for clinical use for the longest time. Four commercial preparations of BoNT-A are available: Botox (Allergan), Dysport (Ipsen), Xeomin (Merz Pharmaceuticals GmbH; only available in Germany) and Hengli, a Chinese form. (Jankovic 2004, Aoki et al. 2006). The type B formulation is known as Myobloc in the United States and as Neurobloc outside the United States. Botox, Dysport and Myobloc/Neurobloc are the preparations used in children with CP (Heinen et al. 2006b). Because the different commercial preparations have different formulations, molecular structures, and purification methods, they are unlikely to be clinically equivalent. The treating physician must understand these differences to ensure that each product is used safely and effectively. Individual dosages should be calculated independently for the preparations, guided by the dosing instructions specific to each product and based on previous response and clinical experience. Fixed dose-conversion factors are not applicable in the treatment of spasticity in children with CP (Heinen et al. 2006b).

The molecular mass of isolated BoNT-A is 150 kDa, composed of a heavy chain and a light chain connected by a disulfide bond. In its native form, the toxin associates with accessory proteins to produce various sized complexes ranging from 150 to 900 kDa. This molecular mass of the complex differs between commercially available botulinum toxin formulations, resulting in different efficacy profiles and safety and therapeutic margins. The heavy chain binds with high affinity and specificity to the presynaptic membranes of the cholinergic motor neurones. When attached to the receptor on the distal axon, the toxin is internalised via receptor-mediated endocytosis, a process by which the plasma membrane of the nerve cell invaginates the toxin-receptor complex, forming a toxin-containing vesicle inside the nerve terminal (Fig. 4.4.1a). After internalization, the light chain of the toxin molecule is released into the cytoplasm of the nerve terminal and BoNT-A blocks acetylcholine release by cleaving SNAP-25, a cytoplasmic protein required for the release of this transmitter (Fig. 4.4.1b). The terminals affected are thereby inhibited from stimulating muscle contraction. Evidence indicates that initial neural recovery occurs by terminal sprouting of new nerve-endings of the affected distal axon. In animal studies this reinnervation through sprouting was recognised at 28 days after injections (Fig. 4.4.1c). At a later stage, definitive repair is established by return of vesicle turnover to the original terminals, the original neuromuscular junction begins to function normally again, and the terminal sprouts gradually regress (Aoki 2001, 2003, Dolly 2003) (Fig. 4.4.1d). The return of synaptic function to the original neuromuscular junction associated with elimination of the sprouts requires approximately 91 days. The period of clinically useful relaxation is usually 12–16 weeks (de Paiva et al. 1999, Aoki 2003, Aoki et al. 2006). The biochemistry of BoNT-A is illustrated for clarity.

Historical perspective
BoNT-A injections were first given therapeutically for strabismus in the early 1980s by Allan Scott in the USA. In the following years, the therapeutic spectrum of BoNT-A has been successively expanding. The treatment has been adopted for other conditions, such as blepharospasm, cervical dystonia, hemifascial spasm, hyperhidrosis, spastic bladder and urethra and migraine headaches (Denislic et al. 1994, Jankovic and Brin 1991). The first clinical trial of BoNT-A for managing spasticity in patients with CP was initiated in 1988 by L. Andrew Koman, Beth Petreson Smith and Amy Goodman, and reported by Koman et al. (1993). At the same time, Cosgrove and Graham showed that BoNT-A, injected during the growth period, allowed normal growth of the muscle of the hereditary spastic mouse (Cosgrove and Graham 1994). Since the first documentation regarding BoNT-A treatment in children with spastic CP, a number of studies have been conducted to investigate the effect of BoNT-A in these patients (Corry et al. 1998, Wissel et al. 1999, Heinen et al. 2006b, Nolan et al. 2006, Papavasiliou 2009).

PHENOL NEUROLYSIS*
BoNT-A was not the first agent used for chemical denervation in spastic muscles. Injections of phenol were used to treat spasticity for several decades before the advent of BoNT-A.

---

*Much of the discussion of phenol neurolysis was contributed by Mark Gormley MD for a previous edition of this book.

(a) Neurotoxin internalized into nerve ending by endocytosis

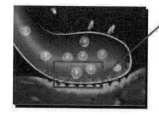

(b) Due to the cleaved SNAP-25 protein, acetylcholine-containing vesicles no longer fuse with the membrane

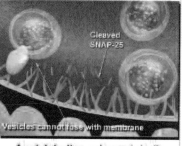

Acetylcholine release into the synaptic cleft is inhibited

(c)

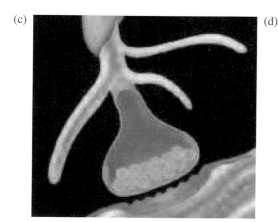

(d)

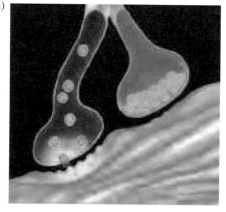

Fig. 4.4.1 Botulinum toxin's mechanism of internalization into a cell. (a) Neurotoxin internalized into nerve ending by endocytosis. (b) Due to the cleaved SNAP-25 protein, acetylcholine-containing vesicles no longer fuse with the membrane. Acetylcholine release into the synaptic cleft is inhibited. (c) After acetylcholine is blocked, collateral axonal sprouts develop. (d) The new sprout establishes a new neuromuscular junction (NMJ). Eventually the original NMJ resumes function and the sprout regresses.

Phenol or carbolic acid can denature protein and cause tissue necrosis in concentrations greater than 5% (Glenn 1990). When phenol is injected on to a motor neuron a chemical neurolysis occurs, thus denervating that particular muscle. This can lead to a reduction in both the efferent and afferent impulses input to a muscle from the muscle spindle, both of which can reduce spasticity. Phenol has been used for many decades to treat spasticity in children (Easton et al. 1984). Because it does not diffuse readily in tissue, phenol must be injected within a few millimeters of a motor neuron. This requires electrical stimulation to adequately localize the target nerve. Phenol can be injected into motor points, which are motor neurons within a muscle, or motor nerves before they innervate a muscle. Localization of the motor neuron needs to very precise and the child needs to be fully cooperative and move minimally during the procedure. Phenol neurolysis can take 10–60 minutes, depending on which and how many nerves are injected. Electrical stimulation can be uncomfortable and the phenol itself can be painful when injected. For these reasons phenol neurolysis in a child typically requires general anesthesia. The lethal dose of injected phenol is approximately 8.5 g in adults (Wood 1978). The recommended maximum dose is less than 1 g for one treatment session (Glenn 1990). Dosing guidelines have not been well established in children, but doses of less than 30mg/per kg of body weight are considered safe (Morrison et al. 1991). This dosing guideline usually will allow treatment of two to four major muscle groups in a given session. For example simultaneous injection of bilateral adductors and hamstrings can be performed using several cubic centimetres of 5%–7% phenol in each muscle group.

The most common side effect of phenol neurolysis is dysesthesias. These typically occur if phenol is injected into a sensory nerve. This can result in a burning sensation and/or a hypersensitivity to touch that can last several weeks. Injections into the distal portion of the upper and lower extremities have the highest risk for dysesthesias, since motor and sensory neurons are in close proximity there. If they occur, dysesthesias can be treated with ibuprofen, gabapentin or carbamazepine. The incidence of dysesthesias in children is typically less than 5%, which is significantly less than the reported incidence of 15% in adults (Glenn 1990). The lower reported incidence of pain in children may just reflect the fact that children tend to complain less about pain than adults.

Phenol blocks are temporary and generally last 3–12 months (Spira 1971). Some cumulative effect can occur with repeat injections, and the duration of the effect may be longer than one year. This increased duration of effect typically occurs in muscles with more easily accessible nerves. For example, the obturator nerve (hip-adductors) and the musculocutaneous nerve (biceps) are typically easy to locate, whereas motor points within the medial hamstrings and distal upper extremity muscles are more difficult to find. However, even though the distal upper extremity motor points may be more difficult to locate, phenol neurolysis in this area can still lead to significant improvement in function.

Perineural injections of phenol into the motor point of selected muscles produce a sustained reduction in limb tone. Both phenol and BoNT-A cause selective and temporary muscular denervation and are thus effective for the treatment of focal spasticity; however, their chemical denervation effects are related to different mechanisms of action. Phenol has been used mainly in adult stroke or brain trauma patients. Despite the fact that phenol has proven effectiveness as a chemical denervation agent, with immediate onset of action, at a low cost and a potential longer duration of effect, phenol has been less popular than BoNT-A in recent decades. This may be due to the technical challenges associated with its administration and concerns about safety and adverse effects (Kolaski et al. 2008). Moreover, phenol, being a nerve block, can be considered as less selective than BoNT-A, with risks for causalgia. In recent years, most chemodenervation in children with spasticity has been performed with BoNT-A. Clinicians who perform phenol injections often do so in combination with BoNT-A because this allows more muscles to be treated without exceeding the dosage recommendations for either agent (Gormley 1999, Kolaski et al. 2008).

Key points
- Children with CP should receive conservative treatment until the motor patterns are matured, usually between 8 and 10 years of age. Delaying surgery is important because the results of early surgery are less predictable and have a higher risk of failure and relapse. There is now evidence that the consequences of persistent increased muscle tone can be limited when conservative therapies such as physical therapy and orthoses are complemented by a selective treatment for the spasticity by BoNT-A injections (Graham et al. 2000, Heinen et al. 2006b, Molenaers et al. 2006, Desloovere et al. 2007)
- Selective tone control treatment by means of BoNT-A, started at a young age, provides a window of opportunity for therapeutic interventions by decreasing muscle tone, and thereby allowing increased range-of-motion, potential to strengthen antagonist muscles, and the opportunity to develop better motor control and balance
- The philosophy underlying, and results seen in single-event multilevel surgery have led to the development of a multilevel treatment approach, in which a number of muscle groups are treated with BoNT-A in the course of one session (Molenaers et al. 1999a, Heinen et al. 2006). It should be emphasized that appropriate techniques are required to apply the multilevel BoNT-A approach safely
- Patient-specific goal setting should guide the multilevel treatment approach
- Within the BoNT-A treatment approach for children with CP, 'reflection' is more important than 'injection', because the use of BoNT-A should be considered as a major therapeutic intervention, and not as a stand-alone treatment (Molenaers et al. 1999a, Heinen et al. 2006b)
- An adequate follow-up treatment including orthotic management, serial casting and intensive physical therapy is of major importance for a maximal profit of the BoNT-A injections.

Indications from patient assessment
BoNT-A treatments in children with CP are usually recommended because of lack of progression in motor development, development of muscle contractures, intolerance of day and night splinting, and/or decrease in functionality. Treatments are appropriate for a variety of diagnoses (predominantly spastic type of hemiplegia, diplegia, triplegia and quadriplegia) and functional levels I–V on the Gross Motor Function Classification System (GMFCS). Children with a wide range of functional abilities, as well as more involved children, can benefit from this treatment as long as the goal settings are adapted to the specific problems. BoNT-A treatment may also be successful for muscular hyperactivity in childhood resulting

from other causes, such as traumatic brain injury (Van Rhijn et al. 2005), hereditary spastic paraplegia and myelomeningocele (Boyd and Graham 1997, Heinen et al. 1997, Graham et al. 2000). BoNT-A treatment has also recently been applied more frequently in the management of upper limb problems in CP (Lowe et al. 2006, Reeuwijk et al. 2006, Wallen et al. 2007).

The main indication is increased muscle tone that adversely affects function and, if untreated, will very likely lead to fixed contracture (Flett 2003). Ideally, therefore, BoNT-A treatment should start at a young age when gait patterns and motor function are still flexible, allowing gross motor function learning during the time window of tone reduction. The optimal timing is often reported to be between 2 and 6 years of age (Boyd and Graham 1997, Wissel et al. 1999, Graham et al. 2000). Older children usually benefit from a more targeted treatment approach. Results are likely to be best in patients with focal spasticity who have adequate selective motor control. The point at which the spasticity is judged as being too 'generalized' is matter of the multidisciplinary discussion. Moreover, BoNT-A may also be used in combination with other treatments such as oral medications and intrathecal baclofen, and may also be used for other purposes such as treatment of upper limb, spastic bladder, drooling, headache etc. (Graham et al. 2000, Tilton 2006). Future challenges will be to organize the BoNT-A treatment for different purposes in the same patient.

The optimum therapeutic approach, and appropriate choice of target muscles to be injected with BoNT-A, must be based on a thorough and complete evaluation of the child. For optimal evaluation, it is crucial to use a combination of validated instruments and methods, focusing clinical assessment parameters, motor capacities (such as gait) and function. As spasticity is velocity dependent, dynamic evaluations, such as observation of gait, are thought to be a decisive factor in the 'fine-tuning' of BoNT-A treatment of ambulant children and, hence, gait analysis plays a crucial role in the identification of target muscles (Desloovere et al. 2001). Objective 3D gait analysis helps to identify the muscles causing pathological motion patterns, provides better insight into the complexity of the motor problems, and makes possible early detection of multi-level problems, the recognition of immaturity of gait, and the impact of primary (neurological) problems on gait. Indications of spasticity can be found in the pathological kinematic patterns, in raw EMG data (reflex activity, walking at different velocities, clonus activity) and in the discrepancy between kinetic data and EMG data (premature and/or prolonged activity). Conclusions from these evaluations, related to the individually defined goal settings, will be crucial for the final selection of the muscles that should be injected. A supplementary clinical evaluation under anesthesia (or sedation with or without mask anesthesia) can provide additional information.

Goals of treatment
Treatment goals for BoNT-A have been expanded in recent times. Because treatment indications extended, and because children with CP are a very heterogeneous group with regard to motor impairment and ability, treatment goals need to be well defined and tailored to the individual needs of the patient. As mentioned before, more involved children, as well as more functional children can benefit from BoNT-A treatment, as long as the goal settings are adapted to the specific problems.

Treatment goals for different indications may be focused on improving function (gait) and thereby influencing the pathological process for the functional child (GMFCS level I–III) and improving balance, control of sitting, positioning and facilitating hygienic care and bracing for non-ambulatory patients (GMFCS level IV–V). More specific goals are listed below (Graham et al. 2000, Boyd et al. 2001, Chambers 2001, O'Brien 2002, Flett 2003, Mall et al. 2006, Rutz et al. 2008):

- facilitation of orthotic management
- continuation of conservative management until maturity of gait is achieved
- evaluation of short-term functional gain providing crucial information for the future treatment plan
- simulation of orthopaedic surgery or neurosurgery
- facilitating training in order to achieve a better condition before going into surgery
- assisting in prevention of hip subluxation by controlling spasticity in hip-adductors and flexors, with hip-abduction brace
- decreasing spasms for patients with highly fluctuating tone in upper and lower limbs
- allowing improved positioning and control of posture
- treatment of pain caused by spasms (spastic–athethoid)
- treatment of back pain due to hyperlordosis, where tone reduction of the psoas muscle can help
- relief of pain postoperatively
- use of BoNT-A as an adjunctive treatment for regional or generalized spasticity.

Treatment options
The first published study using BoNT-A in children with CP used doses of 1–2 units/kg body weight (bw) injected into the gastrocnemius muscle of ambulatory patients with CP to improve equinus gait (Koman et al. 1993). As more information has become available on the safety and efficacy of BoNT-A, the use of BoNT-A to treat spasticity in children with CP has evolved rapidly. Injection techniques have improved, dosage and number of muscles injected have expanded, and the role of optimal aftercare has become clear (Gormley et al. 2001, Heinen et al. 2006b, Molenaers et al. 2006, Desloovere et al. 2007).

MUSCLE SELECTION
Muscle selection should be fine-tuned for each patient individually, based on the results of clinical assessment (with special focus on spasticity, selectivity and strength of agonists and antagonists), gait analysis and evaluation of function. Conclusions from these evaluations, related to individually defined goal setting will be crucial for the final selection of the muscles that should be injected. A supplementary evaluation of muscle tone and length under anesthesia, immediately prior to injection, can provide additional information.

DOSAGE
While BoNT-A produces a dose-dependent chemical denervation, systemic side effects or untoward responses occur as the total dose of BoNT-A increases. Therefore the BoNT-A dose is a crucial determinant of outcome. Individual dosages must be calculated

independently for each of the preparations of BoNT-A. It is important to note that fixed dose-conversion factors between commercial products are not applicable (Heinen et al. 2006b). Referred dosages in this chapter are for Botox. Because several muscles are often injected simultaneously within one treatment session, multilevel treatments may involve a higher total dosage than single-level treatments (Molenaers et al. 1999a, Kinnett 2004). Each dose should be expressed in units/kg muscle. The total dose also has to be expressed in units/kg body weight (U/kg bw). The optimal dosage per muscle depends on the muscle volume, the amount of spasticity and the degree of the muscle's involvement in the pathological motion pattern. The less involved muscle needs a lower dosage, compared with a severely involved muscle that plays a significant role in creating the pathological gait pattern. Appropriate ranges for Botox per muscle group of the lower limbs are indicated below (Table 4.4.1).

Each 100U vial of Botox is usually reconstituted with 1–2 ml saline. Recent study results suggest an improved effect for higher dilutions. A possible explanation for the increased effects of higher dilution compared to lower dilution could be that a larger volume/dilution enables a greater spread of the toxin to neuromuscular junctions, and therefore improved paralysis and reduction in muscle tone (Kawamura et al. 2007).

For each selected muscle, BoNT-A should be injected at multiple sites in order to distribute the amount evenly within the muscle, for a better effect with the product, and to prevent the possible 'overflow' of the toxin into the systematic circulation. Therefore multiple sites should be injected in each selected muscle, to a maximum of 50 U Botox per site, with an intersite distance of minimum 4–5 cm (Sanders et al. 1999, Chell and Hunter 2001). The multisite technique can cover all major zones of muscle groups involved. However, the ideal place of action of BoNT-A is the neuromuscular junction at the motor endplates (MEP). Shaari and Sanders (1993) demonstrated in the rat tibialis anterior muscle that injecting toxin at or near the MEP band is paramount for producing effective paralysis. There is a rapid fall-off in paralysis when the toxin is injected at small distances from the MEP. Unfortunately, information is sparse or non-existent concerning the detailed distribution of the neuromuscular junctions in adult and juvenile human muscles.

In the literature total dosages ranging from 2 to 29 U/kg bw can be found. Because most early studies included only equinus treatment, the dose range referred to most frequently

TABLE 4.4.1
Indications for appropriate ranges for Botox per muscle group of the lower limbs

Muscle group	Dosage (units/kg/body weight)
Gastrocnemius	4–6
Soleus	1–3
Tibialis posterior	1–2
Medial hamstrings (semitendinosis, semimembranosis, gracilis)	3–5
Lateral hamstrings	1–2
Hip-adductors	1–3
Rectus femoris	1–2
Iliopsoas	2–4
Dosage per injection site	Max. of 50 units Botox/site

was 4–8 U/kg bw. When a multilevel treatment was used, the maximal doses in the literature ranged from 10 to 29 U/kg bw. In one study (Awaad et al. 1999, 2000) a dose up to 40 U/kg bw was used within multilevel treatment. These authors concluded that BoNT-A (Botox) treatment at the higher dose is safe. In an overview of the studies that were performed, with the multilevel/multisite technique, on monkeys, Aoki et al. (1997) stated that there were no observable systematic effects at doses below 33 U/kg bw. However there was toxicity progressing to death at doses of 38–42 U/kg bw. Given the fact that there is an upper limit on the total dosage of BoNT-A that can be used, simultaneous use of phenol, for example in the adductors, can allow a more effective dosing of BoNT-A into other muscles.

Safe recommended total dosages recently reported in the literature for children with CP (Heinen et al. 2006b) are as follows:

Botox
Range (U/kg bw): 1–20 (–25)
Max total dose (U): 400 (–600)
Range max dose/site (U): 10–50

Dysport
Range (U/kg bw): 1–20 (25)
Max total dose (U): 500–1000
Range max dose/site (U): 50–250

Neurobloc/Myobloc
Range (U/kg bw): not established
Max total dose (U): not established
Range max dose/site (U): not established

Guidelines indicate that the frequency of injecting should not be more than one session of injections every 3 months. However, one should aim for longer intervals, especially within a high-total-dosage regime. By applying the integrated approach in which BoNT-A injections are combined with casting, orthotic management and intensive physical therapy, the duration of the BoNT-A effect is increased. The averaged duration of effect according to this approach was found to be more than 1 year (Molenaers et al. 2001).

INJECTION TECHNIQUE
Intramuscular BoNT-A injections can be administered under local anesthesia, conscious sedation, or general anesthesia (Graham et al. 2000). If multiple levels are involved, we strongly recommend that BoNT-A is administered under general anesthesia. This also permits an additional clinical evaluation while the child is sleeping.

An accurate localization technique is mandatory. For large muscles, correct needle placement (usually 26 gauge × 23 mm and 22 gauge × 30 mm) for the different muscle groups can be defined by using palpation with the muscle under stretch and by manual testing. By applying a passive motion to the joint, the needle will be moving with the muscle and the correct needle placement can be confirmed. This is particularly interesting for separating biarticular and monoarticular muscle groups. Classic neurophysiological localization methods (electromyography, electrical stimulation) may be helpful to localize the muscles to be injected (Graham et al. 2000, Suputtitada 2000, Willenborg et al. 2002). Ultrasonography is now the most appropriate technique allowing precise and painless identification of any target muscle (Berweck et al. 2002, Westhoff et al. 2003, Heinen et al. 2006b).

In children with CP, the psoas muscle is often involved and should be treated too. This requires an accurate, simple and safe injection technique of the psoas (Molenaers 1999c, Berweck and Heinen 2004).

SIDE EFFECTS

Increasing the dose of BoNT-A brings an increased potential for side effects. However, widespread use supports the safety of high-total-dosage BoNT-A treatments in children with CP, as the total dose is distributed over multiple muscles and over multiple injection sites per muscle (Molenaers et al. 1999a, Desloovere et al. 2001, Heinen et al. 2006a, Goldstein 2006). Significant unwanted side effects are rare (Bakheit et al. 2001, Flett 2003, Naumann and Jankovic 2004, Heinen et al. 2006a, b). Described adverse events tend to be expected consequences of muscle relaxation, such as weakness or initial loss of function, which can occur as patients learn to readjust their postural control in response to altered muscle tone (Koman et al. 2001, Goldstein 2006). Recovery and strengthening exercises and orthoses should rectify these problems. Temporary incontinence has been reported occasionally. However, caution has been expressed about children with severe spastic quadriplegia who have dysphagia, for whom the total dosage should be limited (<18 U/kg bw).

The major factor that can impact on the long-term efficacy of BoNT-A is the development of neutralizing antibodies, which may result from repeated injections of multilevel, high total dosage BoNT-A. Evidence of developing antibodies was mainly investigated in long-term studies on cervical dystonia and was correlated with secondary non-response in earlier studies (Greene et al. 1994, Jankovic and Schwartz 1995, Zuber et al. 1995, Göschel et al. 1997, Dressler 2002, Herrmann et al. 2004). Treatment intervals of approximately 1 year in children with CP when applying the integrated approach (Molenaers et al. 1999a) widely exceed the commonly used reinjection period of at least 3 months to prevent antibody resistance. With mean total dosages that did not increase, and mean intervals between treatments that did not decrease across repeated treatment sessions, recent study results provide evidence for stable response to long-term, high-total-dosage BoNT-A (Botox) treatment in children with CP, thereby indirectly excluding the development of antibodies (Molenaers et al. 2009).

The adverse effect profiles of BTX-B (Neurobloc/Myobloc) and BoNT-A differ considerably. BTX-B, used in dystonic movement disorders in adult patients, produces substantial systemic anticholinergic side effects, such as dry mouth and dysphagia (Schwerin et al. 2004, Dressler and Eleopra 2006). To date, there have been few reports of visual disturbances after treatment with BTX-B (Dubow et al. 2005).

AFTERCARE

Casting and day and night orthoses are used in conjunction with physical therapy to prolong improved muscle length and facilitate carry-over of improved motor control following

BoNT-A injections. The combination of these different conservative treatments is found to be crucial within the integrated approach and should be seen as a continuum in which the treatments are strongly linked to each other, mainly by the use of physical therapy.

Casting

For some time, the general indication for toxin injection was 'the presence of a dynamic contracture, interfering with function, in the absence of a fixed myostatic contracture' (Boyd and Graham 1997). However, in many cases, there are components of both dynamic muscle shortening and early contractures. Various combinations of injections with periods of casting may then be appropriate, and may extend the window of a strict BoNT-A treatment. There is evidence that BoNT-A alone is as effective as casting alone in the management of dynamic equinus, having a similar magnitude of response, but a longer duration (Corry et al. 1998, Flett et al. 1999, Graham et al. 2000). From the work of Molenaers et al. (1999b) and Desloovere et al. (2000) the additional benefits of the combined treatment have become clear. Children that were treated with BoNT-A injections combined with casting showed an improved 2nd ankle-rocker and longer-lasting effects, as compared to children that were treated without casting. From a prospective study, Desloovere et al. (2001) concluded that more benefits, mainly in the proximal joints, were seen for the children who were casted after injections as compared to the children who were casted before injections.

Most of the studies have examined the effects of casting on spastic equinus. However, casting can also be applied for other muscles at other levels. Because of the inconvenience of casting proximal muscles and proximal joints, these casts should be removable and be worn for a part of the day. It should be noted that, although several studies and long-term clinical practice indicated the advantages of combining BoNT-A injections with casting, Blackmore et al. (2007) concluded in their review that there is still no strong and consistent evidence that combining casting and BoNT-A is superior to using either intervention alone, or that either casting or BoNT-A is superior to the other immediately after treatment.

PHYSICAL THERAPY

As previously mentioned, the overall aim is to make functional progress or at least to preserve a status quo in the medium to long-term. A number of studies emphasize the importance of physical therapy combined with BoNT-A treatment (Leach 1997, Boyd et al. 2001, Damiano et al. 2001, Love et al. 2001, Ong et al. 2001, Smedal et al. 2001). Surprisingly, few prospective studies with objective outcome measures of physical therapy in CP have been reported, despite their frequent use in clinical practice (Coleman et al. 1995, Fetters and Kluisick 1996, Law et al. 1997, Reddihough et al. 1998, Boyd et al. 2001), and so far, there are no studies describing the specific aspects of physical therapy pre and post BoNT-A.

At the University Hospital of Pellenberg (Belgium), special treatment plans have been developed for children who were being prepared for BoNT-A treatment, based on general principles of motor training. First, the physical therapist should ensure the child's optimum preparation before the BoNT-A treatment, including definition of goal setting, starting new specific motor training (training new postures and specific movements); warning the child of a possible initial loss of functionality shortly after the injections and as a consequence the need to start a more intensive physical therapy program.

For the children with fairly high functional ability, training the sense of new movements and the full joint amplitude during active motion is especially important. An analytical approach may be used to assist in establishing the balance between agonists, antagonists and synergistic muscles (Hoare and Imms 2004). Converting muscle function into functional activities is also important, because it allows more automatic performance of new motions (for instance by treadmill training), ensuring the carry-over effect. Employing a dynamic approach and building variability into the functional activities will make the learning process more interesting for the child, provide more functional possibilities and help to prevent the child from relapsing to the same posture and movement as before. Intensive post-BoNT-A injection physical therapy starts at the time of the casting period and should focus on (1) analytical therapy by electrostimulation and/or proprioceptive training of, for instance, gluteus medius, specific muscle training in open and closed loops, fast motion exercises and training of specific muscle activities in parts of the active range of motion, such as full hip and knee extension, that are unknown and not used by the child and (2) functional therapy by active gait rehabilitation and use of newly recovered muscle activity in daily life. The long-term physical therapy should then focus on preserving gained muscle length by stretching and the use of orthoses, casts and positioning, continuing strengthening and proprioceptive training of the antagonists and/or agonists and (3) automation of new motor development.

In the more involved child, postural problems caused by muscle contractions and skeletal/joint deformations are of major concern. Through the use of tone controlling injections and rehabilitation, physical therapy stimulates a more symmetrical active posture, with major focus on active trunk control. In addition, these children are stimulated by sitting, standing, and other modalities of treatment such as a walking belt, standing table, sitting aid, pressure splint, and/or body jacket.

ORTHOTIC MANAGEMENT

After BoNT-A injections, the use of night splinting and day orthoses appears to be a critical factor in influencing the long-term effects of BoNT-A treatment (the effects on both preserving muscle length and providing stability to distal joints are thought to be important). This allows selective training of more proximal muscle groups ('target training'). For some children, day splinting contributes to proprioceptive training, and for children who lack selective control of certain muscle groups the day splints are crucial for normalizing gait (for instance, for correcting a drop foot) (Molenaers et al. 1999a). Orthoses supply the appropriate biomechanical alignment to allow practice and ensure functional carry-over outside periods of targeted motor training conducted by the physical therapist. Bilateral leafsprings are common post injection day orthoses. For spastic adductors (with hips at risk) the combination of BoNT-A and use of variable hip abduction orthoses may be indicated (Graham et al. 2000, 2008). At night (or in the evening) fixed ankle–foot orthoses (AFOs) with knee-extension braces and an abduction–external rotation rod are applied (Huenaerts et al. 2004).

Supporting evidence/outcome data

A follow-up gait analysis after BoNT-A treatment allows objective evaluation of the outcome. In the post BoNT-A treatment evaluation we are interested in the *individual's treatment result*, but also in evaluating the *treatment hypothesis*.

The individual's treatment result provides new and interesting information that may be important in the further development or fine-tuning of that child's overall treatment strategy. By carefully evaluating the treatment outcome, we learn how the child develops new motor abilities in therapy, gait and normal daily life. In particular, the functional use of the antagonist and restoration of the agonist/antagonist balance is important in this respect. An objective evaluation after BoNT-A injections can also help to highlight other problems, especially the contributions of weakness, poor balance and inadequate trunk stability. Moreover, post-injection gait analysis data are useful to distinguish between primary gait deviations and coping mechanisms. Differences between the two can be quite subtle; however, by definition, coping mechanisms will disappear spontaneously once the primary gait problems are resolved (Gage 1991). Finally, BoNT-A treatment has a role as a presurgical evaluation method for children in whom the benefits of surgery (orthopaedic or neurosurgery) are difficult to predict, or for whom the fine-tuning of the operation requires more fundamental information about underlying motor problems (Rutz et al. 2008).

The post BoNT-A treatment evaluation can also be used to evaluate the present treatment hypothesis. BoNT-A has a variety of short-term successful outcome parameters such as a reduction of muscle tone (Corry et al. 1998, Wissel et al. 1999), an increased range of joint motion (Corry et al. 1998, Sutherland et al. 1999, Wissel et al. 1999, Koman et al. 2000), an improved gait pattern (Sutherland et al. 1999, Koman et al. 2000), an increased muscle length (Eames et al. 1999) and improved function as assessed by the Gross Motor Function Measure (Scholtes et al. 2006). Different types of assessment tools were used in the studies performed in recent years, which may explain the variety of treatment outcome parameters. Variability in outcome may also be related to crucial factors like dose, antibody formation, aftercare and age (Wissel et al. 1999, Goldstein 2006).

There are only a limited number of studies on the long-term outcome. Molenaers et al. (2006) and Desloovere et al. (2007) demonstrated that BoNT-A treatment, in combination with common conservative treatment options, delays and reduces the frequency of surgical procedures and results in a gait pattern that is less defined by secondary problems (e.g. bony deformities) at 5–10 years of age, minimizing the need for complex surgery at a later age and enhancing quality of life.

Clinical case

An illustration showing the effect of multilevel BoNT-A treatment is found on the accompanying Interactive Disc (Case 2). This case demonstrated treatment according to the integrated/multilevel approach, at a single setting, on the gait of a 6-year-old boy with spastic hemiplegia. Under general anesthesia this boy underwent injections of multiple muscle groups (gastrocnemius, soleus, medial hamstrings, hip adductors and psoas unilaterally) with Botox. The total dosage was 23.5U/kg bw. Following BoNT-A injections,

375

the boy received serial casting and used appropriate day- and night-time orthoses and went to physical therapy three times a week.

REFERENCES

Aoki KR (2001) Botulinum toxin type A and other botulinum toxin serotypes: a comparative review of biochemical and pharmacological actions. *Eur J Neurol* **8**: 21–9.

Aoki KR (2002) Immunologic and other properties of therapeutic botulinum toxin serotypes. In: Brin MF, Hallett M, Jankovic J, editors. *Scientific and Therapeutic Aspects of Botulinum Toxin*. Philadelphia: Lippincott Williams & Wilkins. p 103–13.

Aoki KR (2003) Pharmacology and immunology of botulinum toxin type A. *Clin Dermatol* **21**: 47–80.

Aoki KR, Ismail M, Tang-Lui D, Brar B, Wheeler LA (1997) Botulinum toxin type A: from toxin to therapeutic agent. *Eur J Neurol* **4**: S1–3.

Aoki KR, Ranoux D, Wissel J (2006) Using translational medicine to understand clinical differences between botulinum toxin formulations. *Eur J Neurol* **13**: 10–19.

Awaad Y, Tayem H, Elgamal A, Coyne MF (1999) Treatment of childhood myoclonus with botulinum toxin type A. *J Child Neurol* **14**: 781–6.

Awaad Y, Tayem H, Munoz S (2000) High dose of botulinum toxin type-A (BTX): safety and efficacy in patients with cerebral palsy. *Mov Disord* **15**: 137.

Bakheit AM, Severa S, Cosgrove A, Morton R, Roussounis SH, Doderlein L, Lin JP (2001) Safety profile and efficacy of botulinum toxin A (Dysport) in children with muscle spasticity. *Dev Med Child Neurol* **43**: 234–8.

Berweck S, Heinen F (2004) Use of botulinum toxin in pediatric spasticity (cerebral palsy). *Mov Disord* **19**: S162–7.

Berweck S, Feldkamp A, Francke A, Nehles J, Schwerin A, Heinen F (2002) Sonography-guided injection of botulinum toxin A in children with cerebral palsy. *Neuropediatrics* **33**: 221–223.

Blackmore AM, Boettcher-Hunt E, Jordan M, Chan MD (2007) A systematic review of the effects of casting on equinus in children with cerebral palsy: an evidence report of the AACPDM. *Dev Med Child Neurol* **49**: 781–90. (Review.)

Boyd R, Graham HK (1997) Botulinum toxin A in the management of children with cerebral palsy: indications and outcome. *Eur J Neurol* **4**: S15–22.

Boyd RN, Morris ME, Graham HK (2001) Management of upper limb dysfunction in children with cerebral palsy: a systematic review. *Eur J Neurol* **8**: 150–66.

Chambers HG (2001) Treatment of functional limitations at the knee in ambulatory children with cerebral palsy. *Eur J Neurol* **8**: 59–74.

Chell J, Hunter JB (2001) Urinary incontinence following botulinum toxin A injection in cerebral palsy. Abstract of the 20th EPOS meeting, Montpellier, France, 4–7 April.

Coleman GJ, King JA, Reddihough DS (1995) A pilot evaluation of conductive education based intervention for children with cerebral palsy: the Tongala project. *J Pediatr Child Health* **31**: 412–17.

Corry IS, Cosgrove AP, Duffy CM, McNeill S, Taylor TC, Graham HK (1998) Botulinum toxin A compared with stretching casts in the treatment of spastic equinus: a randomised prospective trial. *J Pediatr Orthop* **18**: 304–11.

Cosgrove AP, Graham HK (1994) Botulinum toxin A prevents the development of contractures in the hereditary spastic mouse. *Dev Med Child Neurol* **36**: 379–85.

Cosgrove A, Corry I, Graham J (1994) Botulinum toxin in the management of the lower limb in cerebral palsy. *Dev Med Child Neurol* 36: 386–96.

Damiano DM, Quinlivan J, Owen BF, Shaffrey M, Abel MF (2001) Spasticity versus strength in cerebral palsy: relationships among involuntary resistance, voluntary torque, and motor function. *Eur J Neurol* **8**: 40–9.

Denislic M, Pirtosek Z, Vodusek DB, Zidar J, Meh D (1994) Botulinum toxin in the treatment of neurological disorders. *Ann NY Acad Sci* **710**: 76–87.

de Paiva A, Meunier FA, Molgó J, Aoki KR, Dolly JO (1999) Functional repair of motor endplates after botulinum neurotoxin type A poisoning: biphasic switch of synaptic activity between nerve sprouts and their paren terminals. *Proc Natl Acad Sci USA* **9**: 3200.

Desloovere K, Molenaers G, Jonkers I, Van Deun S, Nijs J (2000) The effect of combined botulinum toxin injections and serial casting on gait disorders in cerebral palsy. *Gait Posture* **12**: 57.

Desloovere K, Molenaers G, Jonkers I, De Cat J, De Borre L, Nijs J, Eyssen M, Pauwels P, De Cock P (2001) A randomised study of botulinum toxin A and casting in the ambulant child with cerebral palsy using objective measures. *Eur J Neurol* **8**: 75–87.

Desloovere K, Molenaers G, De Cat J, Pauwels P, Van Campenhout A, Ortibus E, Fabry G, De Cock P (2007) Motor function following multilevel botulinum toxin for children with cerebral palsy. *Dev Med Child Neurol* **49**: 56–61.

Dolly O (2003) Synaptic transmission: inhibition of neurotransmitter release by botulinum toxins. *Headache* **43**: S16–24.

Dressler D (2002) Clinical features of antibody-induced complete secondary failure of botulinum toxin therapy. *Eur Neurol* **48**: 26–9.

Dressler D, Eleopra R (2006) Clinical use of non-A botulinum toxins: botulinum toxin type B. *Neurotox Res* **9**: 121–5.

Dressler D, Munchau A, Bhatia KP, Quinn NP, Bigalke H (2002) Antibody-induced botulinum toxin therapy failure: can it be overcome by increased botulinum toxin doses? *Eur Neurol* **47**: 118–21.

Dubow J, Kim A, Leikin J, Cumpson K, Bryant S, Rezak M (2005) Visual system side effects caused by parasympathetic dysfunction after botulinum toxin type B injections. *Mov Disord* **20**: 877–80.

Eames NW, Baker R, Hill N, Graham K, Taylor T, Cosgrove A (1999) The effect of botulinum toxin A on gastrocnemius length: magnitude and duration of response. *Dev Med Child Neurol* **41**: 226–32.

Easton J, Ozel T, Halpern D (1984) Intramuscular neurolysis for spasticity in children. *Arch Phys Med Rehabil* **60**: 156–8.

Fetters L, Kluisick J (1996) The effect of neurodevelopmental treatment versus practice on the reaching of children with spastic cerebral palsy. *Phys Ther* **76**: 346–58.

Flett PJ (2003) Rehabilitation of spasticity and related problems in childhood cerebral palsy. *J Paediatr Child Health* **39**: 6–14.

Flett PJ, Stern LM, Waddy H, Connell TM, Seeger JD, Gibson SK (1999) Botulinum toxin A versus fixed cast stretching for dynamic calf tightness in cerebral palsy. *J Paediatr Child Health* **35**: 71–7.

Gage R (1991) *Gait Analysis in Cerebral Palsy*. London: Mac Keith Press. p 101–31.

Glenn M (1990) Nerve blocks. In: Glenn M, Whyte J, editors. *The Practical Management of Spasticity in Children and Adults*. Philadelphia, PA: Lea and Febiger. p 230.

Goldstein EM (2006) Safety of high-dose botulinum toxin type A therapy for the treatment of pediatric spasticity. *J Child Neurol* **21**: 189–92.

Gormley ME (1999) Management of spasticity in children. Part I. Chemical denervation. *J Head Trauma Rehabil* **14**: 97–9.

Gormley ME, Gaebler-Spira D, Delgado MR (2001) Use of botulinum toxin type A in pediatric patients with cerebral palsy: a three-center retrospective chart review. *J Child Neurol* **16**: 113–18.

Göschel H, Wohlfarth K, Frevert J, Dengler R, Bigalke H (1997) Botulinum A toxin therapy: neutralizing and nonneutralizing antibodies – therapeutic consequences. *Exp Neurol* **147**: 96–102.

Graham HK, Aoki RK, Autti-Rämo I, Boyd RN, Delgado MR, Gaebler-Spira DJ, Gormley ME, Guyer BM, Heinen F, Holton AF, Matthews D, Molenaers G, Motta F, Garcia Ruiz PJ, Wissel J (2000) Recommendations for the use of botulinum toxin type A in the management of cerebral palsy. *Gait Posture* **11**: 67–79.

Graham HK, Boyd R, Carlin JB, Dobson F, Lowe K, Nattrass G, Thomason P, Wolfe R, Reddihough D (2008) Does botulinum toxin A combined with bracing prevent hip displacement in children with cerebral palsy and 'hips at risk'? A randomized, controlled trial. *J Bone Joint Surg Am* **90**: 23–33.

Greene P, Fahn S, Diamond B (1994) Development of resistance to botulinum toxin type A in patients with torticollis. *Mov Disord* **9**: 213–17.

Heinen F, Wissel J, Philipsen A, Mall V, Leititis J-U, Schenkel A, Stücker R, Korinthenberg R (1997) Interventional neuropediatrics: treatment of dystonic and spastic muscular hyperactivity with botulinum toxin A. *Neuropediatrics* **28**: 307–13.

Heinen F, Schroeder AS, Fietzek U, Berweck S (2006) When it comes to botulinum toxin, children and adults are not the same: multi-muscle option for children with cerebral palsy. *Mov Disord* **21**: 2029–30.

Heinen F, Molenaers G, Fairhurst C, Carr LJ, Desloovere K, Chaleat Valayer E, Morel E, Papavassiliou AS, Tedroff K, Ignacio Pascual-Pascual S, Bernert G, Berweck S, Di Rosa G, Kolanowski E, Krägeloh-Mann

I. (2006b) European consensus table 2006 on botulinum toxin for children with cerebral palsy. *Eur J Paediatr Neurol* **10**: 215–25. (Review.)

Herrman J, Geth K, Mall V, Bigalke H, Schulte Mönting J, Linder M, Kirschner J, Berweck S, Korinthenberg R, Heinen F, Fietzek UM (2004) Clinical impact of antibody formation to botulinum toxin A in children. *Ann Neurol* **55**: 732–5.

Hoare BJ, Imms C (2004) Upper-limb injections of botulinum toxin-A in children with cerebral palsy: a critical review of the literature and clinical implications for occupational therapists. *Am J Occup Ther* **58**: 389–97.

Huenaerts C, Desloovere K, Molenaers G, Nijs J, Callewaert B (2004) The effects of ankle–foot orthoses on the gait of children with cerebral palsy after treatment with botulinum toxin A: effects on temporal-spatial parameters and kinematics and kinetics of the proximal joints. *Gait Posture* **20**: S63.

Jankovic J (2004) Botulinum toxin in clinical practice. *J Neurol Neurosurg Psychiatry* **75**: 951–7.

Jankovic J, Brin MF (1991) Therapeutic uses of botulinum toxin. *N Engl J Med* **324**: 1186–94.

Jankovic J, Schwartz K (1995) Response and immunoresistance to botulinum toxin injections. *Neurology* **45**: 1743–6.

Kawamura A, Cambell K, Lam-Damji S, Fehlings D (2007) A randomized controlled trial comparing botulinum toxin A dosage in the upper extremity of children with spasticity. *Dev Med Child Neurol* **49**: 331–7.

Kinnett D (2004) Botulinum toxin A injections in children: technique and dosing issues. *Am J Phys Med Rehabil* **83**: S59–64.

Kolaski K, Ajizian SJ, Passmore L, Pasutharnchat N, Koman LA, Smith BP (2008) Safety profile of multilevel chemical denervation procedures using phenol or botulinum toxin or both in a pediatric population. *Am J Phys Med Rehabil* **87**: 556–66.

Koman LA, Mooney III JF, Smith B, Goodman A, Mulvaney T (1993) Management of cerebral palsy with botulinum A toxin: preliminary investigation. *J Pediatr Orthop* **13**: 489–95.

Koman LA, Mooney III JF, Smith BP, Goodman A, Mulvaney T (1994) Management of spasticity in cerebral palsy with botulinum-A toxin: report of a preliminary, randomized, double-blind trial. *J Pediatr Orthop* **14**: 229–303.

Koman LA, Mooney JF, Smith BP, Walker F, Leon JM (2000) Botulinum toxin type A neuromuscular blockade in the treatment of lower extremity spasticity in cerebral palsy: a randomized, double-blind, placebo-controlled trial. *J Pediatr Orthop* **20**: 108–15.

Koman LA, Brashear A, Rosenfeld S, Chambers G, Russman B, Rang M, Root L, Ferrari E, Garcia de Yebenes Prous J, Smith BP, Turkel C, Walcott JM, Molloy PT (2001) Botulinum toxin type A neuromuscular blockade in the treatment of equinus foot deformity in cerebral palsy: a multicenter, open-label clinical trial. *Pediatrics* **108**: 1062–71.

Law M, Russell D, Pollock N, Rosenbaum P, Walter S, King G (1997) A comparison of intensive neurodevelopmental therapy plus casting and a regular occupational therapy program for children with cerebral palsy. *Dev Med Child Neurol* **39**: 664–70.

Leach J (1997) Children undergoing treatment with botulinum toxin: the role of the physical therapist. *Muscle Nerve* **6**: S194–207.

Love SC, Valentine JP, Blair EM, Price CJ, Cole JH, Chauvel PJ (2001) The effect of botulinum toxin type A on the functional ability of the child with spastic hemiplegia, a randomised controlled trial. *Eur J Neurol* **8**: 50–8.

Lowe K, Novak I, Cusick A (2006) Low-dose/high-concentration localized botulinum toxin A improves upper limb movement and function in children with hemiplegic cerebral palsy. *Dev Med Child Neurol* **48**: 170–5.

Mall V, Heinen F, Siebel A, Bertram C, Hafkeymeyer U, Wissel J, Berweck S, Haverkamp F, Nass G, Döderlein L, Breitbach-Faller N, Schulte-Mattler W, Korinthenberg R (2006) Treatment of adductor spasticity with BTX-A in children with CP: a randomised, double-blind, placebo-controlled study. *Dev Med Child Neurol* **48**: 10–13.

Molenaers G, Desloovere K, Eyssen M, Decat J, Jonkers I, De Cock P (1999a) Botulinum toxin type A treatment of cerebral palsy: an integrated approach. *Eur J Neurol* **6**: S51–7.

Molenaers G, Eyssen M, Desloover K, Jonkers I, de Cock P (1999b) The effect of multilevel botulinum toxin type A treatment combined with short leg casting and orthotic management on the gait of CP children. *Gait Posture* **10**: 74.

Molenaers G, Eyssen M, Desloovere K, Jonkers I, De Cock P (1999c) A multilevel approach to botulinum toxin type A treatment of the (ilio)psoas in spasticity in cerebral palsy. *Eur J Neurol* **6**: S59–62.

378

Molenaers G, Desloovere K, De Cat J, Jonkers I, De Borre L, Pauwels P, Nijs J, Fabry G, De Cock P (2001) Single event multilevel botulinum toxin type A treatment and surgery: similarities and differences. *Eur J Neurol* **8**: 88–97.

Molenaers G, Desloovere K, Fabry G, De Cock P (2006) The effects of quantitative gait assessment and botulinum toxin A on musculoskeletal surgery in children with cerebral palsy. *J Bone Joint Surg Am* **88**: 161–70.

Molenaers G, Schörkhuber V, Fagard K, Van Campenhout A, De Cat J, Pauwels P, Ortibus E, De Cock P, Desloovere K (2009) Long-term use of botulinum toxin type A in children with cerebral palsy: treatment consistency. *Eur J Paediatr Neurol*, in press.

Morrison J, Matthews D, Washington R, Fennessey P, Harrison L (1991) Phenol motor point blocks in children: plasma concentrations and cardiac dysrhythmias. *Anesthesiology* **75**: 359–62.

Naumann M, Jankovic J (2004) Safety of botulinum toxin type A: a systematic review and meta-analysis. *Curr Med Res Opin* **20**: 981–90.

Nolan KW, Cole LL, Liptak GS (2006) Use of botulinum toxin A in children with cerebral palsy. *Phys Ther* **86**: 573–84.

O'Brien CF (2002) Treatment of spasticity with botulinum toxin. *Clin J Pain* **18**: S182–90.

Ong HT, Chong HN, Yap SSP (2001) Comprehensive management of spasticity in cerebral palsy: Role of physical therapy and other adjunctive treatments. *Singapore Pediatr J* **43**: 133–6.

Papavasiliou AS (2009) Management of motor problems in cerebral palsy: a critical update for the clinician. *Eur J Paediatr Neurol*, in press.

Reddihough DS, King J, Coleman G, Catanese T (1998) Efficacy of programs based on conductive education for young children with cerebral palsy. *Dev Med Child Neurol* **40**: 763–70.

Reeuwijk A, Van Schie PE, Becher JG, Kwakker G (2006) Effects of botulinum toxin type A on upper limb function in children with cerebral palsy: a systematic review. *Clin Rehabil* **20**: 375–87.

Rutz E, Hofmann E, Brunner R (2008) Preoperative botulinum toxin to avoid poor surgical results of muscle lengthening in patients with cerebral palsy. *Gait Posture* **28**: S2.

Sanders I, Shaari C, Amirali LAY (1999) The glycogen depletion assay and the measurement of botulinum toxin injections. Abstract from International Conference on basic and therapeutic aspects of botulinum and tetanus toxins, Orlando, FL, 16–18 Nov. p 33.

Scholtes VA, Dallmeijer AJ, Knol DL, Speth LA, Maathuis CG, Jongerius PH, Becher JG (2006) The combined effect of lower-limb multilevel botulinum toxin type A and comprehensive rehabilitation on mobility in children with cerebral palsy: a randomized clinical trial. *Arch Phys Med Rehabil* **87**: 1551–8.

Schwerin A, Berweck S, Fietzek UM, Heinen F (2004) Botulinum toxin B treatment in children with spastic movement disorders: a pilot study. *Pediatr Neurol* **31**: 109–13.

Shaari CM, Sanders I (1993) Quantifying how location and dose of botulinum toxin injections affect muscle paralysis. *Muscle Nerve* **16**: 964–9.

Smedal T, Gjelsvik B, Lygren H, Borgmann R, Waje-Andreassen U, Gronning M (2001) Botulinum toxin A and effect on spasticity. *Tidsskr Nor Laegeforen* **121**: 3277–80.

Spira R (1971) Management of spasticity in cerebral palsied children by peripheral nerve block with phenol. *Dev Med Child Neurol* **13**: 164–73.

Suputtitada A (2000) Managing spasticity in pediatric cerebral palsy using very low dose of botulinum toxin type A: preliminary report. *Am J Phys Med Rehabil* **79**: 320–6.

Sutherland DH, Kaufman KR, Wyatt MP, Chambers HG, Mubarak SJ (1999) Double-blind study of botulinum A toxin injections into the gastrocnemius muscle in patients with cerebral palsy. *Gait Posture* **10**: 1–9.

Terence ES (2001) Clinical utility of botulinum toxin in the treatment of cerebral palsy: comprehensive review. *J Child Neurol* **16**: 37–46.

Tilton AH (2006) Therapeutic interventions for tone abnormailities in cerebral palsy. *NeuroRx* **3**: 217–24.

Van Rhijn J, Molenaers G, Ceulemans B (2005) Botulinum toxin type A in the treatment of children and adolescents with an acquired brain injury. *Brain Inj* **19**: 331–5.

Wallen M, O'Flaherty SJ, Waugh M-CA (2007) Functional outcomes of intramuscular botulinum toxin type A and occupational therapy in the upper limbs of children with cerebral palsy: a randomized controlled trial. *Arch Phys Med Rehabil* **88**: 1–10.

Wenger DR, Rang M (1993) *The Art and Practice of Children's Orthopaedics*. New York: Raven.

Westhoff B, Seller K, Wild A, Jaeger M, Krauspe R (2003) Ultrasound-guided botulinum toxin injection technique for the iliopsoas muscle. *Dev Med Child Neurol* **45**: 829–32.

Willenborg MJ, Shilt JS, Smith BP, Estrada RL, Castle JA, Koman LA (2002) Technique for iliopsoas ultrasound-guided active electromyography-directed botulinum A toxin injection in cerebral palsy. *J Pediatr Orthop* **22**: 165–8.

Wissel J, Heinen F, Schenkel A, Doll B, Ebersbach G, Müller J, Poewe W (1999) Botulinum toxin A in the management of spastic gait disorders in children and young adults with cerebral palsy: a randomized, double-blind study of 'high-dose' versus 'low-dose' treatment. *Neuropediatrics* **30**: 120–4.

Wood K (1978) The use of phenol as a neurolytic agent: a review. *Pain* **5**: 205–29.

Zuber M, Sebald M, Bathien N, de Recondo J, Rondot P (1995) Botulinum antibodies in dystonic patients treated with type A botulinum toxin: frequency and significance. *Neurology* **43**: 1715–18.

Section 5
OPERATIVE TREATMENT

5.1
TREATMENT OF SPASTICITY WITH INTRATHECAL BACLOFEN

Linda E. Krach

Pathophysiology and pharmacology

Spasticity affects approximately 70% of those with cerebral palsy (CP) and is the most common tonal abnormality associated with CP (Matthews and Wilson 1999). Spasticity is defined as velocity-dependent resistance to movement associated with increased deep tendon reflexes and clonus. Dystonia is another common type of increased muscle tone associated with CP. Dystonia is defined as an involuntary alteration in the pattern of muscle activation during voluntary movement characterized by varying tone often increased with intent or emotion and associated with assuming abnormal postures (Sanger et al. 2003). It is assumed that hypertonicity, either spasticity or dystonia, interferes with functional abilities, contributes to the development of bony deformities and contractures, and also results in discomfort. Intrathecal baclofen has been shown to be an effective intervention to reduce both of these tonal abnormalities.

Baclofen has been available for at least 30 years as an oral medication for the treatment of increased muscle tone. Chemically it is 4-amino-3-[p-chlorophenyl] butyric acid and is structurally similar to gamma aminobutyric acid, a significant inhibitory neurotransmitter (Murphy et al. 2002). Baclofen reduces the excitability of primary afferent terminals, increases presynaptic inhibition, inhibits mono- and polysynaptic reflexes, reduces muscle-spindle activity, and reduces gamma motor activity. Its effectiveness orally has been limited, and it has not been uncommon to find that an effective dose has not been reached before the individual begins to experience limiting side effects of sedation and/or dizziness. Baclofen's site of action is at the level of the spinal cord. Therefore it was logical to begin using it as an intrathecal medication when the means was available to deliver it in this manner. When administered intrathecally, it can be given in a lower dose with greater effectiveness, thus avoiding the side effects due to brain exposure to baclofen. It has been reported that with a continuous infusion of intrathecal baclofen (ITB) therapy of 400 μg/day there is a cerebrospinal fluid (CSF) concentration of 380 μg/l and a plasma concentration of less than 5 μg/l. Also, giving baclofen intrathecally rather than orally results in a CSF concentration that is ten times higher (Albright 1995). With a low thoracic or high lumbar catheter tip level, the relative concentration of baclofen in the lumbar area is four times greater than in the cervical area. The half-life of baclofen in the CSF is 4–5 hours, and the pattern of CSF flow and reabsorption results in limited baclofen exposure to the cerebral hemispheres (Albright 2003).

Historical perspective

ITB was first used for spasticity of spinal origin such as spinal cord injury or multiple sclerosis, but more recently has been approved for spasticity of cerebral origin and for use in children. Food and Drug Administration (FDA) approval for these latter indications was obtained in 1996 (Penn 1992, Krach et al. 2006). ITB is currently delivered by implanted drug pump attached to a catheter that is subcutaneously tunneled from the site of pump implantation, generally subcutaneously or subfascially in the abdominal area, to the back where it is introduced into the intrathecal space. Most pump-managing professionals work with a programmable pump so that the dosage can be adjusted without changing the concentration of drug within the pump as is necessary with constant flow rate pumps. The pump is placed surgically and the programmable device that is currently available in the United States (Synchromed II, Medtronic, Inc.) has a projected life of approximately 7 years, requiring surgical explant and replacement in order to continue ITB treatment. ITB requires ongoing management by practitioners experienced in its use and with access to the specialized equipment for refilling and reprogramming the pump. The drug ITB is known to be stable for 6 months, so that depending upon the dose of medication and the concentration of drug being used refills need to be done at least every 6 months, but typically with greater frequency than that. Early after pump implant it is helpful to see the patient in follow up more frequently in order to adjust the dosage of ITB. It can take 6–12 months to reach a stable dose, depending on the frequency of follow up and dose adjustment (Meythaler et al. 2001, Albright and Ferson 2006). Initially after pump implantation it is important to have therapy evaluation to assist with evaluation of equipment for possible modification to avoid pressure over the pump (wheelchair seatbelts, orthoses) and to assure that the individual is able to weight bear for transfers or ambulation if that was a pre-implant functional activity (Krach 2004).

Key points
- ITB reduces spasticity and dystonia
- Management requires experienced professionals
- Significant risks of infection, hardware problem or drug related adverse events
- More research is needed to assess functional changes related to use of ITB in CP.

Indications for use of ITB

Currently, indications for the use of intrathecal baclofen include tone that is thought to interfere with function or the ability to provide care, significantly increased muscle tone (> 3 on 5-point Ashworth scale), and definable goals for spasticity reduction. It has also been advocated for use in those with recurrent deformities due to increased muscle tone. Contraindication to ITB is hypersensitivity to baclofen (Albright and Ferson 2006). A relative contraindication is depression or psychosis. Baclofen, orally or intrathecally, has been reported to increase depression (Sommer and Petrides 1992). Also, since trouble shooting can be an important part of ITB pump management, it is important to be able to obtain a clear history from either the individual with the pump or his/her care givers. There is not a consensus about whether all possible oral medications for the treatment of hyper-tonicity need to be tried prior to considering ITB.

A child's size must be considered prior to pump implantation. The pump must fit between the lower margin of the ribs and the iliac crest lateral to the umbilicus (Albright 2003). Nutrition and the presence of adequate subcutaneous tissue is a consideration, as a pocket needs to be created surgically to accommodate the pump and allow the incision to be closed over the implanted pump without tension.

Another important consideration is whether or not the individual/family will be able to comply with the specialized follow up that is necessary for ITB pump management. The drug is known to be stable within the pump for up to 6 months so refills need to be done at least that frequently. Initially after pump implantation more frequent follow up is needed for dose titration and to ascertain the individual's response to ITB. Subsequent dosing adjustments are based on the individual's responses as they can be quite variable. Having access to an experienced pump management program is also important for trouble shooting when there are suspected difficulties with the system or drug delivery (Albright and Ferson 2006).

Current recommendations are for a trial of ITB prior to implantation, but some providers do not routinely do trial doses. Those who have decided against trial doses note that ITB is almost always effective in the treatment of spasticity, so for those individuals whose major problem is spasticity, a trial is superfluous. Also, the typical trial with a lumbar puncture administered dose of 50 μg does not provide an indication of what an individual's function is likely to be after pump implantation and dose titration. After this initial 50 μg bolus tone is usually reduced to a much greater extent than initially after pump implantation with a constant infusion with a daily dose of 100 μg which is the typical starting dose (Albright and Ferson 2006). A trial infusion can be done for those with mixed tone or dystonia, those with atypical movement disorders, and those in whom evaluation of varying catheter tip levels is desired. The catheter can be placed under anesthesia and tunneled a distance under the skin before being brought to the surface. After it is well stabilized on the skin, it is connected to an external pump that can be programmed for varying doses of ITB (Albright and Ferson 2006). Also, if the catheter tip is initially placed high in the cervical region, the position can be changed by judiciously pulling small lengths of the catheter out and checking the new catheter tip level radiographically. Typically during infusion trials, particularly with high catheter tip levels, oximetry is used to monitor respiratory rate and oxygen saturation. We have seen some individuals who are sensitive to ITB and tolerate only low doses with high catheter tip levels. Although doses can be changed up to twice a day and catheter tip levels daily, it is important not to change both at the same time and to carefully and systematically evaluate the individual at each dose and catheter tip level. Even though this technique gives a better feel for likely function after pump implantation, it is still inexact in that individuals become somewhat tolerant of ITB over time and require dose adjustments. Also, to optimize function it is appropriate to plan for a course of therapy with individualized goals. Catheter infusion trial is contraindicated in individuals who have had previous spinal fusion due to the increased likelihood of CSF leak and infection after trial in these individuals. One drawback of this type of infusion trial is that typically the characteristics of the external pumps are different than the implanted pump, so that the baclofen dose is usually delivered in a larger volume of fluid, which could impact its diffusion characteristics in the intrathecal space. Our center has found it necessary to start with very low infusion rates with cervical catheter tip placement in order to avoid unwanted side effects including bradycardia and nausea.

In general, catheter infusion trial is limited to 5–7 days in order to decrease the likelihood of infection. Individuals are hospitalized during the infusion trial. A positive trial is noted to be a decrease in the Ashworth score of >1.

The ITB pump can be programmed to provide a continuous, constant hourly dose or a dose that varies during the course of the day. Usually initial programming is with the constant dose method. When to try other possible programming has not been systematically evaluated. There have been reports of successful use of varying doses to accommodate predictable changing levels of muscle tone throughout the day and night or to 'optimize' the effect of ITB by providing boluses periodically during the course of 24 hours with a lower dose in between those boluses (Rawlins 2004, Krach et al. 2007). Prospective systematic evaluation of the effect of the different dosing methodologies would be helpful.

Individuals appear to have an idiosyncratic response to ITB. It is important to begin dose adjustment in a conservative fashion, observe the individual's response to the dose, and plan future doses based on that response. In CP typically dose changes are between 5% and 20% of the established dose. Dose does not appear to be dependent upon age or size. Those with ventriculoperitoneal shunts usually require lower doses than those without shunts (Meythaler et al. 2001). The treatment of dystonia appears to require higher doses than spasticity. Also, once a stable dose has been reached, it is unusual to require significant dose adjustments in the future, and if such requirements arise, it is appropriate to evaluate the pump and catheter to assure that there is not a problem with drug delivery. The range of doses required by individuals with CP is quite broad-ranging, from 30 to 1500 µg per day or more (Albright and Ferson 2006).

Goals of treatment

The goals of ITB treatment need to be individualized. The existence of hypertonicity alone is not sufficient to justify a decision to treat abnormal tone. Typical goals for the use of ITB include reducing spasticity and/or dystonia in order to increase comfort, decrease the likelihood of recurrent deformity, to improve the ability to perform activities of daily living, and to improve the ability of others to provide care for the individual receiving the treatment.

Treatment options

A best practices paper regarding surgical implantation has been published (Albright et al. 2006). The authors noted that experience correlated with outcome and recommended that implanting surgeons do 10 or more pump implantations annually to preserve their skills. The pump can be placed either subfascially or subcutaneously. Some note that subfascial placement is associated with less obvious profile of the pump under the skin; however, those followed at our center who have had both subcutaneous and subfascial placement have noted that it takes longer to become comfortable after subfascial placement and refills are somewhat more difficult and painful.

Whether placed subcutaneously or subfascially, the surgeon creates a pocket to accommodate the pump. The pump is secured in the pocket with suture loops or by placing it in a Dacron pouch and suturing that in place. A back incision is made through which a Tuohy needle is inserted into the intrathecal space. The Tuohy needle should be inserted through the fascia using a paramedian approach, approximately 5 mm lateral to midline, and be directed obliquely to penetrate the thecal sac 1–2 levels cephalad to the insertion site. After confirmation of the intrathecal location of the needle, the catheter is introduced through the Tuohy needle, care being taken not to withdraw the catheter within the Tuohy needle at any point during its introduction as this can result in scoring the catheter and contributing to catheter breakage. L2–3 or L3–4 interspace is recommended as there is less movement in the lumbar spine here than at the L4–5 level and therefore less stress on the catheter. A purse string suture is tightened around the catheter where it exits the fascia, the catheter is anchored to fascia or muscle with appropriate hardware, and the catheter is tunneled to the pump pocket and connected to the pump (Albright 2003, Albright et al. 2006, Sgouros 2007).

ITB reduces tone in lower extremities to a greater extent than in the upper extremities. There have been reports of increasing upper-extremity effects by implanting the catheter with a higher catheter tip level, high thoracic or cervical (Grabb et al. 1999). The decision to proceed with this catheter tip level should also include consideration of the effect of decreased truncal tone and whether that has functional or positioning implications. ITB has also been reported to reduce oral/facial musculature tone as well. To date, there has been no systematic evaluation of the effects of catheter tip level.

POTENTIAL COMPLICATIONS

Although ITB treatment is effective in the reduction of hypertonicity, it is not without risks. Risks can relate to the hardware, the surgery to place the hardware, or the drug itself.

Infection can range from a superficial stitch abscess to meningitis. Reported rates of infection are quite variable, ranging from 0% to 24%. It is not unexpected that there is a risk of infection as this procedure involves the implantation of a foreign body within the body. Perioperative antibiotic administration is performed to decrease the likelihood of infection. If infection does develop, it is most likely to develop within 90 days of surgical intervention, although late infections have been reported that are hypothesized to be due to bacteria being introduced at the time of pump reservoir refill. These late infections are not common. If an infection occurs it most frequently is due to skin bacteria but gram negative infections, including meningitis, have been reported. Typically significant infection necessitates pump explantation and a course of intravenous antibiotics. In a few case reports the pump was left in place and the infection treated by adding antibiotic to the reservoir (Campbell et al. 2002, Murphy et al. 2002, Boviatsis et al. 2004, Fitzgerald et al. 2004, Gooch et al. 2004, Guillaume et al. 2005, Albright and Ferson 2006, Krach et al. 2006, Wunderlich and Krach 2006, Sgouros 2007). In addition to treating the infection, explant of the ITB delivery system results in the need to proactively monitor for and treat potential ITB withdrawal.

Wound dehiscence is a possibility after pump implantation. Care must be taken when evaluating surgical candidates to be assured that they are of sufficient size to support a pump and that their nutrition has been optimized. The optimization of nutrition can be challenging in some, as their tone may both be interfering with their ability to eat and be using a significant proportion of their ingested calories so that weight gain can be challenging. It is also recommended that the incision line not be directly over the pump so that it is not causing pressure on the healing wound. The pump pocket should be constructed so that this does not occur. It has also been recommended that the catheter access portion of the pump be positioned medially, again reducing pressure and stress on the skin surrounding this structure.

CSF leaks can occur. In an effort to avoid this, the dura is typically closed around the catheter with a purse string suture and, depending upon the center, patients are on bed rest without elevation of the head for 12–72 hours. Some of these CSF leaks result from occult hydrocephalus, with the entry point of the catheter allowing a tract through which the CSF can escape. The CSF can accumulate either subcutaneously by the back incision or in the pump pocket. If the CSF leak is due to occult hydrocephalus it is likely that the individual will need a ventriculoperitoneal shunt (Murphy et al. 2002, Albright et al. 2005). However, if the CSF leak is not due to occult hydrocephalus conservative measures can be tried including a period of bed rest, cushioned pressure over the pump site (sheepskin and abdominal binder), and/or acetazolamide (Gooch et al. 2003, Fitzgerald et al. 2004). If necessary, a blood patch can be performed. Headaches can occur with significant CSF leaks (Guillaume et al. 2005).

Another potential source of hardware related complication is the catheter. Reported catheter complications have included catheter migration out of the intrathecal space, catheter breakage or a hole, catheter obstruction, catheter detachment from the pump and disconnection at the site of connection for two piece catheters. Again, reported catheter complication rate has been quite variable, ranging from 4% to 20% (Stempien and Tsai 2000, Murphy et al. 2002, Gooch et al. 2003, Albright and Ferson 2006, Kolaski and Logan 2007). Catheter aspiration is a screening tool for catheter dysfunction. Catheter problems are often missed with an injection dye study. This is likely due to the different fluids and delivery mechanics involved. The contrast material is more viscous than ITB and is delivered much more rapidly, likely resulting in its flowing past small holes in the catheter, whereas with the slow rate of ITB delivery the fluid readily leaks out of the hole (Krach and Partington 2008).

The pump itself has also been reported to flip within the pump pocket (Gooch et al. 2003, 2004). This is particularly likely to happen if there is a significant fluid collection in the pump pocket, either CSF or a seroma, resulting in the sutures breaking. This phenomenon is sometimes discovered when those managing the pumps are unable to locate the reservoir port when attempting to refill the pump. A radiograph can confirm the pump orientation and, if needed, one can carefully attempt to flip the pump back to the correct orientation for the refill. If flipping continues, the catheter can become obstructed or be withdrawn from the intrathecal space. If flipping is a chronic problem the pump needs to be surgically re-secured.

Drug-related adverse events are typically dose-related. A potentially avoidable dose related drug adverse event is overdose due to programming error. When changing concentration of drug in the pump it is necessary to program a bolus to account for the lower concentration of drug in the catheter and internal pump tubing. When refilling a catheter after a catheter aspiration, it is necessary to only consider the amount of drug in the catheter. If the internal pump tubing is included as well, this can result in an overdose (Gooch et al. 2003). If a significant overdose occurs, a catheter aspiration can be done to remove 30–40 ml of CSF to reduce the total baclofen load in the CSF and the patient should be monitored closely with resources available to provide respiratory support if necessary (Yeh et al. 2004).

Sometimes, catheter difficulties can result in episodic under-delivery alternating with over-delivery of baclofen and the respective signs and symptoms associated with these conditions (Bardutzky et al. 2003, Krach and Partington 2008).

Decrease in cognitive function, listlessness and fatigue have been reported as a dose dependent adverse event (Gooch et al. 2003, Albright and Ferson 2006).

Constipation has also been reported with ITB (Stempien and Tsai 2000, Albright and Ferson 2006).

There does not appear to be a consistently reported effect of ITB on seizure activity. There are anecdotal reports of increased seizure activity, but a prospective study of children receiving ITB did not report a change in seizure frequency (Gilmartin et al. 2000, Campbell et al. 2002).

Weight gain after initiation of ITB therapy has been noted. This may be beneficial in the typically underweight child with quadriplegic CP, but results in the need for careful monitoring of weight post-pump implant to ensure that weight gain is not excessive (McCoy et al. 2006).

Likewise, there is not a consensus about whether ITB is associated with an increased risk for the development of scoliosis. Recent publications have presented contradictory results. Senaran et al. (2007) and Shilt et al. (2008) found no correlation between ITB treatment and the progression of scoliosis. Ginsburg and Lauder (2007) reported an increased rate of the progression of scoliosis. Further evaluation of this issue is warranted.

Incontinence and urinary retention have both been reported (Guillaume et al. 2005). It is thought that decreasing external sphincter activity could result in stress incontinence while decreasing detrusor activity could result in urinary retention. Dose dependent impotence or decreased duration or rigidity of erection have also been reported in men receiving ITB for spasticity due to spinal cord injury (Denys et al. 1998, Dario et al. 2004). We have also observed dose-dependent impotence in a young adult man with CP at our center.

A potentially life-threatening complication of ITB is the development of ITB withdrawal syndrome. It can occur when delivery of ITB is interrupted for any reason, but does not always occur when this interruption happens. The syndrome consists of rapidly increasing muscle tone and spasms, malaise, agitation, dysesthesias – typically pruritis, hallucinations, diaphoresis – and if untreated can progress to rhabdomyolysis, elevated creatine kinase levels, and multisystem organ failure. Others have reported that ITB withdrawal mimics sepsis or can result in respiratory distress (Reeves et al. 1998, Coffey and Ridgely 2001, Coffey et al. 2002, Greenberg and Hendrickson 2003, Kao et al. 2003, Santiago-Palma et al. 2004). Withdrawal symptoms have been reported to occur with low reservoir volumes resulting in under-delivery of ITB (Rigoli 2004). A prolonged ITB withdrawal syndrome requiring intervention for up to 2 months has also been reported (Douglas et al. 2005, Hansen et al. 2007). Although benzodiazepines, oral baclofen, dantrolene, cyproheptadine, low-dose propofol and other medications have been used to treat ITB withdrawal, the most effective intervention is to restore the delivery of ITB as soon as possible (Khorasani and Peruzzi 1995, Meythaler et al. 2003, Zuckerbraun et al. 2004, Ackland and Fox 2005). This can be done on a temporary basis with placement of a lumbar drain connected to an external pump as is done in trial infusions of ITB (Duhon and MacDonald 2007).

As noted previously, it is important for a team that is experienced with the management of ITB to provide service for these individuals. It can be challenging to troubleshoot and determine if there is a pump or catheter problem or another cause of increased spasticity. One should always keep in mind the possibility of infection, illness, constipation, change in seizure frequency and pain as possible reasons for muscle tone being increased over baseline. It has been suggested that the presence of pruritis can be a method for differentiating ITB withdrawal from other causes of increased muscle tone in an individual with a pump (Smail et al. 2005).

Supporting evidence
As noted previously, a number of reports have noted that ITB reduces hypertonicity and the effect continues long term. Attempts to assess this neurophysiologically have included assessing effect on the H reflex, H/M ratio, flexor reflex, and instrumented evaluation of EMG of stretch reflex. All were reduced (Sgouros and Seri 2002, Stokic et al. 2005, Kolaski and Logan 2008).

Reports have attempted to evaluate ITB use and improvements in function. Some have reported improvements in positioning, activities of daily living, transfers, sleep, oral motor skills, hand use, and comfort (Fitzgerald et al. 2004, Gooch et al. 2004, Krach et al. 2006). Motor function measured by the Gross Motor Function Measure (GMFM), Pediatric Evaluation of Disability Inventory (PEDI), Functional Independence Measure for Children (WeeFIM), and Functional Independence Measure (FIM) has been reported to be improved (Awaad et al. 2003, Krach et al. 2005, Guillaume et al. 2005). Others have found no improvement in the GMFM and PEDI (Campbell et al. 2002). Scores for both satisfaction and performance within the Canadian Occupational Performance Measure have also been noted to improve post-treatment with ITB (Guillaume et al. 2005).

One study described the oral motor, communication and nutritional status of children receiving ITB treatment. The authors found variable results, with some showing improvements and some worsening in the various areas described, but more improvement than worsening was reported in speech, use of assistive technology to communicate, appetite, self feeding, and saliva control. Stool frequency worsened in more of the children than improved (Bjornson et al. 2003). Others have reported improved bowel and bladder function (Stempien and Tsai 2000).

A case report has noted improvement in sleep apnea in an adult with CP after ITB pump implantation allowing discontinuation of continuous positive airway pressure during sleep (Fuller et al. 2001).

Meythaler et al. (2001) reported their findings with a group of adolescents and adults who received ITB for over 12 months. They reported effective and sustained reduction of muscle tone in lower and upper extremities. Two of their group required spinal fusion for scoliosis during this first year after pump implantation. They also reported improvement in activities of daily living and transfer status, improved dysarthria, increased comfort, and improved ability to control power wheelchair and augmentative communication devices. They also noted that post-pump implant, their subjects benefited from a period of intensive rehabilitation. Another reported series of adults with acquired brain injury noted decreased sedation when medications used for tone reduction were able to be discontinued after pump implantation as well as improvements in functional skills including one progressing from wheelchair use to walking with assistive devices, and eased provision of cares for those who were dependent on others (Dario et al. 2002). A review of the use of ITB for adult spasticity due to either spinal or cerebral causes noted that beneficial effects included increased independence, mobility and self-care abilities. Also improved sleep pattern, decreased bladder hyperreflexia, and decreased pain were reported (Hsieh and Penn 2006).

Relatively little has been written about the effect of ITB on gait. A study of gait in seven people with spastic hemiplegia, including one with CP, showed increased maximum walking speed and stride length after ITB bolus. Kinematically minimal knee extension and maximal ankle dorsiflexion were increased. Also, the duration of activity of spastic muscles decreased after ITB (Remy-Neris et al. 2003). Another report of gait in 28 individuals with acquired brain injury after ITB bolus demonstrated significant improvements in stride length. Although the effect on velocity was variable, a majority experienced an increase in velocity (Horn et al. 2005). After stroke Francisco and Boake (2003) reported that of the ten individuals that they saw who had ITB pumps implanted an average of 28.6 months after their stroke, statistically significant improvements in walking speed, functional mobility ratings (based on the locomotion-walking and stairs items of the Functional Independence Measure, the community access item of the Functional Assessment Measure, and two unpublished items – sit to stand and stand to sit) and Ashworth scores were noted an average of 8.9 months after pump implantation. Another report of 24 individuals, 21 of whom had spastic cerebral palsy and the remainder spasticity after traumatic brain injury, noted improvements of one functional level in nine patients, no change in twelve, and worsened gait in three. Functional levels were defined as community, household, non-functional, and non-ambulatory. However, patients and families reported improved walking in 20, unchanged in two and worsened in two (Gerszten et al. 1997).

It is thought that ITB treatment will decrease the need for orthopaedic surgery in individuals with CP. Some orthopaedic surgeons prefer to have spasticity reduction via continuous infusion of ITB prior to performing surgical correction of bony deformities or refer for evaluation for this intervention if bony abnormalities have recurred after prior surgical correction. One study retrospectively reviewed the course of 48 children and adults who had undergone ITB pump implantation and treatment. At the time of pump implantation orthopaedic surgery was planned in 28, but only ten underwent surgery (Gerszten et al. 1998). It has also been suggested that consideration be given to implanting ITB pumps in individuals as they approach their adolescent growth spurt in order to decrease the likelihood of the development of contractures during this time of rapid bone growth. In theory this could be a temporary measure followed by weaning and discontinuing the baclofen after growth is completed.

A few studies have also addressed quality of life in those receiving management of hypertonicity with ITB. One survey of 49 subjects including 30 adults noted that 88% believed that their quality of life had improved with ITB treatment and 8% were not sure whether it had. The most frequently noted positive effects were reduced muscle tone without sedation, ease of care for caregivers, easier positioning, less pain/increased comfort, and improved transfers (Staal et al. 2003). Two studies of adults with spinal cord injury or multiple sclerosis who received ITB for management of their muscle tone reported significant improvement in scores on the Sickness Impact Profile, particularly the physical health, mental health, mobility, and sleep and rest subscales, and the Hopkins Symptom Checklist (Middel et al. 1997, Gianino et al. 1998).

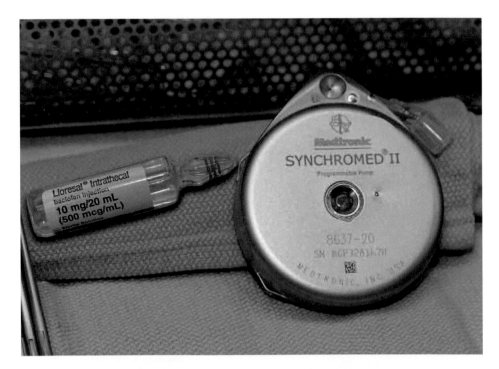

Fig. 5.1.1 A SyncroMed II baclofen pump next to a vial of baclofen. The pump is about the size and thickness of a hockey puck. The battery inside the pump has a life expectancy of approximately 7 years, after which the pump must be replaced.

Cost effectiveness of ITB therapy has been described. Sampson et al. (2002) did a literature review of the effect of ITB on function and quality of life. Outcomes were used to estimate potential gains in quality-adjusted life years. They found an acceptable cost-benefit ratio for this UK study. Another group, looking specifically at spasticity related to CP, found that ITB treatment increased the 5-year cost of treatment in the US by $49,000, but this was accompanied by a gain of 1.2 quality-adjusted life years and the result was within the ratio accepted as being cost-effective (diLissovoy et al. 2007). A third study showed that ITB therapy was more expensive and more effective than standard treatment and that overall it was consistent with the definition of cost-effectiveness in the Netherlands (Hoving et al. 2008).

Despite the potential complications, ITB continues to be a frequently used intervention for hypertonicity. A recent report indicated that over 10,000 pumps have been implanted for spasticity management (Kolaski and Logan 2008). Also, despite complications, the majority of individuals who have pumps indicate that they would still opt for the use of ITB for the management of their abnormal muscle tone (Krach et al. 2006). Treatment with ITB is more effective than oral medications for the treatment of hypertonicity and in contrast to selective dorsal rhizotomy is potentially reversible. (See Case 3 on Interactive Disc.)

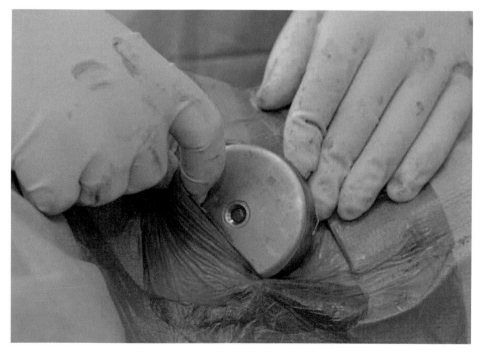

Fig. 5.1.2 A surgical photo of a pump being inserted into a pocket on the right side of the abdomen. The catheter is inserted into the dura through a separate posterior incision and then passed subcutaneously around to the front and attached to the pump.

REFERENCES

Ackland GL, Fox R (2005) Low-dose propofol infusion for controlling acute hyperspasticity after withdrawal of intrathecal baclofen therapy. *Anesthesiology* **103**: 663–5.

Albright AL (1995) Spastic cerebral palsy: approaches to drug treatment. *CNS Drugs* **4**: 14–27.

Albright AL (2003) Neurosurgical treatment of spasticity and other pediatric movement disorders. *J Child Neurol* (Suppl 1) **18**: S67–78.

Albright AL, Ferson SS (2006) Intrathecal baclofen therapy in children. *Neurosurg Focus* 21: E3–8.

Albright AL, Ferson SS, Carlos S (2005) Occult hydrocephalus in children with cerebral palsy. *Neurosurgery* **53**: 93–7.

Albright AL, Turner M, Pattisapu JV (2006) Best-practice surgical techniques for intrathecal baclofen therapy. *J Neurosurg (4 Suppl Pediatr)* **104**: 233–9.

Awaad Y, Tayem H, Munoz S, Ham S, Michon AM, Awaad R (2003) Functional assessment following intrathecal baclofen therapy in children with spastic cerebral palsy. *J Child Neurol* **18**: 26–34.

Bardutzky J, Tronnier V, Schwab S, Meinck H (2003) Intrathecal baclofen for stiff-person syndrome: life-threatening intermittent catheter leakage. *Neurology* **60**: 1976–8.

Bjornson K, McLaughlin J, Loeser J, Novak-Cooperman K, Russel M, Bader K, Desmond S (2003) Oral motor, communication and nutritional status of children during intrathecal baclofen therapy. *Arch Phys Med Rehabil* **84**: 500–6.

Boviatsis EJ, Kouyialis AT, Boutsikakis I, Korfias S, Sakas DE (2004) Infected CNS infusion pumps. Is there a chance for treatment without removal? *Acta Neurochir* **146**: 463–7.

Campbell WM, Ferrel A, McLaughlin JF, Grant GA, Loeser JD, Graubert, C, Bjornson K (2002) Long-term safety and efficacy of continuous intrathecal baclofen. *Dev Med Child Neurol* **44**: 660–5.

Coffey RJ, Ridgely PM (2001) Abrupt intrathecal baclofen withdrawal: management of potentially life-threatening sequelae. *Neuromodulation* **4**: 146.

Coffey RJ, Edgar TS, Francisco GE, Graziani V, Meythaler JM, Ridgely PM, Sadiq SA, Turner MS (2002) Abrupt withdrawal from intrathecal baclofen: recognition and management of a potentially life-threatening syndrome. *Arch Phys Med Rehabil* **83**: 735–41.

Dario A, DiStefano MG, Grossi A, Casagrande F, Bono G (2002) Long-term intrathecal baclofen infusion in supraspinal spasticity of adulthood. *Acta Neurol Scand* **105**: 83–7.

Dario A, Scamoni C, Casagrande F, Tomei G (2004) Pharmacological complications of the chronic baclofen infusion in the severe spinal spasticity: personal experience and review of the literature. *J Neurosurg Sci* **48**: 177–81.

Denys P, Mane M, Azouvi P, Chartier-Kastler E, Thiebaut J, Bussel B (1998) Side effects of chronic intrathecal baclofen on erection and ejaculation in patients with spinal cord lesions. *Arch Phys Med Rehabil* **79**: 494–6.

diLissovoy G, Matza LS, Green H, Werner M, Edgar T (2007) Cost-effectiveness of intrathecal baclofen therapy for the treatment of severe spasticity associated with cerebral palsy. *J Child Neurol* **22**: 49–59.

Douglas AF, Weiner HL, Schwartz DR (2005) Prolonged intrathecal baclofen withdrawal syndrome: case report and discussion of current therapeutic management. *J Neurosurg* **102**: 1133–6.

Duhon BS, MacDonald JD (2007) Infusion of intrathecal baclofen for acute withdrawal: technical note. *J Neurosurg* **107**: 878–80.

Fitzgerald JJ, Tsegaye M, Vloeberghs MH (2004) Treatment of childhood spasticity of cerebral origin with intrathecal baclofen: a series of 52 cases. *Br J Neurosurg* **18**: 240–5.

Francisco GE, Boake C (2003) Improvement in walking speed in poststroke spastic hemiplegia after intrathecal baclofen therapy: a preliminary study. *Arch Phys Med Rehabil* **84**: 1194–9.

Fuller McCarty S, Gaebler-Spira D, Harvey RL (2001) Improvement of sleep apnea in a patient with cerebral palsy. *Am J Phys Med Rehabil* **80**: 540–2.

Gerszten PC, Albright AL, Barry MJ (1997) Effect on ambulation of continuous intrathecal baclofen infusion. *Pediatr Neurosurg* **27**: 40–4.

Gerszten PC, Albright AL, Johnstone GF (1998) Intrathecal baclofen infusion and subsequent orthopedic surgery in patients with spastic cerebral palsy. *J Neurosurg* **88**: 1009–13.

Gianino JM, York MM, Paice JA, Shott S (1998) Quality of life: effect of reduced spasticity from intrathecal baclofen, *J Neurosci Nursing* **30**: 47–54.

Gilmartin R, Bruce D, Storrs BB, Abbott R, Krach L, Ward J, Bloom K, Brooks WH, Johnson DL, Madsen JR, McLaughlin JF, Nadell J (2000) Intrathecal baclofen for management of spastic cerebral palsy: multicenter trial. *J Child Neurol* **15**: 71–7.

394

Ginsburg GM, Lauder AJ (2007) Progression of scoliosis in patients with spastic quadriplegia after insertion of an intrathecal baclofen pump. *Spine* **32**: 2745–50.

Gooch JL, Oberg WA, Grams B, Ward LA (2003) Complications of intrathecal baclofen pumps in children. *Pediatr Neurosurg* **39**: 1–6.

Gooch JL, Oberg WA, Grams B, Ward LA, Walker ML (2004) Care provider assessment of intrathecal baclofen in children. *Dev Med Child Neurol* **46**: 548–52.

Grabb PA, Guin-Renfroe S, Meythaler JM (1999) Midthoracic catheter tip placement for intrathecal baclofen administration in children with quadriparetic spasticity. *Neurosurgery* **45**: 833–7.

Greenberg MI, Hendrickson RG (2003) Baclofen withdrawal following removal of an intrathecal baclofen pump despite oral baclofen replacement. *Clin Toxicol* **41**: 83–5.

Guillaume D, Van Havenbergh A, Vloeberghs M, Vidal J, Roeste G (2005) A clinical study of intrathecal baclofen using a programmable pump for intractable spasticity. *Arch Phys Med Rehabil* **86**: 2165–71.

Hansen CR, Gooch JL, Such-Neibar T (2007) Prolonged, severe intrathecal baclofen withdrawal syndrome: a case report. *Arch Phys Med Rehabil* **88**: 1468–71.

Horn TS, Yablon SA, Stokic D (2005) Effect of intrathecal baclofen bolus injection on temporospatial gait characteristics in patients with acquired brain injury. *Arch Phys Med Rehabil* **86**: 1127–33.

Hoving MA, Evers SMAA, Ament AJHA, van Raak EPM, Vles JSH (2008) Intrathecal baclofen therapy in children with intractable spastic cerebral palsy: a cost-effectiveness analysis. *Dev Med Child Neurol* **50**: 450–5.

Hsieh JC, Penn RD (2006) Intrathecal baclofen in the treatment of adult spasticity. *Neurosurg Focus* **21**: E5–10.

Kao LW, Amin Y, Kirk MA, Turner MS (2003) Intrathecal baclofen withdrawal mimicking sepsis. *J Emerg Med* **24**: 423–7.

Khorasani A, Peruzzi WT (1995) Dantrolene treatment for abrupt intrathecal baclofen withdrawal. *Anesthes Analges* **80**: 1054–6.

Kolaski K, Logan LR (2007) A review of the complications of intrathecal baclofen in patients with cerebral palsy. *NeuroRehabil* **22**: 383–95.

Kolaski K, Logan LR (2008) Intrathecal baclofen in cerebral palsy: a decade of treatment outcomes. *J Pediatr Rehabil Med* **1**: 3–32.

Krach LE (2004) Rehabilitation following spasticity reduction. In: Gage JR, editor. *The Treatment of Gait Problems in Cerebral Palsy*. London: Mac Keith Press. p 305–13.

Krach LE, Partington MD (2008) Injected contrast study fails to demonstrate catheter-pump connector tear: a case report. *J Pediatr Rehabil* **1**: 175–8.

Krach LE, Kriel RL, Gilmartin R, Swift DM, Storrs B, Abbott R, Ward J, Bloom K, Brooks WH, Madsen JR, McLaughlin JF, Nadell J (2005) GMFM 1 year after continuous intrathecal baclofen infusion. *Pediatr Rehabil* **8**: 207–13.

Krach LE, Nettleton A, Klempka B (2006) Satisfaction of individuals treated long-term with continuous infusion of intrathecal baclofen by implanted programmable pump. *Pediatr Rehabil* **9**: 210–18.

Krach LE, Kriel RL, Nugent AC (2007) Complex dosing schedules for continuous intrathecal baclofen infusion. *Pediatr Neurol* **37**: 354–9.

Matthews DJ, Wilson P (1999) Cerebral palsy. In: Molnar GE, Alexander MA, editors. *Pediatric Rehabilitation*, 3rd edn. Philadelpia, PA: Hanley and Belfus. p 193–217.

McCoy AA, Fox MA, Schaubel DE, Ayyangar RN (2006) Weight gain in children with hypertonia of cerebral origin receiving intrathecal baclofen therapy. *Arch Phys Med Rehabil* **87**: 1503–8.

Meythaler JM, Guin-Renfroe S, Law C, Grabb P, Hadley MN (2001) Continuously infused intrathecal baclofen over 12 months for spastic hypertonia in adolescents and adults with cerebral palsy. *Arch Phys Med Rehabil* **82**: 155–61.

Meythaler JM, Roper JF, Brunner RC (2003) Cyproheptadine for intrathecal baclofen withdrawal. *Arch Phys Med Rehabil* **84**: 638–42.

Middel B, Kuipers-Upmeijer H, Bouma J, Staal M, Oenema D, Postma T, Terpstra S, Stewart R (1997) Effect of intrathecal baclofen delivered by an implanted programmable pump on health related quality of life in patients with severe spasticity. *J Neurol Neurosurg Psychiatr* **63**: 204–9.

Murphy NA, Irwin MCN, Hoff C (2002) Intrathecal baclofen therapy in children with cerebral palsy: efficacy and complications. *Arch Phys Med Rehabil* **83**: 1721–5.

Penn RD (1992) Intrathecal baclofen for spasticity of spinal origin: seven years of experience. *J Neurosurg* **77**: 236–40.

Rawlins PK (2004) Intrathecal baclofen therapy over 10 years. *J Neurosci Nurs* **36**: 322–7.

395

Reeves RK, Stolp-Smith KA, Christopherson MW (1998) Hyperthermia, rhabdomyolysis, and disseminated intravascular coagulation associated with baclofen pump catheter failure. *Arch Phys Med Rehabil* **79**: 353–6.

Remy-Neris O, Tiffreau V, Bouilland S, Bussel B (2003) Intrathecal baclofen in subjects with spastic hemiplegia: assessment of the antispastic effect during gait. *Arch Phys Med Rehabil* **84**: 643–50.

Rigoli G (2004) Intrathecal baclofen withdrawal syndrome caused by low residual volume in the pump reservoir: a report of two cases. *Arch Phys Med Rehabil* **85**: 2064–6.

Sampson FC, Hayward A, Evans G, Morton R, Collett B (2002) Functional benefits and cost/benefit analysis of continuous intrathecal baclofen infusion for the management of severe spasticity. *J Neurosurg* **96**: 1052–7.

Sanger TD, Delgado MR, Gaebler-Spira D, Hallett M, Mink JW and the Task Force on Childhood Motor Disorders (2003) Classification and definition of disorders causing hypertonia in childhood. *Pediatrics* **111**: e89–97.

Santiago-Palma J, Hord D, Vallejo R, Trella J, Ahmed SU (2004) Respiratory distress after intrathecal baclofen withdrawal. *Anesthes Analges* **99**: 227–9.

Senaran H, Shah SA, Presedo A, Dabney KW, Glutting JW, Miller F (2007) The risk of progression of scoliosis in cerebral palsy patients after intrathecal baclofen therapy. *Spine* **32**: 2348–54.

Sgouros S (2007) Surgical management of spasticity of cerebral origin in children. *Acta Neurochirurg Suppl* **97**: 193–203.

Sgouros S, Seri S (2002) The effect of intrathecal baclofen on muscle co-contraction in children with spasticity of cerebral origin. *Pediatr Neurosurg* **37**: 225–30.

Shilt JS, Lai LP, Cabrera MN, Frino J, Smith BP (2008) The impact of intrathecal baclofen on the natural history of scoliosis in cerebral palsy. *J Pediatr Orthop* **28**: 684–7.

Smail DB, Hugeron C, Denys P, Bussel B (2005) Pruritus after intrathecal baclofen withdrawal: a retrospective study. *Arch Phys Med Rehabil* **86**: 494–7.

Sommer BR, Petrides G (1992) A case of baclofen-induced psychotic depression. *J Clin Psychiatr* **53**: 211–12.

Staal C, Arends A, Ho S (2003) A self-report of quality of life of patients receiving intrathecal baclofen therapy. *Rehabil Nurs* **28**: 159–63.

Stempien L, Tsai T (2000) Intrathecal baclofen pump use for spasticity: a clinical survey. *Am J Phys Med Rehabil* **79**: 536–41.

Stokic DS, Yablon SA, Hayes A (2005) Comparison of clinical and neurophysiologic responses to intrathecal baclofen bolus administration in moderate-to-severe spasticity after acquired brain injury. *Arch Phys Med Rehabil* **86**: 1801–6.

Wunderlich CA, Krach LE (2006) Gram-negative meningitis and infections in individuals treated with intrathecal baclofen: a retrospective study. *Dev Med Child Neurol* **48**: 450–5.

Yeh RN, Nypaver MM, Deegan TJ, Ayyangar R (2004) Baclofen toxicity in an 8-year-old with an intrathecal baclofen pump. *J Emerg Med* **26**: 163–7.

Zuckerbraun NS, Ferson SS, Albright AL, Vogeley E (2004) Intrathecal baclofen withdrawal: emergent recognition and management. *Pediatr Emerg Care* **20**: 759–64.

5.2
TREATMENT OF SPASTICITY WITH SELECTIVE DORSAL RHIZOTOMY

Joyce P. Trost, Mary E. Dunn, Linda E. Krach, Nelleke G. Langerak, Tom F. Novacheck and Michael H. Schwartz

Key points

1. *Patients suitable for a selective dorsal rhizotomy meet the following criteria:*
   - preterm birth
   - imaging consistent with periventricular leukomalacia
   - primarily spastic tone
   - evidence of fair selective motor control
   - fair strength
   - gait energy inefficiency of greater than two times that of speed-matched control
   - demonstrated ability to cooperate and follow through with rehabilitation program.
2. *Other treatments to consider include the following:*
   - oral medication for a generalized effect
   - botulinum toxin and phenol use for focal/temporary spasticity management
   - intrathecal baclofen for mixed hypertonia
   - orthopaedic surgery for primarily bone deformities.
3. *Surgical technique consistent with good outcomes involves the following:*
   - no preoperative sedation
   - propofol at normal concentrations
   - laminaplasty
   - microdissection with 150–250 rootlets per level
   - no supra-threshold stimulation
   - 25%–45% of rootlets are cut.
4. *Short- and long-term outcomes demonstrate the following:*
   - decreased spasticity
   - improved or unchanged strength
   - improved gait pattern
   - decreased oxygen cost
   - improved overall function including decreased use of walking aids.
5. *More research is needed, including investigation of the following:*
   - who else could benefit from this procedure?
   - what are the specific risk factors for a poor outcome?
   - larger cohort for longitudinal studies.

Although spasticity is one of the primary causes of functional impairment in ambulatory patients with cerebral palsy (CP), its evaluation and management remain varied (Vaughan et al. 1998, Steinbok 2001). Current treatment options include oral medications, physical therapy, bracing, chemodenervation with botulinum toxin or phenol, intrathecal baclofen, orthopaedic surgery, and selective dorsal rhizotomy (SDR) (Gormley et al. 2001, Abbott 2004, Tilton 2004). Treatment may include one or a combination of these procedures. Patient selection for any procedure to treat spasticity plays a pivotal role in its safety and efficacy (Arens et al. 1989a, Vaughan et al. 1998, Gormley et al. 2001).

Review of relevant pathophysiology
Spasticity is the most common muscle tone abnormality of CP and affects approximately 75% of those with CP (Matthews and Wilson 1999, Sanger et al. 2003). Spasticity is defined as a velocity-dependent resistance to stretch with one or both of the following signs: (1) the resistance increases with increasing speed of movement and varies with the direction of joint motion, and (2) resistance to movement rises rapidly above a threshold speed of joint angle (a spastic catch) (Sanger et al. 2003, Ivanhoe and Reistetter 2004). This definition of spasticity implies that it involves both the motor and sensory systems, as the externally imposed movement, different velocities and changing joint angles depend on afferent feedback from the proprioceptive system (Sanger et al. 2003, Ivanhoe and Reistetter 2004). Balanced excitatory and inhibitory influences on the alpha motor neurons result in normal muscle tone (Young 1994, Albright 1995). Inhibitory influences are gamma amino-butyric acid mediated and involve interneurons that synapse with alpha motor neurons. Excitatory influences are glutamate and aspartate mediated afferents from the muscle spindles and Golgi tendon organs (Davidoff 1985, Albright 1995). In CP, damage in the brain results in descending tracts not being able to provide their inhibitory influence, therefore producing an imbalance with an excess of excitatory influence (Davidoff 1985, Young 1994, Albright 1995, Dietz 1999, Burchiel and Hsu 2001, Ivanhoe and Reistetter 2004). For a more thorough discussion of the causes and indications of spasticity, see the detailed discussions in Chapters 2.1 and 2.2. SDR is undertaken to reduce the excitatory input from the afferents to reduce the abnormal, increased muscle tone seen in cerebral palsy (Fig. 5.2.1).

Historical perspective
Division of the posterior roots for children with spastic cerebral palsy was first published by Foerster in 1913, outlining the indication for 'resection of posterior roots in spasticity'. Foerster's technique was not reported by others until the 1960s when Gros in Montpellier, France, performed partial dorsal rhizotomies (Steinbok 2007). Major contributions to the evolution of theory and technique from that point on have been made by Fasano and Peacock (Fasano et al. 1978, 1979, 1980, 1988, Peacock and Arens 1982, Peacock et al. 1987, Peacock and Staudt 1990, 1991).

The SDR procedure has been utilized clinically in the United States for the treatment of spasticity in children with CP for more than 20 years. There are many positive outcome studies that have been published (Privat et al. 1976, Fasano et al. 1978, 1980, Peacock and

Arens 1982, Laitinen et al. 1983, Peacock et al. 1987, Vaughan et al. 1988, Abbott et al. 1989, Arens et al. 1989a, b, Staudt et al. 1990, Giuliani 1991, Abbott et al. 1993, Boscarino et al. 1993, McDonald and Hays 1994, McLaughlin et al. 1994, Abbott 1996, 2004, Subramanian et al. 1998, Vaughan et al. 1998, Steinbok 2001). However, this procedure has been and remains controversial. This is in part because of the risk of peri- and post-operative complications (Abbott 1992, Steinbok and Schrag 1998, Trost et al. 2008). There are concerns about longer-term possibility of crouch gait, spinal deformity, foot deformity, hip subluxation, sensory impairments, and functional weakness (Yasuoka et al. 1982, Landau and Hunt 1990, Greene et al. 1991, Abbott 1992, 2004, Montgomery 1992, Abbott et al. 1993, Payne and DeLuca 1993, McLaughlin et al. 1998, Steinbok and Schrag 1998, Johnson et al. 2004, Molenaers et al. 2004). Others argue that children who are selected to undergo this procedure would do well with any surgical intervention because of good strength, motor control, and ambulation ability (Landau and Hunt 1990). 'The tendency of children to improve coordination and function with increasing age must be distinguished from the effect of treatment' (Paine 1962), 'To what extent are the functional impairments of children with cerebral palsy due to spasticity?' and 'These are the very children who do better with any surgery' are all critiques of this intervention (Landau and Hunt 1990).

Age, severity of cerebral palsy and pre-existing conditions all factor into the risk of iatrogenic complications that feed the skepticism. Even among those who use SDR, opinion regarding the ideal candidate and the appropriate surgical technique has clouded the research into the efficacy of the procedure (Foerster 1913, Cahan et al. 1987, Peacock et al. 1987, Arens et al. 1989b, Cohen and Webster 1991, Peter and Arens 1994, Nishida et al. 1995, Chicoine et al. 1996, Steinbok and Kestle 1996, McLaughlin et al. 1998, 2002, Vaughan et al. 1998, Krach 2000a, Park 2000, van Schie et al. 2005, Kim et al. 2006, Steinbok 2007, Trost et al. 2008). Several authors have reported the safety of the procedure when done correctly (Steinbok 2007, Trost et al. 2008). The incidence of orthopaedic deformities such as hip subluxation is equal to or less than that of natural history (Park et al. 1994, Heim et al. 1995, Hicdonmez et al. 2005). There have been mixed reports on the risks of spinal deformity, dependent on the severity of CP as well as the use of laminoplasty versus laminectomy (Peter et al. 1993, Johnson et al. 2004, Spiegel et al. 2004, Steinbok et al. 2005). Despite the proven safety and efficacy of the procedure if done properly and acknowledgement that it is just one tool that may need to be combined with others in treating children with spastic CP, hesitation to utilize SDR still remains.

Indications from patient assessment
Children with CP have a varied history, etiology, and physical make-up with regard to spasticity, other tonal abnormalities, strength, bone alignment, and selective control of lower-extremity musculature. Each of these characteristics may add to or detract from the success of a SDR procedure. The SDR is generally used in a subgroup of individuals with CP to reduce spasticity as a means of increasing function. The selection criterion for that sub-group varies from place to place, and even within an institution (Vaughan et al. 1998, Steinbok 2001, McLaughlin et al. 2002). A variety of selection criteria and exclusion criteria have been published (Arens et al. 1989b, Boscarino et al. 1993, Thomas et al. 1996, Buckon

et al. 1997, Steinbok et al. 1997, Subramanian et al. 1998, Wright et al. 1998, Graubert et al. 2000, Steinbok 2001, McLaughlin et al. 2002, Mittal et al. 2002, van Schie et al. 2005). These include criteria for age, diagnosis, tone, ambulatory ability, birth history, motor control, specific medical conditions, orthopaedic status, availability of postoperative therapy and intellectual development. In reviewing published investigations regarding outcomes of SDR, it is clear that while general notions of an ideal candidate are discussed, specific selection criteria, practical adherence to the criteria, and the decision process for assessing those criteria have not been adequately stated.

SELECTION PROCESS AND CRITERIA

Children should be seen in a multidisciplinary clinic as part of the evaluation process to determine if their increased tone is problematic, is concerning enough to warrant inter-vention, and if so which treatment would be the best. This evaluation includes physiotherapy (PT) evaluation, computerized gait analysis, social work interview and simultaneous clinic visits with pediatric orthopaedics, pediatric neurosurgery and pediatric rehabilitation medicine physicians. This multidisciplinary evaluation is believed to be an integral part of the decision-making process and is described below.

Prior to seeing the patient in clinic the three physicians (pediatric orthopaedist, pediatric neurosurgeon, and pediatric rehabilitation medicine physician) review and discuss the information available. This typically includes outside records including birth history, imaging reports or studies, and previous interventions. Next, the physical therapy evaluation and gait analysis are reviewed. The physicians pay particular attention to the amount of spasticity, functional use of tone, and presence of dystonia. Consistent and diminished sagittal-plane hip and knee range of motion between walking trials on gait data, in the absence of multilevel contractures, supports the presence of spasticity. Excessive simultaneous hip flexion, knee flexion and ankle dorsiflexion in swing suggest reflexive, patterned movement. Variable sagittal-plane motion between walking trials is suggestive of dystonia. Gross Motor Function Measure (GMFM) subscale scores, comments concerning the child's ability to cooperate, gait video and the rest of the gait analysis information, oxygen consumption, and any notation of child or parent goals are discussed as well.

Within the clinic room itself, the physicians clarify and expand upon the history as necessary, assess the child's muscle tone regarding type and severity, evaluate range of motion and ascertain if any bony deformities are present. In order to assess if the child is making use of tone, functional tasks are observed. For example, while a physician is providing support for safety, the child is asked to go from upright standing to touching the floor and then back to a standing position. This will demonstrate if the child is using total flexion and extension for this task or able to isolate movement. Also, the ability to isolate movement at the hip, knee, and ankle is assessed. The PT and gait analysis videos can also be used for this portion of the evaluation.

After completing their evaluation and integrating the information from PT and the Motion Lab, the three physicians discuss their findings, reach consensus about a recommendation and discuss it with the patient and family. Five factors have been deemed the most relevant in selection of appropriate SDR candidates and are used for this decision

400

making process. These five factors, based on Peacock's original criteria, have been modified for clinical use and have been retrospectively reviewed in an outcome study of 136 subjects seen in clinic at Gillette (Trost et al. 2008). The putative ideal candidate would have the following clinical indications:

Birth history. Preterm birth is defined as less than 36 weeks gestation, along with neuroimaging evidence of periventricular leukomalacia. These two criteria are indicative of a brain insult that typically results in spasticity rather than mixed tone abnormalities (see Chapters 2.1 and 2.2). Preterm birth as the etiology of hypertonia is thought to result in an upper motor neuron lesion resulting in pure spasticity more frequently than mixed spasticity and dystonia associated with term birth CP. In addition to reviewing imaging findings to see if periventricular leukomalacia is present, imaging is reviewed to assure that other findings such as neuronal migration disorders, untreated hydrocephalus, or spinal cord pathology – if history and physical examination are suggestive of that etiology – are not present as they are other potential causes of spasticity.

Tone. Primarily spastic tone should be noted on clinical examination and suggested by computerized gait analysis (repeatable gait pattern between walking trials, limited sagittal-plane range of motion and consistent EMG). There should be minimal evidence of mixed tone on motion assessment physical exam (PE), physical therapist PE, and physicians' PE. Ashworth scores of 2–4 at the rectus, hamstrings, hip-flexors, adductors and plantarflexors must be recorded (Lee et al. 1989). There should be no evidence of rigidity. Children with underlying hypotonia in postural muscles, especially the trunk, coexisting with high-extremity tone are felt to not be optimal candidates for SDR (Nazar et al. 1990).

Selective motor control. Complete or partial ability to isolate movement at the hips, knees and ankles as measured on PE in lying, sitting and standing is also an important factor. Good motor control as noted by an absence of reflexive movement patterns during walking (i.e. exaggerated hip flexion, knee flexion, and ankle dorsiflexion during swing) gives a positive indication of the ability for typical movement patterns. Having the ability to isolate muscle movements such as ankle dorsiflexion without hip flexion, unilateral knee extension, and hip flexion without dorsiflexion suggests that the child has no 'obligate synergies' (Sanger et al. 2006). If they have 'good selective motor control', as defined by Sanger, and are able to regulate muscle control and force, patients will therefore have a greater ability for muscle strengthening during postoperative rehabilitation (Sanger et al. 2003). The Selective Motor Control grading scale that is used at Gillette is described in Chapter 3.1. Children with 0 grade selectivity, showing only patterned movement, do not receive a recommendation for SDR.

Strength. At least antigravity strength at the hip-flexors is needed for good postoperative outcome. Studies have not shown any unmasking of weakness after SDR (Buckon et al. 2002); however, less than antigravity hip-flexor strength would suggest that the child was marginally ambulating prior to surgery. Such marginal ambulators could be making use of spasticity to assist their antigravity efforts and tone reduction could significantly affect their ability to ambulate after SDR. An attempt is also made to determine if there is enough underlying strength so that the reduction in lower-extremity spasticity will be beneficial to the child's ambulatory function rather than detrimental.

Gait inefficiency. Oxygen cost measures the overall efficiency of a child's gait (Schwartz et al. 2006). An oxygen cost value greater than two times that of speed-matched controls is suggestive of spasticity (Schwartz 2001). Often young children are unable to complete this test per protocol (Schwartz 2007). In those cases, this piece is not used in the decision-making process (Trost et al. 2008).

Other important aspects of selection because of their impact on postoperative rehabilitation are cooperation, age, and prior treatments. The availability of postoperative rehabilitation has also been noted to be an important consideration. Cooperation includes motivation and sufficient developmental maturity (Nazar et al. 1990). The ideal age is thought to be 4–10 years old. The history behind this criterion is to decrease the patient's spasticity while they are still young enough to learn new motor patterns. Little has been published about SDR in teens and adults. A report of 30 teenagers and young adults by Peter and Arens (1994) noted all had good tone reduction and a majority demonstrated improved function. Gillette's limited experience in this area is similar, but adults have experienced more pain and progressed with their rehabilitation at a slower rate than children after SDR. Some authors have suggested that prior orthopaedic surgical intervention is a contraindication for SDR (McDonald and Hays 1994). Lengthening of a muscle will result in relative weakness of that muscle and therefore care might need to be taken to minimize the amount of rootlet sectioning at the level of innervations of a previously lengthened muscle.

Goals of treatment

Standard outcome measures can assess success across a group; however, satisfaction for a patient and family is dependent on the goals set prior to intervention. In selecting SDR as a treatment option for children with cerebral palsy, it is imperative to have a well defined set of goals discussed and outlined prior to intervention. Equally important is the discussion that SDR is only one treatment in the overall long-term plan for the child. Patient and family perceptions of the child's problems should be discussed with the clinician. A common understanding of the anticipated outcome must be agreed upon.

Goals will generally fall into the body structures/function and activities levels of the International Classification of Functioning (ICF), Disability and Health framework (Rosenbaum and Stewart 2004). Included in these levels are the outcome categories of spasticity, range of motion, ease of movement, comfort, strength, cosmesis, gait pattern quality, functional walking ability, activities of daily living, and gait efficiency. Goals for the rehabilitation phase as well as both short and long term goals should be defined. Often the goals of the families address the activities of the child in their current life situations, such as wanting them to be able to play more easily on the playground with friends. However, the clinician can help them see that in the future, this 5-year-old will need to be able to maintain the endurance to ambulate long distances for social independence. Both of these perspectives should be discussed.

Treatment options

After assessing the patient and considering the goals, the clinicians may conclude that SDR is not be the best choice for a child because of a selection profile inconsistent with the criteria outlined above, or because the family's goals cannot be met by this intervention. Other treatment options for managing the child's spasticity and improving function could then be discussed. These may include oral medication, injectables such as botulinum toxin or phenol, intrathecal baclofen pump (ITB), or orthopaedic surgery. Oral medications result in a generalized effect and can often cause significant sedation (see Chapter 4.3). Functionally, there may not be sufficient change to warrant the side effects of weakness and sedation for an ambulatory child (Tilton 2003). Botulinum toxin and phenol can be used for local management of spasticity. However, there is a limit to the number of muscles that can receive treatment simultaneously (see Chapter 4.4). Because botulinum toxin's effects are temporary, periodic reinjection is required. Intrathecal baclofen is effective for patients that have multiple forms of hypertonia (Abbott 2004, Steinbok 2007). Studies have shown improvement in tone, spasm, contractures and pain. However, gait and function improvements have not been reported consistently (Gerszen et al. 1997, Gormley et al. 2001, Kan et al. 2008). ITB also has a higher complication rate than SDR (Kolaski and Logan 2007). At Gillette, ambulatory children considered for ITB do not generally meet the criteria for SDR (see Chapter 5.1). As a result, ITB and SDR patients are not comparable at this institution. Orthopaedic surgery is another treatment used for ambulatory children to improve gait efficiency, functional walking ability and gait pathology (Marty et al. 1995, Buckon et al. 2004, Schwartz et al. 2004). Schwartz et al. (2004) found that children who do not undergo SDR before orthopaedic surgery have substantially higher rates of soft-tissue surgery than those who have had SDR. This reinforces the notion that spasticity reduction and orthopaedic surgery are complementary elements of an integrated management approach.

Once the child has been deemed an appropriate candidate, and the goals have been considered, the operative procedure is now of utmost importance. There are varieties of dorsal rhizotomy procedures performed across the world, including selective and non-selective, as well as alternatives in surgical exposure from L1–S1 versus at the level of the conus only. The operative procedure at Gillette is based on that described by Peacock and Fasano with an emphasis on selectivity via electrophysiologic guidance and meticulous dissection (Peacock and Arens 1982, Fasano et al. 1988, Steinbok 2007, Trost et al. 2008).

Operative Procedure

The operative procedure performed at Gillette combines elements of Fasano's and Peacock's approaches with the addition of increased microdissection reaching up to 250 rootlets tested, and anatomic restoration with laminaplasty as opposed to laminoplasty. Approximately 400 such operative procedures have been performed by a group of neurosurgeons at Gillette and the Shriners' Hospital Twin-Cities Unit since 1987. Details of this procedure are as follows.

Preoperative sedation is not administered, as it alters intraoperative neurophysiology (Fasano et al. 1988, Mittal and Farmer 2001). Induction and maintenance of general anesthesia is accomplished using desflurane at 4%–6% or sevoflurane at 1.0–1.5% and a short-acting paralytic agent for endotracheal intubation (no narcotics, benzodiazepines or succinylcholine). The optimal nitrous oxide concentration is 50% because higher concentrations negatively affect stimulation thresholds. Propofol at normal concentrations is used, as it does not interfere with H-reflex activity (Kerz et al. 2001).

The patient is positioned prone. Insulated needle electrodes are placed in the bilateral adductors, quadriceps, medial and lateral hamstrings, tibialis anterior, gastrocnemius, and gluteus medius as well as the anal sphincter to monitor stimulation response.

The dura is exposed by a trap door laminoplasty (Fasano et al. 1988). The dural sac is opened midline and tack up sutures placed to expose the cauda equina. Rhizotomy hooks are placed 1 cm apart and motor stimulation is accomplished using 0.1 mA at 50 Hz for 500 ms (Fig. 5.2.1). Once motor level is established, the roots are divided into motor and sensory divisions. The sensory roots are micro-dissected (as many as 150–250 total rootlets are

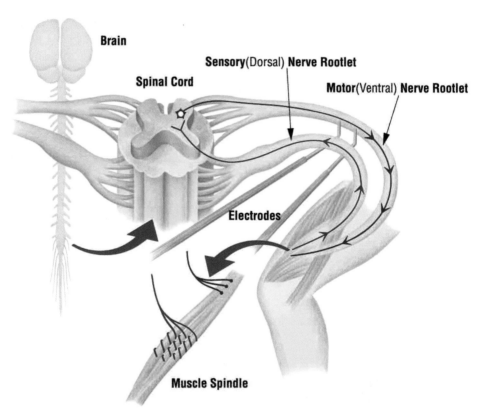

Fig. 5.2.1 SDR is performed at the L1–S2 level of the spinal cord to decrease facilitation. The roots are divided into motor and sensory divisions. The sensory roots are micro-dissected and each component rootlet is stimulated by two electrodes at threshold 0.2–3 mA. Rootlets associated with an abnormal clinical response and abnormal EMG are divided to decrease the sensitivity of the muscle spindle therefore decreasing spasticity.

typically dissected), and each component rootlet is stimulated at threshold, beginning at S1, to establish threshold response. The S1 starting level is chosen since it typically reflects the highest level of spasticity, and elimination of these rootlets with abnormal response impacts electrophysiological recording at subsequent levels. The sensory stimulation for threshold response ranges from 0.2 mA to 3 mA. Care is taken to avoid delivering supra-threshold stimulation.

Electromyographic (EMG) response and clinical observation are recorded for each rootlet. Single twitch, decremental, or squared responses are considered to be normal. Incremental, clonic, multiphasic, sustained, and responses that spread to three or more muscles beyond the primary level of stimulation or the opposite leg are considered abnormal (Fig. 5.2.2). Rootlets with abnormal response are cut. This paradigm is repeated for each sensory root on both sides S1 (or S2) to L1. Rootlets that only produced anal sphincter activity are preserved.

Typically, between 30% and 40% (total) of rootlets are cut. The upper limit (of 45%) is never violated for the patient overall, although at any individual level more than 45% of rootlets may be cut. At a single level, when the overall number of abnormal EMG responses

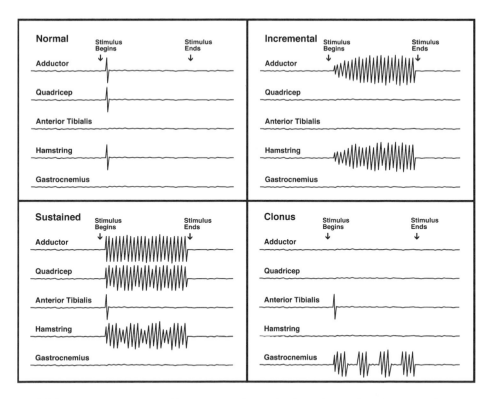

Fig. 5.2.2 Typical electromyographic responses of normal and spastic muscle during threshold stimulation are represented. Incremental, sustained, and clonus are all abnormal responses.

405

exceeds 45%, clinical examination (level where spasticity was interfering most with function), and gait analysis data (the muscles which demonstrated the most deviation from typical) are used to decide which of the rootlets should be cut.

Intravenous narcotics and 0.25% bupivacaine injected into the paraspinals are used intraoperatively for postoperative pain relief. Knee-immobilizers are used to reduce postoperative muscle spasms; ketorolac, narcotics, and muscle relaxants are used for the first 48 hours postoperatively.

Using the surgical technique described above, the rate of intraoperative, perioperative, and postoperative complications is low (Table 5.2.1) and most resolve by the time of discharge (6 weeks postoperatively), indicating a high level of technical safety of the procedure (Steinbok and Schrag 1998). Careful intraoperative monitoring, meticulous hemostasis, and surgical decision-making limiting the percentage of rootlets cut, contribute to the safety and efficacy of the procedure (Trost et al. 2008). Long-term complications have not been studied at Gillette; however the long-term outcome study by Langerak et al. (2008b) described a few of the long-term complications. These outcomes are summarized at the end of this chapter. Several other studies have stressed the importance for orthopaedic follow-up post SDR to treat spinal deformities, hip subluxation, lever arm dysfunction, foot deformities and residual muscle tightness (Carroll et al. 1998, Schwartz et al. 2004, Spiegel et al. 2004) for optimal long-term outcome.

Although many publications of treatment with SDR indicate that surgery is followed by intensive rehabilitation, what constitutes intensive rehabilitation is often not detailed. Some studies note discharge shortly after surgery with varying amounts of outpatient PT and occupational therapy, while others indicate an inpatient stay of 4–6 weeks (Engsberg et al. 1998, Krach 2000b, McLaughlin et al. 2002). Specific outcome studies comparing the variety of postoperative rehabilitation protocols have not been done. No benefit has been found to preoperative intensive physical therapy. At Gillette, rehabilitation protocols are initiated 3 days after surgery. The children remain in the hospital an average of 40 days, participating in an intensive inpatient rehabilitation program including twice daily PT and occupational therapy (OT). The program emphasizes the mastery of lower level motor skills before progressing to higher level skills, strengthening, and selective control (see Chapter 5.4 for details).

TABLE 5.2.1
Short-term complications of 136 subjects included in the outcome study of Trost et al. (2008).

Category	Number	%
Bowel and bladder	11	8
Skin related	9	7
Wound healing	8	6
Headache	6	4
Paresthesias	5	4
Weakness	4	3
Miscellaneous related	5	4
Miscellaneous not related	3	2

Supporting evidence/outcome data

Despite the skepticism and the significant variations between centers in the way the procedure is done, SDR has become a standard neurosurgical procedure that has benefited many children with CP (Steinbok 2007, Trost et al. 2008). Studies with variable levels of evidence, have shown that SDR reduces spasticity, improves range of motion, function, and self-care activities, and normalizes gait patterns (Steinbok 2001). A few researchers have tried to link certain pre-operative factors to poor outcomes. Kim et al. (2006) stated that diagnosis appears to be a strong predictor of poor outcome, and Chicoine et al. (1996) suggested that age, preoperative gait score, voluntary dorsiflexion, and diagnosis were prognostic indicators for ambulatory outcome. No study has been able to make the conclusion that poor selection would result in a poor outcome. In the study published by Trost et al. (2008) an attempt was made to evaluate the risk of poor selection by evaluating the adherence to the previously mentioned selection criteria (Fig. 5.2.3). The study was inconclusive, though the data did seem to suggest that the more patients matched the selection criteria outlined above, the lower the risk of poor outcomes (Trost et al. 2008).

In the study by Trost et al. (2008) 136 children were evaluated retrospectively in a comprehensive manner. A mean of 36% of rootlets were cut (Table 5.2.2a). Patients are not chosen for SDR based on their GMFCS level. However, the relationship between GMFCS level and strength, spasticity, and oxygen cost implicitly results in a predominance of children in GMFCS levels II and III receiving SDR (Table 5.2.2b). A uniform scheme for

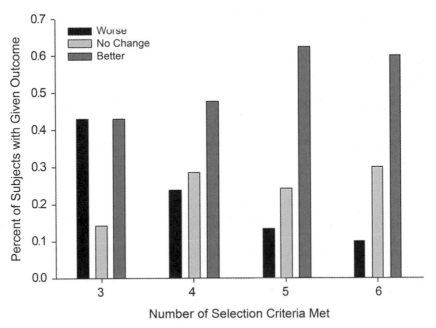

Fig. 5.2.3 Categorical outcomes versus number of selection criteria met. The relationship between number of selection criteria met and the outcome is shown. The more selection criteria that were met by a patient, the less likely was that to have a poor outcome.

TABLE 5.2.2a
Demographic and surgical profiles of the 136 patients included in the study of Trost et al. (2008)

Sex	n	Age (years) Mean	SD	Follow-up time (mo)	Rootlets cut (%)
Female	55	7y 7mo	2y 1mo	19.1 (4.9)	35
Male	81	6y 11mo	2y 0mo	17.8 (4.0)	37
Total	**136**	**7y 3mo**	**2y 1mo**	**18.3 (4.4)**	**36**

TABLE 5.2.2b
Functional profiles of the same patients

Sex	n	GMFCS – before I	II	III	IV	GMFCS – after I	II	III	IV
Female	55	3	25	24	3	13	25	16	1
Male	81	3	39	35	4	16	35	30	0
Total	**136**	**6**	**64**	**59**	**7**	**29**	**60**	**46**	**1**

determining categorical outcomes was used consistently across all outcome measures. The scheme allowed an outcome to be rated as *poor* (worsening or loss from within typical range), *neutral* (no change or maintenance within typical limits), or *good* (improvement or correction to within typical limits). Multiple domains of outcome showed a high level of efficacy for SDR performed in the manner described above, and on participants meeting the selection criteria described above (Fig. 5.2.4, Table 5.2.3). The SDR was shown to be effective in reducing spasticity (Ashworth scale), improving gait quality (GGI), improving gait efficiency (oxygen cost) and improving overall ambulatory function (Gillette Functional Assessment Questionnaire – FAQ) (Lee et al. 1989, Novacheck et al. 2000, Schutte et al. 2000, Romei et al. 2005, Schwartz et al. 2006).

Spasticity decreased substantially at the major muscle groups (Table 5.2.4). A large percentage of muscle groups with preoperative spasticity had complete correction (postoperative Ashworth score 1): hip-flexor (83%), adductor (72%), hamstring (84%), and rectus femoris (74%). Complete correction of plantarflexor spasticity was not as common (41%). While it may be possible to reduce spasticity further by sectioning a higher percentage of rootlets, it appears that low levels of residual spasticity in children with mildly impaired motor control may be functionally beneficial for joint stabilization and power production. Relief of spasticity is not an end in itself, but rather a means to improve function. In other outcome studies published, there is very strong evidence that SDR results in a decrease in lower extremity spasticity both in the short term and in the long term (Steinbok et al. 1997, Engsberg et al. 2002, 2006, Farmer and Sabbagh 2007).

Muscle strength has shown either no change or improvement in the lower extremities following SDR (Engsberg et al. 1998, 2002, 2006, Steinbok 2001, Buckon et al. 2002).

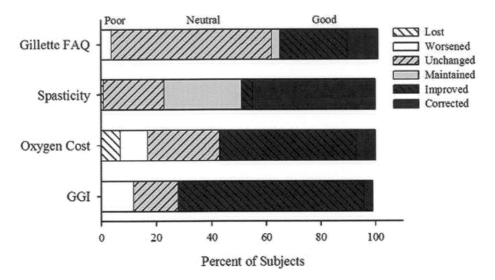

Fig. 5.2.4 Categorical outcomes for the spectrum of measures included in this study are shown. These include measures of overall function (FAQ), spasticity (Ashworth scores), gait efficiency (Oxygen Cost), and gait pattern pathology (GGI). The good outcomes range from around 30% (FAQ) to 70% (GGI). There is a very low rate of poor outcomes (~10%).

Other studies have addressed strength indirectly through functional and self-care gains such as the measured on the GMFM and on the PEDI or WeeFIM. Several have shown improvement, but only two have shown improvement greater than with therapy alone on the GMFM (Steinbok et al. 1997, Wright et al. 1998). There are several prospective case series that show improvements in self-care (Nishida et al. 1995, Loewen et al. 1998, Mittal et al. 2002, van Schie et al. 2005).

Positive changes in gait pattern, as defined by the GGI, were about 7.5 times more likely than poor ones in the Gillette study (Trost et al. 2008). Good outcomes were seen in 71% of patients, while 16% had a neutral response, and 12% poor (Table 5.2.5). The changes in GGI were largely due to improvements in the sagittal plane (Fig. 5.2.5). Some improvements were in range of motion and/or modulation, while others were manifest as normalization in timing of key gait events. Mixed results were seen at the pelvis, with an improvement in the 'double bump' pattern, but a worsening in mean tilt. Hip range-of-motion and maximum extension improved, as did the knee-flexion/extension curve (initial contact, loading response, maximum extension, range-of-motion, peak swing). At the ankle there was significant reduction of equinus and improved consistency of kinematic patterns. These post-SDR improvements are believed to be attributable to the reduction in spasticity. It should be noted that even post-SDR, the GGI remained significantly elevated compared with unimpaired gait. Orthopaedic deformity, weakness, and deficits in motor control contribute to the residual gait pathology.

An elevated oxygen cost is common in children with CP. The net non-dimensional oxygen cost, which reflects overall gait efficiency, decreased for the Gillette group as a

TABLE 5.2.3

Comprehensive outcome measures of the 136 subjects included in the outcome study by Trost et al. (2008)

Measure	Subjects (n)	% participants	Mean before (SD)	Mean after (SD)	Typical	Change mean (SD)	Possible gain	p	Test
GGI	136	100	242 (123)	180 (128)	15	−62 (105)	27%	<0.001	Paired t
FAQ	121	89	7.3 (1.7)	8.2 (1.3)	10	0.9 (1.5)	33%	<0.001	Wilcoxon
Oxygen cost (% typical)	96	71	343 (149)	291 (142)	100	−53 (132)	22%	<0.001	Paired t
Dimensionless walking speed	96	71	0.26 (0.11)	0.29 (0.09)	0.43	0.03 (0.07)	27%	<0.001	Paired t
Ashworth Scores	*Sides (n)*								
Hip-flexors	133	98	1.6 (0.8)	1.1 (0.3)	1	0.5 (0.8)	83%	<0.001	Wilcoxon
Hip-adductors	134	99	2.8 (0.8)	1.3 (0.6)	1	1.4 (0.7)	78%	<0.001	Wilcoxon
Hamstrings	135	99	2.1 (0.7)	1.1 (0.4)	1	1.0 (0.8)	91%	<0.001	Wilcoxon
Rectus femoris	135	99	2.5 (1.1)	1.3 (0.6)	1	1.2 (1.1)	80%	<0.001	Wilcoxon
Plantarflexors	135	99	3.0 (0.8)	1.6 (0.6)	1	1.3 (0.9)	65%	<0.001	Wilcoxon

TABLE 5.2.4
Spasticity outcomes (Ashworth Scores) listed by preoperative selective dorsal rhizotomy values for five major lower-extremity muscle groups (gray boxes signify a neutral outcome. Positive outcomes lie above the gray boxes and negative outcomes lie below)

TABLE 5.2.4a
Hip-flexors Ashworth Score

		Pre SDR					Total
		1	2	3	4	5	
Post SDR	1	90	9	26			125
	2	1	2	4			7
	3			1			1
	4						0
	5						0
	Total	91	11	31	0	0	133

TABLE 5.2.4b
Adductors Ashworth Score

		Pre SDR					Total
		1	2	3	4	5	
Post SDR	1	5	40	42	10		97
	2	1	6	15	7		29
	3			1	6		7
	4			1	1		1
	5						0
	Total	6	46	58	24	0	134

TABLE 5.2.4c
Hamstrings Ashworth Score

		Pre SDR					Total
		1	2	3	4	5	
Post SDR	1	26	58	31	1		116
	2	1	10	5	1		17
	3			1	0		1
	4						0
	5						0
	Total	27	68	37	2	0	134

TABLE 5.2.4d
Rectus Femoris Ashworth Score

		Pre SDR					Total
		1	2	3	4	5	
Post SDR	1	23	44	20	14	3	104
	2	2	12	6	4	2	26
	3		2	1	1	1	3
	4			1		1	2
	5						0
	Total	26	56	28	19	7	135

411

TABLE 5.2.4e
Plantarflexors Ashworth Score

		Pre SDR					Total
		1	2	3	4	5	
Post SDR	1		16	26	12		54
	2	2	16	39	16	1	74
	3		2	3	1		6
	4						0
	5						0
	Total	2	34	68	29	1	134

TABLE 5.2.5
Comprehensive outcome measures of the 136 subjects (Trost et al. 2008) by GMFCS level

Measure	Pre-op group	Good outcome		Neutral outcome		Poor outcome	
		Corrected	Improved	Maintained	Unchanged	Worse	Lost
Speed	GMFCS I			4	1		
	GMFCS II	7		33	1	1	1
	GMFCS III	10	12	9	9	3	2
	GMFCS IV	1	1		1		
O$_2$ cost	GMFCS I		4		1		
	GMFCS II	6	23		10	3	1
	GMFCS III	1	20		13	8	3
	GMFCS IV		1		1		1
GGI	GMFCS I		3			3	
	GMFCS II	4	44		12	4	
	GMFCS III		43		10	6	
	GMFCS IV		3			4	
FAQ	GMFCS I	1		3	2		
	GMFCS II	10	9		35	1	
	GMFCS III	2	16		31	4	
	GMFCS IV		5		2		
GMFCS	GMFCS I	N/A	N/A	6	N/A	N/A	
	GMFCS II	22	N/A	N/A	40	2	N/A
	GMFCS III	1	20	N/A	38		N/A
	GMFCS IV		6	N/A	1		N/A

Numbers of study participants with outcomes in respective categories

whole (Table 5.2.3). The same was true for dimensionless speed (defined as speed/ [gravity*leg length]$^{0.5}$) (Table 5.2.3). However, there was heterogeneity of the response (Fig. 5.2.6). The predominant response was one of increased speed and decreased oxygen cost. Improved energy efficiency was seen in over half of the participants (Table 5.2.5). Spasticity, weakness, orthopaedic deformity and impaired motor control also contribute to energy inefficiency. These factors probably account for the 25% of patients who

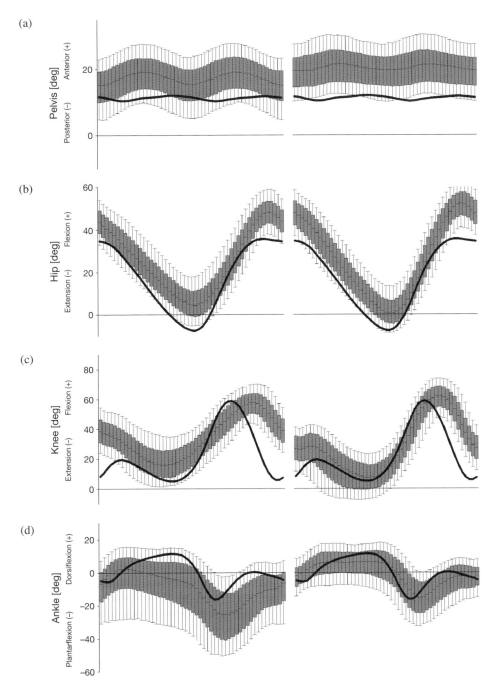

Fig. 5.2.5 Sagittal-plane kinematics show the most noticeable changes in gait pattern preoperatively to postoperatively. The box plots show the 25th–75th centile range (bars) and the 5th–95th centile range (whiskers). The mean typical value (control) is shown with a heavy line.

413

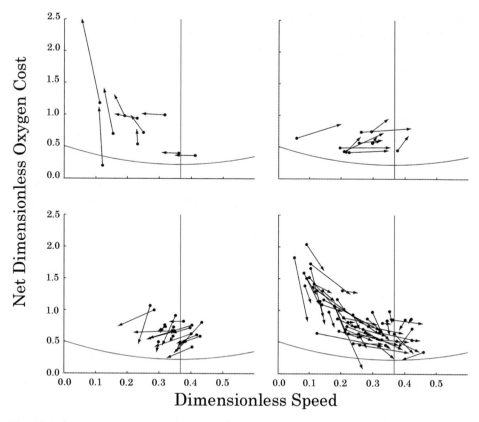

Fig. 5.2.6 The arrows begin at the preoperative speed-cost value, and terminate at the postoperative speed-cost value. The control cost versus speed is shown (parabola), along with the control free speed (vertical line). The four quadrants show responses that were poor – slower and less efficient (a), mixed – faster and less efficient (b), mixed – slower and more efficient (c), and those that were good – faster and more efficient (d).

showed no change in oxygen cost, as well as the residual elevated energy cost in many participants.

Overall ambulatory function (FAQ) improves after SDR. Participants who were limited community ambulators demonstrated a mix of neutral and good responses with many becoming good functional community ambulators (FAQ level 8 or 9) (Table 5.2.5). Participants who had a preoperative FAQ of 8 or higher had predominantly neutral responses owing to a ceiling effect, and the fact that a 1-level improvement was categorized as 'unchanged'. The only way for these participants to achieve a 'good' outcome was to reach FAQ level 10.

Children who used assistive devices preoperatively (GMFCS levels III/IV) had an equal or better likelihood of a good outcome for gait (GGI and speed respectively) and ambulatory function (FAQ) (Table 5.2.5). Of the children who used assistive devices preoperatively, 32% no longer used devices postoperatively. Conversely, only 3% moved from independent to device-dependent walking. Children who used assistive devices for community ambulation were more likely to show improvements in speed postoperatively than their independent ambulating counterparts, in part because the independent ambulators walked faster preoperatively.

LONG-TERM OUTCOMES

There may be patients who could benefit from SDR but who did not receive treatment because they did not meet the strict selection criteria at Gillette. This is a group to be followed longitudinally and compared to those who did receive SDR. We may be able to determine if the selection criteria can be widened, or what aspects of it are valid by collaborative research groups. Future studies must also examine data from patients who were considered for, accepted, but for some reason did not undergo an SDR. Trost et al. (2008) showed that for the short term, SDR is safe and effective when performed in the manner described here, on patients that match the stated selection criteria. At this time, however, the question 'What will happen when these children are adults?' can best be answered by the data of Langerak et al. (2007). Since SDR was introduced in Cape Town in the early 1980s this research group is in the best position to give an impression of the long-term outcomes of SDR.

In line with 1-, 3- and 10-year follow-up gait studies, Langerak and colleagues conducted a 20-year follow-up study (Vaughan et al. 1988, 1991, Langerak et al. 2008a). The patient cohort of this study was based on 14 children with spastic diplegia who were ambulant before they received SDR by Warwick Peacock at Red Cross Children's Hospital in 1985. All of them (six women, eight men; mean age 27 years and range 22–33 years) were tracked down in 2005. Patients were required to walk barefoot, without any orthoses, and their own customary gait on a walkway of at least 11 meters. Outcome measures included (1) angular kinematics: knee and hip range of motion, and knee and hip mid-range values (MRV); and (2) temporal-distance parameters: dimensionless cadence and step length as normalized by Hof (1996). Since one patient was not able to walk 20 years after SDR, 13 patients were included in this gait study. For comparison purposes, at each point in the study a control group of 12 age-matched healthy volunteers was included.

Figures 5.2.7 and 5.2.8 provide an overview of the changes in gait parameters before and at 1, 3, 10 and 20 years after SDR (Langerak et al. 2008a). The angular kinematic data show a major increase during the first years after SDR, followed by a decrease and then stabilization in the joint angles. Dimensionless cadence appears to be affected minimally after SDR, which results in no significant changes after SDR except for 20 years postoperatively. The changes in dimensionless step length values are comparable to the changes as shown in knee range of motion after SDR. During the first 3 years a significant increase in step length is shown, then it deteriorates slightly, before stabilizing 10 and 20 years after SDR.

In addition to the gait follow-up study the Cape Town research group performed (with the same patient cohort) neuromuscular and functional assessments 1 year (Berman 1989, Berman et al. 1990) and 20 years (Langerak et al. 2008b) after SDR. Outcome measures included muscle tone, joint stiffness, and voluntary and functional movements as described by Berman (1989). Results of this study were comparable with the long-term gait follow-up study; patients showed an improvement in their neuromuscular and functional status 1 year after surgery, which was maintained or further improved 20 years after SDR. These outcomes were in line with the changes as shown in levels of the Gross Motor Function Classification System (GMFCS) during the years.

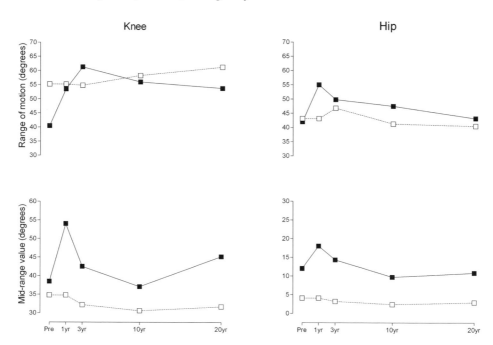

Fig. 5.2.7 Hip and knee range of motion and mid-range outcomes. Median values of knee and hip angular kinematic data (joint range of motion and mid-range values) of patients with spastic diplegia (black squares) and age-matched healthy controls (open squares) before and 1, 3, 10 and 20 years after SDR. (Graphs are adapted from Langerak et al. 2008.)

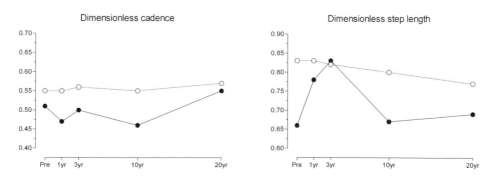

Fig. 5.2.8 Speed and cadence outcomes. Median values of dimensionless temporal-distance parameters (step frequency and step length) of patients with spastic diplegia (black circles) and age-matched healthy controls (open circles) before and 1, 3, 10 and 20 years after SDR. (Graphs adapted from Langerak et al. 2008.)

In addition to the 20-year follow-up studies, Langerak and colleagues (2007, 2008a, b) requested the 14 adults with spastic diplegia (SDR group) to complete a questionnaire. Andersson and Mattsson (2001) published a descriptive study with emphasis on locomotion in adults with CP who did not receive SDR (no-SDR group). Table 5.2.6 shows a comparable selection of outcomes for both studies. The SDR group shows better walking ability, with 79% of them who did not use walking aids in and/or outdoors 20 years after SDR, compared to 48% in the no-SDR group. In line with this outcome, 86% of the SDR group never used a wheelchair, which is in contrast with 12% of the no-SDR group. However, the SDR group received less physical training and visited a physical therapist at the same frequency as the no-SDR group.

When the SDR group was asked what their feelings were about the SDR operation, 12 of them answered positively while two of them had mixed feelings. Although all patients received intense physical therapy years before and after SDR, these two adults experienced

TABLE 5.2.6
Physical activity of adults with spastic diplegia 20 years after SDR compared to patients who did not receive SDR.

Characteristics	SDR group[a] (%)	No SDR group[b] (%)
Walking ability		
Without walking aids	79	48
With walking aids	14	32
Not walking	7	20
Use of wheelchair		
Never	86	12
Very seldom	7	6
Walk and use of wheelchair	0	44
Always	7	21
No answer	0	17
Physical training		
Never	71	31
Organized sports	0	16
Weight training	0	9
Home training	0	6
Combination	14	14
Other	14	21
No answer	0	3
Received physiotherapy		
Never	64	55
Occasionally	21	14
Once a month	0	1
Once a week	7	17
Several times a week	0	5
Every day	0	0
Varies	7	4
No answer	0	4

Outcomes are based on (a) 20-year follow-up study after SDR of Langerak et al. 2007, 2008 (n = 14); and (b) a descriptive study by Andersson and Mattsson 2001 (n = 77).

417

problems with muscle weakness postoperatively. One of them had become dependent on a wheelchair during the previous few years. In addition, 20 years after SDR all the patients had relatively poor balance and more than half of the cohort had problems with back pain, which logically had an influence on the patients' physical activities.

The 20-year follow-up studies of Langerak and colleagues (2008a, b) give a clear impression of the long-term outcomes of SDR in patients with spastic diplegia. However, the authors acknowledge that this study had a limited sample size and did not include a control group of adults with CP who did not receive SDR. Future research should include long-term follow-up studies which compare outcomes in all dimensions of the ICF-model (Rosenbaum and Stewart 2004) for patients with CP. Ideally, these studies should compare SDR patients with other treatments for spasticity.

Case study (see Case 4 on Interactive Disc)
To further illustrate the patient selection and treatment outcome, a case study is included with information on the pre-SDR visit, post-SDR/pre-orthopaedic visit, and 7 years post-SDR. Full videos and more graphs are included on the Interactive Disc.

INITIAL EVALUATION
BC, a girl aged 4 years 10 months, with a diagnosis of diplegic CP, was referred for a gait analysis with concerns regarding increased muscle tone and orthopaedic deformity.

Selection criteria
- Birth history. Met criteria: BC was born preterm with a birthweight of 2 pounds, 4 ounces.
- Tone. Met criteria: no documentation of mixed tone. Ashworth scores between 2 and 4 for lower-extremity hypertonicity.
- Selectivity. Met criteria: isolated or partially isolated movement observed.
- Strength. Met criteria: hip-flexor strength greater than fair grade.
- Gait inefficiency. Met criteria: normalized O_2 consumption of 0.16 at dimensionless speed of 0.26. This is equivalent to 265% speed-matched control value.

Previous medical history
BC's early motor milestones were delayed, with the onset of walking using a walker and solid ankle–foot orthoses occurring at 2 years 6 months.

BC has not had any past orthopaedic surgery, but has had two treatments of botulinium toxin to bilateral hamstrings, and four treatments to bilateral gastrocnemius in the 2 years prior to this evaluation.

Gait by observation (GBO) (Fig. 5.2.9; see Case 4 on the Interactive Disc for complete GBO): BC is an independent limited community ambulator with the use of hinged ankle–foot orthoses. She requires handheld assist in crowds and on uneven surfaces. Barefoot gait pattern is characterized by high toe walking bilaterally. Foot-progression angles are internal bilaterally. At the knees, she enters the walking cycle with slight increased knee flexion and maintains knee flexion throughout stance phase. Her swing phase knee

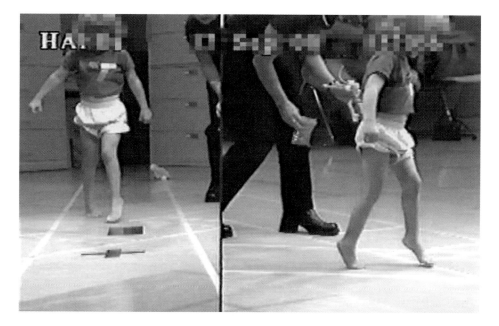

Fig. 5.2.9 Pre-SDR barefoot gait of Case Example 4 at 4 years 10 months.

motion is decreased and delayed. Thighs are internal bilaterally. She has an increased pelvic tilt with increased hip flexion at initial contact and decreased hip extension in terminal stance. There appears to be excessive pelvic range of motion throughout the walking cycle.

Physical examination
She demonstrates generalized lower-extremity spasticity (between 2 and 4 on the Ashworth scale for all major muscle groups with no evidence of mixed tone). On evaluation of her range of motion, she had bilateral hip flexion contracture of 20°, a right knee-flexion contracture of 10°, and bilateral gastrocnemius and soleus contractures. On evaluation of her motor selectivity, she had isolated to partially isolated motor control throughout her lower extremities with strength that ranged from fair to good.

Bone measurements include bilateral femoral anteversion of 70°, internal tibial torsion on the left of 15°, right forefoot adductus and a limb-length inequality with the right side 1.5cm longer than the left.

Interpretation of computerized gait analysis
The pertinent data are illustrated in Figure 5.2.10 and 5.2.11. The video of the case contains additional data. Dynamic EMG demonstrates excessive activity of all muscle groups. Her kinematics are consistent from trial to trial, which is an indication of spasticity as opposed to mixed tone. Limitations to range of motion and spasticity relate to decreased range of motion including hip, knee and ankle. Femoral anteversion relates to excessive internal hip rotations bilaterally. Limb-length inequality appears to be related to a pelvic obliquity.

419

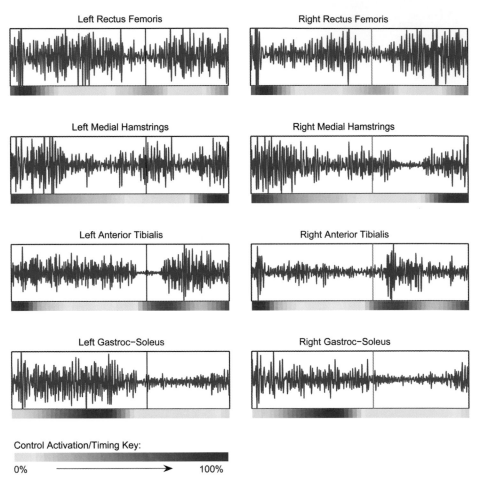

Left Rectus Femoris

Right Rectus Femoris

Left Medial Hamstrings

Right Medial Hamstrings

Left Anterior Tibialis

Right Anterior Tibialis

Left Gastroc–Soleus

Right Gastroc–Soleus

Control Activation/Timing Key:

0% → 100%

Fig. 5.2.10 Pre-SDR EMG.

Muscle weakness around the hips is related to excessive hip ab/adduction. An increased pelvic tilt with a double bump pattern is consistent with hip-flexor tightness and spasticity, and hip-extensor weakness found on the physical examination. She tends to walk with her right side carried back and down.

Preoperative summary

BC has a combination of bony malrotations, soft-tissue tightness and spasticity affecting her gait. There is some decreased motor control, which is also affecting her walking. The plan was to proceed with SDR. A 40% SDR was completed L1–S2. The planned rhizotomy

420

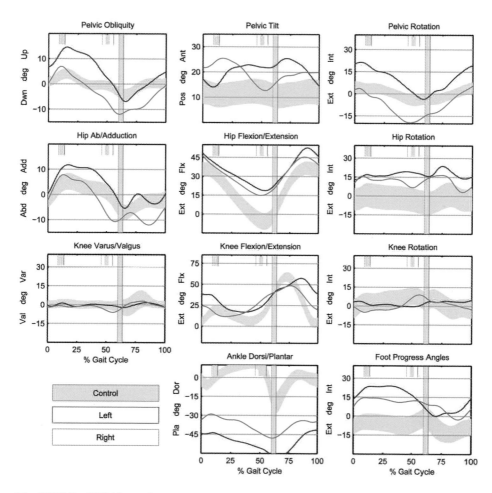

Fig. 5.2.11 Pre-SDR kinematics.

will not correct bony deformities (lever-arm dysfunction) and she will probably need correction of femoral anteversion and foot deformities in the future.

FOLLOW-UP EVALUATION 1 YEAR AFTER SDR

BC's parents are extremely satisfied with the outcome of the SDR. She is now able to walk in the community and keep up with peers. She can now go up and down stairs and curbs without holding onto a railing, can run with good control, and jump off a single step without falling (Table 5.2.7).

TABLE 5.2.7
Comprehensive outcome measures of case study (BC) prior to rhizotomy and at
1 and 7 years post-SDR.

	Pre-SDR	Post-SDR	7 years post-SDR
GMFCS	II	II	II
FAQ	6	9	8 (pain)
GDI	58	75.5	75.5
Oxygen consumption	256%	202%	159%
Spasticity (Ashworth) (average LE)	2.8	1.4	1.2

Orthopaedic procedures were done to correct lever-arm dysfunction at one year post-SDR.

Gait by observation (Fig. 5.2.12; see Case 4 on Interactive Disc for complete GBO)
BC is an independent community ambulator with the use of hinged ankle–foot orthoses. She
is independent in crowds and on uneven surfaces. Barefoot gait pattern is characterized by
footflat initial contact on the left and low heel strike on the right. Foot-progression angles
are internal bilaterally. At the knees, she enters the walking cycle with slight increased knee
flexion and maintains slight increased knee flexion throughout stance phase on the right.
Her swing-phase knee motion is good but slightly delayed. Her thighs are internally rotated
bilaterally. She has an increased pelvic tilt with increased hip flexion at initial contact and
slightly decreased hip extension in terminal stance. In static standing she is able to stand
with her feet plantargrade with mild pes planovalgus foot deformities. Her hindfoot does
not correct with toe-raising (Root sign).

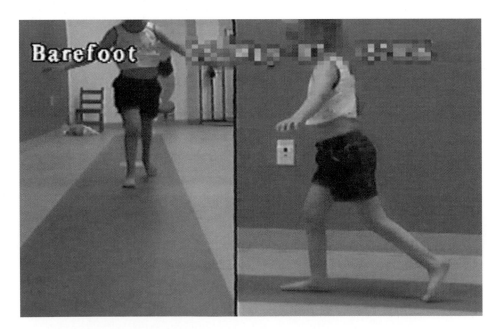

Fig. 5.2.12 1 year post-SDR barefoot gait of Case Example 4 at 4 years 10 months.

Bone measurements include femoral anteversion, and pes valgus foot deformities. Muscle findings are hip-flexor tightness, mild hip-abductor weakness, and mild gastrocnemius tightness on the left. Spasticity has been significantly decreased with mild plantarflexor spasticity still present. Selectivity is isolated to partially isolated, and she has good to fair grade strength.

Interpretation of computerized gait analysis (Fig. 5.2.13; see Interactive Disc for more data)

BC is consistent from trial to trial. She has limitations to pelvic range of motion related to mild decreased hip extension in stance and an increased pelvic tilt. Femoral anteversion

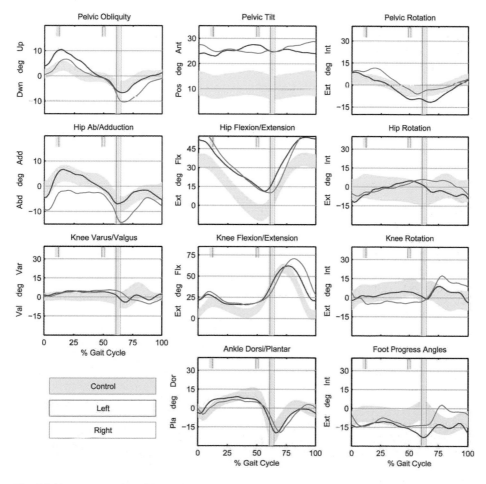

Fig. 5.2.13 1 year post-SDR kinematics.

423

related to internal hip rotations bilaterally. Muscle weakness around the hips is also related to excessive hip adduction in stance.

Post-rhizotomy summary (see outcome Table 5.2.7)
The decision was that she needed further treatment to include bilateral femoral osteotomies, bilateral os calcis lengthenings, bilateral Strayer gastrocnemius recessions, and bilateral psoas lengthening at the pelvic brim. If you are interested in the final result following the orthopaedic procedures, see Case 4 on the Interactive Disc for a full discussion.

ACKNOWLEDGEMENT

The authors gratefully acknowledge the work of the following researchers who conducted the long-term outcome research cited in this chapter: Christopher L. Vaughan PhD, Hyman Goldberg Professor of Biomedical Engineering, and Director: MRC/UCT Medical Imaging Research Unit, Department of Human Biology, Faculty of Health Sciences, University of Cape Town, Observatory, Western Cape 7925, South Africa; Robert P. Lamberts MSc, MRC/UCT Medical Imaging Research Unit, Department of Human Biology, Faculty of Health Sciences, University of Cape Town, Observatory, Western Cape 7925, South Africa; A. Graham Fieggen FCS, Division of Paediatric Neurosurgery, Red Cross Children's War Memorial Hospital, Rondebosch, Western Cape, South Africa; Jonathan C. Peter FRCS, Division of Paediatric Neurosurgery, Red Cross Children's War Memorial Hospital, Rondebosch, Western Cape, South Africa; Lize van der Merwe PhD, Biostatistics Unit, South African Medical Research Council, Tygerberg, Western Cape, South Africa; and Warwick J. Peacock FRCS, Department of Neurological Surgery, University of California, San Francisco, USA.

REFERENCES

Abbott R (1992) Complications with selective posterior rhizotomy. *Pediatr Neurosurg* **18**: 43–7.
Abbott R (1996) Sensory rhizotomy for the treatment of childhood spasticity. *J Child Neurol* **11** (Suppl 1): S36–42.
Abbott R (2004) Neurosurgical management of abnormal muscle tone in childhood. *Pediatr Clin N Am* **51**: 457–75.
Abbott R, Forem SL, Johann M (1989) Selective posterior rhizotomy for the treatment of spasticity: a review. *Childs Nerv Syst* **5**: 337–46.
Abbott R, Johann-Murphy M, Shiminski-Maher T, Quartermain D, Forem SL, Gold JT, Epstein FJ (1993) Selective dorsal rhizotomy: outcome and complications in treating spastic cerebral palsy. *Neurosurg* **33**: 851–7.
Albright AL (1995) Spastic cerebral palsy: approaches to drug treatment. *CNS Drugs* **4**: 17–27.
Andersson C, Mattsson E (2001) Adults with cerebral palsy: a survey describing problems, needs, and resources, with special emphasis on locomotion. *Dev Med Child Neurol* **43**: 76–82.
Arens LJ, Peacock WJ, Peter J (1989a) Selective posterior lumbar rhizotomy: criteria for selection of cases. *Physiother* **45**: 97–9.
Arens LJ, Peacock WJ, Peter J (1989b) Selective posterior rhizotomy: a long-term follow-up study. *Child's Nerv Syst* **5**: 148–52.
Berman B (1989) Selective posterior rhizotomy? Does it do any good? *Neurosurg: State Art Rev* **4**: 431–44.

424

Berman B, Vaughan CL, Peacock WJ (1990) The effect of rhizotomy on movement in patients with cerebral palsy. *Am J Occup Ther* **44**: 511–16.

Boscarino LF, Õunpuu S, Davis RB 3rd, Gage JR, DeLuca PA (1993) Effects of selective dorsal rhizotomy on gait in children with cerebral palsy. *J Pediatr Orthop* **13**: 174–9.

Buckon CE, Thomas S, Pierce R, Piatt JH Jr, Aiona MD (1997) Developmental skills of children with spastic diplegia: functional and qualitative changes after selective dorsal rhizotomy. *Arch Phys Med Rehabil* **78**: 946–51.

Buckon CE, Thomas SS, Harris GE, Piatt JH Jr, Aiona MD, Sussman MD (2002) Objective measurement of muscle strength in children with spastic diplegia after selective dorsal rhizotomy. *Arch Phys Med Rehabil* **83**: 454–60.

Buckon CE, Thomas SS, Piatt JH Jr, Aiona MD, Sussman MD (2004) Selective dorsal rhizotomy versus orthopedic surgery: a multidimensional assessment of outcome efficacy. *Arch Phys Med Rehabil* **85**: 457–65.

Burchiel KJ, Hsu FPK (2001) Pain and spasticity after spinal cord injury. *Spine* **26**: S146–60.

Cahan LD, Kundi MS, McPherson D, Starr A, Peacock W (1987) Electrophysiologic studies in selective dorsal rhizotomy for spasticity in children with cerebral palsy. *Appl Neurophysiol* **50**: 459–62.

Carroll KL, Moore KR, Stevens PM (1998) Orthopedic procedures after rhizotomy. *J Pediatr Orthop* **18**: 69–74.

Chicoine MR, Park TS, Vogler GP, Kaufman BA (1996) Predictors of ability to walk after selective dorsal rhizotomy in children with cerebral palsy. *Neurosurgery* **38**: 711–14.

Cohen AR, Webster HC (1991) How selective is selective posterior rhizotomy? *Surg Neurol* **35**: 267–72.

Davidoff RA (1985) Antispasticity drugs: mechanisms of action. *Ann Neurol* **17**: 107–16.

Dietz V (1999) Supraspinal pathways and the development of muscle-tone dysregulation. *Dev Med Child Neurol* **41**: 708–15.

Engsberg JR, Olree KS, Ross SA, Park TS (1998) Spasticity and strength changes as a function of selective dorsal rhizotomy. *J Neurosurg* **88**: 1020–6.

Engsberg JR, Ross SA, Wagner JM, Park TS (2002) Changes in hip spasticity and strength following selective dorsal rhizotomy and physical therapy for spastic cerebral palsy. *Dev Med Child Neurol* **44**: 220–6.

Engsberg JR, Ross SA, Collins DR, Park TS (2006) Effect of selective dorsal rhizotomy in the treatment of children with cerebral palsy. *J Neurosurg* **105**: 8–15.

Farmer JP, Sabbagh AJ (2007) Selective dorsal rhizotomies in the treatment of spasticity related to cerebral palsy. *Childs Nerv Syst* **23**: 991–1002.

Fasano VA, Broggi G, Barolat-Romana G, Sguazzi A (1978) Surgical treatment of spasticity in cerebral palsy. *Childs Brain* **4**: 289–305.

Fasano VA, Barolat-Romana G, Zeme S, Squazzi A (1979) Electrophysiological assessment of spinal circuits in spasticity by direct dorsal root stimulation. *Neurosurgery* **4**: 146–51.

Fasano VA, Broggi G, Zeme S, Lo Russo G, Sguazzi A (1980) Long-term results of posterior functional rhizotomy. *Acta Neurochir Suppl (Wien)* **30**: 435–9.

Fasano VA, Broggi G, Zeme S (1988) Intraoperative electrical stimulation for functional posterior rhizotomy. *Scand J Rehabil Med Suppl* **17**: 149–54.

Foerster O (1913) On the indications and results of the excision of posterior spinal nerve roots in men. *Surg Gynecol Obstet* **16**: 463–75.

Gerszten PC, Albright AL, Barry MJ (1997) Effect on ambulation of continous intrathecal baclofen infusion. *Pediatr Neurosurg* **27**: 40–4.

Giuliani CA (1991) Dorsal rhizotomy for children with cerebral palsy: support for concepts of motor control. *Phys Ther* **71**: 248–59.

Gormley ME, Krach LE, Piccini L (2001) Spasticity management in the child with spastic quadriplegia. *Eur J Neurol* **8**: 127–35.

Graubert C, Song KM, McLaughlin JF, Bjornson KF (2000) Changes in gait at 1 year post-selective dorsal rhizotomy: results of a prospective randomized study. *J Pediatr Orthop* **20**: 496–500.

Greene WB, Dietz FR, Goldberg MJ, Gross RH, Miller F, Sussman MD (1991) Rapid progression of hip subluxation in cerebral palsy after selective posterior rhizotomy. *J Pediatr Orthop* **11**: 494–7.

Heim RC, Park TS, Vogler GP, Kaufman BA, Noetzel MJ, Ortman MR (1995) Changes in hip migration after selective dorsal rhizotomy for spastic quadriplegia in cerebral palsy. *J Neurosurg* **82**: 567–71.

Hicdonmez T, Steinbok P, Beauchamp R, Sawatzky B (2005) Hip joint subluxation after selective dorsal rhizotomy for spastic cerebral palsy. *J Neurosurg* **103**: 10–16.

Hof AL (1996) Scaling data to body size. *Gait Posture* **4**: 222–3.

Ivanhoe CB, Reistetter TA (2004) Spasticity: the misunderstood part of the upper motor neuron syndrome. *Am J Phys Med Rehabil* **83** (Suppl): S3–9.

Johnson M, Goldstein L, Sienko Thomas S, Piatt JH, Aiona MD, Sussman MD (2004) Spinal deformity after selective dorsal rhizotomy in ambulatory patients with cerebral palsy. *J Pediatr Orthop* **24**: 529–36.

Kan P, Gooch J, Amini A, Ploeger D, Grams B, Oberg W, Simonsen S, Walker M, Kestle J (2008) Surgical treatment of spasticity in children: comparison of selective dorsal rhizotomy and intrathecal baclofen pump implantation. *Childs Nerv Syst* **24**: 239–43.

Kerz T, Hennes HJ, Feve A, Decq P, Filipetti P, Duvaldestin P (2001) Effects of propofol on H-reflex in humans. *Anesthesiology* **94**: 32–7.

Kim HS, Steinbok SP, Wickenheiser D (2006) Predictors of poor outcome after selective dorsal rhizotomy in treatment of spastic cerebral palsy. *Childs Nerv Syst* **22**: 60–6.

Kolaski K, Logan LR (2007) A review of the complications of intrathecal baclofen in patients with cerebral palsy. *Neurorehabilitation* **22**: 383–95.

Krach LE (2000) Selective dorsal rhizotomy in the treatment of cerebral palsy. *Phys Med Rehabil: State of the Art Rev* **14**: 263–74.

Laitinen LV, Nilsson S, Fugl-Meyer AR (1983) Selective posterior rhizotomy for treatment of spasticity. *J Neurosurg* **58**: 895–9.

Landau WM, Hunt CC (1990) Dorsal rhizotomy, a treatment of unproven efficacy. *J Child Neurol* **5**: 174–8.

Langerak NG, Lamberts RP, Fieggen AG, Peter JC, Peacock WJ, Vaughan CL (2007) Selective dorsal rhizotomy: long term experience from Cape Town. *Childs Nerv Syst* **23**: 1003–6.

Langerak NG, Lamberts RP, Fieggen AG, Peter JC, van der Merwe L, Peacock WJ, Vaughan CL (2008) A prospective gait analysis study in patients with diplegic cerebral palsy 20 years after selective dorsal rhizotomy. *J Neurosurg Pediatr* **1**: 180–6.

Lee KC, Carson L, Kinnin E, Patterson V (1989) The Ashworth Scale: a reliable and reproducible method of measuring spasticity. *J Neurorehabil* **3**: 205–9.

Loewen P, Steinbok P, Holsti L, MacKay M (1998) Upper extremity performance and self-care skill changes in children with spastic cerebral palsy following selective posterior rhizotomy. *Pediatr Neurosurg* **29**: 191–8.

Marty GR, Dias LS, Gaebler-Spira D (1995) Selective posterior rhizotomy and soft-tissue procedures for the treatment of cerebral diplegia. J Bone Joint Surg Am **77**: 713–18.

Matthews DJ, Wilson, P (1999) Cerebral palsy. In: Molnar GE, Alexander MA, editors. *Pediatric Rehabilitation,* 3rd edn. Philadelphia, PA: Hanley & Belfus. p 193–217.

McDonald CM, Hays RM (1994) Selective dorsal rhizotomy: Patient selection, intraoperative electrophysiologic monitoring, and clinical outcome. *Phys Med Rehabil: State Art Rev* **8**: 579–603.

McLaughlin JF, Bjornson KF, Astley SJ, Hays RM, Hoffinger SA, Armantrout EA, Roberts TS (1994) The role of selective dorsal rhizotomy in cerebral palsy: critical evaluation of a prospective clinical series. *Dev Med Child Neurol* **36**: 755–769.

McLaughlin JF, Bjornson KF, Astley SJ, Graubert C, Hays RM, Roberts TS, Price R, Temkin N (1998) Selective dorsal rhizotomy: efficacy and safety in an investigator-masked randomized clinical trial. *Dev Med Child Neurol* **40**: 220–32.

McLaughlin J, Bjornson K, Temkin N, Steinbok P, Wright V, Reiner A, Roberts T, Drake J, O'Donnell M, Rosenbaum P, Barber J, Ferrel A (2002) Selective dorsal rhizotomy: meta-analysis of three randomized controlled trials. *Dev Med Child Neurol* **44**: 17–25.

Mittal S, Farmer J (2001) Reliability of intraoperative electrophysiologic monitoring in selective posterior rhizotomy. *J Neurosurg* **95**: 67–75.

Mittal S, Farmer JP, Al-Atassi B, Montpetit K, Gervais N, Poulin C, Benaroch TE, Cantin MA (2002) Functional performance following selective posterior rhizotomy: long-term results determined using a validated evaluative measure. *J Neurosurg* **97**: 510–18.

Molenaers G, Desloovere K, De Borre L, Pauwels P, De Cat J, Eyssen M, De Cook P, Nuttin B, Nijs J (2004) Effect of selective dorsal rhizotomy on gait in children with CP: the risk of including soleus and gluteus rootlets in the SDR procedure. *Eur Soc for Movement Analysis in Adults and Children* 23–5 Sept: 130.

426

Montgomery PC (1992) A clinical report of long-term outcomes following selective posterior rhizotomy: implications for selection, follow-up and research. *Phys Occup Ther Pediatr* **12**: 69–88.

Nazar GB, Linden RD, Badenhausen W (1990) The role of functional dorsal rhizotomy for the treatment of children with spastic dorsal rhizotomy. *J Ky Med Assoc* **88**: 483–7.

Nishida T, Thatcher SW, Marty GR (1995) Selective posterior rhizotomy for children with cerebral palsy: a 7-year experience. *Childs Nerv Syst* **11**: 374–80.

Novacheck TF, Stout JL, Tervo R (2000) Reliability and validity of the Gillette Functional Assessment Questionnaire as an outcome measure in children with walking disabilities. *J Pediatr Orthop* **20**: 75–81.

Paine RS (1962) On the treatment of cerebral palsy:The outcome of 177 patients, 74 totally untreated. *Pediatrics* **29**: 605–16.

Park TS (2000) Selective dorsal rhizotomy: an excellent therapeutic option for spastic cerebral palsy. *Clin Neurosurgery* **47**: 422–39.

Park TS, Vogler GP, Phillips LH 2nd, Kaufman BA, Ortman MR, McClure SM, Gaffney PE (1994) Effects of selective dorsal rhizotomy for spastic diplegia on hip migration in cerebral palsy. *Pediatr Neurosurg* **20**: 43–9.

Payne LZ, DeLuca PA (1993) Heterotopic ossification after rhizotomy and femoral osteotomy. *J Pediatr Orthop* **13**: 733–8.

Peacock WJ, Arens LJ (1982) Selective posterior rhizotomy for the relief of spasticity in cerebral palsy. *S Afr Med J* **62**: 119–24.

Peacock WJ, Staudt LA (1990) Spasticity in cerebral palsy and the selective posterior rhizotomy procedure. *J Child Neurol* **5**: 179–85.

Peacock WJ, Staudt LA (1991) Functional outcomes following selective posterior rhizotomy in children with cerebral palsy. *J Neurosurg* **74**: 380–5.

Peacock WJ, Arens LJ, Berman B (1987) Cerebral palsy spasticity. Selective posterior rhizotomy. *Pediatr Neurosci* **13**: 61–6.

Peter JC, Arens LJ (1994) Selective posterior lumbosacral rhizotomy in teenagers and young adults with spastic cerebral palsy. *Br J Neurosurg* **8**: 135–9.

Peter JC, Hoffman EB, Arens LJ (1993) Spondylolysis and spondylolisthesis after five-level lumbosacral laminectomy for selective posterior rhizotomy in cerebral palsy. *Childs Nerv Syst* **9**: 285–8.

Privat JM, Benezech J, Frerebeau P, Gros C (1976) Sectorial posterior rhizotomy, a new technique of surgical treatment for spasticity. *Acta Neurochir* **35**: 181.

Romei M, Galli M, Motta F, Schwartz M, Crivellini M, diMilano P (2005) Reply letter to the editor. *Gait Posture* **22**: 378.

Rosenbaum P, Stewart D (2004) The World Health Organization International Classification of Functioning, Disability, and Health: a model to guide clinical thinking, practice and research in the field of cerebral palsy. *Semin Pediatr Neurol* **11**: 5–10.

Sanger TD, Delgado MR, Gaebler-Spira D, Hallett M, Mink JW (2003) Classification and definition of disorders causing hypertonia in chilhood. *Pediatrics* **111**: 89–97.

Sanger TD, Chen D, Delgado MR, Gaebler-Spira D, Hallett M, Mink JW, Taskforce on Childhood Motor Disorders (2006) Definition and classification of negative motor signs in childhood. *Pediatr* **118**: 2159–67.

Schutte LM, Narayanan U, Stout JL, Selber P, Gage JR, Schwartz MH (2000) An index for quantifying deviations from normal gait. *Gait Posture* **11**: 25–31.

Schwartz MH (2001) The effect of gait pathology on the energy cost of walking. *Gait Posture* **13**: 260.

Schwartz MH (2007) Protocol changes can improve the reliability of net oxygen cost data. *Gait Posture* **26**: 494–500.

Schwartz MH, Viehweger E, Stout J, Novacheck TF, Gage JR (2004) Comprehensive treatment of ambulatory children with cerebral palsy: an outcome assessment. *J Pediatr Orthop* **24**: 45–53.

Schwartz MH, Koop SE, Bourke JL, Baker R (2006) A nondimensional normalization scheme for oxygen utilization data. *Gait Posture* **24**: 14–22.

Spiegel DA, Loder RT, Alley KA, Rowley S, Gutknecht S, Smith-Wright DL, Dunn ME (2004) Spinal deformity following selective dorsal rhizotomy. *J Pediatr Orthop* **24**: 30–6.

Staudt LA, Peacock WJ, Oppenheim WL (1990) The role of selective posterior rhizotomy in the management of cerebral palsy. *Infants Young Children* **2**: 48–58.

Steinbok P (2001) Outcomes after selective dorsal rhizotomy for spastic cerebral palsy. *Childs Nerv Syst* **17**: 1–18.

Steinbok P (2007) Selective dorsal rhizotomy for spastic cerebral palsy: a review. *Childs Nerv Syst* **23**: 981–90.

Steinbok P, Kestle JR (1996) Variation between centers in electrophysiologic techniques used in lumbosacral selective dorsal rhizotomy for spastic cerebral palsy. *Pediatr Neurosurg* **25**: 233–39.

Steinbok P, Schrag C (1998) Complications after selective posterior rhizotomy for spasticity in children with cerebral palsy. *Pediatr Neurosurg* **28**: 300–13.

Steinbok P, Reiner AM, Beauchamp R, Armstrong RW, Cochrane DD, Kestle J (1997) A randomized clinical trial to compare selective posterior rhizotomy plus physiotherapy with physiotherapy alone in children with spastic diplegic cerebral palsy. *Dev Med Child Neurol* **39**: 178–84.

Steinbok P, Hicdonmez T, Sawatzky B, Beauchamp R, Wickenheiser D (2005) Spinal deformities after selective dorsal rhizotomy for spastic cerebral palsy. *J Neurosurg* **102**: 363–73.

Subramanian N, Vaughan CL, Peter JC, Arens LJ (1998) Gait before and 10 years after rhizotomy in children with cerebral palsy spasticity. *J Neurosurg* **88**: 1014–19.

Thomas SS, Aiona MD, Pierce R, Piatt JH 2nd (1996) Gait changes in children with spastic diplegia after selective dorsal rhizotomy. *J Pediatr Orthop* **16**: 747–52.

Tilton AH (2003) Approach to the rehabilitaion of spasticity and neuromuscular disorders in children. *Neurol Clin N Am* **21**: 853–81.

Tilton AH (2004) Management of spasticity in children with cerebral palsy. *Semin Pediatr Neurol* **11**: 58–65.

Trost JP, Schwartz MH, Krach LE, Dunn ME, Novacheck TF (2008) Comprehensive short-term outcome assessment of selective dorsal rhizotomy. *Dev Med Child Neurol* **50**: 765–71.

Turi M, Kalen V (2000) The risk of spinal deformity after selective dorsal rhizotomy. *J Pediatr Orthop* **20**: 104–7.

van Schie PE, Vermeulen RJ, van Ouwerkerk WJ, Kwakkel G, Becher JG (2005) Selective dorsal rhizotomy in cerebral palsy to improve functional abilities: evaluation of criteria for selection. *Childs Nerv Syst* **21**: 451–7.

Vaughan CL, Berman B, Staudt LA, Peacock WJ (1988) Gait analysis of cerebral palsy children before and after rhizotomy. *Pediatr Neurosci* **14**: 297–300.

Vaughan CL, Berman B, Peacock WJ (1991) Cerebral palsy and rhizotomy. A 3-year follow-up evaluation with gait analysis. *J Neurosurg* **74**: 178–84.

Vaughan CL, Subramanian N, Busse ME (1998) Selective dorsal rhizotomy as a treatment option for children with spastic cerebral palsy. *Gait Posture* **8**: 43–59.

Wright FV, Sheil EM, Drake JM, Wedge JH, Naumann S (1998) Evaluation of selective dorsal rhizotomy for the reduction of spasticity in cerebral palsy: a randomized controlled tria. *Dev Med Child Neurol* **40**: 239–47.

Yasuoka S, Peterson HA, MacCarty CS (1982) Incidence of spinal column deformity after multilevel laminectomy in children and adults. *J Neurosurg* **57**: 441–45.

Young RR (1994) Spasticity: a review. *Neurology* **44**: S12–20.

5.3
NEUROSURGICAL TREATMENT OF DYSTONIA

Leland Albright

Dystonia, the involuntary sustained muscle contractions that cause twisting and abnormal postures, particularly in people with cerebral palsy (CP), is the second most common movement disorder (after spasticity) in CP, and is greatly underrecognized. Diagnosis and treatment of dystonia is important to orthopaedists treating individuals with CP. Otherwise, as one pediatric orthopaedist quipped, 'Dystonia is when the orthopaedic surgeon does an operation and it doesn't work.'

Review of relevant pathophysiology
Dystonia appears to be caused by excessive excitation of the premotor and supplementary motor cortices because of an abnormality in the two neural circuits connecting them with the basal ganglia. The resultant abnormal output from the primary motor cortex travels down the corticospinal tract and out via the ventral roots to cause the dystonic muscle contractions. Treatment could thus be targeted at the excessively stimulated cortex, the dysfunctional neural loops between the basal ganglia and the cortex, or the nerves innervating dystonic muscles.

Historical perspective
Dystonia was treated – ineffectively – in the first half of the 20th century by ablation of the motor cortex and premotor cortex. In the 1950s, Cooper made lesions in the globus pallidus and thalamus and reported improvement in 70% of patients but similar results have not been replicated by others (Cooper 1969). Thalamotomies, operations that made lesions in the ventrolateral thalamus, improved dystonia in approximately 25% of patients, but results were unpredictable and delayed for several months (Andrew et al. 1983). Bilateral thalamic and globus pallidus lesions are often complicated by trouble speaking and swallowing, and are no longer done. Focal dystonia causing torticollis has been treated since the mid-1970s by selective denervation of C1–5, the Bertrand procedure (Bertrand 1993).

Key points
- Dystonia must be distinguished from spasticity and athetosis, with which it may be associated.
- Unless dystonia is treated, the dystonic muscle contractions it causes will increase the likelihood that the orthopaedic release of a dystonic muscle contracture will be unsuccessful.

Indications from patient assessment

It is essential to determine whether the patient's dystonia is primary (in which case it will probably respond well to deep brain stimulation), dopa-responsive (in which case dopa – e.g. Sinemet – is virtually curative), heredo-degenerative (in which case the treatment should be one whose effects can be adjusted as the disease progresses), or secondary – the consequence of cerebral palsy, trauma, or other structural lesions. The vast majority of the cases of dystonia that orthopaedists will encounter are secondary dystonia, in persons with cerebral palsy, where it may be focal, regional, hemidystonic or generalized. The most common form by far (~ 90%) is generalized.

Neurosurgical treatment of dystonia can be considered if the patient has not responded satisfactorily to oral medications and/or botulinum toxin injections. The dystonic movements impede function and caregiving, and cause discomfort. Sustained dystonic muscle contractions occasionally lead to the development of muscle contractures, particularly of the plantarflexors and posterior tibial muscles. Because dystonic muscle contractions are usually somewhat migratory and not sustained for long periods of time, musculoskeletal contractures are much less common than in people with spasticity.

Goals of treatment

The primary goals of treatment are most often to increase patient comfort and to facilitate care. Severe dystonia causes painful muscle spasms: individuals arch their neck forcibly backward and break the headrest on their wheelchair; they extend their trunk backward – making seating in a wheelchair difficult without a lap bar; and they extend the legs and feet tonically downward, breaking the wheelchair footrest.

Improving function is not often a primary goal of neurosurgical intervention, particularly in dystonic cerebral palsy. Although function may improve after treatment of primary dystonia, it improves less often in people with secondary dystonia – on average, in one-third. Prevention of musculoskeletal contractures is almost never a treatment goal in dystonia, in contradistinction to treating spasticity.

Treatment options

Treatment modalities for dystonia include oral medications, intramuscular medications, intrathecal medications, nerve transection, and deep brain stimulation. *Oral medications* are used mainly for generalized dystonia in younger children, e.g. 2–8 years of age, and are mildly helpful. The common oral medications are baclofen, trihexyphenidyl (Artane), and levodopa-carbidopa (Sinemet). The use of a GABA agonist (baclofen), an anticholinergic (trihexyphenidyl), and a dopa-agonist (levodopa-carbidopa) indicates that no single neurotransmitter abnormality is at work in dystonia. Baclofen doses are usually 10–30 mg t.i.d., trihexyphenidyl doses 3–7 mg t.i.d., and levodopa-carbidopa doses 25/100mg 1–3 times a day. Oral tizanidine and dantrolene have been used less often. On average, 26% of individuals have a beneficial response to oral medications (Chuang et al. 2002). Combination therapy appears to be more beneficial than monotherapy.

The *intrathecal medication* is almost always baclofen; intrathecal use of clonidine for dystonia is rare. Intrathecal baclofen (ITB) may affect dystonia at a cortical level by inhibiting the excessively stimulated premotor and supplementary motor cortex. The site of action is uncertain, however. Electrophysiological data including motor-evoked potentials and H reflex have indicated a spinal site of action (Dachy and Dan 2004). It is quite possible that both cortical and spinal sites are affected. ITB involves the implantation of a programmable pump to continuously infuse baclofen via an intrathecal catheter (Fig. 5.3.1). ITB may be infused in a continuous rate or a variable rate, e.g. 200 μg every 4 hours. There are no criteria to determine if a continuous or variable rate is better; if children do not respond to continuous infusion of 800–1000 μg/day, intermittent boluses can be tried.

Nerve transections such as peripheral neurectomies, ramisectomies and rhizotomies are operations that divide motor components of nerves innervating dystonic muscles. These procedures have been used far more often in Europe, India and developing countries than in the USA, and used more often to treat focal spasticity than focal dystonia, but because they divide motor roots or fascicles, they treat both spasticity and dystonia. They will be discussed in greater detail below.

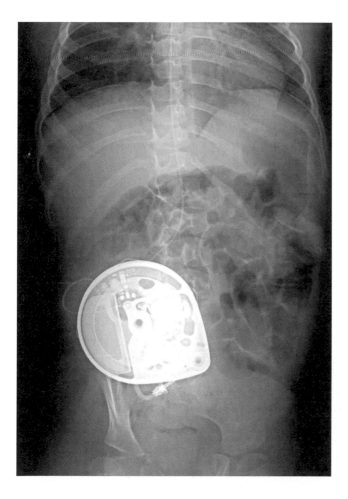

Fig. 5.3.1 Infusion pump and intrathecal catheter.

431

Deep brain stimulation (DBS) involves the stereotactic implantation of electrodes into the basal ganglia (usually the internal globus pallidus) and an implantable, programmable, pulse generator (Fig. 5.3.2). The electrodes may be implanted according to coordinates calculated from magnetic resonance (MR) scans or by supplementing those coordinates with data from microelectrode recording. In the latter, microelectrodes are inserted to a depth approximately 2.5 cm above the target, then advanced in sub-millimeter increments while recording the electrical discharges of individual neurons. Neurons in the putamen, external globus pallidus and internal globus pallidus have characteristic patterns of discharging; those patterns can be observed on an oscilloscope and heard on an amplifier. When the best target is identified by the microelectrode recording, the microelectrode is removed and a permanent electrode is inserted and connected via extension wires to the pulse generator, which is implanted subcutaneously in the infraclavicular region. Postoperatively, programming often requires several months to identify the optimal stimulation parameters. Programming is complex, adjusting voltage, pulse width, stimulation frequency, and contacts in either monopolar or bipolar modes. Programming DBS is far more complex than programming ITB.

FOCAL DYSTONIA

Oral medications are used infrequently for focal dystonia. Intramuscular injections of botulinum toxins (serotype A – Botox, and serotype B – Myobloc) are the primary nonsurgical treatment and may be effective for several years. The American Academy of Neurology recently reviewed the published literature about botulinum toxin and found seven class I studies of its usefulness for cervical dystonia, one class I study and three class II studies for focal upper-extremity dystonia, and one class II study for focal lower-extremity dystonia (Simpson et al. 2008). Doses of botulinum toxin needed to treat dystonia are often higher than those required to treat spasticity.

Neurosurgical procedures are indicated when botulinum toxin is ineffective or a more permanent therapy is desired. Although peripheral neurectomies are often appropriate for focal extremity spasticity, they are infrequently used for focal dystonia in the upper extremities because they partially denervate the limb and never improve function. However, sometimes partial denervation and the consequent limp limb is a significant improvement over a severely dystonic limb. Focal cervical dystonia (causing some variant of torticollis) can be treated with division of the posterior rami of C1–5, a modification of the original Bertrand procedure (Bouvier and Molina-Negro 2004). Focal extremity dystonia in non-functional children, or in sites where ITB and DBS are not available, can be treated with ventral rhizotomies, dividing approximately 85% of the ventral roots innervating the dystonia muscles. That degree of denervation does not paralyze the muscle but markedly decreases the severity of dystonic muscle contractions. If the dystonia coexists with spasticity in the same extremity, a dorsal rhizotomy can be done at the same time to treat the spasticity (Albright and Tyler-Kabara 2007).

We have used epidural motor cortex stimulation (EMCS) to treat three young adults with focal secondary dystonia of the upper extremity. EMCS involves the implantation of an epidural strip electrode over the motor cortex innervating the dystonic upper extremity

432

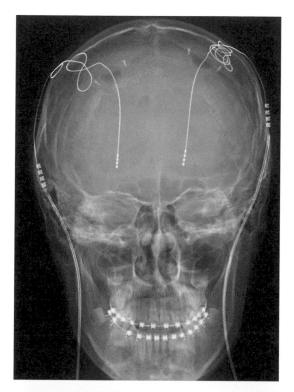

Fig. 5.3.2 Anteroposterior radiograph (top) and coronal MRI (bottom) showing bilateral DBS electrodes in the internal globus pallidus.

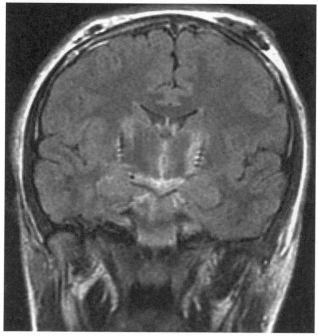

433

(Priori and Lefaucheur 2007) (Fig. 5.3.3). The electrode is connected by extension wires to the same type pulse-generator that is used in DBS. We obtained sustained mild improvement in dystonia in one of the three patients but only transient improvement in the other two. EMCS has the potential to treat focal upper-extremity dystonia with considerably less complexity than is involved with DBS but its use is in its infancy.

HEMIDYSTONIA

The typical appearance of a person with hemidystonic CP is demonstrated in Figure 5.3.4. The appearance is different from that of an individual with spastic hemiparesis – lacking the characteristic flexion at multiple joints – and muscle bulk in dystonia is typically accentuated because of the sustained 'isometric' muscle contractions. As shown in the figure, muscle contractures develop and require orthopaedic releases. However, recurrence of the contractures is likely if the dystonia is not addressed, analogous to the recurrence of contractures if significant spasticity is not addressed.

Hemidystonia is usually secondary to a structural lesion in the basal ganglia or thalamus and may be treated by either ITB or deep brain stimulation if it is refractory to oral medications. No comparisons of the outcomes of ITB and DBS have been done. ITB is a simpler treatment for hemidystonia than DBS. As an initial neurosurgical step, it is

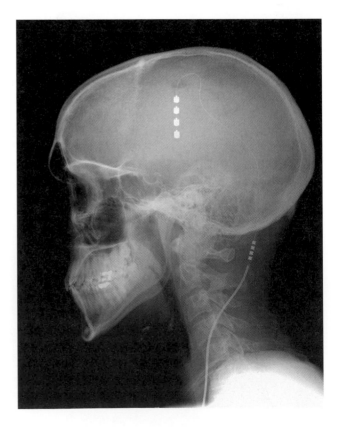

Fig. 5.3.3 Strip electrode used for epidural motor cortex stimulation.

reasonable to evaluate the response of hemidystonia to ITB by a continuous infusion screening trial.

In such a trial, an intrathecal catheter is inserted and connected to an external micro-infusion pump. ITB is infused continuously, beginning at 200 μg/day and increasing in increments of 50 μg every 8 hours until improvement of the dystonia is evident, adverse side effects occur, or a total daily dose of 900 μg/day is given without reduction in the dystonia. Too few patients with hemidystonic CP have been treated to know accurately how effective it is; extrapolation from data about ITB for generalized dystonia would indicate improvement in 85%–90%. Ideally, dystonia is graded before the trial and at intervals during it by a physical therapist. Grading can be with either of two validated scales, the Barry–Albright Dystonia (BAD) scale or the Burke–Fahn–Marsden (BFM) scale (Barry et al. 1999). The BAD scale was developed to grade secondary dystonia in children, the BFM scale to grade primary dystonia in adults.

DBS has been used to treat hemidystonia in a small number of patients. In Zhang et al.'s (2006) series of nine patients with secondary dystonia, two patients with hemidystonia were treated by DBS of the subthalamic nucleus. One had slight improvement and the other had less stiffness of his shoulder and mildly improved posture. Loher et al. (2000) used DBS of the internal globus pallidus to treat a 24-year-old with hemidystonia secondary to a head

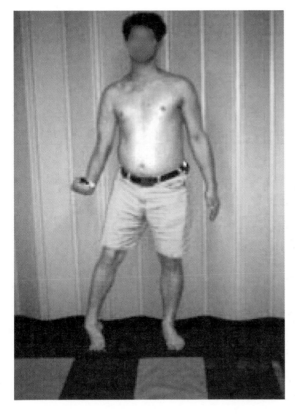

Fig. 5.3.4 Characteristic hemidystonic posture.

injury at age 15 with sustained improvement in dystonia, pain and posture after 4 years of follow-up.

GENERALIZED DYSTONIA

Perhaps 90% of dystonia in persons with CP is generalized; most of these are non-ambulatory and in Gross Motor Function Classification System (GMFCS) levels IV and V. Neurosurgical intervention is appropriate if they have failed oral medications, but is also appropriate if their dystonia is severe, since the likelihood that it can be effectively treated with oral medications, even multiple oral medications, is small.

ITB is the initial treatment for severe generalized dystonic CP. We used continuous ITB infusion screening trials in the first hundred or more patients and found that 90% or more responded to the infusion with significant reductions in dystonia, and now no longer do the screening trials. The intrathecal catheters are positioned higher, e.g. C1–4, when treating dystonia than when treating spastic quadriparesis. In general, ITB doses needed to treat dystonia are twice or more the doses needed to treat spasticity (where the site of action is clearly at the spinal cord level). Recently intraventricular baclofen (IVB) has been used to treat generalized dystonic CP (Albright 2009). IVB is particularly useful in children with fused spines who need infusion into spinal fluid. IVB doses needed to obtain satisfactory improvement in dystonia appear to be lower than when the infusion is intrathecal.

In our 2001 report of ITB in the first 89 cases with dystonia treated for 1 year or longer, we found that dystonia scores on the BAD scale improved significantly, from a mean score of 18 (out of a maximum possible of 32) pre-ITB, to 13 at 3 months, 10 at 6 months, and 7 at 12 months postoperatively, p < 0.001 (Albright et al. 2001). 92% of the patients retained their improvement during 2 years of follow-up. Patients and caregivers reported that quality of life improved in 85%, ease of care increased in 86%, speech improved in 33%, and extremity function improved in 34/36% (upper/lower extremities). Since that publication, other authors have reported benefit of ITB for individuals with secondary dystonia (Dachy and Dan 2004, Woon et al. 2007, Motta et al. 2008). Motta et al. (2008) evaluated the effects of ITB in children in level V of the Gross Motor Function Classification Sysyem (GMFCS) by its effects on their BFM and BAD scores at 3, 6 and 12 months after ITB. Scores were significantly decreased on both scales, to approximately the same extent.

The use of ITB in dystonia appears to be associated with a higher frequency of complications than are seen when treating spasticity. In our 2001 publication, surgical complications occurred in 36% of patients and included CSF leaks in 8%, infections in 14% and catheter problems in 21% (Albright et al. 2001). Several patients had more than one complication. However, the complication rate has decreased substantially since then. The infection rate has decreased with better antimicrobial therapy, including prepping with chlorhexidine and other modalities listed in a recent publication about best practices in ITB therapy (Albright et al. 2006). The currently available intrathecal catheters are far better than the ones used prior to the 2001 publication, and have been associated with complication rates in the 5% range in the past 2 years.

For patients with generalized secondary dystonia who do not respond adequately to ITB, DBS should be considered. DBS is the treatment of choice for primary dystonia but for secondary generalized dystonia it is generally used only if ITB is found to be ineffective. To treat generalized dystonia, electrodes are usually inserted bilaterally into the internal globus palllidus (GPi) (Starr et al. 2006). Electrodes have been inserted recently into the subthalmic nucleus; data are not available to know which of the two sites is better.

It seems clear that the response of secondary dystonia to DBS is substantially less than the response of primary dystonia. Cif et al. (2003) reported DBS of GPi in 21 patients. At a mean follow-up of 23 months, their Burke–Fahn–Marsden (BFM) scores were decreased by 31%. Alterman and Tagliati (2007) treated five children with secondary dystonia with DBS of the internal globus pallidus and observed 33% reductions in their BFM scores one year postoperatively. Zhang et al. (2006) treated nine patients who had secondary dystonia with DBS, primarily of the subthalamic nucleus, and reported only mild improvement. Of the six patients reported by Eltahawy et al. (2004) with DBS of the GPi, patients had either mild or no improvement in their dystonia and no functional improvement.

Summary

The treatment of dystonia in individuals with CP has improved substantially in the past decade. Focal dystonia is being treated with peripheral neurectomies or ventral rhizotomies. Hemidystonic CP is being treated with ITB or DBS, although which procedure is better is unknown. Generalized dystonic CP, the most common form, can be substantially improved in most individuals with ITB, and for those who do not respond sufficiently to ITB, DBS may be helpful. Although the improvement of dystonia by DBS is only 30%–35% or so, that improvement may be of substantial clinical significance in persons with severe dystonia who have been refractory to oral medications, botulinum toxin injections and ITB.

REFERENCES

Albright AL, Ferson, SS (2009) Intraventricular baclofen for dystonia; techniques and outcomes. *J Neurosurg Pediatr* 3: 11–14.
Albright AL, Tyler-Kabara EC (2007) Combined ventral and dorsal rhizotomies for dystonic/spastic extremities. *J Neurosurg Pediatr* 107: 324–7.
Albright AL, Barry MJ, Shafron DH, Ferson SS (2001) Intrathecal baclofen for generalized dystonia. *Dev Med Child Neurol* 43: 652–7.
Albright AL, Turner M, Pattisapu JV (2006) 'Best practice' surgical techniques for intrathecal baclofen therapy. *J Neurosurg Pediatr* 104: 233–9.
Alterman RL, Tagliati M (2007) Deep brain stimulation for torsion dystonia in children. *Childs Nerv Syst* 23: 1033–40.
Andrew J, Fowler CJ, Harrison MJG (1983) Stereotaxic thalamotomy in 55 cases of dystonia. *Brain* 106: 981–7.
Barry MJ, Van Swearingen, Albright AL (1999) Reliability and responsiveness of the Barry–Albright Dystonia Scale. *Dev Med Child Neurol* 41: 404–11.
Bertrand CM (1993) Selective peripheral denervation for spasmodic torticollis: surgical technique, results and observations in 260 cases. *Surg Neurol* 40: 96–103.
Bouvier G, Molina-Negro P (2004) Selective peripheral denervation for spasmodic torticollis. In: Winn HR, editor. *Youman's Neurological Surgery*, 5th edn. Philadelphia: W.B. Saunders. p 2891–9.
Burke RE, Fahn S, Marsden CD, Bressman SB, Moskowitz C, Friedman J (1995) Validity and reliability of a rating scale for the primary torsion dystonias. *Neurology* 35: 73–7.
Chuang C, Fahn S, Frucht SJ (2002) The natural history and treatment of acquired hemidystonia: report of 33 cases and review of the literature. *J Neurol Neurosurg Psychiatry* 72: 57–67.

Cif L, El Fertit H, Vayssiere N, Hemm S, Hardouin E, Gannau A, Tuffery S, Coubes P (2003) Treatment of dystonic syndromes by chronic electrical stimulation of the internal globus pallidus. *J Neurosurg Sci* **47**: 52–5.

Cooper IS (1969) *Involuntary Movement Disorders*. New York: Harper & Row. p 131–292.

Dachy B, Dan B (2004) Electrophysiological assessment of the effect of intrathecal baclofen in dystonic children. *Clin Neurophysiol* **115**: 774–8.

Eltahawy HA, Saint-Cyr J, Giladi N, Lang AE, Lozano AM (2004) Primary dystonia is more responsive than secondary dystonia to pallidal interventions: outcome after pallidotomy or pallidal deep brain stimulation. *Neurosurgery* **54**: 610–21.

Loher TJ, Hasdemir MG, Burgunder J-M, Krauss JK (2000) Long-term follow-up study of chronic globus pallidus internus stimulation for posttraumatic hemidystonia. *J Neurosurg* **92**: 457–60.

Motta F, Stignani C, Antonello CE (2008) Effect of intrathecal baclofen on dystonia in children with cerebral palsy and the use of functional scales. *J Pediatr Orthop* **28**: 213–17.

Priori A, Lefaucheur J-P (2007) Chronic epidural motor cortical stimulation for movement disorders. *Lancet Neurol* **6**: 279–86.

Simpson DB, Blitzer A, Brashear A, Comella C, Dubinsky R, Hallett M, Jankovic J, Karp B, Ludlow CL, Miyasaki JM, Naumann M, So Y (2008) Assessment: botulinum neurotoxin for the treatment of movement disorders (an evidence-based review): report of the Therapeutics and Technology Assessment Subcommittee of the American Academy of Neurology. *Neurol* **70**: 1699–706.

Starr PA, Turner RS, Rau G, Lindsey N, Heath S, Volz M, Ostrem JL, Marks WJ (2006) Microelectrode-guided implantation of deep brain stimulators into the globus pallidus internus for dystonia: techniques, electrode locations, and outcomes. *J Neurosurg* **104**: 488–501.

Woon K, Tsegaye M, Vloeberghs MH (2007) The role of intrathecal baclofen in the management of primary and secondary dystonia in children. *Br J Neurosurg* **21**: 355–8.

Zhang J-G, Zhang K, Wang Z-C, Ge M, Ma Y (2006) Deep brain stimulation in the treatment of secondary dystonia. *Chin Med J* **119**, 2069–74.

5.4
REHABILITATION FOLLOWING SPASTICITY REDUCTION

Linda E. Krach

Reduction of hypertonicity is only one part of what should be a coordinated approach to care involving multiple specialties that is customized for the individual patient (Petropoulou et al. 2007). There is a general consensus that it is appropriate to have individuals participate in an intensified rehabilitation program after they undergo spasticity reduction, but there has not been a systematic evaluation of rehabilitation interventions for this purpose. It has been suggested, however, that reduction of muscle tone allows increased voluntary muscle activation, which might increase the effectiveness of a strengthening program (van Doornik et al. 2008). Reports have appeared that include descriptions of a variety of rehabilitation programs.

It is important to remember that spasticity is only one of the impairments that can be associated with cerebral palsy. Even after the reduction of muscle tone, deficits in balance, motor control, strength, coordination, and sensation can be present and impact rehabilitation potential. Secondary problems can exist as well including bony deformities and contractures (McDonald 1991). The correction of bony deformities resulting from abnormal muscle pull on growing bones is often indicated as well. The degree of these deformities can also impact the ability to effectively rehabilitate an individual. If the deformity is severe it can interfere with the appropriate biomechanical action of the muscle and make it difficult to effectively strengthen the muscle. After tone reduction it may be easier to stretch contractures, decreasing the need for surgical intervention.

Overall, the post-tone reduction rehabilitation program is impacted by the goals that were established prior to intervention. If an intrathecal baclofen pump is placed for comfort and to ease the provision of care it is most likely that an evaluation of post-procedure status and equipment needs will suffice. However, if the goal is to improve ambulation a more intensive program of strengthening, stretching and motor practice is likely to be undertaken.

Selective dorsal rhizotomy

Most commonly, selective dorsal rhizotomy (SDR) is performed on children who tend to be relatively functional, typically in Gross Motor Function Classification System levels I–III, so their goals often relate to ambulation (Chan et al. 2008). Immediately after SDR there is a dramatic decrease in muscle tone. Often children and parents interpret this as weakness, as they are used to using their hypertonicity to assist them with activities. It is logical that children would need a course of rehabilitation services to assist them with strengthening, stretching, relearning how to move with less muscle tone (Giuliani 1991). Reports of post-SDR rehabilitation programs in the literature have varied widely. It is common to keep the children at bed rest without elevation of their heads for 48–96 hours after surgery. This is to allow sufficient time for the dura to seal and to avoid the development of a cerebrospinal fluid leak. During bed rest, therapists can begin working with children, building a rapport and providing gentle passive range of motion. Once children are comfortable, more active intervention can begin. After this time period, some allow children to return to their usual activities with an outpatient therapy program while others have advocated a prolonged inpatient rehabilitation course of up to 3 months followed by outpatient therapies as well (McDonald 1991, Buckon et al. 2002, Krach 2004, Chan et al. 2008). Chan et al. (2008) described their intensive physical therapy program through 12 months after SDR, including objectives, location and intensity. Their program involves a 4-week inpatient stay with 5 hours of therapy per day, and then continues with 3–6 hours of outpatient therapy per week throughout the remainder of the first 12 months after SDR. Although they carefully document therapy intervention, they did not include the rationale for this specific protocol. There is a general consensus that intensive therapy services, either inpatient and outpatient, or only outpatient need to continue for a period of time after SDR. This is generally thought to be 6–12 months (Oppenheim 1990, Bleck 1993, Nishida et al. 1995, Steinbok et al. 1997, McLaughlin et al. 1998, Wright et al. 1998, Olree et al. 2000).

Programs restrict passive hamstring stretching for varying periods of time. This is hypothesized to allow dural healing before providing a stretch to neural bundles that can be transmitted to the dura. Typically this restriction ranges from 3 to 6 weeks (McDonald 1991, Krach 2004). Our institution also limits passive trunk rotation, allowing active pain-free trunk rotation, for the first 6 weeks after surgery.

Knee-immobilizers are placed on the children after the conclusion of the surgery to assist with positioning. In our experience this has not only assisted with beginning work on hamstring stretching, but also has decreased the hip- and knee-flexor spasms that are sometimes seen post-SDR. Once the period of flat bed rest is over, the children also work on prone positioning, prone on elbows and prone on extended arms, to assist with hip-flexor stretching and to work on neck, upper back, and shoulder girdle strength and stability (Krach 2004).

Early post-SDR is often a good time to institute a serial casting program if ankle plantarflexion contractures are present. Since the tone has been reduced, the stretching is often much more effective than any attempts prior to surgery. Typically casts can be changed every 7–10 days. Accomplishing the casting in the shortest amount of time possible is helpful to allow the progression of activities during the active rehabilitation phase. Weightbearing casts can be used as appropriate (Krach 2004). This is important since goals of SDR are usually to improve ambulation, particularly since FDA approval of intrathecal baclofen for children and spasticity of cerebral origin.

Tailoring the intervention for the individual child and maintaining a flexible approach over the course of the postoperative rehabilitation experience is imperative. As the children increase both their range of motion and strength it is common that needs for assistive devices for ambulation and orthoses change. Typically less supportive devices are needed over time until improvements plateau. This is particularly true of assistive devices if the children are able to strengthen hip-extensors and abductors sufficiently (Krach 2004).

Some clinicians have expressed concerns about continuing weakness after SDR. This has been investigated by several groups. Quantitative muscle strength assessment has shown improvement in absolute knee-extensor strength, knee-flexor strength, and ankle dorsiflexion strength 8–12 months post-SDR. Ankle plantarflexion strength did not change (Steinbok et al. 1995, Engsberg et al. 1998, 2000, Buckon et al. 2002). However, it should be noted that growth is also common after SDR and these reports did not consistently state whether they normalized strength for the child's size. Buckon et al. (2002) did note that although absolute strength increased they did not see a significant change in strength when values were normalized for the significant increase in height and weight.

The approach to therapy after SDR tends to be an eclectic one, including aspects of neurodevelopmental therapy, proprioceptive neuromuscular facilitation and the incorporation of principles of motor control. Use of an assistive device for ambulation during rehabilitation can be helpful in slowing the child to allow more conscious practice of an improved movement pattern. Integrating a more normal movement pattern can take a significant period of time (Peacock et al. 1987, Wright et al. 1998).

It is also important to include upper extremity activities, including fine-motor skills, and to work on increasing independence in activities of daily living as part of the post-SDR rehabilitation program. Usually children can more easily reach their feet after SDR and have success in increasing dressing skills (McDonald 1991, Nishida et al. 1995, Krach 2004).

Changes 1 year after SDR in upper-extremity strength, range of motion, fine-motor coordination, and activities of daily living were reported for a group of 26 children (Buckon et al. 1995). Grasp strength and manipulation patterns improved significantly. Also a significant improvement was seen in the ability to perform toileting skills, dressing and undressing. Albright et al. (1995) reported improvements in hand function and ability to perform activities of daily living after SDR. Another report looked at fine-motor skills 3–5 years after SDR (Mittal et al. 2002). In this series children received an intensive 6-week inpatient rehabilitation program including both occupational and physical therapies and continuing services on an outpatient basis after discharge from the hospital. Their subjects showed significant improvement in fine-motor skills.

Another group evaluated the effect of intensive therapy prior to SDR. Although the therapists believed that the children made more rapid gains early after surgery, there was no difference between the groups at 2 years after surgery (Steinbok and McLeod 2002).

Intrathecal baclofen
Little has been written about the need for rehabilitation after ITB pump implantation. This intervention tends to be used for individuals with greater motoric impairment and therefore frequently goals of treatment are directed to ease of care provision and comfort. In individuals whose goals include ease of care provision, ITB pump implantation often results in the need to change seating systems (Steinbok and McLeod 2002). It is helpful to assess wheelchair seatbelt position and other equipment that could cause pressure over a pump prior

to discharge from the hospital after pump implantation (Krach 2004). When it is mentioned, authors indicate that rehabilitation programs need to be customized for the individual patient (Awaad et al. 2003, Krach 2004, Marra et al. 2007).

One important thing that regular therapy after ITB pump implantation provides is increased feedback to the pump managing provider about the effects of dose changes on tone and function and the need for further dose titration (Krach 2004).

There is not a consensus about pursuing inpatient or outpatient therapy after pump implantation. One published report noted a small improvement in functional skills with an increase in outpatient physical therapy for 1–3 months after pump implantation (Scheinberg et al. 2001). Meythaler et al. (2001) stated that inpatient rehabilitation is important to allow individuals to have optimal benefit from both the reduction in tone and apparent increase in motor control seen after implantation of an ITB pump.

When the patient should engage in a rehabilitation program is another controversial topic. Achieving the optimal dose of ITB for tone reduction can take weeks to several months. Should therapy await dose optimization or begin during the process of dose titration (Krach 2004)?

The frequency of therapy can vary depending on the goal of tone reduction (Albright 1996). If the pump has been implanted with improvement in function as a major goal, therapy should be directed toward achieving this improvement. The use of the Canadian Occupation Performance Measure (COPM) after ITB pump implantation has been reported to assist with patient and caregiver participation in the selection of goals (Guillaume et al. 2005). This study also reported significant improvement in COPM scores 3 and 12 months after pump implantation. Therapy programs were not specified.

If the patient had been bearing weight on lower extremities prior to pump implantation, it is important to assure that they are able to do so after pump implantation. It might initially be necessary to allow some residual spasticity to be present to facilitate this. This can be important for both those who do assisted standing pivot transfers and those who are ambulating with or without assistive devices (Krach 2004, Dones 2007).

Many aspects of 'routine care' for those with severe motoric impairment should be reevaluated after ITB pump implantation. Sometimes tone or spasms have been beneficial for pressure relief in both bed and wheelchair. Patients should be evaluated to ascertain if different cushions or pressure relief routines are required to preserve skin integrity. Also, if orthosis use or position had been limited by dynamic contractures as opposed to fixed contractures, orthoses should be reevaluated and potentially modified or refitted (Krach 2004). If severely motorically impaired patients have volitional movement and it is improved after tone reduction by ITB management, it is appropriate to reevaluate them for the potential to make use of switches for communication, environmental controls, or mobility devices (Krach 2004).

Conclusions

Careful consideration of goals of tone reduction and the likely need for rehabilitation intervention should occur at the time of assessment for these interventions. It is important to remember that cerebral palsy involves more than just abnormal muscle tone and the possible problems with motor control, strength, balance, and weakness, as well as secondary impairments such as contractures or bony deformity, need to be considered both during goal-setting and in designing the rehabilitation program.

Many questions concerning the optimal type and timing of rehabilitation programs after spasticity reduction remain. Current literature is mostly anecdotal with poor descriptions of actual rehabilitation programs undertaken.

REFERENCES

Albright AL (1996) Intrathecal baclofen in cerebral palsy movement disorders. *J Child Neurol* **11** (Suppl 1): S29–35.

Albright AL, Barry MJ, Fasick MP, Janosky J (1995) Effects of continuous intrathecal baclofen infusion and selective posterior rhizotomy on upper extremity spasticity. *Pediatr Neurosurg* **23**: 82–5.

Awaad Y, Tayem H, Munoz S, Ham S, Michon AM, Awaad R (2003) Functional assessment following intrathecal baclofen therapy in children with spastic cerebral palsy. *J Child Neurol* **18**: 26–34.

Bleck E (1993) Posterior rootlet rhizotomy in cerebral palsy. *Arch Dis Child* **68**: 717–19.

Buckon CE, Thomas SS, Aiona MD, Piatt JH (1995) Assessment of upper-extremity function in children with spastic diplegia before and after selective dorsal rhizotomy. *Dev Med Child Neurol* **38**: 967–75.

Buckon CE, Thomas SS, Harris GE, Piatt JH, Aiona MD, Sussman MD (2002) Objective measurement of muscle strength in children with spastic diplegia after selective dorsal rhizotomy. *Arch Phys Med Rehabil* **83**: 454–60.

Chan SH, Yam KY, Yiu-Lau BP, Poon CY, Chan NN, Cheung HM, Wu M, Chak WK (2008) Selective dorsal rhizotomy in Hong Kong: multidimensional outcome measures. *Pediatr Neurol* **39**: 22–32.

Dones I (2007) Intrathecal baclofen for the treatment of spasticity. *Acta Neurochir Suppl* **97**: 185–8.

Engsberg JR, Olree KS, Ross SA, Park TS (1998) Spasticity and strength changes as a function of selective dorsal rhizotomy. *J Neurosurg* **88**: 1020–6.

Engsberg JR, Ross SA, Olree KS, Park TS (2000) Ankle spasticity and strength in children with spastic diplegic cerebral palsy. *Dev Med Child Neurol* **42**: 42–7.

Giuliani C (1991) Dorsal rhizotomy for children with cerebral palsy: support for concepts of motor control. *Phys Ther* **71**: 248–59.

Guillaume D, Van Havenbergh A, Vloeberghs M, Vidal J, Roeste G (2005) A clinical study of intrathecal baclofen using a programmable pump for intractable spasticity. *Arch Phys Med Rehabil* **86**: 2165–71.

Krach LE (2004) Rehabilitation following spasticity reduction. In: Gage JR, editor. *The Treatment of Gait Problems in Cerebral Palsy*. London: Mac Keith Press. p 305–313.

Marra GA, D'Aleo G, Di Bella P, Bramanti P (2007) Intrathecal baclofen therapy in patients with severe spasticity. *Acta Neurochir Suppl* **97**: 173–80.

McDonald CM (1991) Selective dorsal rhizotomy: a critical review. *Phys Med Rehabil Clin N Am* **2**: 891–915.

McLaughlin JF, Bjornson KF, Astley SJ, Graubert C, Hays RM, Roberts TS, Price R, Temkin N (1998) Selective dorsal rhizotomy: efficacy and safety in an investigator-masked randomized clinical trial. *Dev Med Child Neurol* **40**: 220–32.

Meythaler JM, Guin-Renfroe S, Law C, Grabb P, Hadley MN (2001) Continuously infused intrathecal baclofen over 12 months for spastic hypertonia in adolescents and adults with cerebral palsy. *Arch Phys Med Rehabil* **82**: 155–61.

Mittal S, Farmer J, Al-Atassi B, Montpetit K, Gervais N, Poulin C, Benaroch TE, Cantin MA (2002) Impact of selective posterior rhizotomy on fine motor skills: long-term results using a validated evaluative measure. *Pediatr Neurosurg* **36**: 133–41.

Nishida T, Thatcher SW, Marty GR (1995) Selective posterior rhizotomy for children with cerebral palsy: a 7-year experience. *Childs Nerv Syst* **11**: 374–80.

Olree KS, Engsberg JR, Ross SA, Park TS (2000) Changes in synergistic movement patterns after selective dorsal rhizotomy. *Dev Med Child Neurol* **42**: 297–303.

Oppenheim WL (1990) Selective posterior rhizotomy for spastic cerebral palsy. *Clin Orthop Rel Res* **253**: 20–9.

Peacock WJ, Arens LJ, Berman B (1987) Cerebral palsy spasticity. Selective posterior rhizotomy. *Pediatr Neurosci* **13**: 61–6.

443

Petropoulou KB, Panourias IG, Rapidi C, Sakas DE (2007) The importance of neurorehabilitation to the outcome of neuromodulation in spasticity. *Acta Neurochir Suppl* **97**: 243–50.

Scheinberg AM, O'Flaherty S, Chaseling R, Dexter M (2001) Continuous intrathecal baclofen infusion for children with cerebral palsy: a pilot study. *J Paediatr Child Health* **37**: 283–8.

Steinbok P, McLeod K (2002) Comparison of motor outcomes after selective dorsal rhizotomy with and without preoperative intensified physiotherapy in children with spastic diplegic cerebral palsy. *Pediatr Neurosurg* **36**: 142–7.

Steinbok P, Gustavsson B, Kestle JR, Reiner A, Cochrane DD (1995) Relationship of intraoperative electrophysiological criteria to outcome after selective functional posterior rhizotomy. *J Neurosurg* **83**: 18–26.

Steinbok P, Reiner AM, Beauchamp R, Armstrong RW, Cochrane DD (1997) A randomized clinical trial to compare selective posterior rhizotomy plus physiotherapy with physiotherapy alone in children with spastic diplegic cerebral palsy. *Dev Med Child Neurol* **39**: 178–84.

van Doornik J, Kukke S, McGill K, Rose J, Sherman-Levine S, Sanger TD (2008) Oral baclofen increases maximal voluntary neuromuscular activation of ankle plantar flexors in children with spasticity due to cerebral palsy. *J Child Neurol* **23**: 635–9.

Wright FV, Sheil EMH, Drake JM, Wedge JH, Naumann S (1998) Evaluation of selective dorsal rhizotomy for the reduction of spasticity in cerebral palsy: a randomized controlled trial. *Dev Med Child Neurol* **40**: 239–47.

5.5
ORTHOPAEDIC TREATMENT
OF MUSCLE CONTRACTURES

Tom F. Novacheck

Key points
- The treatment algorithm presented in this book is based on the idea of optimizing joint moment generating capacity via spasticity management and correction of bone malalignments. Surgical lengthening of musculotendinous contractures is a consideration of last resort
- Biarticular muscles are primarily affected by the neurological impairments of cerebral palsy. Therefore they are more commonly contracted than are the monoarticular muscles
- Accurate estimation of dynamic biarticular muscle lengths and velocities (lengthening rate) would be the optimal information to guide clinical decision-making for soft tissue lengthening or transfer. While some musculoskeletal models provide this information, further advances are necessary to achieve this goal for all the muscles in question. In the meantime, kinematic and kinetic data must be integrated to guide clinical decision-making
- Although occasionally indicated, isolated soft tissue lengthening is rarely effective and/or useful. Typically these procedures are integrated into a single-event multilevel surgery (SEMLS).

Review of relevant pathophysiology
As mentioned in Chapter 2.4, the neuropathology of cerebral palsy selectively targets the two-joint muscles, such as the psoas, rectus femoris, hamstrings and gastrocnemius. The one-joint muscles are typically not affected by spasticity. In addition, related to the growth pattern and biomechanics of movement in cerebral palsy gait, the one-joint musculo-tendinous units seldom become shortened. In fact, if crouch gait develops, they are typically excessively long.

It is too simplistic to say that the primary pathology in cerebral palsy is hypertonia (spasticity and dystonia) alone. Other primary impairments include poor balance, weakness, and lack of selective motor control. Delays in attaining normal gross motor milestones and atypical walking patterns lead to further bone and joint deformity.

Muscle function during gait is markedly more complicated than what is learned in physiology classes in college and medical schools. Muscles contribute joint moments not only through active muscular contraction but also through the passive properties of the musculotendinous unit (Chapter 2.5) (Delp et al. 1995). Both components of muscle force generation (passive and active) are affected by the length of the structure when the joints and body segments are in functional positions. Sarcomere lengths, muscle fiber-type ratios, muscle fiber length and flexibility can all be adversely affected by cerebral palsy (Shortland et al. 2002). Induced acceleration models make it increasingly clear that dynamic muscle function during gait has important local and remote effects, with some biarticular muscles functioning in a paradoxical manner (Chapter 3.6) (Kimmel and Schwartz 2006).

When we discuss and consider musculotendinous contracture, we should not focus only on the contractures of the two-joint muscles. We must also direct attention to the one-joint muscles, which may be over-elongated either iatrogenically or as a result of the pathological walking pattern. Certainly this consideration should include the avoidance of lengthening these tissues surgically. In addition, increasing emphasis must be placed on re-tensioning (tightening) the one-joint stance-phase stabilizers. Patellar advancement is an example of this that is already successfully implemented (see Chapter 5.11) (Stout et al. 2008). We have also successfully tightened the hip-abductor musculature that is either too weak or over-elongated by advancing the greater trochanter. Hopefully, similar advances can be made with positive benefit for other one-joint muscles such as the gluteus maximus and the soleus.

Historical perspective
The history of the orthopedic management of children with cerebral palsy has been focused on muscle lengthening procedures (Fig. 5.5.1; Video 5.5.1a, b available on the Interactive Disc). Procedures were performed in isolation with children often requiring frequent trips back to the operating room (coined the 'birthday syndrome' by Mercer Rang because of its virtually annual schedule). The focus of the algorithm outlined in this textbook is to potentiate muscle function by relieving or minimizing the damaging affects of hypertonia (see Chapters 4.3, 4.4, 5.1 and 5.2) and optimizing the skeletal lever arms on which they work (see Chapters 5.6–8). Spasticity causes excessive tension and reflexive contractions at inappropriate times during function. Over the years of a child's growth and development, contractures result. Heel cord, hamstring, and adductor lengthening have been the primary targets of surgical lengthening traditionally, with the frequent development of crouch gait and hyperlordosis.

In addition, there has been an inadequate recognition of the differential effect of cerebral palsy on the one- and two-joint muscles. Therefore lengthening of the tendo-Achilles (a significant component of this tissue's function is from the one-joint muscle, the soleus) was a common operation. Similarly, a release of the iliopsoas tendon at the lesser trochanter also ignores this distinction and when it was done in the past, excessive weakening of the hip-flexors was the result (Bleck 1971). The adductors (longus, brevis and magnus) represent a third group of single-joint muscles that have been blamed excessively for the pathology of cerebral palsy gait, and as a result have historically been inappropriately or over-lengthened.

Until the 1970s and 80s, correction of torsional deformities of the femur and tibia (now a mainstay of the treatment algorithm presented in this book) were not typically considered.

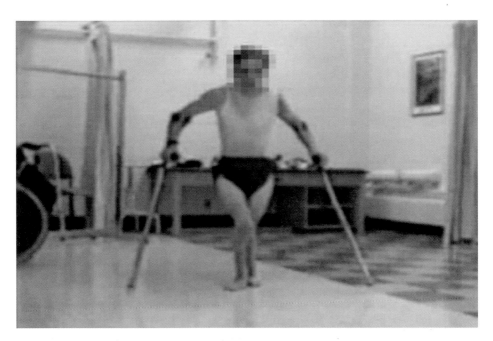

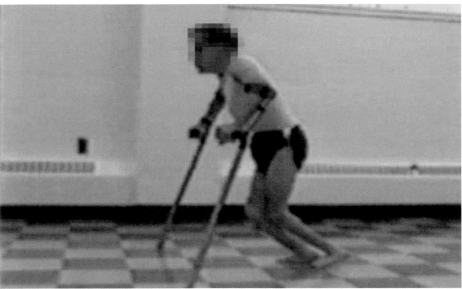

Fig. 5.5.1 Adolescent with diplegic cerebral palsy treated with a series of soft-tissue lengthening procedures through the course of his childhood without any correction of lever-arm deformity. His legs have stiffness, weakness, and malalignment. He lacks strength to support body weight and power for propulsion. Thus he is heavily dependent on his arms for these functions. To avoid this result, the emphasis for surgical management is on spasticity management and correction of lever arm malalignment. The frequency and amount of soft tissue lengthening is thereby minimized. (See Video 5.5.1a and 5.5.1b available on the Interactive Disc.)

Indications from patient assessment

PHYSICAL EXAMINATION

Psoas
Hip-flexion contracture is identified by the Thomas test (Chapter 3.1). The position of the pelvis must be standardized as a reference point for hip joint range of motion with the anterior superior and posterior superior iliac spines positioned in a line that is vertically directed. The existence of lumbar hyperlordosis, when the child is lying in a supine position, is suggestive of hip-flexor tightness. Finally, identifying a difference between the unilateral and bilateral popliteal angle is an indication of hip-flexor tightness on the opposite side. For example, a difference between the popliteal angles with pelvic position corrected and not corrected on the left side indicates a right-sided hip flexion deformity. Because normal walking requires hip extension of 7° in terminal stance, even small degrees of hip-flexion deformity can adversely affect walking function. The presence of hip-flexor spasticity compounds this further.

Adductors
The finding of limited hip abduction range of motion on physical examination is rarely an indication for surgical lengthening of the adductors unless the limitation is severe. Normal hip ad/abduction range of motion during gait is from 10° abduction to 10° adduction. An adduction contracture that allows only 15° hip abduction (with the hip and knee in extension) is therefore fully compatible with normal gait dynamics, unless spasticity is also present.

Hamstrings
The hamstrings have often been implicated as a cause of crouch gait in cerebral palsy. Traditional treatments have focused on hamstring lengthening. However, gait analysis data have shown no correlation between popliteal angle by physical examination and crouch gait (Delp et al. 1996, Thompson et al. 2001, Desloovere et al. 2006, Louis et al. 2008). As a result, static measures should be given limited weight in the decision-making process for the hamstrings. The hamstrings have also been excessively lengthened in situations when anterior pelvic tilt has limited the available hamstring length (Hoffinger et al. 1993, Arnold et al. 2006). While the unilateral popliteal angle (see Chapter 3.1) is more representative of the configuration of the body at the time when maximum hamstring length is needed, the bilateral popliteal angle is more indicative of available hamstring length if other treatments are successful at correcting excessive anterior pelvic tilt during gait. It would be rare to consider a bilateral popliteal angle of less than 30° as being problematic.

Distinguishing knee-joint contracture from hamstring contracture is essential as these physical examination findings point towards different pathologies requiring different treatments.

Rectus femoris
Limited knee-flexion range of motion in the prone position and/or rectus femoris spasticity are indicative of rectus femoris pathology. These are the only physical examination findings specific for the rectus femoris.

Gastrocnemius

The Silverskjøld test is the physical examination test to differentiate soleus from gastrocnemius contracture. In children with diplegia and quadriplegia, there is almost always a clear distinction between them. Contracture of the gastrocnemius is common. Contracture of the soleus is rare. In the hemiplegic population, it is more common to find contractures of both, but even in this condition the gastrocnemius is the more contracted of the two.

As described in Chapter 3.1, it is crucially important that the hindfoot and midfoot be held in the proper position to accurately assess gastrocnemius length. As indicated in Chapter 3.2, examination of the foot in the subtalar neutral position is pivotal for this assessment. If the foot cannot be corrected to subtalar neutral, then surgical correction of the foot deformity could be required first to bring the foot to proper position. Then gastrocnemius and soleus length can be assessed under anesthesia to allow a final decision regarding the need for lengthening.

Differentiation of spasticity from contracture

Range of motion can be restricted by both spasticity and contracture. Care must be taken during the physical examination to differentiate between them (see Chapter 3.1). An examination under anesthesia may be required for some or all of these soft-tissue structures if the patient is uncooperative during physical examination or if spasticity is severe. Under anesthesia, spasticity is eliminated and the physical examination is more specific for restricted musculotendinous length.

IMAGING

Currently, a supine anteroposterior (AP) pelvis radiograph is the only imaging that may be helpful for assessing musculotendinous contractures (see Chapter 3.4). Pelvic obliquity with the femur in an adducted position suggests hip-adductor contracture. An anteriorly tilted pelvis can indicate hip-flexion contracture. On the other hand, malpositioning at the time of radiographic evaluation could be caused by spasticity. These radiographic indicators would never be the sole criterion for surgical intervention. Hip-adduction or flexion contractures can be correlated with hip dysplasia which would be identifiable only radiographically. Posterior pelvic tilting (outlet view of the pelvis, altered projection of the obturator foraminae) can be an indication of severe hamstring contracture. Weightbearing radiographs of the feet can underscore the malpositioning of the calcaneus in an equinus position due to gastrocnemius contracture.

In the future, soft-tissue imaging – ultrasonography or magnetic resonance elastography, for example – may be a helpful adjunct for making decisions regarding musculotendinous contractures (Shortland et al. 2002) (see Chapter 2.5). Intraoperative laser diffraction has been used to assess sarcomere length to guide tensioning of soft tissues intraoperatively to optimize active force generation capacity in a functional position (Lieber and Friden 2002).

OBSERVATIONAL GAIT ANALYSIS

It is difficult to assess pelvic position and pelvic range of motion visually, but with experience, excessive sagittal plane pelvic motion can be accurately identified. This finding would be suggestive of psoas or hamstring contracture. A pelvic tilt that becomes progressively more anterior during mid- to terminal stance, when the hip is going into maximum extension, would suggest restricted flexibility of the psoas. Progressive posterior tilting in terminal swing could indicate hamstring contracture.

In the past a scissoring gait pattern was attributed to adductor pathology, but this is almost always a visual misconception arising from the combination of excessive hip and knee flexion combined with excessive internal hip malrotation. A fixed oblique position of the pelvis could be caused by adductor contracture but also could be due to multiple other etiologies such as leg-length discrepancy, hip dysplasia, and hip-abductor insufficiency.

Stiff-knee gait is a common pattern in children with cerebral palsy. Rectus femoris pathology is one of the most common causes of this pattern. Inadequate power production resulting in decreased knee-flexion velocity in preswing and at toe-off (hip-flexors, knee-flexors, and the ankle plantarflexors) and slow walking speed are also causes (see Chapter 3.6) (Goldberg et al. 2004).

Tight hamstrings can cause a flat back, posterior pelvic tilt, short step length, and poor extension of the knee in late swing. However, other causes of shortened step length include poor stance-phase stability on the opposite side and impaired central balance mechanisms.

It can be difficult to visually differentiate 'true' equinus from 'apparent' equinus on the basis of observation alone. In both cases initial contact occurs on the forefoot instead of the hind-foot and the heel rise occurs too early in mid-stance. In apparent equinus, the pathology is proximal to the ankle. A lack of knee extension leads to a lower leg position that does not allow initial contact with the hindfoot. Apparent equinus has been the cause for many inappropriate heel cord lengthenings because of the misperception based on visual observation. Finally, while a drop-foot in swing phase can be caused by gastrocnemius contracture, it can also be caused by dysfunction of the ankle dorsiflexors.

A variety of observational gait scales have been developed and validated that could be used if the practitioner does not have access to a gait lab. These scales can be used to rate gait quality and could be used for comparisons between visits. Some have been validated against the Gillette Gait Index, and cross-validation studies suggest reliability (Mackey et al. 2003, Maathuis et al. 2005, Wren et al. 2007, Brown et al. 2008).

Quantitative Gait Analysis

A comprehensive review of quantitative gait data interpretation is beyond the scope of any single chapter in this book. Numerous other chapters include aspects of this topic (see Chapters 1.3, 2.6, 3.5, and most of the chapters in this section). Gait interpretation courses and extensive training are required to master these complexities. Since each of the following findings could be caused by other pathologies, caution must be exercised in interpreting the following discussion as it applies to individual patient data to avoid oversimplification. Spasticity and contracture of each of these tissues will manifest themselves at the subphase of the gait cycle when maximum elongation rate and total length attainment occur. Therefore understanding this timing is crucial to quantitative gait data interpretation as it applies to soft-tissue lengthening surgery.

Psoas
Common findings suggestive of hip-flexor dysfunction include the following:

- excessive anterior pelvic tilt
- excessive pelvic tilt range of motion with a double bump pelvic pattern for diplegia and quadriplegic patients, and a single bump pelvic pattern for hemiplegic patients
- diminished extension of the hip in mid- and terminal stance
- a delay in the transition from a hip-extensor moment to a hip-flexor moment (typically occurs at 25% of the gait cycle), referred to as a hip-extensor dominance pattern
- diminished, blunted, or irregular hip-flexor power burst.

Adductors
Diminished abduction in swing phase is perhaps the only reliable finding indicative of hip-adduction contracture. During stance, excessive adduction can be caused by hip-joint pathology, hip-abductor insufficiency, or leg-length discrepancy.

Hamstrings
During the second half of swing, the hamstrings must elongate to allow the hip to remain flexed and for the knee to extend without progressive posterior tilting of the pelvis. The hamstrings must achieve their longest length and must also elongate the most rapidly at this period of the gait cycle. Therefore terminal swing phase is the best time during the gait cycle to identify hamstring contracture (and/or spasticity). This is in sharp distinction to traditional teaching that links crouch gait with hamstring pathology. Numerous factors affect knee position in mid-stance (see Chapter 5.11), making it impossible to identify hamstring pathology during this phase of the gait cycle. When the extremity is unloaded, one can better isolate the effects of the hamstrings.

Rectus femoris
Diminished or delayed peak swing-phase knee flexion associated with pre-swing rectus femoris electromyographic (EMG) activity has been the accepted indication for rectus femoris transfer (Gage et al. 1987, Perry 1987). Over the past few years, this decision-making paradigm has been scrutinized since some patients benefit from the procedure while others do not. Hip flexion power at toe off (H3) and ankle-plantarflexor power generation in pre-swing (A2) are responsible for propelling the limb into swing. Hip and knee flexion result if the hamstrings and gastrocnemius unlock the knee from its position of extension in stance. Deficits in the function of any of these can also lead to inadequate hip and knee flexion in swing. In addition, excessive knee extension moments generated by the vasti during late stance to compensate for a crouch gait position could lead to diminished knee-flexion velocity at toe-off (Goldberg et al. 2004, Reinbolt et al. 2008). Advanced musculoskeletal modeling and statistical modeling and simulation are helping to further refine our understanding of rectus femoris pathology and will likely improve our decision-making regarding specific indications for rectus femoris transfer (see Chapter 3.6).

Gastrocnemius

The primary indicators for soft-tissue lengthening of the gastrocnemius include the following:

- excessive plantarflexion from initial contact through mid-stance or during mid-swing
- delayed or diminished movement of the ankle into dorsiflexion during second rocker
- absent first rocker (immediate onset of a plantarflexion moment at initial contact)
- double bump ankle moment pattern, and
- inappropriate mid-stance ankle plantarflexor power generation.

Two important confounding factors must be kept in mind. First, many of the findings in the above list can also be seen in 'apparent equinus'. Secondly, the effects of midfoot breakdown through the talonavicular joint can mask many of them. Because of the restrictive effects of spasticity and contracture on motion of the calcaneus, the gastrocnemius contributes to the development of this type of foot deformity. If the ankle cannot dorsiflex satisfactorily, then the excessive and premature forefoot loading leads to increased stresses in the midfoot and the development of excessive range of motion (dorsiflexion and abduction) through the talonavicular joint (see Chapter 3.2). Because of these confounding factors, decision-making for gastrocnemius lengthening cannot be based solely on quantitative gait data. Two other factors are also important. First, many different combinations of patterns of kinematics and kinetics can be seen for subjects with gastrocnemius contractures. Second, the simplistic one segment foot model (see Chapters 3.2 and 5.8) limits the utility of quantitative gait data. The ankle may appear to dorsiflex adequately when in actuality, the dorsiflexion is occurring through the talonavicular joint. Finally, one must remember that during second rocker the gastrocnemius must achieve its greatest length as the ankle achieves maximum dorsiflexion at the same time that the knee is maximally extended. Therefore gastrocnemius contracture can contribute to excessive knee flexion in mid-stance (crouch).

Goals of treatment

In general, the goal of lengthening musculotendinous contractures (or transfer in the case of the rectus femoris) is to allow the joints to achieve satisfactory joint position during gait without restriction. If this is not possible, compensatory movement patterns develop. When considering tendon lengthenings, the surgeon must remember that the musculotendinous units are the generators of the forces required to propel body segments and to exert the joint moments necessary to oppose gravitational forces. If musculotendinous length is not satisfactory for the joints to achieve a normal position, then surgical treatment of the musculotendinous unit is necessary. However, careful consideration must be given to the other potential causes of abnormal joint position or range of motion to avoid lengthening a musculotendinous unit whose length is not restrictive. In addition, in order for a muscle to function well on the length vs tension curve, the muscle must be functioning at appropriate length with proper tension in the functional position of the joints and body segments (Fig. 5.5.2). If this is not the case, then judicious muscle lengthening can be safe and appropriate.

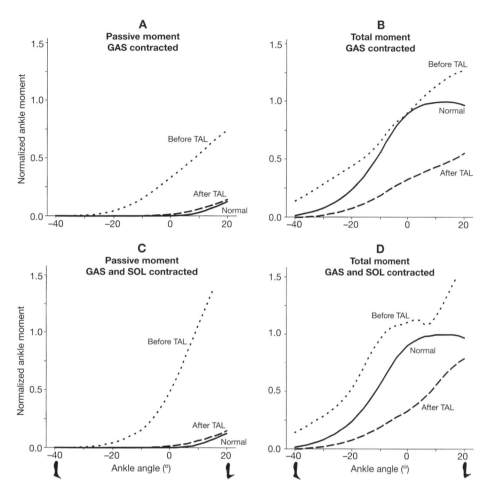

Fig. 5.5.2 The effect of tendo-Achilles lengthening. Ankle moment versus ankle angle before and after simulated Achilles tendon lengthening (TAL) with isolated gastrocnemius (GAS) contracture (A and B) and with contracture of both the gastrocnemius and the soleus (SOL) (C and D). After Achilles tendon lengthening, the passive moment developed by the triceps surae is restored to approximately normal (A and C); however, the total moment is substantially less than normal (B and D). The data suggest that Achilles tendon lengthening should not be used to treat isolated gastrocnemius contracture because doing so may decrease the strength of the plantarflexors greatly (Delp et al 1995).

Treatment options

Since musculoskeletal contractures develop in cerebral palsy primarily due to the effects of abnormal muscle tone, the initial treatment algorithm is focused on non-operative management (Chapters 4.1, 4.2) at young ages followed by tone management (Chapters 4.3, 4.4, 5.1–3) at slightly older ages. If patients are of appropriate age and are candidates for focal or global spasticity management, then typically those treatments are pursued first. If

TABLE 5.5.1
Specific goals of musculotendinous lengthening/transfer surgery in cerebral palsy

Psoas	• attain adequate length to allow normal hip extension without increasing anterior pelvic tilt
Adductors	• improve the balance between the contracted adductors in the face of weak hip-abductors (primarily in stance phase)
	• allow adequate hip abduction during swing to avoid a clearance problem as the swinging limb passes the opposite leg
Hamstrings	• allow extension of the knee in terminal swing without progressive posterior pelvic tilting in order to improve step length
Rectus femoris	• improve peak swing-phase knee flexion and timing in order to improve swing phase clearance
	• convert the rectus femoris from a hip-flexor/knee-extensor to hip-flexor/knee-flexor
Gastrocnemius	• eliminate its deforming effects on the midfoot
	• improve stance phase stability by allowing a plantigrade foot position with the knee in full extension

those treatments are effective, the need for soft-tissue surgery is minimized. For example, hamstring lengthening and rectus femoris transfer are less frequently required following selective dorsal rhizotomy (Schwartz et al. 2004, Trost et al. 2008). If a patient is not a candidate for tone management or contractures develop despite it, then soft-tissue surgery is considered.

PSOAS (SEE INSTRUCTIONAL VIDEO 'PSOAS LENGTHENING AT THE PELVIC BRIM')
Psoas lengthening at the pelvic brim is the treatment of choice. A variety of techniques have been described (Skaggs et al. 1997, Sutherland et al. 1997, Novacheck et al. 2002).

Technique
1. The author's preferred incision is a 3–4 cm oblique incision along the inguinal ligament starting at the anterior superior iliac spine and directed inferomedially (Novacheck et al. 2002). Surgeons less comfortable with dissecting the abdominal musculature near the inguinal ligament prefer a more proximal incision at the iliac crest with the abdominal musculature taken off the subcutaneous border of the ilium. The psoas tendon is approached at the same level (the pelvic brim) and therefore the exposure of the tendon is more difficult from this more proximal incision. Sutherland et al. (1997) preferred an exposure distal to the inguinal ligament. All approaches use the same deep-tissue plane underneath (lateral to) the iliacus muscle belly (Fig. 5.5.3).
2. The external oblique fascia is identified and divided just above its attachment on the inguinal ligament.
3. Blunt dissection through the internal oblique and transversus abdominus just medial and adjacent to the anterior superior iliac spine allows access to the inner table of the ilium extraperiosteally. The lateral femoral cutaneous nerve typically crosses the surgical wound and is identified and protected, but sometimes is medial and not encountered.

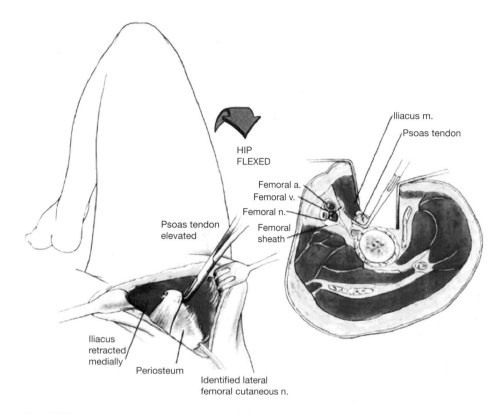

HIP FLEXED

Iliacus m.

Psoas tendon

Femoral a.

Femoral v.

Femoral n.

Psoas tendon elevated

Femoral sheath

Iliacus retracted medially

Periosteum

Identified lateral femoral cutaneous n.

Fig. 5.5.3 Psoas tendon lengthening at the pelvic brim. The femoral neurovascular structures are protected and the psoas tendon is visualized by retracting the iliacus medially with an Army–Navy retractor. A right-angle clamp is passed around the psoas tendon. By isolating it from the surrounding muscle, the structure is confirmed to be the psoas tendon.

4. With the hip flexed, a finger is passed down along the superior pubic ramus underneath the iliacus and psoas to identify the psoas tendon by palpation. The psoas tendon is visualized by retracting the iliacus medially with an Army–Navy retractor.

5. A right-angle clamp is passed around the psoas tendon. By isolating it from the surrounding muscle, the structure is confirmed to be the psoas tendon. The femoral neurovascular structures are only 2–3 mm away (Skaggs et al. 1997). Caution should be exercised. In fact, some surgeons prefer to use a nerve stimulator to confirm the anatomy.

6. Muscle fibers are retracted and the tendon is divided with electrocautery, leaving the muscle intact. Any inflexible (tendinous or myofascial tissues) should be divided. Note that many patients have a psoas minor tendon which must also be identified and divided. Leave muscular tissues intact to maintain hip-flexor function.

ADDUCTORS (SEE INSTRUCTIONAL VIDEO 'ADDUCTOR LONGUS TENOTOMY' ON INTERACTIVE DISC)

For the management of ambulatory problems due to adductor contracture, typically the lengthening is only of the adductor longus. One should keep in mind the gracilis is also an adductor. If the physical examination shows more restriction of abduction range of motion with the knee in extension, then the gracilis may be a primary contributor to the pathology. Distal lengthening as part of a medial hamstring lengthening (see next subsection) could be considered. Otherwise, if adductor longus tenotomy is planned, then proximal fascial release of the gracilis can be accomplished through the same incision. For GMFCS III and IV patients, lack of strength and motor control leads to greater dependence on the adductors for pelvifemoral stabilization. Lengthening of the adductors in these situations should be done with great caution not only regarding the decision to perform the procedure, but also how much lengthening to do. If adductor lengthening is required in an ambulator, simple adductor longus tenotomy is typically all that is required. See Chapter 5.7 for surgical considerations if hip dysplasia is present.

Technique
- A short transverse (typical) or longitudinal incision over the palpable origin of the adductor longus is used
- The adductor longus tendon is separated from the surrounding tissues (pectineus laterally, gracilis medially, and adductor brevis and anterior branch of the obturator nerve deep)
- The adductor longus tendon is divided as proximal as possible. For ambulatory patients, this is typically the only tissue that should be lengthened.

HAMSTRINGS (SEE INSTRUCTIONAL VIDEO 'MEDIAL HAMSTRING LENGTHENING' ON INTERACTIVE DISC)

The most common treatment for the hamstrings is medial lengthening. Because of the concern for anterior pelvic tilt, lateral hamstring lengthening is rarely performed (although it may safely be considered in the case of a posterior pelvic tilt). If medial and lateral hamstring lengthening is performed, there may be a role for an isolated transfer of the semitendinosus to the adductor magnus insertion to protect the hip-extensor function of the hamstrings. If performed, care should be taken to avoid overtightening the transfer leading to a shortened step length. The role and indications for this procedure are ill-defined and debatable. We have attempted to review our results with this procedure, but the confounding effects of other procedures performed simultaneously made it difficult to assess the direct contribution of this procedure to the patients' outcome. Complete transfer of the hamstrings to the femur is now of historical interest only and should be avoided (Eggers 1952).

Technique
- A posterior incision along the medial hamstring insertion just above the popliteal crease is used
- The medial hamstrings are isolated from surrounding soft tissues
- The semitendinosus can be intramuscularly lengthened leaving the muscle intact if the tendon is not too long. Otherwise, it is Z-lengthened

- The semimembranosus is lengthened via fascial striping oblique to the long axis of the muscle. The number of stripes (typically one or two) depends on the amount of lengthening necessary. The muscle is left intact
- The gracilis can be intramuscularly lengthened if rectus transfer is not going to be performed. In most cases, rectus transfer is performed simultaneously. In this case, the intramuscular tendon of the gracilis is dissected free of the muscle belly. The tendon is transected proximally and left attached distally. A heavy nonresorbable suture is placed in the proximal end
- By dissecting deeper, the medial intermuscular septum is identified and opened longitudinally to enter the anterior compartment. The vastus medialis is visualized. The suture and the gracilis tendon stump are then passed through the intermuscular septum to lie next to the vastus medialis. It is then available for transfer to the rectus femoris later
- The amount of lengthening is decided intraoperatively by achieving a popliteal angle of 30°.

RECTUS FEMORIS (SEE INSTRUCTIONAL VIDEO 'RECTUS FEMORIS TRANSFER' ON INTERACTIVE DISC)

The pathophysiology of cerebral palsy neuromuscular dysfunction is obvious if one considers the quadriceps. The one joint vasti are weak and elongated while the two joint rectus femoris is short and spastic. Rectus femoris transfer was first performed by Gage et al. (1987). The idea for the procedure was the result of personal communication between him and Dr Jacqueline Perry with the advent of more sophisticated gait analysis techniques in the 1980s (Perry 1987). Inappropriate swing phase rectus femoris activity was found to be associated with stiff knee gait. Since then, the procedure has been widely performed and reported (Gage 1990, Sutherland et al. 1990, Novacheck 1996, McMulkin et al. 2001). Surgical techniques vary, yet there have been a paucity of detailed reports of actual technique. Initially, the transfers were performed to the sartorius. While still widely used, in the past 10–15 years, we typically perform the transfer to the intramuscular gracilis tendon. The semimembranosus, semitendinosus, biceps femoris, and iliotibial band have also been used as transfer sites without evidence of superiority of one transfer site over another (Õunpuu et al. 1993a). Simple release of the rectus femoris has been shown to not be as effective as transfer (Sutherland et al. 1990, Õunpuu et al. 1993b). There seems to be a consensus of opinion that the important thing is that it is transferred.

Technique
- An oblique incision starting near the superior pole of the patella is extended proximally and medially
- The quadriceps tendon and the distal end of the rectus femoris muscle are exposed
- The interval between the rectus femoris and the remaining quadriceps is developed proximally and extended distally. A partial thickness extension of the rectus is developed from the quadriceps tendon down to the superior pole of the patella and divided at the patellar insertion.
- A nonresorbable Krackow stitch is placed in the end of the tendon
- The partial thickness quadriceps defect is repaired

- The rectus is dissected proximally to allow it to rest more medially and in a straight line following the transfer
- Subfascial dissection on the medial side of the vastus medialis is performed to the medial intermuscular septum. It is opened, and the gracilis tendon is identified intramuscularly. The tendon is separated from the muscle as described in the hamstring lengthening surgical technique. If hamstring lengthening was performed first, the gracilis tendon stump and the suture are identified in this interval
- A side-to-side repair of the rectus femoris to the gracilis is performed with nonresorbable suture. The tension is set with the knee in 30° flexion. Full knee extension should still be possible after the transfer.

GASTROCNEMIUS (SEE INSTRUCTIONAL VIDEO 'STRAYER GASTROCNEMIUS RECESSION' ON INTERACTIVE DISC)

Numerous methods of lengthening of the gastrocnemius have been described (Strayer, Baumann, Vulpius). Outcome studies have not shown any clear differences between different methods of gastrocnemius recession. Again, a clear distinction in the pathology between the two-joint gastrocnemius (short, spastic) and one-joint soleus (weak, elongated) is recognized. Musculoskeletal modeling has shown that a one centimeter lengthening of the soleus results in a 50% loss of its force generation capacity (Delp et al. 1995). The soleus is particularly sensitive to lengthening because of its bipinnate muscle fiber orientation and its short muscle fiber lengths. In children with diplegic or quadriplegic cerebral palsy, the soleus rarely requires lengthening. The gastrocnemius is much less sensitive to lengthening and is typically the only one that requires lengthening. In hemiplegia, the soleus may also require lengthening. Fortunately, the risk of overcorrection is lower in hemiplegia than in diplegia or quadriplegia. Baker lengthening is more conservative than tendo-Achilles lengthening (TAL) and can be considered (Borton et al. 2001). In late presenting cases, TAL may be the only option to achieve the necessary amount of lengthening (rare if a child has been cared for in a coordinated, multidisciplinary center).

Technique (Strayer, the author's usual method of choice)
- A 4 cm posterior mid-calf incision exposes the musculotendinous junction of the gastrocnemius. The sural nerve emerging from the interval between the medial and lateral heads of the gastrocnemius is identified and protected
- The interval between the gastrocnemius and soleus is bluntly developed transversely underneath the gastrocnemius (typically easier working from medial to lateral)
- The gastrocnemius tendon is divided just distal to the caudal end of the muscle and just proximal to its blending with the soleus fascia
- It is recessed by extending the knee and dorsiflexing the ankle to neutral
- If ankle dorsiflexion remains restricted regardless of knee position, the soleus is contracted. Its fascia can be striped at this level allowing it to gape open (usually about 1 cm)
- The gastrocnemius tendon is attached to the underlying soleus fascia with interrupted nonresorbable sutures. The amount of recession needed to achieve this position is typically about 2 cm.

Contraindications

The main problems with soft-tissue surgery in cerebral palsy have been the following:

- A lack of recognition that contractures occur primarily due to the effects of spasticity. Therefore spasticity management should be the primary consideration. While options were not available in the past, many are today. Tendon surgery should be deferred as much as possible
- Inappropriate surgical indications due to misconceptions regarding the cause of gait pathology. Adductor lengthening for scissoring gait is a good example. As mentioned previously, the adductors have been inappropriately blamed for scissoring gait. 3D gait analysis differentiates true hip-adduction deformity from the usual cause of scissoring gait (simultaneous flexion of the hip and knee with internal rotation of the lower extremity due to excessive femoral anteversion)
- Inappropriate lengthening of one joint muscles leading to weakness. TAL and release of the iliopsoas tendon at the lesser trochanter are two examples
- Undertreatment due to difficulty identifying pathology. The psoas is a prime example. The combination of incorrect physical examination technique (underdiagnosis) and concerns about post-surgical weakness (a residual from the days of complete release of the tendon from the trochanter) has led to undertreatment
- Overly aggressive surgery to isolated structures. TAL, combined medial and lateral hamstring lengthening, complete transfer of all of the hamstrings to the femur (Eggers), obturator neurectomy, and iliopsoas release at the lesser trochanter are all examples. These procedures are rarely (if ever) indicated for the treatment of gait dysfunction
- Single-level surgery leading to joint imbalance and the need for numerous trips to the operating room.

Postoperative care concerns

The specifics of the rehabilitation protocols for these procedures can be found in Chapter 5.9. The concepts of early mobility to avoid stiffness and early strengthening programs to avoid weakness are important for all procedures. Of particular importance is to avoid postoperative positioning that can negate the effects of surgical lengthening. Two notable examples are psoas lengthening and rectus transfer. Postoperative positioning of the hip in a flexed position following psoas surgery can result in a hip contracture that is no better and possibly worse than preoperatively. Following rectus femoris transfer promoting early range of motion is essential to allow the transferred tendon to develop free passage through its new, non-anatomical area. Long leg casting should not be done.

Complications

- The primary concern following psoas lengthening at the pelvic brim is femoral neurovascular injury. The proximity of the femoral nerve and artery to the psoas tendon has been well documented (Skaggs et al. 1997)
- Pelvifemoral instability following adductor surgery in patients in Gross Motor Functional Classification System (GMFCS) III/IV was mentioned earlier

459

- Inappropriate lengthening of the hamstrings leads to poor pelvic outcomes (worsened anterior pelvic tilt) (Arnold et al. 2006)
- Persistent knee stiffness following rectus femoris transfer can be avoided by using the postoperative rehabilitation protocols provided in Chapter 5.9
- Crouch gait is more common after TAL (Dietz et al. 2006, Filho et al. 2008).

Outcome data

Because lower-extremity surgical intervention is seldom performed in isolation, analysis of overall alignment and function following multilevel surgery has been done. It has been shown to be effective (Schwartz et al. 2004, Gough et al. 2004, Rodda et al. 2006, Thomason et al. 2008).

Psoas

Recession of the iliopsoas tendon to the hip joint capsule causes excessive weakness (Bleck 1971). To assess outcome, multivariate tools (such as the hip-flexor index, HFI) should be considered as no single kinematic or kinetic variable completely describes hip-flexor function (Schwartz et al. 2000). Correlated variables and redundancy make it difficult to report meaningful statistics. Benefit and safety with psoas lengthening at the pelvic brim have been shown (Matsuo et al. 1987, Chung et al. 1994, Skaggs et al. 1997, Sutherland et al. 1997, Novacheck et al. 2002, Filho et al. 2006). Improvements in anterior pelvic tilt are seen when performed in conjunction with femoral derotational osteotomy (Novacheck et al. 2002). On the other hand, others have noted that psoas lengthening surgery does not improve anterior pelvic tilt (DeLuca et al. 1998). Variations in surgical indications may be the explanation for this difference, being more restrictive at some centers (DeLuca et al. 1998) than at others (Novacheck et al. 2002). Hip-flexor power generation as measured by the H3 power burst and by functional outcomes measures has not shown any impairment following psoas lengthening at the pelvic brim, i.e. the procedure is both effective and safe (Novacheck et al. 2002).

Adductors

There are no recent reports regarding the appropriateness and outcomes of adductor surgery in ambulatory cerebral palsy. Reports prior to 1990 documented only improvements in hip-abduction range of motion (impairment level) without any indication of dynamic changes in hip-adductor function based on gait analysis or its effect on function in the community (functional level). Therefore there is little literature of value to report.

Hamstrings

Most reports of hamstring lengthening since the advent of gait analysis have focused on the improvements in stance phase knee extension (Gage 1990, Sutherland and Davids 1993, Kay et al. 2002). The combination of medial with lateral hamstring lengthening carries the possibility of greater improvements in stance-phase knee extension, but also places the patient at an increased risk of knee hyperextension (Kay et al. 2002). Hamstring contractures certainly do affect knee position during stance, but so do many other factors (see

Chapter 5.11). The focus for outcomes assessment for hamstring lengthening has been shifting over the last 10 years to muscle-length data during swing when the hamstrings must elongate rapidly to their maximum dynamic length (see Chapter 3.6) (Delp et al. 1996, Arnold et al. 2006). Improvements in knee extension during late swing occur when decisions regarding hamstring lengthening are made consistent with muscle length and velocity data (Arnold et al. 2006). When hamstrings are lengthened in cases of normal hamstring function (normal muscle length and velocity in swing), excessive anterior pelvic tilt and pelvic range of motion may develop.

RECTUS FEMORIS

The addition of rectus femoris transfer surgery to the treatment algorithm for children with stiff knee gait due to cerebral palsy has led to improvement in swing-phase knee flexion (Gage et al. 1987, Sutherland et al. 1990). There is no doubt that rectus femoris transfer has helped many individuals with stiff knee gait. But many questions remain. Why do some patients have a poor outcome? Does the surgery achieve its goal of converting the rectus to a knee-flexor? Are the indications correct? Do all children with 'stiff-knee gait' have a 'stiff knee' due to rectus femoris pathology? Could a lack of propulsive power fail to generate the momentum to propel the limb into flexion during swing? Could the crouch position during stance lead to knee extension moments that restrict knee flexion velocity at toe-off? These important questions are addressed in Chapter 3.6, under the heading 'Muscle-driven forward-dynamic simulations of stiff-knee gait'.

No apparent adverse functional effects of performing the rectus femoris transfer have been documented. There has been no evidence that it exacerbates knee-extension weakness. The rectus femoris is an important muscle for controlling knee flexion during more rapid walking speeds and for running. There has been some conjecture that a rectus femoris transfer in a high-functioning patient who is able to run could lead to difficulty with running, but this also has not been documented.

GASTROCNEMIUS

Gastrocnemius recession has been studied by numerous authors and has been shown to decrease the double bump moment pattern, improve 2nd rocker, and decrease abnormal power generation in mid-stance (Saraph et al. 2000). The ankle power burst in late stance is preserved or enhanced (Rose et al. 1993). However, these studies have been short term follow-ups. Seemingly safe in the short term, the risk of overcorrection (calcaneus deformity) is higher following TAL than proximal aponeurotic lengthening (Baker procedure) over the longer term (Borton et al. 2001). Given the previously noted reduction in force-generating capacity following soleus lengthening (computer simulation) (Delp et al. 1995) and the importance of the soleus in providing stance phase support (Winter 1991, Gage and Schwartz 2004), TAL may promote crouch due to impairments of the plantarflexion/knee-extension couple (see Chapter 2.4). While this has not been proven, two recent studies report that the incidence of crouch gait is higher in adolescence in children who have undergone prior TAL (Dietz et al. 2006, Filho et al. 2008). It is widely held that the gastrocnemius is a significant contributor to foot deformity. Unlike rectus femoris transfer and hamstring lengthening, gastrocnemius recession has not been less common following selective dorsal rhizotomy (Schwartz et al. 2004).

Case study (see Case 5 on Interactive Disc)
This 10-year-old with spastic diplegic cerebral palsy is an independent community ambulator without the use of assistive devices or orthoses (GMFCS II). At 1 year of age, he had undergone bilateral TAL and plantar fascia release.

Gait by observation shows toe-toe initial contact bilaterally, worse on the right (Fig. 5.5.4, Video 5.5.2 on Interactive Disc). Bilateral knee hyperextension in mid-stance and bilateral internal foot-progression angles are apparent.

Physical examination shows mild hip flexion contractures (5°), bilateral hamstring and rectus femoris contractures, bilateral femoral anteversion (40°, right and 50°, left), a mild left internal tibial torsion, and bilateral equinus contractures (right greater then left). Motor control is good and strength is rated 3–4/5 in general. Spasticity is felt to be mild at the hips and knees and moderate at the ankle plantarflexors.

Kinematics of the transverse plane demonstrate excessive bilateral internal hip rotation, worse on the right, but with a more severe internal foot progression angle on the left (Figs 5.5.5, 6). These findings suggest contributions from excessive femoral anteversion bilaterally and internal tibial torsion on the left.

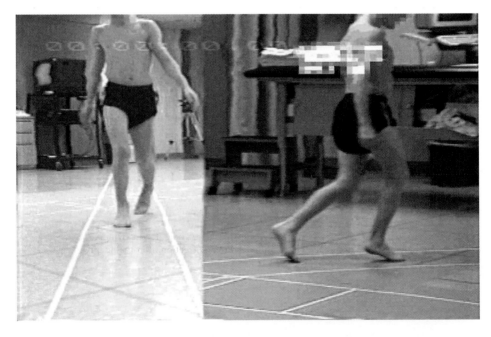

Fig. 5.5.4 10-year-old boy with spastic diplegic cerebral palsy. Preoperative gait pattern shows forefoot initial contact, excessive knee flexion at initial contact, mild stiff knee gait, inward knee rotation, and in-toeing. (See pre-op video of Case 5 on Interactive Disc.)

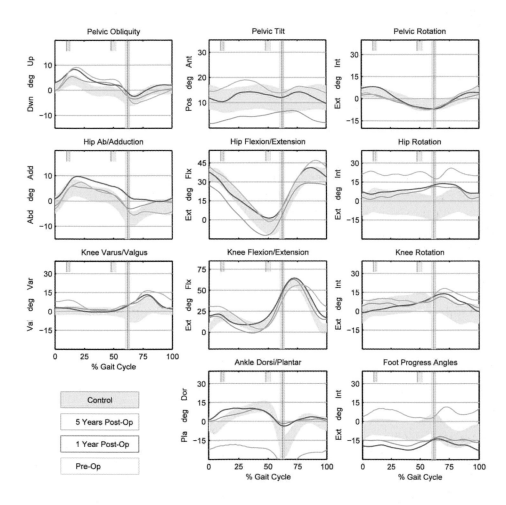

Fig. 5.5.5 Kinematic analysis, right. Preoperative data (light blue) show equinus, diminished knee extension in late swing with excessive knee flexion at initial contact and during loading response, mildly limited swing-phase knee flexion, mildly restricted hip extension in terminal stance associated with increasing anterior pelvic tilt (double bump), excessive internal hip rotation leading to in-toeing. One year postoperative data (dark blue) show correction of equinus, improvement of knee extension in late swing, improved knee modulation in stance, improved knee flexion in swing, diminished double bump pelvic pattern, improved hip rotation, and overcorrection of in-toeing. Five year postoperative data (green) show the results are maintained with the exception of slight posterior pelvic tilt probably due to hamstring tightness.

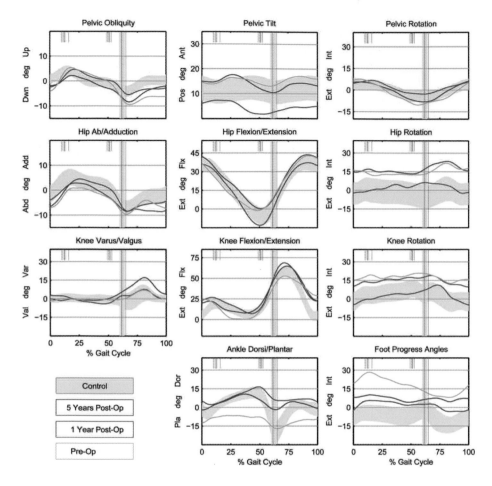

Fig. 5.5.6 Kinematic analysis, left. Preoperative data (light blue) shows similar findings to the right side except equinus is not as severe and intoeing is more severe. One year postoperative data (dark blue) and 5-year postoperative data (red) show similar improvements compared to the right side except that in-toeing is mildly persistent due to mild internal tibial torsion.

Sagittal-plane kinematics are consistent with multilevel spasticity/contracture. He has a double-bump pelvic pattern, restriction of hip extension in terminal stance, excessive knee flexion at initial contact, diminished peak swing phase knee flexion, restricted knee extension in late swing, mild genu recurvatum in mid-stance, and equinus bilaterally (worse on the right than the left).

Coronal-plane findings are normal with the exception of pelvic obliquity (right side elevated) and excessive adduction of the right hip. This is felt to be a compensation for the functional leg length discrepancy caused by the asymmetric equinus deformity (again, worse on the right).

464

Sagittal-plane kinetics show a lack of 1st rocker, a very abnormal and early ankle moment, lack of power generation for push-off at the ankle, excessive knee-flexion moments bilaterally (secondary to excessive plantarflexion/knee-extension couples), and prolonged hip-extension moments in stance (hip-extensor dominance pattern) (Figs 5.5.7, 8). Hamstring muscle length is short in terminal swing, indicating contracture, but the rate of elongation is normal, indicating no spasticity (Fig. 5.5.9). Stride length and walking speed are diminished (approximately 0.75 times normal) (Table 5.5.2). Gillette Gait Index is 114 (Schutte et al. 2000). FAQ walking level is 7 (*Walks outside the home for community distances, is able to get around on curbs and uneven terrain in addition to level surfaces, but usually requires minimal assistance or supervision for safety*) (Novacheck et al. 2000). He is able to perform 18/22 higher-level skills.

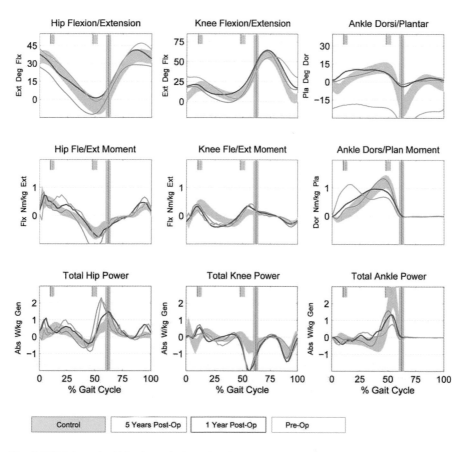

Fig. 5.5.7 Right sagittal kinetic analysis. Using the same coloring convention (see Fig. 5.5.5) preoperative double bump ankle moment is corrected one year postoperatively with restoration of 1st rocker at final follow-up. Ankle plantar-flexor push-off power is improved, and hip flexion power at toe-off is preserved.

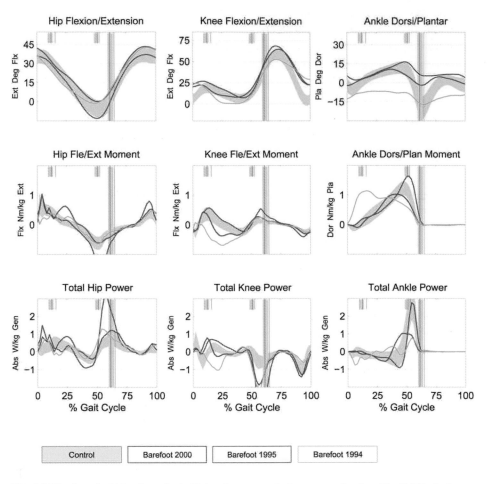

Fig. 5.5.8 Left sagittal kinetic analysis. Using the same coloring convention (see Fig. 5.5.6) similar improvements are seen on the left. At 5 years postoperatively, ankle plantarflexion push-off power is normalized.

Even though many of these kinematic and kinetic findings could be due to multilevel spasticity, the findings of multilevel contractures by physical examination and only a mild elevation of oxygen consumption (1.51 × normal, just outside the normal range) suggest that spasticity is not severe enough to consider selective dorsal rhizotomy and would not address the musculotendinous contractures. Motor control and strength are quite good making this patient a good candidate for rehabilitation following multiple lower extremity surgery to correct multiple contractures and bone deformities bilaterally. It is felt that the left internal tibial torsion is not severe enough to warrant surgical correction. On the basis of this information, the surgeries included the following:

(1) bilateral intertrochanteric femoral derotational osteotomies
(2) bilateral psoas lengthenings at the pelvic brim
(3) bilateral medial hamstring lengthenings
(4) bilateral rectus femoris transfers to the gracilis
(5) bilateral Strayer gastrocnemius recessions
(6) right soleus fascial striping.

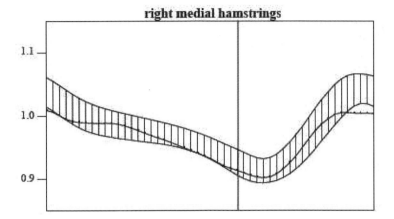

Fig. 5.5.9 Hamstring muscle length. Over one gait cycle, control hamstring length (vertical hatched area) varies from approximately 103% (range ±1 SD, 101–6%) of anatomic resting length at initial contact to an average of 93% in in early swing. The rate of elongation of the hamstrings is greatest during swing phase to maximum length attainment in late swing (average 104%). This patient's data (only right side is shown, left side was similar) suggest hamstring contracture in late swing (unable to achieve normal length), but no evidence of spasticity (normal rate of elongation in midswing).

TABLE 5.5.2
Linear parameters of patient in case study

	Control	Preoperative		1 year postoperative		5 years postoperative	
		Left	Right	Left	Right	Left	Right
Opposite foot off (%)	9.8	10.0	11.5	12.2	10.0	15.8	12.3
Opposite foot contact (%)	49.6	50.0	51.9	51.0	48.0	52.6	47.4
Foot off (%)	59.0	62.0	61.5	61.2	62.0	64.9	63.2
Single support (%)	39.7	40.0	40.4	38.8	38.0	36.8	35.1
Stride length (cm)	117	78	84	96	96	121	119
Stride time (seconds)	0.99	0.83	0.87	0.82	0.83	0.95	0.95
Cadence (steps/minute)	122	72	69	73	72	63	63
Spced (cm/second)	118	94	97	117	114	127	126
Double support (%)	19.3	22.0	21.2	22.4	24.0	28.1	28.1

Walking speed is normalized at 1 year postoperatively and is maintained at final follow-up. Stride length and stride time are normalized at final follow-up. Slow cadence persists.

Postoperative analysis was performed 10 months later. Because of the focus of this chapter, only the sagittal-plane findings will be described. Improved walking pattern is apparent (Fig. 5.5.10, Video 5.5.2 on Interactive Disc). Pelvic tilt, pelvic tilt double bump pattern, and slope of hip extension are improved (attributable to psoas surgery) (Figs 5.5.5, 6). Knee extension in preparation for and at initial contact is improved (attributable to hamstring surgery). Knee hyperextension is resolved with normal knee extension in midstance with no evidence of crouch gait (attributable to improved muscular balance of hamstrings and gastrocnemius). The magnitude of peak swing phase knee flexion is improved because of rectus femoris transfer. The equinus contracture is resolved (attributable to gastrocsoleus surgery).

Ankle moment is improved bilaterally (Figs 5.5.7, 8). Power generation at the ankle is improved because of increased ankle motion. The knee flexion moment in stance on the left is normalized. The hip-extensor dominance pattern persists.

Oxygen consumption is now in the normal range (1.22 × normal). Speed and stride length are improved (Table 5.5.2). The postoperative Gillette Gait Index shows significant improvement to 35, a 70% change. His functional ambulation is improved to level 8 (*Walks outside the home for community distances, easily gets around on level ground, curbs, and uneven terrain, but has difficulty or requires minimal assistance or supervision for safety*). While there are no gains in the number of higher-level skills that he is able to accomplish, his ability to do them improved in 16 of the 18. The family felt that he has improved strength and endurance and is better able to keep up with peers. Other observations by parent report

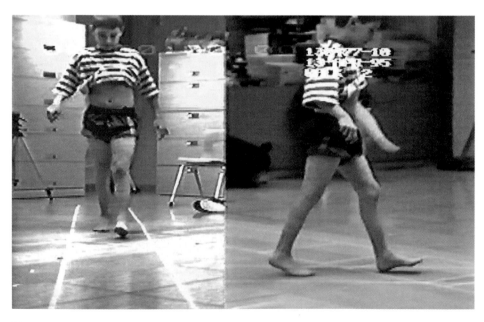

Fig. 5.5.10 Boy with spastic diplegic cerebral palsy, 1 year postoperative. Heel strike is restored, knee extension is improved at initial contact, and inward knee rotation is corrected. Trunk alignment is improved. (See one-year video of Case 5 on Interactive Disc.)

468

include the following: reciprocal stair climbing has been achieved, there is better balance with fewer falls, walking speed is increased, and gait is more natural. Femoral implants are removed.

Follow-up after the adolescent growth spurt at age 16 (over 5 years postoperative) reveals a nearly normal gait appearance (Fig. 5.5.11, Video 5.5.2 on Interactive Disc). No botulinum toxin has been used, and no other surgery has been performed. Some stretching has been done at home, but no formal physical therapy is ongoing. Recreational activities include golfing. Some hamstring contracture and mild gastrocnemius tightness are apparent by physical examination.

Kinematics are in the normal range in the sagittal plane (Figs 5.5.5, 6). In particular, hip extension is normal in terminal stance, knee modulation is normal, there is no equinus, and hindfoot initial contact is normal. The hip, knee and ankle moments are in the normal range (Figs 5.5.7, 8). Power production of the hip-flexors at toe-off and ankle plantarflexors in preswing is increased. This assessment shows no losses with growth despite having gone through the adolescent growth spurt (significant, because the natural history of untreated cerebral palsy is typically characterized by worsening) (Bell et al. 2002, Gough et al. 2004). Gait efficiency (oxygen consumption) remains normal. Walking speed and stride length are normal (Table 5.5.2).

The Gillette Gait Index shows only slight deterioration to 49. This patient still maintains a 57% improvement in gait pattern compared to preoperative status (seven years earlier) despite growth during adolescence. Ambulatory function is now rated higher

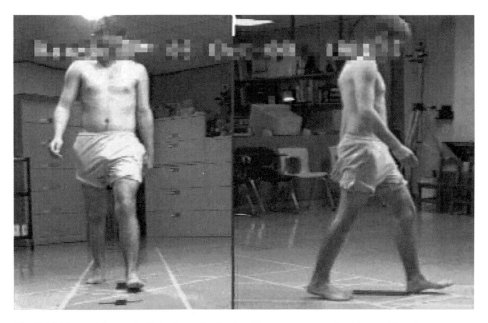

Fig. 5.5.11 Boy with spastic diplegic cerebral palsy, 5 years postoperative. At age 16, gait improvements are maintained following the adolescent growth spurt. (See 5-year pre-op video of Case 5 on Interactive Disc.)

at FAQ level 10, an increase of 2 more levels above the one level increase seen postoperatively.

REFERENCES

Arnold AS, Liu MQ, Schwartz MH, Õunpuu S, Delp SL (2006) The role of estimating muscle-tendon lengths and velocities of the hamstrings in the evaluation and treatment of crouch gait. *Gait Posture* **23**: 273–81.

Bell KJ, Õunpuu S, DeLuca PA, Romness MJ (2002) Natural progression of gait in children with cerebral palsy. *J Pediatr Orthop* **22**: 677–82.

Bleck EE (1971) Postural and gait abnormalities caused by hip-flexion deformity in spastic cerebral palsy. Treatment by iliopsoas recession. *J Bone Joint Surg Am* **53**: 1468–88.

Borton DC, Walker K, Pirpiris M, Nattrass GR, Graham HK (2001) Isolated calf lengthening in cerebral palsy: Outcome analysis of risk factors. *J Bone Joint Surg Br* **83**: 364–70.

Brown CR, Hillman SJ, Richardson AM, Herman JL, Robb JE (2008) Reliability and validity of the Visual Gait Assessment Scale for children with hemiplegic cerebral palsy when used by experienced and inexperienced observers. *Gait Posture* **27**: 648–52.

Chung CY, Novacheck TF, Gage JR (1994) Hip function in cerebral palsy – the kinematic and kinetic effects of psoas surgery. *Gait Posture* **2**: 61.

Delp SL, Statler K, Carroll NC (1995) Preserving plantar flexion strength after surgical treatment for contracture of the triceps surae: a computer simulation study. *J Orthop Res* **13**: 96–104.

Delp SL, Arnold AS, Speers RA, Moore CA (1996) Hamstrings and psoas lengths during normal and crouch gait: implications for muscle-tendon surgery. *J Orthop Res* **14**: 144–151.

DeLuca PA, Ounpuu S, Davis RB, Walsh JH (1998) Effect of hamstring and psoas lengthening on pelvic tilt in patient with spastic diplegia cerebral palsy. *J Pediatr Orthop* **18**: 712–18.

Desloovere K, Molenaers G, Feys H, Huenaerts C, Callewaert B, Van de Walle P (2006) Do dynamic and static clinical measurements correlate with gait analysis parameters in children with cerebral palsy? *Gait Posture* **24**: 302–13.

Dietz FR, Albright JC, Dolan L (2006) Medium term follow-up of achilles tendon lengthening in the treatment of ankle equinus in cerebral palsy. *Iowa Med J* **26**: 27–31.

Eggers GWN (1952) Transplantation of hamstring tendons to femoral condyles in order to improve hip extension and to decrease knee flexion in cerebral spastic paralysis. *J Bone Joint Surg Am* **34**: 827–30.

Filho MC, de Godoy W, Santos, CA (2006) Effects of intramuscular psoas lengthening on pelvic and hip motion in patients with spastic diparetic cerebral palsy. *J Pediatr Orthop* **26**: 260–4.

Filho MC, Kawamura C, Kanaji P, Juliano Y (2008) Relation between triceps surae lengthening and crouch gait in patients with cerebral palsy. *Dev Med Child Neurol* **50** (Suppl. 4): 13.

Gage JR (1990) Surgical treatment of knee dysfunction in cerebral palsy. *Clin Orthop Relat Res* **253**: 45–54.

Gage JR, Schwartz MH (2004) Pathological gait and lever arm dysfunction. In: Gage JR, editor. *The Treatment of Gait Problems in Cerebral Palsy*. London: Mac Keith Press. p 180–204.

Gage JR, Perry J, Hicks RR, Koop S, Werntz JR (1987) Rectus femoris transfer to improve knee function of children with cerebral palsy. *Dev Med Child Neurol* **29**: 159–66.

Goldberg SR, Anderson FC, Pandy MG, Delp SL (2004) Muscles that influence knee flexion velocity in double support: implications for stiff-knee gait. *J Biomech* **37**: 1189–96.

Gough M, Eve LC, Robinson RO, Shortland AP (2004) Short-term outcome of multi-level surgical intervention in spastic diplegic cerebral palsy compared with natural history. *Dev Med Child Neurol* **46**: 91–7.

Hoffinger SA, Rab GT, Abou-Ghaida H (1993) Hamstrings in cerebral palsy crouch gait. *J Pediatr Orthop* **13**: 722–6.

Kay RM, Rethlefsen SA, Skaggs D, Leet A (2002) Outcome of medial versus lateral hamstring lengthening surgery in cerebral palsy. *J Pediatr Orthop* **22**: 169–72.

Kimmel SA, Schwartz, MH (2006) A baseline of dynamic muscle function during gait. *Gait Posture* **23**: 211–21.

Lieber RL, Friden J (2002) Spasticity causes a fundamental rearrangement of muscle–joint interaction. *Muscle Nerve* **25**: 265–70.

Louis ML, Viehweger E, Launay F, Loundou AD, Pomero V, Jacquemier M, Jouve JL, Bollini G (2008) Informative value of the popliteal angle in walking cerebral palsy children. *Rev Chir Orthop Reparatrice Appar Mot* **94**: 443–8.

Maathuis KGB, van der Schans CP, van Iperen A, Rietman HS, Geertzen JHB (2005) Gait in children with cerebral palsy: observer reliability of Physician Rating Scale and Edinburgh Visual Gait Analysis Interval Testing Scale. *J Pediatr Orthop* **25**: 268–72.

Mackey AH, Lobb GL, Walt SE, Stott NS (2003) Reliability and validity of the Observational Gait Scale in children with spastic diplegia. *Dev Med Child Neurol* **45**: 4–11.

Matsuo T, Hara H, Tada S (1987) Selective lengthening of the psoas and rectus femoris and preservation of the iliacus for flexion deformity of the hip in cerebral palsy patients. *J Pediatr Orthop* **17**: 690–8.

McMulkin M, Barr KM, Ferguson R, Caskey P, Baird G (2001) Outcomes of extensive rectus femoris release surgeries compared to transfers. *Gait Posture* **13**: 251.

Novacheck TF (1996) Surgical intervention in ambulatory cerebral palsy. In: Harris GF, Smith PA, editors. *Human Motion Analysis: Current Applications and Future Directions.* Piscataway, NJ: IEEE Press. p 231–54.

Novacheck TF, Stout JL, Tervo R (2000) Reliability and validity of the Gillette Functional Assessment Questionnaire as an outcome measure in children with walking disabilities. *J Pediatr Orthop* **20**: 75–81.

Novacheck TF, Trost JP, Schwartz MH (2002) Intramuscular psoas lengthening improves dynamic hip function in children with cerebral palsy. *J Pediatr Orthop* **22**: 158–64.

Õunpuu S, Muik E, Davis III RB, Gage JR, DeLuca PA (1993a) Rectus femoris surgery in children with cerebral palsy. Part I: The effect of rectus femoris transfer location of knee motion. *J Pediatr Orthop* **13**: 325–30.

Õunpuu S, Muik E, Davis III RB, Gage JR, DeLuca PA (1993b) Rectus femoris surgery in children with cerebral palsy. Part II: A comparison between the effect of transfer and release of the distal rectus femoris on knee motion. *J Pediatr Orthop* **13**: 331–5.

Perry J (1987) Distal rectus femoris transfer. *Dev Med Child Neurol* **29**: 153–8.

Reinbolt JA, Fox MD, Arnold AS, Õunpuu S, Delp SL (2008) Importance of preswing rectus femoris activity in stiff-knee gait. *J Biomech* **41**: 2362–9.

Rodda JM, Graham HK, Nattrass GR, Galea MP, Baker R, Wolfe R (2006) Correction of severe crouch gait in patients with spastic diplegia with use of multilevel orthopaedic surgery. *J Bone Joint Surg Am* **88**: 2653–64.

Rose SA, DeLuca PA, Davis RB, Õunpuu S, Gage JR (1993) Kinematic and kinetic evaluation of the ankle following lengthening of the gastrocnemius fascia in children with cerebral palsy. *J Pediatr Orthop* **13**: 727–32.

Saraph V, Zwick EB, Uitz C, Linhart W, Steinwender G (2000) The Baumann procedure for fixed contracture of the gastrosoleus in cerebral palsy. Evaluation of function of the ankle after multilevel surgery. *J Bone Joint Surg Br* **82**: 535–540.

Schutte LM, Narayanan U, Stout JL, Selber P, Gage JR, Schwartz MH (2000) An index for quantifying deviations from normal gait. *Gait Posture* **11**: 25–31.

Schwartz MH, Novacheck TF, Trost JP (2000) A tool for quantifying hip flexor function during gait. *Gait Posture* **12**: 122–7.

Schwartz MH, Viehweger E, Stout J, Novacheck TF, Gage JR (2004) Comprehensive treatment of ambulatory children with cerebral palsy: an outcome assessment. *J Pediatr Orthop* **24**: 45–53.

Shortland AP, Harris CA, Gough M, Robinson RO (2002) Architecture of the medial gastrocnemius in children with spastic diplegia. *Dev Med Child Neurol* **44**: 158–63.

Skaggs DL, Kaminsky CK, Eskander-Rickards E, Reynolds RA, Tolo VT, Bassett GS (1997) Psoas over the brim lengthenings. Anatomic investigation and surgical technique. *Clin Orthop Relat Res* **339**: 174–9.

Stout JL, Gage JR, Schwartz MH, Novacheck TF (2008) Distal femoral extension osteotomy and patellar tendon advancement to treat persistent crouch gait in cerebral palsy. *J Bone Joint Surg Am* **90**: 2470–84.

Sutherland DH, Davids JR (1993) Common gait abnormalities of the knee in cerebral palsy. *Clin Orthop Relat Res* **288**: 139–47.

Sutherland DH, Santi M, Abel MF (1990) Treatment of stiff-knee gait in cerebral palsy: a comparison by gait analysis of distal rectus femoris transfer versus proximal rectus release. *J Pediatr Orthop* **10**: 433–41.

Sutherland DH, Zilberfarb JL, Kaufman KR, Wyatt MP, Chambers HG (1997) Psoas release at the pelvic brim in ambulatory patients with cerebral palsy: operative technique and functional outcome. *J Pediatr Orthop* **17**: 563–70.

Thomason P, Baker R, Taylor N, Dodd K, Graham K (2008) Trajectory of change following single event multilevel surgery in children with spastic cerebral palsy in the context of a randomized controlled trial. *Dev Med Child Neurol* **50** (Suppl. 4): 12.

471

Thompson NS, Baker RJ, Cosgrove AP, Saunders JL, Taylor TC (2001) Relevance of the popliteal angle to hamstring length in cerebral palsy crouch gait. *J Pediatr Orthop* **21**: 383–7.

Trost JP, Schwartz MH, Krach LE, Dunn ME, Novacheck TF (2008) Comprehensive short-term outcome assessment of selective dorsal rhizotomy. *Dev Med Child Neurol* **50**: 765–71.

Winter DA (1991) *The Biomechanics and Motor Control of Human Gait: Normal, Elderly, and Pathological*, 2nd edn. Waterloo, Ontario: University of Waterloo Press. p 75–85.

Wren TA, Do KP, Hara R, Dorey FJ, Kay RM, Otsuka NY (2007) Gillette Gait Index as a gait analysis summary measure: comparison with qualitative visual assessments of overall gait. *J Pediatr Orthop* **27**: 765–8.

5.6
ORTHOPAEDIC TREATMENT OF LONG BONE TORSIONS

James R. Gage

Key points
- The long bones constitute the levers upon which the muscles act
- Femoral anteversion is present from birth and nearly universal in these children; tibial torsion is also a common deformity but is acquired and comes later
- Abnormal torsions of the long bones and the disabilities they produce are under-recognized and, if function is to be optimized, need to be corrected.

Review of relevant pathophysiology
Torsional lever-arm dysfunction (LAD) is discussed in Chapter 2.4, where it is pointed out that torsional LAD adversely affects the normal joint moments in two ways:

1. The desired moment, e.g. knee extension in mid-stance, is reduced in magnitude.
2. Unwanted secondary moments are introduced. In the case of 'miserable malalignment syndrome', for example, a valgus moment is exerted at the knee and an external torsional moment on the foot and tibia. With time and growth, these abnormal moments will produce further malalignment of bone as well as unwanted gait compensations (see Figs 2.4.11, 12).

To understand why torsional deformities of bone are common and how torsional deformities of bone interfere with normal function, the reader will need to review Chapters 1.3 and 2.4. As Somerville pointed out, femoral anteversion is universal at birth, but normally remodels rapidly in the first few years of life. As discussed in Chapter 1.3, this occurs because as the child begins standing and walking in an erect posture, the force of the ilio–femoral (Bigalow's) ligament is imposed against the cartilaginous femoral head and neck (Somerville 1957). Because of delayed onset of walking, abnormal muscle forces, and the fact that these children walk with their hips in excessive flexion, femoral anteversion does not remodel normally. Consequently, these children have persistent fetal alignment (Fabry et al. 1973, Bobroff et al. 1999). Furthermore, Delp et al. (1999) and Arnold et al. (1997) have shown that when individuals walk with their hips in excessive flexion, the anterior gluteal muscles (gluteus minimus and tensor fascia lata) act as strong internal rotators of the femur, which in a growing child will induce further internal rotation moments on the growing bone (Fig. 5.6.1). In addition, weakness of the tibialis posterior coupled

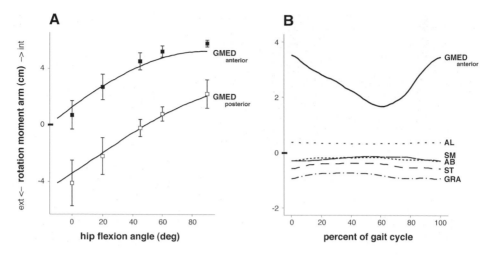

Fig. 5.6.1 Hip rotation moment arms of the anterior and posterior portions of the gluteus medius versus hip-flexion angle and gait cycle (A), which suggests that internal rotation gait may be a result of excessive hip flexion. Internal rotation moment arms of the anterior compartment of the gluteus medial (GMED) during walking (B), computed with an image-based model of a subject with cerebral palsy are approximately four times larger than the rotational moment arms of the medial hamstrings or adductors. (Reproduced from Delp et al. 1999, by permission.)

with relative contracture of the gastrocnemius (both common features in diplegia) lead to breakdown of the longitudinal arch of the foot with resultant talonavicular subluxation and forefoot abduction. This results in external rotation of the foot relative to the knee. Weightbearing on the externally rotated foot places the ground reaction force lateral to the knee, which in turn induces an external torsional torque on the tibia. In a growing child this will generate external tibial torsion, in accordance with the Arkin and Katz postulates, discussed in Chapters 1.3 and 2.4 (Arkin et al. 1956). External tibial torsion is compounded by the fact that these children commonly have 'foot-drag' in swing, which allows the floor to exert an additional external rotation torque on the foot during swing-phase. These same forces, coupled with the inherent weakness of the tibialis posterior, will also produce pes valgus (hindfoot valgus, talonavicular subluxation in the midfoot, and forefoot varus). Consequently, in spastic diplegia or quadriplegia, the usual torsional outcome is femoral anteversion, external tibial torsion, and pes valgus – the so-called 'miserable malalignment syndrome' (Bruce et al. 2004) (Fig. 5.6.2, Video 5.6.1). Although miserable malalignment syndrome affects function at both ends of the lower extremity, it has its greatest deleterious effects at the knee. Since the knee is the pivot point upon which the shank rotates to clear the foot during swing phase, it should be readily apparent that if the axis of the knee is 20° or more out of plane, as is often the case, normal function cannot occur. This combination of internal femoral and external tibial torsion is often mistaken for 'scissoring gait' by the uninitiated, which in turn frequently results in unnecessary lengthening of the hip-adductors.

Torsional deformities in hemiplegia behave differently than in diplegia or quadriplegia. Because standing and walking in children with the milder types of hemiplegia (types I and

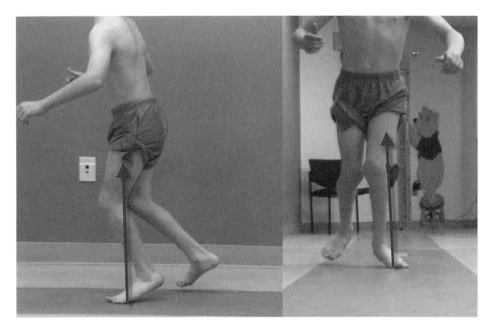

Fig. 5.6.2 Young man with 'malignant malalignment syndrome', which features the combination of internal femoral torsion in conjunction with external tibial torsion and/or pes valgus. Since the knee and foot are malaligned to the plane of progression, a normal plantarflexion/knee-extension (PF/KE) couple can not occur. Consequently, there is no way to restore the normal PF/KE couple without first correcting the malalignments of the femur and tibia, which will require derotational osteotomies of both bones. (To see him in motion, see Video 5.6.1 on Interactive Disc.)

II) are only slightly delayed, persistent fetal alignment is less likely to develop. In addition, the usual foot deformity is equinovarus, which tends to align the foot internally to the knee. Consequently, tibial torsion is more variable. Children with the more severe types of hemiplegia do have significant delays in standing and walking, however, so children with hemiplegia types III and IV commonly have persistent fetal alignment (femoral anteversion) in addition to variable abnormal tibial torsion on the hemiplegic side. Consequently, these children typically walk with pelvic retraction on the anteverted side to compensate both their hemiplegia and the ipsilateral anteversion (Winters et al. 1987, Graham et al. 2005, Dobson et al. 2006, Riad et al. 2007). With time and growth, children with types III and IV hemiplegia often develop a compensatory external tibial torsion on the non-involved side. The compensatory external tibial torsion progression on the sound side enables a normal foot progression angle in the face of the femoral anteversion and pelvic retraction on the hemiplegic side (Fig. 5.6.3, Video 5.6.2). When planning a correction of anteversion and/or tibial torsion on the affected side of a child with types III and IV hemiplegia, it is important to look for external tibial torsion on the sound side, as it needs to be corrected as well. In my personal experience, despite the fact that femoral anteversion and/or tibial torsion were corrected on the affected side, failure to correct the external tibial torsion on the sound side leads to persistent pelvic retraction on the hemiplegic side post-surgery. I think the reason

(a)

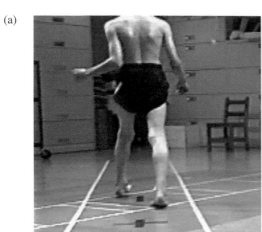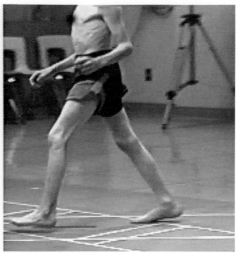

(b)

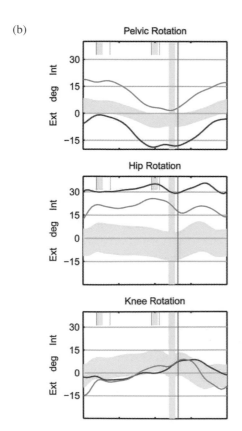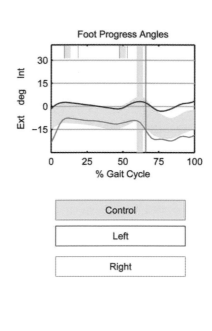

Fig. 5.6.3 opposite (a) Young man with (left) spastic hemiplegia, type 1V. Although it is not readily apparent by looking at the video, he is compensating his left femoral anteversion by retracting his pelvis on the affected side (See Video 5.6.2 on Interactive Disc). (b) The compensation is readily apparent on the kinematic graphs of the transverse plane. The pelvic graph demonstrates that the left side of the pelvis is persistently externally rotated and the right side internally rotated throughout the gait cycle, whereas the left hip is internally rotated throughout the cycle. Frequently, there is an accompanying external tibial torsion on the sound side, which is also the case in this boy. The patient will often key his walking to the foot on the sound side, so it is important to correct abnormal tibial torsion on the unaffected side as well.

for this is that the individual keys his/her walking alignment to the foot on the sound (non-involved) side. Consequently, if the compensatory external rotation of that foot is not corrected, the pelvis will remain retracted on the affected side and the individual will continue to walk with relative external rotation of the affected hemiplegic limb, since correction of the anteversion now has aligned the limb to the pelvis, which remains retracted. On the other hand, if all torsional malalignments are corrected on both the sound and affected limb, the individual usually walks with his/her pelvic in a more neutral position postoperatively (Aminian et al. 2003). In the more severe types of hemiplegia, however, some pelvic retraction on the affected side is likely to remain. Consequently, it is important not to overcorrect the femoral anteversion on the hemiplegic side. In fact, I tend to slightly undercorrect the anteversion, particularly in the older child who is close to the end of growth.

Historical perspective
Sometimes a look into the past will provide insight into present practice. When dealing with gait abnormalities in cerebral palsy, modern day orthopaedists tend to concentrate on muscle surgery and, unless hip subluxation is present, ignore torsional deformities of bone. This, I believe, is a result of about two generations of 'primacy'.

Prior to World War II, antibiotics and/or adequate internal fixation were not available. Consequently, when surgery was contemplated, infection and/or failure of internal fixation were feared. These facts, coupled with the knowledge that long anesthesias were dangerous, militated against bone surgery. Furthermore, in that era the majority of children with cerebral palsy had quadriplegic involvement, since preterm infants rarely survived and diplegia is largely associated with preterm birth. Because of the magnitude and type of cerebral insult, quadriplegic patients usually have poor balance and selective motor control as compared to children with diplegia. Therefore ambulation usually was not a realistic goal. As such, the primary treatments of that time were bracing and physical therapy. If muscle contractures became severe enough to prevent bracing, then a short surgical intervention (usually hip-flexor or hamstring tenotomies and/or a tendo-Achilles lengthening) was indicated to allow resumption of orthotic wear. The practice then was to brace first and use tenotomy or lengthening of muscle only if the child became unbraceable. Osteotomies were avoided because of the high risk of complications. That practice has carried down to the present day, despite the fact that we now have safe anesthesia, reliable internal fixation, good antibiotics, and a preponderance of children with diplegia, who have excellent potential for community ambulation.

477

Patient assessment

To determine the cause of abnormal gait, careful patient assessment is required. This includes the standard history and physical examination plus appropriate imaging. However, because gait is dynamic and the deformities are complex, sagittal- and coronal-plane videos, which can be run in slow motion and repeatedly viewed, are extremely useful. Three-dimensional motion analysis will also provide a great deal of information, if it is available.

Once an examiner is aware of LAD and its implications, it is fairly easy to diagnose. For example in an individual with relatively normal body weight, the clinical examination, as outlined in Chapter 3.1, will often provide a fairly accurate assessment of the degree of anteversion (Ruwe et al. 1992, Davids et al. 2002, Kerr et al. 2003). Tibial torsion also can be estimated from physical examination, but impeding factors such as severe foot deformity and/or fixed ankle equinus may make assessment of tibial torsion difficult or unreliable. Advanced imaging techniques such as computer-augmented tomography are helpful in this regard, but expensive (Davids et al. 2003). In addition, since our primary interest is in the extent to which torsional deformities are interfering with function, slow-motion video and quantitative gait analysis are extremely useful as well. In our laboratory at Gillette Children's Hospital, we are able to do dynamic joint centering, which greatly improves the measurement accuracy of both femoral and tibial torsion (Schwartz and Rozumalski 2005). It is important to remember, however, that femoral rotation measured during gait analysis is not the same as femoral anteversion (Aktas et al. 2000, Kerr et al. 2003, O'Sullivan et al. 2006). The former just tells us the degree of internal rotation of the knee relative to the pelvis during gait, whereas the latter denotes the true amount of rotation in the bone. Severe femoral anteversion demands gait compensations, but those compensations can be accomplished with either internal femoral torsion and/or anterior pelvic tilt. Consequently, it is not unusual to see an individual with severe femoral anteversion and good motor control (GMFCS I or II) walk with relatively neutral rotation of the femora. Finally, the examination under anesthesia at the time of the surgical correction is very useful. If there is a question as to the degree of femoral anteversion present, a percutaneous Steinman pin can be passed down the center of the femoral neck easily and with little or no morbidity at the time of surgery. This allows femoral anteversion to be measured directly by simply comparing the angle of the pin to the angle of the tibia with the knee in 90° of flexion. Similarly, with respect to the tibia, it becomes much easier to reliably assess torsion once the foot and fixed equinus deformities have been corrected.

Indications for treatment

LAD, which is discussed in Chapter 2.4, is a significant component of orthopaedic deformity in that LAD disrupts normal joint moments. That is, it alters (reduces or malaligns) the normal transmission of muscle and/or ground reaction forces to the joints. Long bone torsions (femoral and/or tibial torsion) are particularly problematic in that not only do they reduce the magnitude of the normal moment; they also introduce valgus or rotational joint moments, which are not supposed to be present at all (see Figs 2.4.11, 12). Since growing bones are biologically plastic and derive their future form from the moments acting upon them, these abnormal moments further alter the shape and/or rotation of future growth of both the long bones and feet. Thus, in the short term, long bone torsions impede function. For example, since the greater trochanter is rotated out of plane, femoral anteversion can produce functional weakness of the hip abductors (Arnold et al. 1997, Gage and Schwartz 2004). In the long term, however, they not only impede function but also contribute to further growth deformity. Consequently, over the long term LAD can be devastating to the point of leading to a complete cessation of ambulation (see Case 6 on Interactive Disc, at ages 5, 11 and 16 years).

Goals of treatment

The major goals of any treatment are improvement of comfort, function and cosmesis in both the short and long term. In my experience, in the absence of a significant functional problem, children rarely have discomfort. In other words, functional problems might lead to discomfort and/or pain, but pain in isolation is uncommon in children. For example, a malformed foot eventually may lead to a painful bunion, but a painful bunion is not usually seen until late in adolescence. Therefore most of our treatment in children is directed towards improvement of function.

When treating these individuals, it is important to remember that joints are moved by moments (a force acting on a lever), and that even if the muscle and ground reaction forces were normal, lever-arm deformity would prevent normal moments from occurring. In neuromuscular conditions, it is difficult to correct abnormal muscle function, whereas it is fairly easy to correct abnormal levers. Unfortunately, since many orthopaedic surgeons were not taught the basic mechanics of LAD and its resultant effects, mal-rotation of the long bones in ambulatory patients with cerebral palsy may be recognized but ignored, since it often is considered to be a cosmetic problem and its long-term consequences are not understood.

In the treatment of femoral anteversion, the functional goals are:

(1) restoration of normal lever arms, which will improve the joint moments and thereby allow restoration of more normal function at the hip and knee
(2) elimination of gait compensations, which will result in both functional and cosmetic benefits. Examples of this might be:
  • elimination of lateral trunk sway in stance, which is a compensation for an inadequate hip-abductor moment
  • correction of internal rotation gait, which is often mistaken for scissoring
  • reduction of anterior pelvic tilt, which is a mechanism used to cover the anteriorly directed femoral head and neck.

Correction of excessive internal or external tibial torsion and/or foot deformity will promote the following benefits:

• increase the magnitude of the knee-extension moment, which may result in better knee extension in terminal stance (Hicks et al. 2007)

- restore foot stability and alignment, which results in better distribution of weightbearing forces (often with associated relief of pain and/or callus formation)
- in the long term, reduce the likelihood of recurrent growth deformity. For example, unless external foot rotation is corrected, bunion deformity (hallux valgus) will invariably recur since the individual will continue to push-off on an externally rotated foot thereby thrusting the hallux back into valgus with each step.

Treatment options

Clinical decision-making for the management of torsional deformities in children with cerebral palsy is based on the outcomes of the patient assessment utilizing the tools discussed earlier in this chapter. As knowledge and clinical experience grow, the treating surgeon will become more aware of the importance of correcting torsional bone deformities.

Some minor torsional anomalies will remodel spontaneously. For example, children are born with a minor amount of internal tibial torsion and this does tend to remodel, even in an individual with spastic diplegia. Similarly, minor degrees of femoral anteversion in a very functional, young child (GMFCS I or II involvement) may remodel, particularly if the individual's spasticity has been reduced via a selective dorsal rhizotomy. External tibial torsion, however, is always pathologic and generally worsens with time. Similarly, it has been shown that femoral anteversion normally does not remodel in children who have cerebral palsy, and in fact, tends to worsen over time (Fabry et al. 1973, Bobroff et al. 1999). Dr Cary's goals for the treatment of any child with a neuromuscular disability were outlined at the beginning of this section in my *Introduction and Overview of Treatment Philosophy*. They will not be reiterated here, except to say that in a child, a future problem is a problem and if ignored, time and growth will amplify both the problem's magnitude and its effects.

Non-Operative Treatment

Well-molded orthoses (UCBLs, SMOs, AFOs) are useful for controlling supple foot deformities, particularly in a young child. For example, they can prevent collapse of the valgus foot into external rotation and by so doing maintain better dynamic alignment of the limb during gait. They also allow delay of surgery until a more optimal age when the bones of the feet are larger and there is less future growth to generate recurrent deformity. Even in the older child with cerebral palsy in whom surgery is done, however, orthoses are usually necessary to maintain the correction until the growth is complete. This is because the muscle imbalance that generated the deformity persists throughout the years of growth, and so correction must be maintained until maturity to prevent recurrent deformity.

Braces such as a Denis–Browne bar and/or twister cables generally have very little application in the presence of bony deformity. Twister cables may prove useful, as a training device (to maintain dynamic alignment during walking in children who persist in an abnormal gait pattern following surgical correction of their torsion), but they are encumbering and there is no evidence that they act to unwind tibial or femoral torsion.

With modern internal fixation, surgical correction of torsional deformities has improved a great deal. At our Center, with rare exceptions, children are not placed in spica casts. For example, a child who has had bilateral femoral and tibial osteotomies generally is placed in splinted Robert Jones dressings for the first 3 days. On the 3rd postoperative day, bilateral short leg casts are applied, which are tied together with a removable Denis–Browne bar (see Fig. 5.9.3). The parents are instructed to leave the bar on during the hours of sleep and when doing transfers. Prior to discharge from the hospital, the parents are taught to remove the bar to do passive range-of-motion exercises of the hips and knees, which are carried out multiple times daily from the 3rd postoperative day onward. The Denis–Browne bar is discarded 3 weeks post-surgery and weight bearing is begun as tolerated. Details of our rehabilitation program are discussed in Chapter 5.9. In my personal experience, surgical correction of torsional deformities is best corrected prior to adolescence when the child is still small enough to be toileted easily. Once adolescence has begun, rehabilitation takes longer and emotional issues are much more of a problem. In fact, in an adolescent who is mature or nearing maturity, I generally stage the procedures and correct the more involved limb first leaving the other limb for weightbearing. In that way, down-time is minimized and the individual may be able to perform activities of daily living independently.

So far as the specifics of surgery are concerned, we here at Gillette Children's Specialty Healthcare prefer to do the femoral osteotomies in the intertrochanteric region with the child in the prone position using the approach described by Root and Siegal (1980). This approach provides excellent access to the femur as well as precise assessment of anteversion both pre- and post-correction (Fig 5.6.4). Correcting the deformity above the lesser trochanter allows the lesser trochanter to be rotated anteriorly by an amount equal to the magnitude of the derotation. This not only normalizes the position of the lesser trochanter anatomically, but also relatively lengthens the psoas by reducing the distance between the muscle's origin and insertion (Schutte et al. 1997) (Fig. 5.6.5). In my personal opinion, this is a more physiologic way to correct the deformity. Jenkins et al. (2003) provided further evidence for this by demonstrating that femoral anteversion can be modeled geometrically as occurring proximal to the lesser trochanter. However, articles comparing intertrochanteric osteotomies to those done more distally have not been able to demonstrate a significant difference between the two methods (Kay et al. 2003, Pirpiris et al. 2003).

With respect to the tibia, unless there is a significant component of coxa vera or valga, the correction is best done distally, as there is less risk of compartment syndrome and/or stretch paralysis of the deep peroneal nerve (Davis et al. 1998, Mueller and Farley 2003, Selber et al. 2004, Dilawaiz Nadeem et al. 2005). Tibial derotation alone is usually sufficient, except in the older child in whom it is difficult to maintain tibial alignment without cutting the fibula (Ryan et al. 2005). At our Center, internal fixation is usually achieved with a single, straight, four or five-hole plate, although a variety of fixation methods have been used with success by multiple authors (Selber et al. 2004, Ryan et al. 2005). Since metaphyseal bone heals more rapidly, the osteotomy is done as close to the distal tibial epiphysis as is possible without risk of injury. The tibial osteotomy can be done with the patient either

(a)

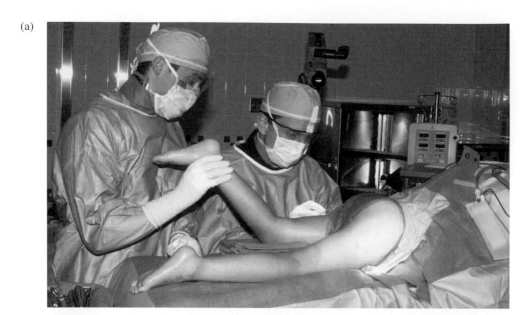

(b)

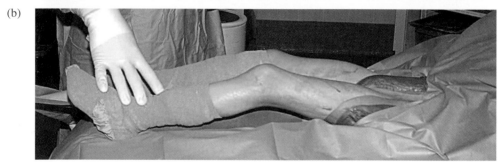

Fig. 5.6.4 Single-event multilevel surgery. An illustration demonstrating surgical draping just prior to surgery. (a) Beginning in the prone position, both lower extremities are draped free to allow full access to the lower extremities. Proximally all of the edges of the drapes are taped with Steri-drape" to lessen the chance of contamination of the surgical field. All foot procedures, long bone osteotomies, and posterior muscle surgery are done with the patient in this position. (b) The patient is then turned into the supine position and re-prepped and draped for intramuscular psoas lengthening, adductor tenotomies, rectus femoris transfers, and/or patellar tendon advancements if any or all of these procedures are indicated. Distal femoral extension osteotomies may be done from either position, but are usually done with the patient supine. (see Instructional Video on femoral osteotomy on Interactive Disc.)

prone or supine, although I personally feel it is easier to assess alignment with the patient prone. Until the foot is corrected, however, it is difficult to assess tibial torsion accurately. Therefore we usually start with the patient prone and with a sterile tourniquet on the limb. The foot deformities are then corrected first, since it is difficult to accurately assess tibial torsion until after the integrity of the foot has been restored. Both varus and valgus foot deformities can be corrected easily with the patient prone. Access to the dorsal aspect of the foot is obtained by simply flexing the knee to about 130°.

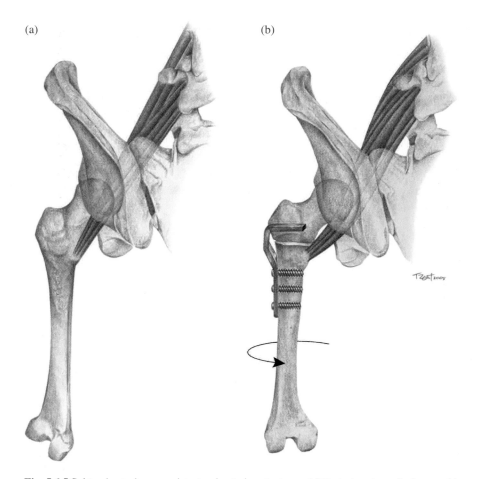

Fig. 5.6.5 Subtrochanteric versus intertrochanteric osteotomy. (a) Posterior view of a femur with about 50° of femoral anteversion. Studies indicate that most of the anteversion occurs proximal to the lesser trochanter, so the iliopsoas insertion is actually rotated 50° posteriorly to the axis of the femoral neck. (b) If an intertrochanteric osteotomy were to be done, the lesser trochanter would now be included with the distal segment and would rotate externally with the knee. Post-surgery, therefore, when the patient walks with his knees in the plane of progression, the trochanter would be in its anatomically correct position, which results in relative lengthening of the psoas. If, on the other hand, the derotation was done in the subtrochanteric region, the malrotation between the femoral head and lesser trochanter would be unchanged and the psoas insertion would now be on the posterior aspect of the femur.

Once the foot is corrected, contractures of the triceps surae are addressed. After these deformities have been corrected, tibial torsion can be accurately assessed using the foot–thigh angle or the 2nd toe test (see Chapter 3.1). With the patient prone and the knee in 130° of flexion, the surgeon has excellent access to the anterior tibia and the tibial osteotomy can be done without difficulty (Fig. 5.6.6, Instructional Video 'Tibial osteotomy' on Interactive Disc). Although pins in the proximal and distal segments can be used to assess rotation, I generally just attach the plate to the distal segment with a single screw in

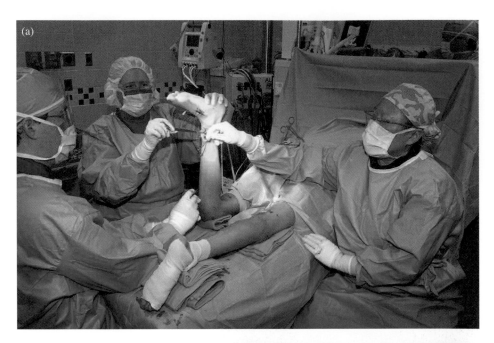

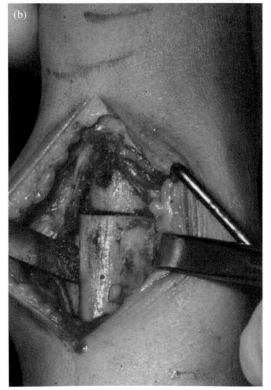

Fig. 5.6.6 Tibial osteotomy from the prone position. (a) With the knee flexed to about 120° and the surgeon seated, s/he has easy access to the anterior surface of the distal tibia to perform the osteotomy. Foot surgery also is accomplished easily using the same technique. (b) Surgical view of the tibial osteotomy in the prone position. The foot is above and the knee below. The plate had been previously attached to the distal segment through the screw hole and removed. The empty screw hole can be seen just proximal to the osteotomy. (See Instructional Video 'Tibial osteotomy' on Interactive Disc.)

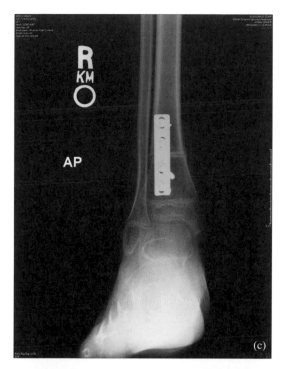

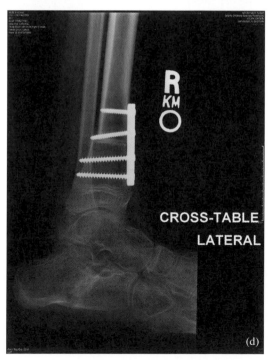

Fig. 5.6.6 continued(c, d) AP and lateral radiographs taken 6 weeks post-surgery of a patient who has had both a distal tibial osteotomy and an os calcis lengthening. Internal fixation is accomplished with a 4-hole straight plate placed close to the distal tibial epiphysis. The bone wedge used for the calcaneal lengthening can be seen as well. It is usually stable without additional internal fixation. At our Center, os calcis lengthening is done with autograft from the bone bank to avoid the necessity of obtaining a bone graft from the pelvis. We have had no difficulties relating to healing of the osteotomy and/or incorporation of the allograft.

the most distal hole, and then swivel the plate 90° to the plane of the tibia while I do the osteotomy. The plate can then be realigned to the tibia and the foot and distal tibial segment rotated in the appropriate direction until the foot–thigh angle and 2nd toe test are normal. I then maintain the alignment while my assistant anchors the proximal end of the plate to the proximal tibial segment. If fibular osteotomy is necessary to obtain adequate alignment, it is usually done at a higher level through a small separate incision (roughly at the junction of the middle and distal thirds) without internal fixation. Again in my personal experience of 30 years doing this procedure, I can recall only one instance of fibular nonunion that required bone grafting.

Supporting evidence

Bioengineering studies can provide good theoretical evidence of the benefits of correction of lever arm dysfunction (see Chapter 3.6). There is convincing evidence of the effects of excessive femoral anteversion based on musculoskeletal modeling (Arnold et al. 1997, Delp et al. 1999, Hicks et al. 2007). Arnold et al. (1997) found that anteversion and valgus deformities of the femur can decrease the abduction moment arm of the gluteus medius substantially. Delp et al. (1999) noted that the functional position of the joint during ambulation significantly altered the rotational effects of the anterior gluteal musculature, such that if an individual walked with his/her hips in excessive flexion, the anterior gluteals functioned as strong internal rotators of the femur. Hicks et al. (2007) reported on the effect of excessive tibial torsion on the capacity of muscles to extend the knee in single stance and concluded that tibial torsion may be a significant contributor to crouch gait.

Long-term evidence of the benefits of correction of abnormal torsion is just starting to appear. Õunpuu et al. (2002) reported evidence of improved function with correction of femoral anteversion in 20 patients followed with clinical examination and 3-dimensional gait analysis at 1 and 5 years post-surgery. Anteversion was reduced from a mean of 63° pre-surgery to 26° at 1 year and 31° at 5 years. Clinical benefits were also maintained. Tylkowski et al. (1980) reported good results in surgical correction of anteversion at a mean of about 3 years in 32 children with cerebral palsy (hip subluxation or dislocation in 18 and severe anteversion with in-toeing in 14) with 'few and minor' complications. Murray-Weir et al. (2003) reported excellent results in 37 individuals at 1 year. Pirpirus et al. (2003) noted excellent short term results with 3-dimensional gait analysis in 28 ambulatory children with spastic diplegia who had bilateral derotational femoral osteotomies done at either a proximal or distal level. Excellent correction of hip rotation and foot rotation was noted regardless of the level of the osteotomies. Kim et al. (2005) studied 30 children with 45 femurs and noted that although correction was achieved in all following surgery, there was significant recurrence of deformity in 15 femurs at 5 years post-surgery. Patients who underwent surgery prior to age 10 were more likely to show recurrence.

Stefko et al. (1998) studied the effects of tibial derotation on a group of 10 ambulatory children with 3-dimensional gait analysis. They stated that derotational tibial osteotomy was a safe, reliable, and effective procedure, which produced significant improvement of foot rotation with a trend toward normal moment data. Ryan et al. (2005) reported on 46 children with 72 distal tibial osteotomies without concomitant fibular osteotomy. They reported eight perioperative complications (11%) with three delayed unions, three superficial wound dehiscences, one pin-tract infection, and one case of osteomyelitis. There were no malunions or nonunions.

Finally, Bruce and Stevens (2004) identified 14 non-cerebral palsy patients with 27 limbs, all of whom had femoral anteversion, external tibial torsion, and patellofemoral pain. Each of the limbs was realigned with a combination of derotational femoral and tibial osteotomies. All of the patients reported full satisfaction with their surgery and outcomes.

Consequently, it is reasonable to assume that although a child with cerebral palsy may tolerate rotational abnormalities with little complaint or sense of limitation, these problems, left untreated, will be poorly tolerated in adult life when body mass is much greater and secondary arthritic changes begin to appear. It is our expectation, therefore, that correction of torsional problems during childhood may well prevent much of the arthritis and joint pain, which we are currently seeing in our adult patients who have not had torsional correction of long bone deformities.

Case example (see Case 7 on Interactive Disc)

The benefits of correction of long bone torsions can probably be best demonstrated with a case example (Fig. 5.6.7, Case 7 on Interactive Disc).

This patient initially presented to our Center at the age of 2½. She was the first-born twin. The twins were born vaginally. Birth was induced at approximately 6½ weeks before the due date due to decreased size of the other twin. At birth, her Apgar scores were 7 and 8 at 1 and 5 minutes respectively. Later, she became floppy and eventually required mechanical ventilation. An ultrasound at that time revealed a left-sided ventricular hemorrhage. She spent approximately 2½ weeks in the NICU. Following her hospital discharge, Molly did quite well. Because of delayed motor milestones she was diagnosed as having a mild spastic triplegia, with the right side being the hemiparetic side, at about 9 months of age. Cognitively she was completely normal. She had no seizures or other associated problems of cerebral palsy.

She began walking at approximately 18 months. By the time she was initially seen at our Center at age 2½, she could run. Her mother stated that Molly's right side was more affected than the left. She wore bilateral UCBLs to control her pes valgus.

Physical examination: She had a fairly typical toddler gait except for fairly severe bilateral pes valgus and when excited or trying to move rapidly she went up onto her toes. Her gait was characterized by internal rotation bilaterally (right side > left) secondary to femoral anteversion. She had a full range of motion of her hips bilaterally but with excessive total rotation (hip internal rotation was 80° and external rotation 40° bilaterally). Femoral anteversion was palpated at 45° on the left and 70° on the right. Her knees were fully mobile and her hamstrings had full range bilaterally. Duncan–Ely signs were negative. Examination of her ankles demonstrated increased tone of the entire right lower extremity, which was most evident at the ankle. There was bilateral hindfoot valgus on standing (right worse than left). Physical examination also demonstrated generalized (inherited) ligamentous laxity.

(a)

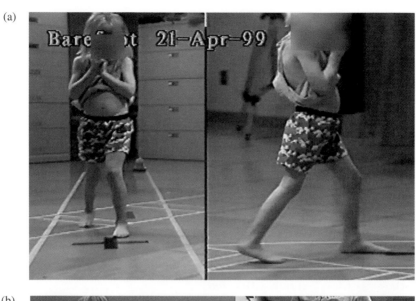

(b)

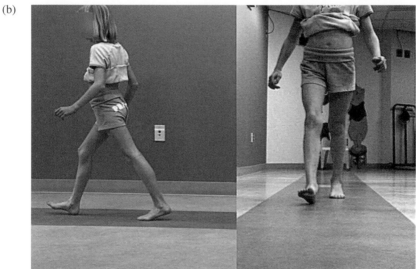

Fig. 5.6.7 Video capture illustration of MJK at age 4½, just prior to surgical correction of her skeletal malalignments. These included bilateral femoral anteversion, right external tibial torsion, and bilateral pes valgus. Note the bilateral pes valgus and internal rotation of her knees secondary to femoral anteversion. Tibial alignment appears normal on the left, but on the right side external tibial torsion is producing a malrotation of about 35° between the knee and the foot. In addition there is premature activity of the gastrocnemius in mid-stance on the right side only. (For a dynamic illustration of this patient, see Case 7 on Interactive Disc.) (b) A video capture illustration of the same girl 5 years later at age 10. She has had no further surgery in the interim. The premature activity of the gastrocnemius, which was seen in the preoperative video, was corrected at the time of the initial surgery by means of a Strayer-type gastrocnemius recession. Her alignment is now normal and she walks with bilateral heelstrike.

Radiographs: An anteroposterior (AP) radiograph of her pelvis revealed the hips to be located with no evidence of subluxation. Weightbearing, AP and lateral radiographs of her feet demonstrated pes valgus with mild talonavicular subluxation bilaterally.

Diagnosis and course of treatment: On the basis of this examination, she was felt to have cerebral palsy subtype right triplegia (GMFCS I) with inherited ligamentous laxity, femoral anteversion, and pes valgus.

Over the next several years, the child was maintained in her orthoses and on a program of physical therapy. During that time she was seen by a pediatric physiatrist on two occasions for botulinum toxin type A injection into her gastrocnemii. Each time botulinum toxin type A was administered, it was followed by a course of stretching casts. At the age of 4½, because of lordotic gait with persistent internal rotation and pes valgus, she was referred for gait analysis. Clinical examination and gait analysis at that time revealed the following:

(1) cerebral palsy, subtype right spastic triplegia with good selective motor control and balance
(2) severe bilateral femoral anteversion (right > left) with lordotic gait (hamstrings at normal length)
(3) bilateral pes valgus (right > left)
(4) premature gastrocnemius activity bilaterally with mild contracture (right>left)
(5) external rotation deformity of the right leg (between knee and foot) secondary to external tibial torsion in conjunction with pes valgus.

Surgery: Just prior to surgery her walking ability was assessed as GMFCS II (level 9/10 on the Functional Classification System with the ability to do 15 of the 22 functional skills). Then the following procedures were performed in September 1999:

(1) bilateral intertrochanteric derotational femoral osteotomies using AO plate fixation
(2) bilateral os calcis lengthening using tricortical allograft
(3) right supramalleolar derotational tibial osteotomy using plate fixation
(4) right Baker-type gastrosoleus lengthening
(5) injection of soleus muscle with 50 units of botulinum toxin.

Outcome: Molly was discharged 5 days post-surgery in bilateral short leg casts tied together with a Denis–Browne bar. She was maintained non-weightbearing for 3 weeks. She then returned as an outpatient for cast change, molding for bilateral UCBL orthoses, and a session of physical therapy. From that point on she was allowed to bear weight as tolerated. At 6 weeks post-surgery, the casts were removed and her orthoses were fitted. She had a second session of physical therapy and instructions for physical therapy at an incidence of 2–3 times a week were sent from our therapist to Molly's home therapist. This was to include some pool therapy.

She returned for plate removal 9 months post-surgery. At that time we assessed her walking at GMFCS I (level 10/10 on the Functional Classification System with the ability to do 20 out of 22 functional skills). The hardware was removed without incident during the course of an overnight admission. She resumed ambulation as soon as she was comfortable enough to do so, but she was maintained on Loftstrand crutches for 4 weeks following the procedure as a precaution against fracture of the plate removal sites. Over the next several years she continued wearing the UCBLs in her school shoes. She was maintained on a daily home program of exercise, which was supervised on a monthly basis by her physical therapist. She was followed over the next several years with no further inventions. When last seen she was 12½ years old and doing well. She was involved in many physical activities and was to be starting 7th grade in the fall. She was planning to participate on the volleyball team at school. She had been riding horses avidly over the summer. Her mother stated that occasionally she noticed that Molly walked with her toes pointing a little bit inwards; however, she was not concerned about this, as it has not been affecting any of her functionality. She had no pain or discomfort in either of her lower extremities. The scars on the lateral aspects of her thighs and right ankle were cosmetically acceptable and Molly indicated that she had no concerns about them. She continued to wear UCBLs in her school shoes. She was in the midst of her adolescent growth spurt and had grown 9.5 cm since the last time was seen in the clinic. Physical examination at that time revealed symmetric anteversion bilaterally of approximately 10°. She had a full range of motion of her hips, knees, and ankles. Examination of her feet revealed well-formed arches with no deformity. Her standing alignment was normal. As she walked she demonstrated occasional mild in-turning of her left foot. Since she was doing so well, she was given an 'as needed' appointment to return to clinic if future problems or difficulties should arise.

REFERENCES

Aktas S, Aiona MD, Orendurff M (2000) Evaluation of rotational gait abnormality in the patients cerebral palsy. *J Pediatr Orthop* **20**: 217–20.

Aminian A, Vankoski SJ, Dias L, Novak RA (2003) Spastic hemiplegic cerebral palsy and the femoral derotation osteotomy: effect at the pelvis and hip in the transverse plane during gait. *J Pediatr Orthop* **23**: 314–20.

Arkin AM, Katz JF (1956) The effects of pressure on epiphyseal growth. *J Bone Joint Surg Am* **38**: 1056–76.

Arnold AS, Komattu AV, Delp SL (1997) Internal rotation gait: a compensatory mechanism to restore abduction capacity decreased by bone deformity. *Dev Med Child Neurol* **39**: 40–4.

Bobroff ED, Chambers HG, Sartoris DJ, Wyatt MP, Sutherland DH (1999) Femoral anteversion and neck-shaft angle in children with cerebral palsy. *Clin Orthop Rel Res* **364**: 194–204.

Bruce WD, Stevens PM (2004) Surgical correction of miserable malalignment syndrome. *J Pediatr Orthop* **24**: 392–6.

Davids JR, Benfanti P, Blackhurst DW, Allen BL (2002) Assessment of femoral anteversion in children with cerebral palsy: accuracy of the trochanteric prominence angle test. *J Pediatr Orthop* **22**: 173–8.

Davids JR, Marshall AD, Blocker ER, Frick SL, Blackhurst DW, Skewes E (2003) Femoral anteversion in children with cerebral palsy: assessment with two and three-dimensional computed tomography scans. *J Bone Joint Surg Am* **85**: 481–8.

Davis CAMD, Maranji KMD, Frederick NMS, Dorey FPD, Moseley CFMD (1998) Comparison of crossed pins and external fixation for correction of angular deformities about the knee in children. *J Pediatr Orthop* **18**: 502–7.

Delp SL, Hess WE, Hungerford DS, Jones LC (1999) Variation of rotation moment arms with hip flexion. *J Biomech* **32**: 493–501.

Dilawaiz Nadeem R, Quick TJ, Eastwood DM (2005) Focal dome osteotomy for the correction of tibial deformity in children. *J Pediatr Orthop* **14**: 340–6.

Dobson F, Morris ME, Baker R, Wolfe R, Graham H (2006) Clinician agreement on gait pattern ratings in children with spastic hemiplegia. *Dev Med Child Neurol* **48**: 429–35.

Fabry G, MacEwen GD, Shands AR Jr (1973) Torsion of the femur. A follow-up study in normal and abnormal conditions. *J Bone Joint Surg Am* **55**: 1726–38.

Gage JR, Schwartz M (2004) Pathological gait and lever-arm dysfunction. In: Gage JR, editor. *The Treatment of Gait Problems in Cerebral Palsy*. London: Mac Keith Press. p 180–204.

Graham HK, Baker R, Dobson F, Morris ME (2005) Multilevel orthopaedic surgery in group IV spastic hemiplegia. *J Bone Joint Surg Br* **87**: 548–55.

Hicks J, Arnold A, Anderson F, Schwartz M, Delp S (2007) The effect of excessive tibial torsion on the capacity of muscles to extend the hip and knee during single-limb stance. *Gait Posture* **26**: 546–52.

Jenkins SEM, Harrington ME, Zavatsky AB, O'Connor JJ, Theologis TN (2003) Femoral muscle attachment locations in children and adults, and their prediction from clinical measurement. *Gait Posture* **18**: 13–22.

Kay RM, Rethlefsen SA, Hale JM, Skaggs DL, Tolo VT (2003) Comparison of proximal and distal rotational femoral osteotomy in children with cerebral palsy. *J Pediatr Orthop* **23**: 150–4.

Kerr AM, Kirtley SJ, Hillman SJ, van der Linden ML, Hazlewood ME, Robb JE (2003) The mid-point of passive hip rotation range is an indicator of hip rotation in gait in cerebral palsy. *Gait Posture* **17**: 88–91.

Kim H, Aiona M, Sussman M (2005) Recurrence after femoral derotational osteotomy in cerebral palsy. *J Pediatr Orthop* **25**: 739–43.

Mueller KLMD, Farley FAMD (2003) Superficial and deep posterior compartment syndrome following high tibial osteotomy for tibia vara in a child. *Orthopedics* **26**: 513–14.

Murray-Weir M, Root L, Peterson M, Lenhoff M, Daly L, Wagner C, Marcus P (2003) Proximal femoral varus rotation osteotomy in cerebral palsy: a prospective gait study. *J Pediatr Orthop* **23**: 321–9.

O'Sullivan R, Walsh M, Hewart P, Jenkinson A, Ross LA, O'Brien T (2006) Factors associated with internal hip rotation gait in patients with cerebral palsy. *J Pediatr Orthop* **26**: 537–41.

Õunpuu S, DeLuca P, Davis R, Romness M (2002) Long-term effects of femoral derotation osteotomies: an evaluation using three-dimensional gait analysis. *J Pediatr Orthop* **22**: 139–45.

Pirpiris M, Trivett A, Baker R, Rodda J, Nattrass GR, Graham HK (2003) Femoral derotation osteotomy in spastic diplegia. Proximal or distal? *J Bone Joint Surg Br* **85**: 265–72.

Riad J, Haglund-Akerlind Y, Miller F (2007) Classification of spastic hemiplegic cerebral palsy in children. *J Pediatr Orthop* **27**: 758–64.

Root L, Siegal T (1980) Osteotomy of the hip in children: posterior approach. *J Bone Joint Surg Am* **62**: 571–5.

Ruwe PA, Gage JR, Ozonoff MB, DeLuca PA (1992) Clinical determination of femoral anteversion. A comparison with established techniques. *J Bone Joint Surg Am* **74**: 820–30.

Ryan DD, Rethlefsen SA, Skaggs DL, Kay RM (2005) Results of tibial rotational osteotomy without concomitant fibular osteotomy in children with cerebral palsy. *J Pediatr Orthop* **25**: 84–8.

Schutte LM, Hayden SW, Gage JR (1997) Lengths of hamstrings and psoas muscles during crouch gait: effects of femoral anteversion. *J Orthop Res* **15**: 615–21.

Schwartz MH, Rozumalski A (2005) A new method for estimating joint parameters from motion data. *J Biomech* **38**: 107–16.

Selber P, Filho ER, Dallalana R, Pirpiris M, Nattrass GR, Graham HK (2004) Supramalleolar derotation osteotomy of the tibia, with T plate fixation: technique and results in patients with neuromuscular disease. *J Bone Joint Surg Br* **86**: 1170–5.

Somerville EW (1957) Persistent foetal alignment of the hip. *J Bone Joint Surg* **39B**: 106–13.

Stefko RM, de Swart RJ, Dodgin DA, Wyatt MP, Kaufman KR, Sutherland DH, Chambers HG. (1998) Kinematic and kinetic analysis of distal derotational osteotomy of the leg in children with cerebral palsy. *J Pediatr Orthop* **18**: 81–7.

Tylkowski CM, Rosenthal RK, Simon SR (1980) Proximal femoral osteotomy in cerebral palsy. *Clin Orthop* **151**: 183–92.

Winters TF Jr, Gage JR, Hicks R (1987) Gait patterns in spastic hemiplegia in children and young adults. *J Bone Joint Surg Am* **69**: 437–41.

5.7
ORTHOPAEDIC TREATMENT OF
HIP PROBLEMS IN CEREBRAL PALSY

Henry G. Chambers

Key points
- The hip is frequently affected by the increased tone of cerebral palsy
- The problems seen at the hip, from loss of flexibility to dysplasia and dislocation, are linked to the severity of functional impairment
- Assessment by careful examination, radiographs and special imaging, and motion analysis will result in the most effective treatment plan
- Interventions are based on the degree to which muscle and bone changes have evolved in the face of altered neurological function
- Best outcomes are obtained with concentric articulation and minimal contracture.

To understand the hip of a child with cerebral palsy we must understand the hip of a typical infant. This is discussed in Chapter 1.3. Then we must understand the consequences of hypertonia, loss of selective motor control, and unbalanced activity in the muscles that surround the hip joint. Altered motor function in cerebral palsy has important consequences for hip development. Increased muscle tone leads to reduced muscle elasticity and decreased ability to stretch the hip joint through a full arc of motion. Muscle growth is reduced yielding decreased muscle length and failure to resolve the infantile hip-flexion contracture (or actual worsening of the contracture). These changes affect the hip-flexor and adductor muscles more than the extensors and abductors.

The muscle changes of cerebral palsy result in atypical, unbalanced application of stress to the femoral head and acetabulum. Infantile anteversion not only fails to resolve, but may actually increase with time. The relationship between the femoral head and neck and the femoral shaft becomes more vertical (coxa valga). Excessive anteversion and coxa valga change the position of the greater trochanter and reduce the efficiency of abductor muscle function. The proximal femoral physis, aligned perpendicular to the net vector of stress at the hip, reflects the imbalance in muscle activity by becoming more horizontal. With incomplete extension and persistent adduction and medial rotation of the thigh, the medial portion of the femoral head and the lateral portion of the acetabulum experience increased compression stress. Following the Heuter–Volkmann principle (see Chapter 1.3) (Sauser et al. 1986) they demonstrate reduced bone growth. The result is an aspherical femoral head (with flattening of the medial surface) and an acetabulum with an underdeveloped bony lateral rim (reflected in the increased acetabular angle). The floor or medial wall of the acetabulum experiences reduced compression stress and increases its growth (demonstrated by widening of the medial 'teardrop'). No longer cup-like, the acetabulum loses its ability to contain the femoral head. The femoral head progressively loses contact with the acetabulum (subluxation) until it dislocates and moves proximally along the outer cortex of the ilium. Dislocation of the femoral head accentuates the flexion and adduction contracture and creates leg length inequality. The nutrition of the articular cartilage is disturbed and the cartilage deteriorates. All of this is compounded by greater motor dysfunction on one side of the body. The progressive hip flexion and adduction contracture leads to pelvic obliquity and windswept posture in which the femur is flexed, adducted and internally rotated while the opposite femur is flexed, abducted and externally rotated.

The risk of experiencing this cascade of hip pathology is not shared equally by children with cerebral palsy. The Gross Motor Functional Classification System (GMFCS) serves as an index of severity of involvement of cerebral palsy (see Chapters 2.4, 2.5 and 6.1). The biarticular muscles in the distal portion of the lower extremity are the most disturbed in children with mild involvement (GMFCS I). This creates problems with motor control and spasticity principally in the muscles of the ankle and foot. As the severity of cerebral palsy increases so does the involvement of more proximal joints. This is the basis for the classification of hemiplegia by Winters and colleagues (1987) discussed in Chapter 2.5. Soo et al. (2006) and Hagglund et al. (2007) have shown that children who function at GMFCS level I have almost no chance of hip subluxation (Figs 5.7.1, 2). Children

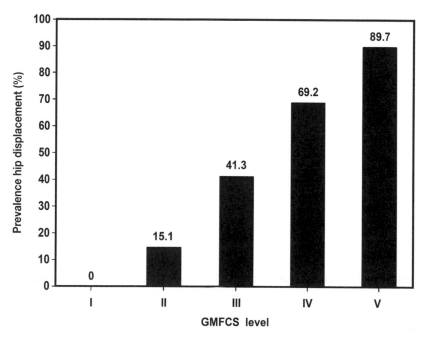

Fig. 5.7.1 The relationship between Gross Motor Function Classification System level and the prevalence of hip dysplasia in cerebral palsy (Soo et al. 2006).

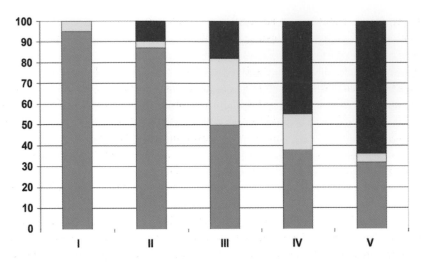

Fig. 5.7.2 The relationship between Gross Motor Function Classification level and migration percentage in cerebral palsy (Hagglund et al. 2007). y axis = migration %.

at a GMFCS level V have a 70%–90 % chance of hip dysplasia, with the overall incidence of hip dysplasia in cerebral palsy in the study of Soo et al. (2006) being 35%. As the GMFCS level increases the degree of hip pathology increases while the ability to walk decreases.

Patient assessment
It is critical to appreciate all of the different problems that affect hip development in a child with cerebral palsy. A complete history includes information about past and current ambulation skills, oral medications, and treatments such as physical therapy, bracing, botulinum toxin, phenol, and surgery (musculoskeletal and neurological). It is very helpful to apply validated assessment tools whose results may serve as a reference point for judging the outcome of future interventions. The GMFCS, Functional Assessment Questionnaire (FAQ) and Functional Mobility Scale (FMS) are excellent methods by which to assess ambulatory patients (see Chapters 2.5, 3.1 and 6.1).

A complete physical examination includes several components: the musculoskeletal and neurological systems and analysis of the child's gait. The key components of physical examination of the hip will be reviewed here. Gait analysis is the subject of this book and is covered in detail elsewhere (see Chapter 3.6).

EXAMINATION OF THE HIP

Musculoskeletal examination
The general musculoskeletal examination was discussed in Chapter 3.1. At the hip it is important (but not always possible) to distinguish between a fixed muscle contracture and a dynamic (neurologic) restriction in hip range of motion.

Hip flexion. The child is placed in a supine position, one leg is kept on the surface of the examination table, and the opposite hip is flexed. The process is then reversed for the two legs.

Hip extension. In the Thomas test both hips are flexed until the lumbar lordosis of the spine is removed and the lumbar spine is flat on the table. Then one hip at a time is extended until the end range. This angle from the table is measured. Staheli (1977) found this method unreliable in cerebral palsy due to inconsistent reduction of lordosis. He proposed a prone hip-extension test in which the hips are flexed over the end. Each hip is then extended and when the end range is reached, the angle between the table and the thigh is measured (Fig. 5.7.3). Some children find this position intolerable.

Hip internal and external rotation. This test is best done while the patient is in the prone position.

Assessment of femoral anteversion. Ruwe et al. (1992) described a clinical method to assess femoral anteversion. They placed the patient in a prone position, palpated the anterior surface of the greater trochanter and when the anterior surface was parallel to the table after internally rotating the thigh they estimated femoral anteversion by measuring the angle formed by the tibia and the surface of the examination table. They termed this the trochanteric prominence angle test (TPAT). Davids et al. (2003) compared this test to anteversion assessment by CT and found that the TPAT significantly overestimated anteversion in 26% of subjects and underestimated the femoral anteversion in more than 50% of subjects. Bobroff et al. (1999) described a method using intraoperative fluoroscopy that correlated well with the CT scan. Thus physical examination provides a good approximation of anteversion but imaging studies are more precise and may be needed to plan surgery (Fig. 5.7.4).

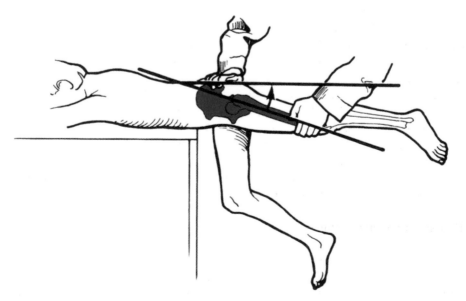

Fig. 5.7.3 The Staheli prone extension test (Staheli 1977).

495

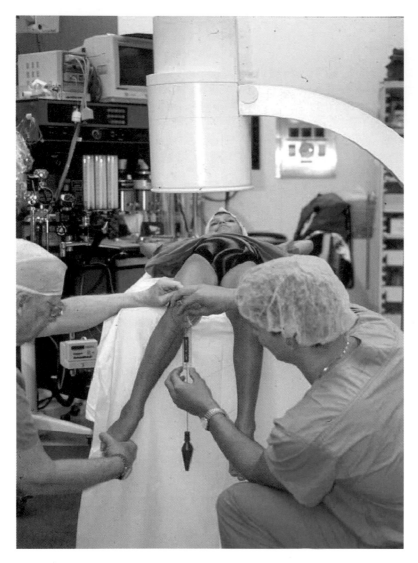

Fig. 5.7.4 Assessment of femoral anteversion by fluoroscopy as performed by Dr David Sutherland.

Neurological examination

A very important component of cerebral palsy is muscle weakness, which is often overlooked. Strength testing should be attempted in all patients. It is difficult to assess strength in the presence of muscle contracture, hypertonia, and poor selective motor control. Adductor and flexor muscles often are found to be stronger than the extensors and abductors. A complete neurological examination also includes assessment of tone: spasticity, dystonia, athetosis or chorea, and rigidity (see Chapters 2.2 and 2.3). Management of motor abnormalities should be part of any musculoskeletal intervention.

Imaging

Physical examination is not a reliable method for detection of mild hip instability or monitoring the behavior of instability. A supine anteroposterior radiograph of the pelvis (performed with neutral leg rotation and alignment) provides important information about femoral head position and the development of the femur and acetabulum. Radiographic changes may be seen as early as 18 months of age, particularly in children with greater neurologic involvement (GMFCS IV and V) or significantly decreased hip abduction (<30°). The first radiograph should be obtained by 24–30 months in nearly all children. It should be repeated every 12 months for children at GMFCS IV and V. For children at GMFCS I or II, a second radiograph should be obtained by age 6–8 years or before any lower extremity surgical interventions. Several measurements are possible but the migration percentage described by Reimers (1980) is particularly important. A classification system has been proposed to characterize the severity of dysplasia (Robin et al. 2009). In more advanced dysplasia CT provides essential information about the location of acetabular deficiency (Kim and Wenger 1997). See Chapter 3.4 for an extensive discussion of bone imaging (Figs 5.7.5, 6).

Computer models

Computer modeling using cadaveric derived models coupled with gait analysis data is an important research tool to gain insight into complex biological problems. These models may enable one to determine if a specific surgery will lead to the desired results. Delp and colleagues have written several thought-provoking articles in this arena (Delp et al. 1999, Arnold et al. 2000, Arnold and Delp 2001). Such computer models have been used to evaluate internal rotation gait and its treatment, the effect of hip flexion on moment arms, and the effect of knee flexion in crouch gait on hip extension. This tool has improved our understanding of biomechanical forces at the hip but has not been used to create individualized treatment plans for actual patients. This is certainly the hope and promise of this technology.

Specific hip problems in cerebral palsy

Problems at the hip will be reduced to individual components knowing that there are combinations and interactions between all of the components. In this artificial construct it is important to remember the effects of problems at other areas such as the foot and ankle, knee, pelvis, trunk and the upper extremities.

The goals of treatment for individuals with cerebral palsy who are able to walk (GMFCS levels I–III) are different than the goals for individuals who have extreme limitations or are unable to walk (GMFCS IV or V). At GMFCS levels I–III the goals are to maintain or improve walking ability, improve efficiency, decrease the use of assistive devices (canes, crutches or walker), and minimize the small risk of hip subluxation and dislocation. At GMFCS levels IV and V the goals are to maintain concentric painless hip articulation and prevent contractures that interfere with perineal care (inadequate abduction), standing (inadequate extension), or sitting with a level pelvis (windswept deformity and scoliosis). To reach these goals it is necessary to restore muscle flexibility and balance and restore

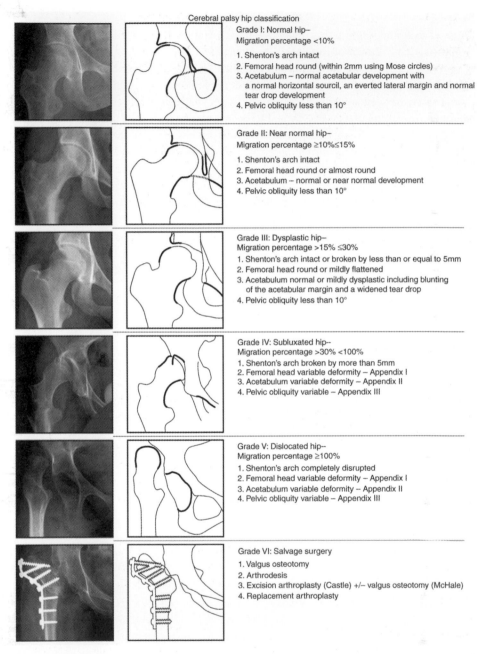

Cerebral palsy hip classification

Grade I: Normal hip–
Migration percentage <10%

1. Shenton's arch intact
2. Femoral head round (within 2mm using Mose circles)
3. Acetabulum – normal acetabular development with a normal horizontal sourcil, an everted lateral margin and normal tear drop development
4. Pelvic obliquity less than 10°

Grade II: Near normal hip–
Migration percentage ≥10%≤15%

1. Shenton's arch intact
2. Femoral head round or almost round
3. Acetabulum – normal or near normal development
4. Pelvic obliquity less than 10°

Grade III: Dysplastic hip–
Migration percentage >15% ≤30%

1. Shenton's arch intact or broken by less than or equal to 5mm
2. Femoral head round or mildly flattened
3. Acetabulum normal or mildly dysplastic including blunting of the acetabular margin and a widened tear drop
4. Pelvic obliquity less than 10°

Grade IV: Subluxated hip–
Migration percentage >30% <100%

1. Shenton's arch broken by more than 5mm
2. Femoral head variable deformity – Appendix I
3. Acetabulum variable deformity – Appendix II
4. Pelvic obliquity variable – Appendix III

Grade V: Dislocated hip–
Migration percentage ≥100%

1. Shenton's arch completely disrupted
2. Femoral head variable deformity – Appendix I
3. Acetabulum variable deformity – Appendix II
4. Pelvic obliquity variable – Appendix III

Grade VI: Salvage surgery

1. Valgus osteotomy
2. Arthrodesis
3. Excision arthroplasty (Castle) +/– valgus osteotomy (McHale)
4. Replacement arthroplasty

Fig. 5.7.5 A progressive radiographic classification system for hip dysplasia in cerebral palsy (Robin et al. 2008).

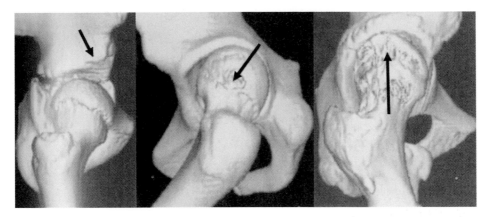

Fig. 5.7.6 Three-dimensional CT reconstruction demonstrating the location of acetabular insufficiency associated with femoral head subluxation. (Reproduced from Kim et al, 1997, by permission)

skeletal integrity (correct femoral anteversion and coxa valga, and correct hip subluxation and acetabular dysplasia).

INCREASED HIP ADDUCTION

Typical clinical presentation
In GMFCS levels I–III, adduction across midline may occur in mid-stance or during swing phase. Many of these individuals also have increased femoral anteversion and it is important to distinguish increased adduction caused by inappropriate muscle activity from internal rotation and adduction that is secondary to femoral anteversion. That is, are the knees crossing one another as a result of adductor spasticity, or does the femoral anteversion make the legs appear to be adducted? Individuals may have increased tripping or difficulty advancing their limbs through the gait cycle because of this problem

Examination
It is important to determine if reduced abduction is due to increased tone or contracture. In the presence of contracture, abduction will be decreased whether the hip is flexed or extended. When the hip and knees are flexed the hamstring muscles are relaxed and abduction of the hip usually increases.

Gait analysis findings
The pelvic rotation, pelvic obliquity and hip abduction and adduction kinematic graphs are very important. Relative hip adduction is seen throughout the gait cycle and, depending on the presence of asymmetric tone, contracture or anteversion pelvic obliquity and pelvic rotation may be seen (Fig. 5.7.7).

Fig. 5.7.7 Motion analysis data in the coronal plane demonstrating adduction.

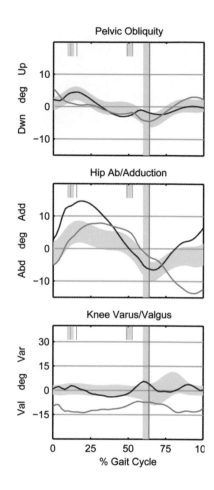

Non-operative treatment

Physical therapy, and abduction splinting during sleep, may be used to prevent contracture. Placement of botulinum toxin A in the muscle components of the hip adductors (including medial hamstrings) or injection of 6% phenol at the motor points of the anterior branch of the obturator nerve will reduce spasticity for several weeks or months, thereby reducing dynamic adduction. These medications appear to have little or no ability to stop progressive hip subluxation (Graham et al. 2008).

Operative treatment

Lengthening of the hip-adductors is done when muscles no longer respond to botulinum toxin or phenol or when radiographs demonstrate progressive hip subluxation. Muscle surgery for subluxation will be discussed in the section on that problem. In hips without subluxation but with less than 30° of abduction (or unresponsive dynamic adduction), a limited adductor procedure can be performed. A small oblique incision is made over the proximal prominence of the adductor longus. The adductor fascia is longitudinally split and the adductor longus tendon and the underlying anterior branch of the obturator nerve are identified. Using electrocautery the tendon is divided, carefully preserving the nerve. The gracilis is often contracted and this muscle is identified as well and divided as a myotomy. If abduction remains less than 45° then lengthening of the adductor brevis muscle is performed. It is important to not lengthen muscles excessively and very important, especially in ambulatory children, to not perform an anterior branch obturator neurectomy.

Complications of treatment
Muscle scarring can contribute to recurrent adduction contracture. Anterior-branch obturator neurectomy may lead to significant hip-abduction contractures. This operation should be reserved for individuals who are at GMFCS IV or V and have recurrent hip-adduction contracture or are undergoing bone surgery for hip dysplasia. Individuals with fixed abduction contractures have marked difficulty ambulating or sitting in a wheelchair. A fixed abduction contracture can be improved by a varus femoral osteotomy but prevention should be stressed rather than treatment.

Postoperative concerns
Significant pain and spasms are common after surgery. Postoperative analgesia (by caudal block, epidural catheter, local anesthetic injection, and/or intravenous narcotics) should be supplemented by spasm control (such as intravenous diazepam). Botulinum toxin, administered at least 1–2 weeks before surgery, may decrease postoperative pain and spasms. Some method of splinting or bracing should be employed to maintain hip abduction in the weeks after surgery. Physical therapy (stretching of adductors and strengthening of abductors) should begin as soon as possible.

Outcomes
Recurrent spasticity and contracture are common, particularly when surgery is performed early (less than 4 years old). Even with stretching therapy and prolonged postoperative bracing, secondary surgeries are common.

Increased Hip Flexion

Typical clinical presentation
Children with increased hip flexion usually present as part of an overall gait pattern of a *jump gait* (increased hip flexion, increased knee flexion, and increased ankle plantarflexion) or *crouch gait* (increased hip flexion, increased knee flexion and increased ankle dorsiflexion). While jump gait is the natural pattern of spastic diplegia, crouch gait is often iatrogenic, caused by isolated lengthening, or overlengthening, of the gastrocsoleus complex. Individuals with increased hip flexion may lean forward or they may develop increased lumbar lordosis since the psoas muscle, a strong hip-flexor, originates from the lumbar spine. Individuals at GMFCS IV and V often develop fixed contractures of their hip-flexors as a consequence of lengthy intervals of sitting.

Examination

As with adduction, increased hip flexion can be multifactorial. It may be the result of spasticity or contracture. The Thomas test and the Staheli prone extension test can be used to detect contracture but it may not be possible to fully assess contracture until the patient is under general anesthesia.

Gait analysis findings

The sagittal kinematic graphs may demonstrate increased anterior pelvic tilt and increased hip flexion throughout the gait cycle. Hicks et al. (2008) demonstrated, using gait analysis data and computer modeling, that crouch gait may decrease the extension ability of the posterior gluteus medius, soleus and vasti to less than 50% of normal. This may explain why this gait is so laborious and why, over time, this gait pattern progressively worsens (Fig. 5.7.8).

Non-operative treatment

There is little role for physical therapy or bracing. Since the psoas, one of the main hip-flexors, is attached to the lumbar spine, it is not possible to 'stretch' the muscle. In those children who have dynamic increased hip flexion, chemodenervation of the psoas is possible and has led to good results. This is best done under general anesthesia using ultrasound to identify the muscle and guide needle placement.

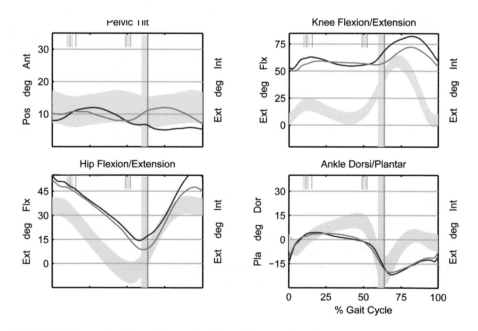

Fig. 5.7.8 Motion analysis data in the sagittal plane demonstrating flexion.

Operative treatment

There are many hip-flexors, including the psoas, iliacus, rectus femoris, sartorius, gracilis, and tensor fascia femoris. The rectus femoris muscle crosses the hip joint as a flexor and the knee joint as an extensor. As a result it was thought that proximal rectus lengthening might improve hip extension in stance and knee flexion during swing phase. It has been shown to have little effect on the stiff-knee gait and almost no effect on the hip or pelvis variables (DeLuca et al. 1998).

The psoas and iliacus are major contributors to hip-flexion deformity in cerebral palsy. They can be lengthened in several different locations: above the pelvic brim, at the pelvic brim or at the lesser trochanter. Novacheck et al. (2002) described a procedure in which the psoas tendon is identified proximal to the inguinal ligament (above the pelvic brim in the substance of the iliacus) and divided at that level. They reported good but mixed results concerning long-term improvement in hip range of motion. Sutherland et al. (1997) described a technique in which the psoas is identified just distal to the inguinal ligament at the pelvic brim. After identifying the femoral nerve, the psoas tendon is isolated and lengthened. They found this procedure was most effective in decreasing excessive hip flexion and anterior pelvic tilt when performed before 10 years of age.

Complications of treatment

The iliacus and psoas tendons combine as they approach their insertion at the lesser trochanter. Iliopsoas tenotomy at the lesser trochanter in individuals who walk may result in weakness that impairs ability to climb stairs. Lengthening or tenotomy at the lesser trochanter in nonambulatory individuals may result in femoral head avascular necrosis (due to injury of the medial femoral circumflex vessel) and has been associated with heterotopic ossification in the psoas tendon sheath (Manjarris and Mubarak 1984).

Postoperative concerns

Children who have iliopsoas procedures should not be immobilized. They should have physical therapy and prone positioning as much as possible to maintain the lengthening effect.

Outcomes

Psoas lengthening remains a controversial procedure. Some authors have demonstrated little change in hip flexion after lengthening of the muscle. The degree of contracture that needs treatment, the best age for surgery, and the type of lengthening remain unclear. However, lengthening should be considered in a child with increased hip flexion and increased anterior pelvic tilt as part of single-event multilevel surgery for individuals with gait disturbances or hip subluxation or dislocation and acetabular dysplasia.

Typical clinical presentation
Walking occurs with an internal foot-progression angle. This is often associated with increased hip adduction and may be misdiagnosed as contracted adductor muscles.

Examination
There are several causes of internal rotation. The gluteus medius and minimus, adductors, tensor fascia femoris and semitendinosus are all hip internal rotators. However, bio-mechanical studies suggest that these muscles have little effect on the excessive internal rotation of the hip in children with cerebral palsy. The most common cause of increased hip rotation is persistent femoral anteversion. There will be increased internal rotation in the prone position with an increase in the trochanteric prominence angle. Observational gait analysis will demonstrate that there is an internal foot progression. Younger children may have internal tibial torsion, which accentuates the internal foot progression angle. Older children may have developed a compensatory external tibial torsion. This improves the foot progression angle but the femur still rotates internally and the knee may have a rotational valgus thrust.

Gait analysis findings
Internal thigh rotation is assessed in the transverse plane graphs. The position of the pelvis in the transverse plane during walking should be considered when interpreting medial thigh rotation and foot progression angles. Significant asymmetry in neurologic impairment (such as hemiplegia) is often associated with pelvic malrotation in which the more impaired side is consistently posterior to the less impaired side. In such a circumstance internal thigh rotation due to increased anteversion may result in a neutral foot-progression angle (Fig. 5.7.9).

Non-operative treatment
No effective non-operative treatment exists for increased hip rotation. In very young children twister cables and taping techniques have been used but have not been found to be helpful long term. There is no role for chemo-denervation or nerve blocks to improve hip internal rotation.

Operative treatment
Lengthening of muscles around the hip does not improve hip medial rotation. The only proven treatment is femoral rotational osteotomy. The osteotomy may be performed just proximal to the lesser trochanter, in the diaphysis, or at the distal junction of diaphysis and metaphysis. Correction of coxa valga requires a proximal osteotomy. This is best accomplished with a blade plate in order to avoid lateral displacement of the femoral shaft (Beauchesne et al. 1992). If correction of coxa valga is not necessary then other options are available. A proximal osteotomy might be fixed with a compression screw and side plate device, but this usually results in a more distal osteotomy and lateral translation of the

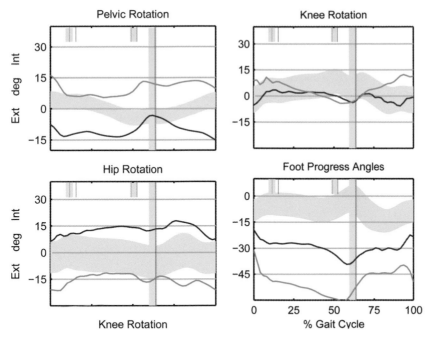

Fig. 5.7.9 Motion analysis data in the transverse plane demonstrating internal rotation.

femoral shaft. Good results with a diaphyseal osteotomy fixed with an intramedullary rod (Gordon et al. 2005, Ferri-de-Barros et al. 2006). Since this device is inserted near the greater trochanter there is a risk of avascular necrosis in the femoral head or disturbance of growth at the trochanteric apophysis. Intramedullary devices should be avoided in young children (<11 years old). Distal osteotomy for anteversion should be fixed with a blade plate rather than threaded Kirschner wires in order to avoid the need for a cast.

Complications of treatment
It is critical that accurate measurements are made prior to performing any of these osteotomies. CT scans can provide an accurate assessment of anteversion but may be difficult to interpret in the presence of coxa valga. Therefore it is important to use physical examination information and gait analysis data with imaging studies to determine the amount of rotation to be performed at the time of surgery. There is a small risk of delayed or non-union. Immobilization with a body cast increases the risk of fracture during early rehabilitation. Intramedullary devices introduced through the greater trochanter are associated with avascular necrosis of the femoral head and should be avoided in younger children (< 11 years old). Two studies evaluating whether the osteotomy should be performed proximally or distally did not show any differences (Kay et al. 2003, Pirpiris et al. 2003).

Postoperative concerns

Usually the fixation strength of a femoral osteotomy is sufficient and no postoperative immobilization is needed. Some children benefit from knee immobilizers for comfort. A short leg cast with a rotation-controlling boot, or bilateral short leg casts with a removable bar to control rotation can be used to simplify limb positioning. Some children do not have solid fixation and require spica cast immobilization for a short period until healing callus is noted on the radiograph.

Outcomes

Õunpuu et al. (2002) evaluated 27 patients at least 5 years after femoral derotation osteotomy. Using gait analysis, they found good long-term outcomes from this surgery. However, Kim et al. (2005) followed 30 children with 45 femurs and found recurrent anteversion in 15 femurs followed at least 5 years after surgery. They had no recurrences when surgery was performed after 10 years of age.

HIP SUBLUXATION AND DISLOCATION

Typical clinical presentation

Children at GMFCS I and II rarely develop progressive hip dysplasia. The likelihood of this problem increases at GMFCS III and it is most common in children at GMFCS IV and V. Pain is uncommon with this problem in younger children. Pain usually does not usually occur until the late teen and early adult period.

Examination

Decreased hip abduction, increased flexion and increased internal rotation rotation are present in most children who have subluxation, but not all. On occasion gentle abduction performed when a child is quiet and tone is minimal will result in palpable translation of a subluxated or dislocated femoral head. Radiographic findings were described earlier in this chapter.

Gait analysis findings

Children with subluxation who are able to walk for gait analysis have findings of increased hip adduction and flexion, increased femoral internal rotation, and increased pelvic tilt.

Non-operative treatment

As stated in the section on increased hip adduction, there is little evidence that long-term bracing, physical therapy, botulinum toxin or phenol have any long-term effect on hip subluxation.

Operative treatment

Surgical planning is linked to how far a child's hip has progressed along the cascade of evolving hip pathology. While it is unclear whether focal tone management will alter hip subluxation once it has started (particularly if the migration percentage is >50%), global efforts to ameliorate tone are valuable. Tone reduction may reduce the number of children who experience hip dysplasia and will ease surgical recovery while reducing the likelihood of recurrent contracture and subluxation.

Soft-tissue surgery usually consists of the adductor lengthening described previously in this chapter in combination with lengthening of the iliopsoas (particularly if a flexion contracture is present). There is no consensus about the role of anterior branch obturator neurectomy in this problem but this procedure should be avoided in all but the most refractory cases (Matsuo et al. 1986).

Bone procedures become more common when the migration percentage exceeds 50%. The surgeon must decide if a proximal femoral varus rotational osteotomy combined with soft-tissue lengthening will result in concentric reduction. If not, open reduction and capsular tightening and a pelvic osteotomy or acetabular augmentation procedure may be necessary. Soft-tissue procedures and femoral osteotomies should be performed for both hips. There is some controversy about this but symmetrical range of motion and similar limb lengths are fundamental to a good sitting position.

The proximal femoral varus derotational osteotomy (VDRO) is performed similar to the technique employed in derotational osteotomies. The amount of rotation and varus is decided preoperatively, and can be verified using fluoroscopy during surgery. The goal is to achieve 15° of femoral anteversion and a 110° neck-shaft angle. There are several devices that can be used for fixation: simple plates and screws, Kirschner wires, external fixators, hip screw and side plates, and various blade plates.

There are many approaches to the pelvic osteotomy to provide hip coverage and containment. As noted earlier in this chapter, the direction of femoral head displacement is variable. Ambulatory children with this problem (usually GMFCS III) have anterior or mid-lateral subluxation while children with greater impairment (GMFCS IV and V) have posterior displacement as they are usually sitting. CT scans, with 3-dimensional formatting, are the best way to determine the direction of hip displacement. This knowledge is essential to plan the correct pelvic osteotomy. It cannot be determined by physical examination or plain radiographs.

The Salter and the Pemberton osteotomies provide excellent anterior coverage but may not be appropriate for subluxations and acetabular deficiencies that are mid-lateral and posterior. The true Dega osteotomy provides anterior coverage similar to the Pemberton osteotomy and good results have been reported. The best method of coverage of the femoral head for children with cerebral palsy is a periacetabular osteotomy that permits improved coverage where it is needed. There are several variations on the method, but essentially it involves making an osteotomy around the acetabulum and placing bone graft in the appropriate position (either from the iliac crest or from the wedge that is removed from the femoral osteotomy site) (McNerney et al. 2000) (Fig. 5.7.10). The Steel triple innominate and Bernese periacetabular osteotomies have been utilized when the triradiate cartilage is closed (Pope et al. 1994, Dutoit and Zambelli 1999). The slotted acetabular augmentation has been used in children with significant acetabular deficiency. The Chiari osteotomy should be used as a salvage procedure when restoration of articular surfaces is not possible (Debnath et al. 2006) (Fig. 5.7.11).

507

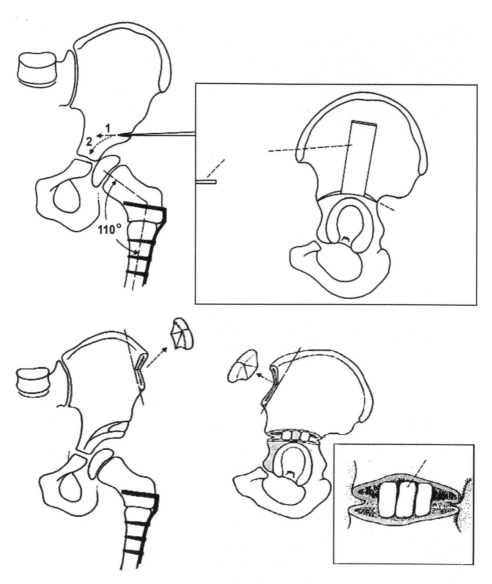

Fig. 5.7.10 The San Diego hip reconstruction technique (McNerney et al. 2000).

Complications of treatment

Children who have bilateral procedures including pelvic osteotomies often require blood transfusions and treatment in an intensive care unit for respiratory problems. Tis et al. (2006) found a 24% major complication rate in this population (blood loss, infection and recurrent dysplasia). Technical complications may occur during surgery including nerve or vascular injury and there is a risk of avascular necrosis of the femoral head. Fracture may occur after postoperative immobilization.

(a)

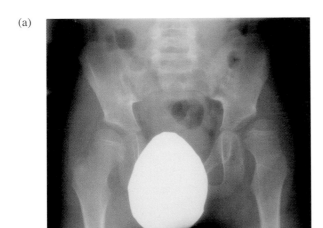

Fig. 5.7.11 (a) Preoperative radiograph of a 10-year-old girl with bilateral hip dysplasia, which is more severe on the left side. (b) Postoperative radiograph of the same child 6 months after bilateral intertrochanteric, varus, derotational femoral osteotomies and left acetabuloplasty using the San Diego technique. (c) Postoperative radiograph of the same girl 5½ years after surgery at age 15½, which demonstrates an excellent final result.

(b)

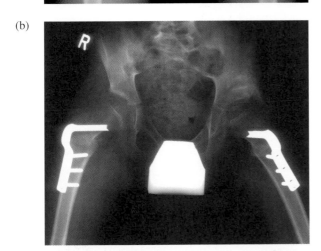

(c)

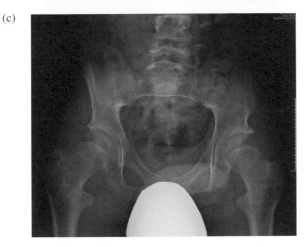

Postoperative concerns

Postoperative pain management is very important. Analgesia through an epidural catheter supplemented with intravenous diazepam for control of muscle spasms can be very effective (see Chapter 4.3). Intravenous analgesia (such as a continuous infusion pump) is an alternative method of pain control. There is a fine line between ineffective pain control and excessive sedation that results in pulmonary compromise.

Immobilization in a hip spica cast for 2–6 weeks after this surgery is common although many institutions begin immediate mobilization and physical therapy. A hip spica cast for 2 weeks provides pain relief, eases transfers and transportation and allows early bone healing. The posterior portion of the cast may then be used as a mold for a custom fabricated splint, which the child wears for 2 months full time except for range of motion exercises and bathing. The splint is then used for at night for 6 months. Immobilization may not be needed if pelvic osteotomy was not performed unless the quality of femoral fixation is poor due to poor bone quality (osteopenia). Schaefer et al. (2007) found that early weightbearing was associated with earlier return to full activities.

Outcomes

The effect of soft-tissue surgery on hip subluxation is difficult to determine. Several factors influence the outcome: the severity of neurologic involvement, the age at surgery, the degree of dysplasia, the type of surgery performed, and the postoperative care. The best outcomes are obtained when the migration percentage is less than 50% and when symmetric surgery is performed for both hips.

Recurrent contractures and persistent or recurrent femoral or acetabular dysplasia are common. Mazur et al. (2004) found that VDRO prior to age 4 had a high level of recurrence of coxa valga. Inan et al. (2006 a, b) reported heterotopic ossification after hip osteotomies in 16% of 219 patients. This was most common in spastic quadriplegia. Schmale et al. (2006) demonstrated that 77% of patients treated with isolated VDRO required reoperation due to inadequate acetabular remodeling. Settecerri and Karol (2000) found that isolated VDRO performed at a mean age of 7.7 years resulted in a stable pain-free hip in 84% of patients at 5-year follow-up. However, by their criteria 56% had fair or poor outcomes based on the radiographs. The long term outcome of these patients is not clear. Mubarak et al. (1992) reported 75 children (104 hips) who underwent VDRO, open reduction and capsulorrhaphy, and periacetabular osteotomy (San Diego technique). Their patients had a 95% good to excellent radiographic outcome with no redislocations after 6.9 year follow-up (McNerney et al. 2000). Long-term follow-up for these patients is not yet available.

Recovery can be prolonged and families should be informed about the magnitude of surgery and the length of the rehabilitation period. Stasikelis et al. (2003) demonstrated that all of the children returned to their preoperative ambulatory status within 30 months of the surgery. Most of the community and household ambulators returned to their preoperative status at 7 months, and the more involved children took 10 months. They also found that those patients who had regular physical therapy recovered much sooner than those who did not.

CHRONIC HIP PAIN

Typical clinical presentation
Many studies demonstrate that approximately 50% of adolescents and young adults with cerebral palsy and chronic hip dislocation experience pain. Communication problems often make it difficult to assess pain in this group (GMFCS IV and V) and there may be other sources for chronic pain. Noonan et al. (2004) attempted to determine if hip dislocation was the source of pain in 77 adults with subluxated or dislocated hips. They could find no correlation between the hip radiographic abnormality and the severity of pain. Nonetheless, individuals with chronic hip dysplasia do experience pain that interferes with their well-being.

Examination
These patients often have severe contractures. Many have windswept hips (one hip adducted and internally rotated, the other hip abducted and externally rotated). They may have pain during movement of their hips and they may have decubitus ulcers over bone prominences (ischium, coccyx or greater trochanter) due to poor position when sitting or recumbent.

Non-operative treatment
Nonsteroidal anti-inflammatory medications can reduce pain but may be contraindicated because of reflux and stomach pain. Intra-articular steroid injection has variable success but can reduce pain for weeks or months. Modifications of seating arrangements and sleep surfaces can relieve pressure over bone prominences and may improve joint pain. Frequent changes in position may be helpful. Botulinum toxin A or phenol injections in muscles about the hip (gluteus medius, maximus, tensor fascia femoris, quadriceps, hamstrings and adductors) may reduce tone and pain (Barwood et al. 2000). This must be repeated every 4–6 months.

Operative treatment
Surgical options include the Chiari pelvic osteotomy (to cover the displaced femoral head), valgus femoral osteotomy (to improve femoral position for sitting and perineal care), hip fusion, proximal femoral resection (Castle procedure), and total hip replacement (Castle and Schneider 1978, Buly et al. 1993, Dietz and Knutson 1995). None of these provide a satisfactory answer to the problems of chronic hip dysplasia in cerebral palsy. Each has technical challenges and complications. The results of all of these procedures are mixed and many patients still have pain after the surgeries. For this reason it seems wise to prevent dysplasia starting at an early age.

Conclusion
Hip problems are common in children with cerebral palsy. These problems begin with the altered neurologic function that creates hypertonia, loss of selective motor control, and unbalanced activity in the muscles that surround the hip joint. Muscles lose flexibility and joint motion is altered. The stress-sensitive bones of the hip (femur and pelvis) respond

with growth and development changes that can lead to disruption of the joint. The result is loss of function. The best approach to this complexity is to break the problem down into individual components that can be studied by focused physical examination, radiographic evaluation and gait analysis. Remember: the hip is just part of entire body involvement in cerebral palsy and should not be treated in isolation.

REFERENCES

Arnold AS, Delp SL (2001) Rotational moment arms of the medial hamstrings and adductors vary with femoral geometry and limb position: implications for the treatment of internally rotated gait. *J Biomech* **34**: 437–47.

Arnold AS, Asakawa DJ, Delp SL (2000) Do the hamstrings and adductors contribute to excessive internal rotation of the hip in persons with cerebral palsy? *Gait Posture* **11**: 181–90.

Barwood S, Baillieu C, Boyd R, Brereton K, Low J, Nattrass G, Graham HK (2000) Analgesic effects of botulinum toxin A: a randomized, placebo-controlled clinical trial. *Dev Med Child Neurol* **42**: 114–21.

Beauchesne R, Miller F, Moseley C (1992) Proximal femoral osteotomy using the AO fixed-angle blade plate. *J Pediatr Orthop* **12**: 735–40.

Bobroff ED, Chambers HG, Sartoris DJ, Wyatt MP, Sutherland DH (1999) Femoral anteversion and neck-shaft angle in children with cerebral palsy. *Clin Orthop Rel Res* **364**: 194–204.

Buly RL, Huo M, Root L, Binzer T, Wilson Jr PD (1993) Total hip arthroplasty in cerebral palsy. Long-term follow-up results. *Clin Orthop Rel Res* **296**: 148–53.

Castle ME, Schneider C (1978) Proximal femoral resection-interposition arthroplasty. *J Bone Joint Surg Am* **60**: 1051–4.

Davids JR, Marshall AD, Blocker ER, Frick SL, Blackhurst DW, Skewes E (2003) Femoral anteversion in children with cerebral palsy. Assessment with two and three-dimensional computed tomography scans. *J Bone Joint Surg Am* **85**: 481–8.

Debnath UK, Guha AR, Karlakki S, Varghese J, Evans GA (2006) Combined femoral and Chiari osteotomies for reconstruction of the painful subluxation or dislocation of the hip in cerebral palsy. A long-term outcome study. *J Bone Joint Surg Br* **88**: 1373–8.

Delp SL, Hess WE, Hungerford DS, Jones LC (1999) Variation of rotation moment arms with hip flexion. *J Biomech* **32**: 493–501.

Deluca PA, Õunpuu S, Davis RB, Walsh JH (1998) Effect of hamstring and psoas lengthening on pelvic tilt in patients with spastic diplegic cerebral palsy. *J Pediatr Orthop* **18**: 712–18.

Dietz FR, Knutson LM (1995) Chiari pelvic osteotomy in cerebral palsy. *J Pediatr Orthop* **15**: 372–80.

Dutoit M, Zambelli PY (1999) Simplified 3D-evaluation of periacetabular osteotomy. *Acta Orthop Belg* **65**: 288–94.

Ferri-de-Barros F, Inan M, Miller F (2006) Intramedullary nail fixation of femoral and tibial percutaneous rotational osteotomy in skeletally mature adolescents with cerebral palsy. *J Pediatr Orthop* **26**: 115–18.

Gordon JE, Pappademos PC, Schoenecker PL, Dobbs MB, Luhmann SJ (2005) Diaphyseal derotational osteotomy with intramedullary fixation for correction of excessive femoral anteversion in children. *J Pediatr Orthop* **25**: 548–53.

Graham HK, Boyd R, Carlin JB, Dobson F, Lowe K, Nattrass G, Thomason P, Wolfe R, Reddihough D (2008) Does botulinum toxin A combined with bracing prevent hip displacement in children with cerebral palsy and 'hips at risk'? A randomized, controlled trial. *J Bone Joint Surg Am* **90**: 23–33.

Hagglund G, Lauge-Pedersen H, Wagner P (2007) Characteristics of children with hip displacement in cerebral palsy. *BMC Musculoskelet Disord* **8**: 101.

Hicks JL, Schwartz MH, Arnold AS, Delp SL (2008) Crouched postures reduce the capacity of muscles to extend the hip and knee during the single-limb stance phase of gait. *J Biomech* **41**: 960–7.

Inan M, Chan G, Dabney K, Miller F (2006a) Heterotopic ossification following hip osteotomies in cerebral palsy: incidence and risk factors. *J Pediatr Orthop* **26**: 551–6.

Inan M, Senaran H, Domzalski M, Littleton A, Dabney K, Miller F (2006b) Unilateral versus bilateral peri-ilial pelvic osteotomies combined with proximal femoral osteotomies in children with cerebral palsy: perioperative complications *J Pediatr Orthop* **26**: 547–50.

512

Kay RM, Rethlefsen SA, Hale JM, Skaggs DL, Tolo VT (2003) Comparison of proximal and distal rotational femoral osteotomy in children with cerebral palsy. *J Pediatr Orthop* **23**: 150–4.

Kim HT, Wenger DR (1997) Location of acetabular deficiency and associated hip dislocation in neuromuscular hip dysplasia: three-dimensional computed tomographic analysis. *J Pediatr Orthop* **17**: 143–51.

Kim H, Aiona M, Sussman M (2005) Recurrence after femoral derotational osteotomy in cerebral palsy. *J Pediatr Orthop* **25**: 739–43.

Manjarris JF, Mubarak S (1984) Avascular necrosis of the femoral heads following bilateral iliopsoas and adductor releases via the medical approach to the hip. *J Pediatr Orthop* **4**: 109–10.

Matsuo T, Tada S, Hajime T (1986) Insufficiency of the hip adductor after anterior obturator neurectomy in 42 children with cerebral palsy. *J Pediatr Orthop* **6**: 686–92.

Mazur JM, Danko AM, Standard SC, Loveless EA, Cummings RJ (2004) Remodeling of the proximal femur after varus osteotomy in children with cerebral palsy. *Dev Med Child Neurol* **46**: 412–15.

McNerney NP, Mubarak SJ, Wenger DR (2000) One-stage correction of the dysplastic hip in cerebral palsy with the San Diego acetabuloplasty: results and complications in 104 hips. *J Pediatr Orthop* **20**: 93–103.

Mubarak SJ, Valencia FG, Wenger DR (1992) One-stage correction of the spastic dislocated hip. Use of pericapsular acetabuloplasty to improve coverage. *J Bone Joint Surg Am* **74**: 1347–57.

Noonan KJ, Jones J, Pierson J, Honkamp NJ, Leverson G (2004) Hip function in adults with severe cerebral palsy. *J Bone Joint Surg Am* **86**: 2607–13.

Novacheck TF, Trost JP, Schwartz MH (2002) Intramuscular psoas lengthening improves dynamic hip function in children with cerebral palsy. *J Pediatr Orthop* **22**: 158–64.

Õunpuu S, Deluca P, Davis R, Romness M (2002) Long-term effects of femoral derotation osteotomies: an evaluation using three-dimensional gait analysis. *J Pediatr Orthop* **22**: 139–45.

Pirpiris M, Trivett A, Baker R, Rodda J, Nattrass GR, Graham HK (2003) Femoral derotation osteotomy in spastic diplegia. Proximal or distal? *J Bone Joint Surg Br* **85**: 265–72.

Pope DF, Bueff HU, Deluca PA (1994) Pelvic osteotomies for subluxation of the hip in cerebral palsy. *J Pediatr Orthop* **14**: 724–30.

Reimers J (1980) The stability of the hip in children. A radiological study of the results of muscle surgery in cerebral palsy. *Acta Orthop Scand Suppl* **184**: 1–100.

Robin J, Graham HK, Baker R, Selber P, Simpson P, Symons S, Thomason P (2009) A classification system for hip disease in cerebral palsy. *Dev Med Child Neurol* **51**: 183–92.

Ruwe PA, Gage JR, Ozonoff MB, Deluca PA (1992) Clinical determination of femoral anteversion. A comparison with established techniques. *J Bone Joint Surg Am* **74**: 820–30.

Sauser DD, Hewes RC, Root L (1986) Hip changes in spastic cerebral palsy. *Am J Roentgenol* **146**: 1219–22.

Schaefer MK, McCarthy JJ, Josephic K (2007) Effects of early weight bearing on the functional recovery of ambulatory children with cerebral palsy after bilateral proximal femoral osteotomy. *J Pediatr Orthop* **27**: 668–70.

Schmale GA, Eilert RE, Chang F, Seidel K (2006) High reoperation rates after early treatment of the subluxating hip in children with spastic cerebral palsy. *J Pediatr Orthop* **26**: 617–23.

Settecerri JJ, Karol LA (2000) Effectiveness of femoral varus osteotomy in patients with cerebral palsy. *J Pediatr Orthop* **20**: 776–80.

Soo B, Howard JJ, Boyd RN, Reid SM, Lanigan A, Wolfe R, Reddihough D, Graham HK (2006) Hip displacement in cerebral palsy. *J Bone Joint Surg Am* **88**: 121–9.

Staheli LT (1977) The prone hip extension test: a method of measuring hip flexion deformity. *Clin Orthop Rel Res* **123**: 12–15.

Stasikelis PJ, Davids JR, Johnson BH, Jacobs JM (2003) Rehabilitation after femoral osteotomy in cerebral palsy. *J Pediatr Orthop* **12**: 311–14.

Sutherland DH, Zilberfarb JL, Kaufman KR, Wyatt MP, Chanmbers HG (1997) Psoas release at the pelvic brim in ambulatory patients with cerebral palsy: operative technique and functional outcome. *J Pediatr Orthop* **17**; 563–70.

Tis JE, Sharif S, Shannon B, Dabney K, Miller F (2006) Complications associated with multiple, sequential osteotomies for children with cerebral palsy. *J Pediatr Orthop* **15**: 408–13.

Winters TF, Gage JR, Hicks R (1987) Gait patterns in spastic hemiplegia in children and young adults. *J Bone Joint Surg Am* **69**: 437–41.

513

5.8
ORTHOPAEDIC TREATMENT OF FOOT DEFORMITIES

Jon R. Davids

Key points

- Foot deformities in children with cerebral palsy (CP) are a consequence of dynamic muscle imbalance
- These deformities may disrupt shock absorption and lever function of the foot during stance phase
- The foot is best considered to consist of three segments and two columns
- The most common foot deformities in children with CP are equinus, equinoplanovalgus, and equinocavovarus
- Surgical correction of foot deformities is performed to improve lever function of the foot by optimizing foot shape and improve shock absorption function by optimizing intra-and intersegmental motion
- When necessary, osteotomy is preferred over arthrodesis to restore foot skeletal segmental alignment.

Pathophysiology

Deformity of the foot in children with CP is usually the result of a dynamic imbalance between the extrinsic muscles of the calf that control segmental foot and ankle alignment. This imbalance may be a consequence of spasticity, disrupted motor control, and/or impaired balance function. Typically, the ankle-plantarflexor muscles are overactive, and the ankle dorsiflexor muscles are ineffective. Variable imbalance patterns may be seen between the foot and ankle supination and pronation muscle groups. These motor imbalances result in three common coupled foot and ankle segmental malalignment patterns in children with spastic type CP (the linkage between the underlying neurological deficits and foot segmental malalignment is less consistent in children with dyskinetic types of CP, in which abnormalities of motor control and balance, rather than spasticity, are most significant) (Davids et al. 1999, 2007). Equinus is characterized by plantarflexion malalignment of the hindfoot relative to the ankle, with normal midfoot and forefoot alignment. Equinoplanovalgus is characterized by equinus deformity of the hindfoot, coupled with pronation deformities of the midfoot and forefoot. The lateral column of the foot is initially functionally shorter than the medial column, and may become structurally shorter with increasing age. Equinocavovarus is characterized by equinus deformity of the hindfoot, coupled with supination deformity of the midfoot and variable malalignment of the forefoot.

The lateral column is initially functionally longer than the medial column. Other more complex or uncoupled segmental alignments may occur, but are much less common. The common segmental malalignments of the foot and ankle are frequently supple and correctible on manipulation in younger children with less severe CP. With increasing age and growth, the muscles develop fixed shortening or myostatic deformity, the bones develop permanent structural accommodations to the malalignment pattern, and the foot and ankle deformities become rigid and uncorrectable on manipulation (Sutherland 1993, Mosca 1998). In all three segmental malalignment patterns, heel strike at initial contact does not occur, disrupting the first rocker and shock absorption function in loading response (Perry 1992). Equinus and equinocavovarus malalignment patterns disrupt the second rocker by blocking ankle dorsiflexion, compromising stability function in midstance (Perry 1992). Equinoplanovalgus malalignment maintains the midfoot and forefoot segments in an 'unlocked' alignment, compromising stability function in midstance, which may result in excessive loading of the plantar, medial portion of the midfoot. All three segmental malalignments may compromise the ability of the ankle plantarflexor muscles to generate an adequate internal plantarflexion moment during third rocker (Sutherland et al. 1980, Gage 1995). The hindfoot malalignment associated with equinus and equinocavovarus malalignment patterns shortens the length of the plantarflexor muscles, compromising their ability to generate tension, as described by the length-tension curve for skeletal muscle (Lieber 1986, Foran et al. 2005). With equinoplanovalgus, the moment generating capacity of the ankle-plantarflexor muscles is further compromised by the malalignment of mid- and forefoot segments, which effectively shortens the lever arm available to this muscle group during the third rocker. In addition, increased external tibial torsion, which may be associated with equinoplanovalgus segmental malalignment, may contribute to an external foot-progression angle, further compromising the lever arm available to the ankle-plantarflexor muscles in terminal stance. All three segmental malalignment patterns of the foot and ankle may inhibit ankle dorsiflexion in swing phase, compromising clearance in midswing and proper positioning of the foot and ankle in terminal swing.

Historical overview
Treatment principles for the surgical management of foot deformities in children with CP were developed from earlier clinical experience in the management of children with poliomyelitis (Davids 2006). Although foot deformities associated with both disease processes may appear to be similar, the pathophysiology, impairment, and associated disability are actually distinct. As a result, many of the treatment principles from poliomyelitis management, where deformities are the consequence of dynamic muscle imbalance due to selective flaccid paralysis and contractures, are not appropriate for the management in CP, where deformities are more commonly the consequence of dynamic muscle imbalance due to spasticity and disrupted motor control (Rang and Wright 1989).

Surgical management strategies carried over from poliomyelitis and applied to CP include dynamic muscle balancing and skeletal stabilization. Muscle balancing is achieved by lengthening or transfer of muscle tendon units. Skeletal stabilization is achieved by arthrodesis of joints in the hindfoot, midfoot and forefoot. When applied to children with

CP, these soft-tissue procedures frequently result in excessive weakness or the development of subsequent deformities. Skeletal procedures stiffened the foot excessively, disrupting shock absorption function and creating dynamic overload of joints proximal or distal to the segment that had been fused.

Current surgical management strategies favor the early management of spasticity by pharmacologic, neurosurgical, and orthotic interventions, to avoid the development of fixed deformities of the muscle-tendon unit (Gage and Novacheck 2001). Selective surgical lengthening techniques that minimize the subsequent weakness of the muscle tendon unit are favored (Rose et al. 1993). When possible, osteotomy is preferred over arthrodesis to restore foot skeletal segmental alignment and maintain intra- and intersegmental motion, in order to optimize both shock absorption and lever functions of the foot (Mosca 1998).

Indications from patient assessment

Clinical decision making for the management of foot deformities in children with CP is based upon the collection and integration of data from a variety of sources, including the clinical history, physical examination, plain radiographs, observational gait analysis, kinematic/kinetic analyses, dynamic electromyography (EMG), and dynamic pedo-barography (Davids et al. 2004).

The most common complaints related to foot deformity in children with CP, as determined from the *clinical history*, are pain with ambulation, shoe wear, or use of orthoses; tripping due to poor clearance in swing phase; and in-toeing or out-toeing. The *physical examination* should include an assessment of foot segmental alignment when weightbearing and non-weightbearing, intra- and intersegmental flexibility, active and passive range of motion, and individual muscle strength and selective control. The plantar and medial margins of the foot should be examined for the presence of inadequate or excessive skin callus formation, which are indicative of disrupted loading patterns or problems with shoe or orthotic wear.

Plain radiographs utilized for the analysis of foot deformity in children with CP should include three weightbearing views: standing anteroposterior (AP) and lateral (LAT) views of the foot, and mortise view of the ankle. Identification and classification of foot deformities from the plain radiographs by segmental analysis are performed by dividing the foot into three segments and two columns, then determining the relative alignment of each segment and the relative length of each column (Fig. 5.8.1). The alignment of each segment may be determined relative to a global reference frame (e.g. the floor, calcaneal pitch), relative to the location of an adjacent segment (e.g. hindfoot relative to the tibia, tibiocalcaneal angle), or relative to the alignment between bones within the same segment (e.g. the talocalcaneal angle). A comprehensive technique of quantitative segmental analysis of the ankle and foot has been developed, based upon qualitative techniques derived from the foot model originally developed by Inman and colleagues (Inman et al. 1981, Davids et al. 2005). This technique of quantitative segmental analysis utilizes ten radiographic measurements to determine the alignment of the three segments and the lengths of the two columns of the ankle and foot. After establishing intra- and interobserver reliability, normative values and ranges were determined from a cohort of 60 normal feet in children between the ages of

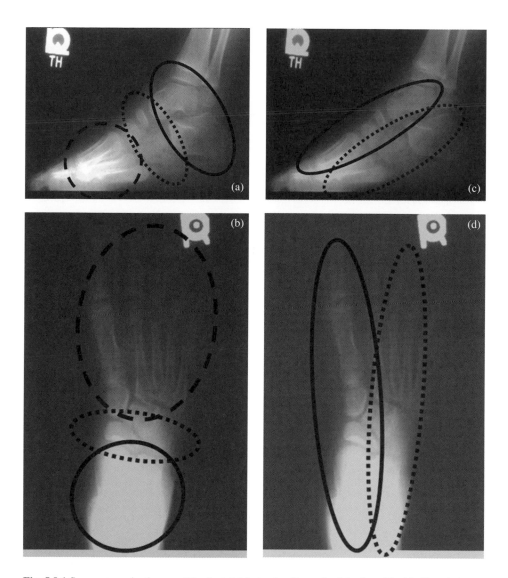

Fig. 5.8.1 Segments and columns of the foot. (a) Lateral radiograph of the foot. The hindfoot (talus and calcaneus) is outlined by the solid circle. The midfoot (navicular and cuboid) is outlined by the dotted circle. The forefoot (cuneiforms, metatarsals and phalanges) is outlined by the dashed circle. (b) Anteroposterior radiograph of the foot. The hindfoot (talus and calcaneus) is outlined by the solid circle. The midfoot (navicular and cuboid) is outlined by the dotted circle. The forefoot (cuneiforms, metatarsals and phalanges) is outlined by the dashed circle. (c) Lateral radiograph of the foot. The medial column (talus, navicular, cuneiforms, great toe metatarsal and phalanges) is outlined by the solid circle. The lateral column (calcaneus, cuboid, lesser toe metatarsals and phalanges) is outlined by the dotted circle. (d) Anteroposterior radiograph of the foot. The medial column (talus, navicular, cuneiforms, great toe metatarsal and phalanges) is outlined by the solid circle. The lateral column (calcaneus, cuboid, lesser toe metatarsals and phalanges) is outlined by the dotted circle.

517

5 and 17 years. Individual measures that fall beyond one standard deviation of the normal mean value are considered to be abnormal and can be utilized to describe segmental malalignment patterns (Table 5.8.1).

Observational gait analysis is helpful in determining the significance of foot deformities appreciated on the clinical examination and plain radiograph analysis. The static standing alignment of the foot should be assessed from the front, behind, and both sides. The segmental alignment of the hindfoot, midfoot and forefoot can be described. Ambulation should be observed from multiple viewpoints in the coronal and sagittal planes, by having the subject walk towards, away, and past the examiner. The principle elements of dynamic foot function that may be appreciated on observational gait analysis include foot position at initial contact (heel strike, flat foot, or toe strike), foot alignment in midstance (varus or valgus in the coronal plane; internal or external in the transverse plane, described as the foot-progression angle), foot alignment at toe off (varus or valgus in the coronal plane, dorsiflexed or plantarflexed in the sagittal plane), and foot clearance in swing phase (Perry 1992).

The calculation of foot and ankle *kinematics and kinetics* involves modeling assumptions and approximations concerning the relationship between the skin markers and the underlying skeletal anatomy (Davis et al. 1991, Gage 1995, Gage et al. 1996). The standard ankle and foot model most commonly used in clinical gait analysis was developed in the early 1980s (Davis et al. 1991, 2007). In this model, the orientation of the tibia is determined by the location of a vector between the calculated knee and ankle joint centers (as determined from distal femoral condylar markers and medial and lateral malleoli markers respectively). The orientation of the foot is defined by a vector that passes from the calculated ankle joint center (medial and lateral malleoli markers) to the space between the 2nd and

TABLE 5.8.1
Radiographic measurements: quantitative and categorical definitions (modified from Davids et al. 2005)

	Normal mean (SD)	Abnormal high value (> mean + 1 SD)	Abnormal low value (< mean – 1 SD)
Hindfoot			
Tibiotalar angle (°)	1.1 (3.75)	Eversion	Inversion
Calcaneal pitch (°)	17 (6.0)	Calcaneus	Equinus
Tibiocalcaneal angle (°)	69 (8.4)	Equinus	Calcaneus
Talocalcaneal angle (°)	49 (6.9)	Eversion	Inversion
Midfoot			
Naviculocuboid overlap (%)	47 (13.8)	Pronation	Supination
Talonavicular coverage angle (°)	20 (9.8)	Abduction	Adduction
Lateral talo–1st metatarsal angle (°)	13 (7.5)	Pronation	Supination
Forefoot			
Anteroposterior talo–1st metatarsal angle (°)	10 (7.0)	Abduction	Adduction
Metatarsal stacking angle (°)	8 2.(9)	Supination	Pronation
Columns			
Mediolateral column ratio	0.9 (0.1)	Abduction	Adduction

518

3rd metatarsals (a single dorsal forefoot marker). In this single segment foot model, it is assumed that the foot segment is relatively rigid from the hindfoot to the forefoot. Ankle motion in the sagittal plane is calculated from the location of the foot axis relative to the tibial axis. Any motion between the forefoot marker and the malleolar markers in the sagittal plane is described by the computer as ankle dorsiflexion or plantarflexion. Any movement between the primary segments of the foot (e.g. hindfoot to midfoot, midfoot to forefoot) that occurs between these two marker groups will be captured by this simple foot model and described as ankle motion. Significant measurement artifact occurs when the integrity of the foot segmental alignment is compromised (e.g. equinoplanovalgus foot malalignment seen in children with CP). This creates apparent discrepancies between the data derived from the physical examination, observational gait analysis, and quantitative gait analysis, which may result in confusion for clinicians and compromise clinical decision-making.

Advances in marker, camera, and computer technologies now support improved spatial measurement resolution, potentially allowing more markers to be placed and tracked on a small limb segment like the foot. This has created the opportunity to develop more sophisticated, multi-segment foot models that more accurately approximate the complex anatomy and biomechanics of the foot (MacWilliams et al. 2003). The majority of these more advanced models have been developed for adult feet with easily identifiable skeletal landmarks that facilitate accurate marker placement. Unfortunately, children with conditions such as CP typically have very small feet (intermarker distances are reduced beyond the ranges of resolution), that are deformed (segmental malalignment may obscure anatomical landmarks and compromise accurate marker placement). An appropriate model should generate information that is useful for clinical decision-making for children regarding orthotic prescriptions, surgical planning, and post-intervention outcome assessment (Davis et al. 2007).

Dynamic EMG may be helpful in the evaluation of specific foot deformities such as equinocavovarus segmental malalignment (Sutherland 1993). By utilizing surface and fine wire EMG it is possible to sort out the relative activity of the tibialis anterior and posterior muscles during the various phases of the gait cycle. This information can guide clinical decision making in selecting a particular muscle-tendon unit for lengthening or transfer.

Dynamic pedobarography is the measurement of the spatial and temporal distribution of force over the plantar aspect of the foot during the stance phase of the gait cycle (Schaff 1993). Pedobarography provides quantitative information regarding dynamic foot function, consisting of foot contact patterns, pressure distribution and magnitude, and progression of the center of pressure (Jameson et al. 2008). In children with CP, foot dysfunction during gait is primarily a consequence of skeletal segmental malalignment that compromises the shock absorption function during 1st rocker, compromises stability during 2nd rocker, and diminishes the moment arm available to the plantarflexor muscles during the 3rd rocker in the stance phase of gait (Gage and Novacheck 2001). This biomechanical disruption has been termed lever-arm deficiency, and is best characterized by the center of pressure progression (COPP) relative to the foot.

Dynamic pedobarography has been used to document the location and duration of the COPP relative to the hindfoot, midfoot and forefoot segments of the foot in 23 normal children between the ages of 6 and 17 years (Jameson et al. 2008). Based upon the values determined from these normal children, deviation in the location and duration of the COPP relative to the segments of the foot can be used to describe common abnormal loading patterns (Fig. 5.8.2). Displacement of the COPP medially in a particular segment of the foot describes a valgus loading pattern, which might be the consequence of a everted, abducted, or pronated segmental malalignment of the foot segment. Displacement of the COPP laterally in a particular segment of the foot describes a varus loading pattern, which might be the consequence of an inverted, adducted, or supinated segmental malalignment of the foot segment. Prolonged duration of the COPP in the forefoot segment describes an equinus foot loading pattern. Prolonged duration of the COPP in the hindfoot segment describes a calcaneus loading pattern. This standardized approach to the determination of foot loading patterns, based upon normative data, should facilitate the characterization of abnormal foot loading patterns, clinical decision-making, and the assessment of outcome following a variety of interventions.

Goals of treatment

Surgical interventions to address foot deformities in children with CP are all designed to improve foot shape. It is presumed that surgically improved foot shape can restore the stability function of the foot in mid-stance and the skeletal lever arm function of the foot in terminal stance. Unfortunately, increased foot stiffness associated with many surgical

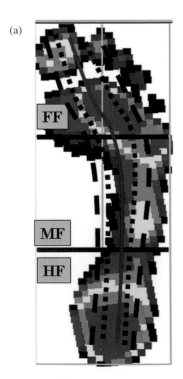

(a)

Fig. 5.8.2 and opposite Qualitative display of pedobarographic data. (a) Normal pediatric pedobarograph. Higher pressures are shown in pink, lower pressures in blue. The foot contact pattern is divided into three segments by the horizontal solid black lines; the hindfoot (HF), midfoot (MF), and forefoot (FF). The mean value for the normal center of pressure progression (COPP) is shown by the solid red line. The 1 S.D. for the mean value of the COPP is shown by the dotted black line. The 2 S.D. for the mean value of the COPP is shown by the dashed black line. (b) Pedobarograph of a child with CP and equinoplanovalgus segmental malalignment. The COPP (solid red line) is deviated medially, indicating a valgus loading pattern. (c) Pedobarograph of a child with CP and equinocavovarus segmental malalignment. The COPP (solid red line) is deviated laterally, indicating a varus loading pattern. (d) Pedobarograph of a child with CP and isolated equinus segmental malalignment. The COPP (solid red line) is deviated distally, indicating an equinus loading pattern. (e) Pedobarograph of a child with CP and calcaneoplanocavus segmental malalignment. The COPP (solid red line) is deviated proximally, indicating a calcaneus loading pattern.

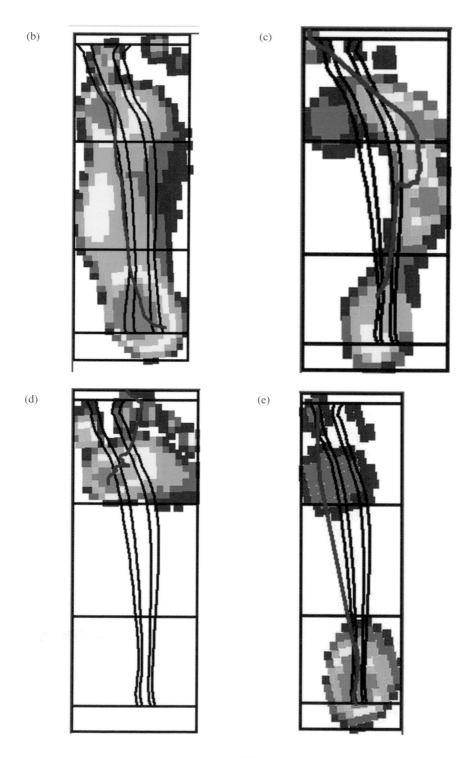

procedures (e.g. arthrodesis) utilized to improve foot shape may compromise shock absorption function of the foot in loading response.

Cosmetic improvements following foot reconstruction are related to improved visual assessment of static standing foot alignment (particularly restoration of the medial longitudinal arch and toe alignment) and improved foot progression angle during stance phase.

Pain associated with foot deformities in children with CP is usually related to poor alignment and instability in stance phase. Equinoplanovalgus segmental malalignment of the foot results in excessive loading of medial midfoot in midstance, leading to the development of painful callosities that may compromise orthosis and shoe wear (Mosca 1996). Equinocavovarus segmental malalignment of the foot results in excessive loading of the lateral mid- and forefoot segments, resulting in instability in mid- and terminal stance, which may lead to frequent inversion injuries of the ankle and hindfoot (Sutherland 1993, Mosca 2001). It is presumed that surgically improved foot shape can correct pain by improving foot loading and stability in stance phase.

Children with CP may tolerate mild or moderate foot deformities, with little complaint of pain or sense of impairment. However, such deformities may be poorly tolerated in adult life, where the magnitude of the abnormal loading is much greater (due to increased body mass), and the cumulative effect over time results in premature degenerative changes of the articular cartilage of the joints of the foot and ankle. It is presumed that surgery to improve foot shape in childhood will improve the loading of the foot and decrease the possibility of early degenerative arthritis in adulthood.

Surgical treatment options

Mild foot deformities, in which the segmental malalignments are flexible and correctable on manipulation, are best treated with soft-tissue (i.e. muscle-tendon unit) surgery. Soft-tissue surgical options include release, lengthening, partial or split transfer, and complete transfer. Moderate and severe foot deformities, in which the segmental malalignments are fixed and not correctable on manipulation, are best treated with a combination of soft-tissue and skeletal surgeries. Skeletal surgical options include osteotomy and arthrodesis. These procedures may correct deformity by addition (i.e. lengthening), subtraction (i.e. shortening), angulation or rotation. When correcting moderate or severe foot deformities, soft-tissue and skeletal procedures are performed in a sequential fashion to restore or optimize foot segmental alignment. Soft-tissue surgeries require immobilization for 2–4 weeks after surgery, with subsequent protection in an ankle–foot orthosis for 4–6 months. Skeletal surgeries may require internal fixation, followed by 6 weeks of immobilization after surgery.

Equinoplanovalgus segmental malalignment: The primary procedure utilized to correct moderate or severe equinoplanovalgus foot segmental malalignment is lateral column lengthening (Mosca 1995, Yoo et al. 2005) (Fig. 5.8.3). This may be performed at the neck of the calcaneus, through the calcaneocuboid joint, or in the body of the cuboid. This procedure may achieve adequate correction of all three segments of the foot, presumably due to ligamentotaxis (Sangeorzan et al. 1993) (Fig. 5.8.4). Sequential correction of equinoplanovalgus segmental malalignment may be divided into four stages:

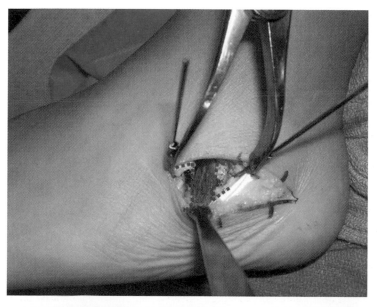

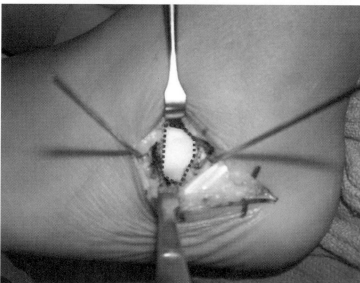

Fig. 5.8.3 Intraoperative photographs of lateral column lengthening of the left foot in a child with CP and equinoplanovalgus segmental malalignment. *Top*: Lateral view of the left hindfoot. The osteotomy has been performed through the neck of the calcaneus. Pins are placed into the proximal and distal fragments, and distraction is applied with a cannulated lamina spreader. The margins of the proximal and distal calcaneal fragments are outlined by the dotted red lines. The medioplantar intrinsic muscles are seen in the depths of the osteotomy. *Bottom*: Lateral view of the left hindfoot. A contoured patellar allograft (outlined by dotted red circle) has been placed into the distracted calcaneal osteotomy. The allograft is usually stable and requires no further fixation. (See Instructional Video, 'Os calcis lengthening', on Interactive Disc.)

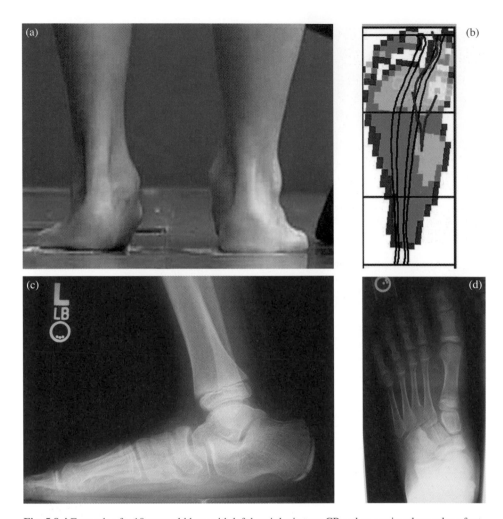

Fig. 5.8.4 Example of a 10-year-old boy with left hemiplegic type CP and an equinoplanovalgus foot segmental malalignment. (a) Preoperative clinical photograph of both feet. Note the valgus alignment of the hindfoot and the collapsed medial arch on the left side. (b) Pedobarograph of the left foot. The COPP is deviated distally and medially, indicating an equinovalgus loading pattern. (c) Preoperative lateral radiograph of the left foot. Note the equinoplanovalgus segmental malalignment. (d) Preoperative anteroposterior radiograph of the left foot. Note the talonavicular uncoverage. (e) Intraoperative stress lateral radiograph of the left foot. Gastrocsoleus muscle group recession and lateral column lengthening through the neck of the calcaneus have been performed. Note the greatly improved foot segmental alignment. (f) Intraoperative stress anteroposterior radiograph of the left foot. Note the talonavicular coverage is greatly improved. (g) Postoperative clinical photograph of both feet 1 year after left side gastrocsoleus recession and lateral column lengthening surgery. Note the improved alignment of the hindfoot and restoration of the medial arch on the left foot. (h) Postoperative pedobarograph of the left foot. The COPP is located in the central zone for each segment of the foot, indicating normalization of the loading pattern. (i) Postoperative lateral radiograph of the left foot. Note the greatly improved alignment of all three segments of the foot. (j) Postoperative anteroposterior radiograph of the left foot. Talonavicular coverage is greatly improved.

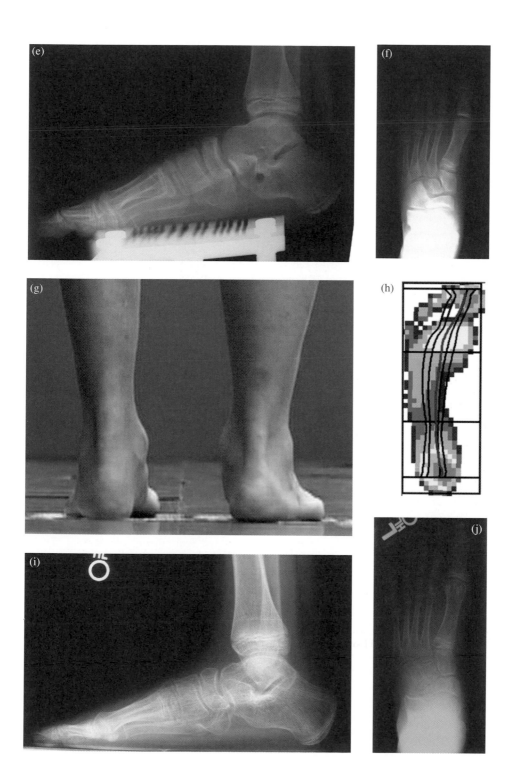

525

1. Correct hindfoot soft tissue contractures. The triceps surae muscle group usually has fixed, or myostatic shortening. The goal is to achieve 5° of ankle dorsiflexion when the knee is extended. When 15° or less of correction is required, lengthening at the myotendinous junction is preferred. When greater than 15° of correction is required, lengthening at the conjoined tendon (tendo-Achilles) level is necessary (Rose et al. 1993). Occasionally there is significant contracture of the peroneus brevis muscle, which is best corrected by lengthening at the myotendinous junction (proximal to the lateral malleolus).

2. Lengthen the lateral column. In children 10 years of age and younger, lateral column lengthening is best performed through the neck of the calcaneus (addition osteotomy) (Mosca 1995). The lengthening is usually between 1 and 2 cm, and interposition grafting with tricortical iliac crest or patella allograft is preferred. The graft itself is usually stable, but longitudinal pin fixation may be used to control the calcaneocuboid joint subluxation that can occur during lateral column lengthening.

   In children over 10 years of age, lateral column lengthening may also be performed through the calcaneocuboid joint (addition arthrodesis) (Danko et al. 2004). The lengthening is usually between 1.5 and 2.5 cm, requiring a larger graft. The graft itself is usually stable, but internal fixation with a 1/3 tubular plate may be performed to minimize the possibility of graft collapse during the absorption and incorporation phases of healing.

3. Assess the medial column. In some cases, lateral column lengthening alone will result in adequate correction of all three segments of the foot. If there is residual forefoot varus deformity, or the medial column (i.e. great toe metatarsal) is judged to be hypermobile in the sagittal plane, then a plantar-based closing wedge (i.e. plantarflexion) osteotomy is performed, through the medial cuneiform or at the base of the great toe metatarsal (when the proximal physis has closed). If there is residual forefoot abduction deformity (i.e. persistent talonavicular subluxation), as determined by palpation of the medial column or intraoperative radiographs of the foot, then a talonavicular arthrodesis is performed (Fig. 5.8.5, Instructional Video, '1st cuneiform osteotomy', on Interactive Disc).

4. If lengthening of the lateral column fails to correct the hindfoot deformity, which is unusual, then subtalar, calcaneocuboid, and talonavicular arthrodeses (i.e. triple arthrodesis) will be required to achieve optimal realignment of the foot. Triple arthrodesis for equinoplanovalgus foot segmental malalignment is best performed through lateral and medial incisions (the latter is required to adequately visualize the talonavicular joint). Triple arthrodesis may be combined with lateral column lengthening through the calcaneocuboid joint to minimize the need for medial column shortening (Horton and Olney 1995).

Equinocavovarus segmental malalignment. Correction of moderate or severe equinocavovarus foot segmental malalignment is fundamentally different, as there is no single skeletal procedure (i.e. that is analogous to the lateral column lengthening) that can achieve adequate correction of all three segments of the foot. Therefore sequential correction of individual segments of the equinocavovarus segmental malalignment, utilizing both soft-tissue and skeletal procedures is preferred (Fig. 5.8.6) and may be divided into three stages, as follows.

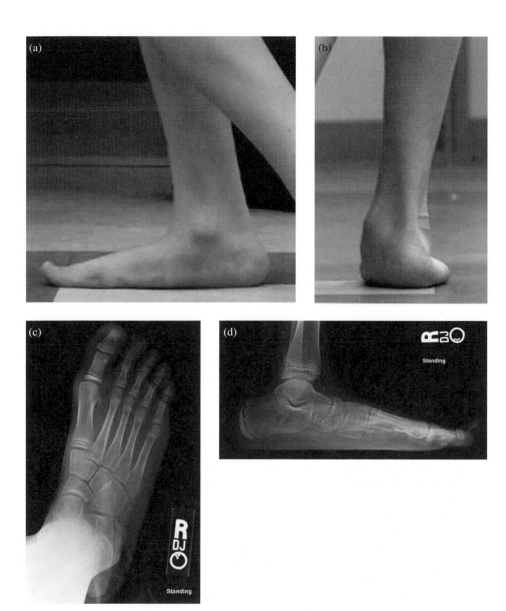

Fig. 5.8.5 Example of a 12-year-old boy with diplegic CP, GMFCS type III who has a neutral hindfoot and forefoot varus in NWB subtalar joint neutral with a hypermobile midfoot. He has poor motor control distally at the foot and ankle. In weightbearing, the foot collapses into an equinoplanovalgus foot deformity. Following os calcis lengthening and gastrocnemius recession, there is residual forefoot abduction deformity, so a talonavicular arthrodesis was performed.
(a) Preoperative clinical photograph of the right foot. Note the collapsed medial arch. (b) Note the valgus alignment of the hindfoot and abduction of the forefoot. (c) Preoperative anteroposterior radiograph. Note the talonavicular uncoverage. (d) Preoperative lateral radiograph. Note the equinoplanovalgus segmental malalignment.

527

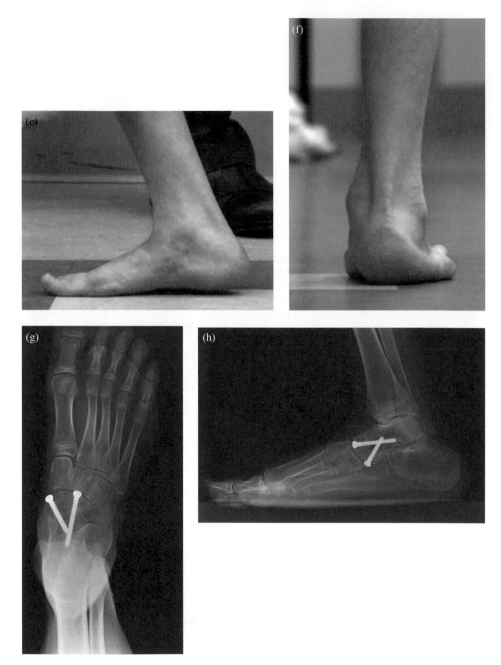

Fig. 5.8.5 continued (e) Postoperative clinical photograph 1 year after os calcis lengthening, gastrocnemius recession, and talonavicular arthrodesis. Note the restoration of the medial arch. (f) Note the improved alignment of the hindfoot. (g) Postoperative anteroposterior radiograph shows restoration of medial column alignment. Talonavicular joint is fused. (h) Postoperative lateral radiograph. Note the greatly improved alignment of all three segments of the foot.

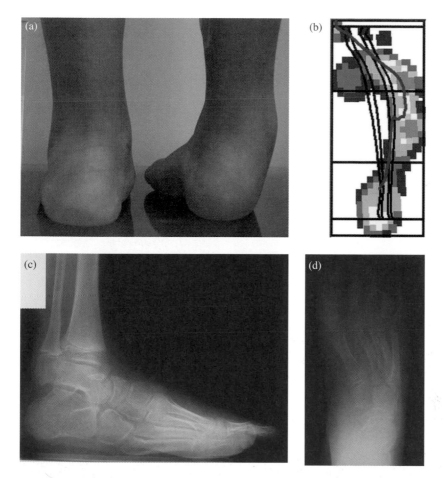

Fig. 5.8.6 Example of an 11-year-old boy with right hemiplegic type CP and an equinocavovarus foot segmental malalignment. (A) Preoperative clinical photograph of both feet. Note the varus alignment of the hindfoot and the increased medial arch on the right side. (B) Pedobarograph of the right foot. The COPP is deviated distally and laterally, indicating an equinovarus loading pattern. (C) Preoperative lateral radiograph of the right foot. Note the equinocavovarus segmental malalignment. (D) Preoperative anteroposterior radiograph of the right foot. There is significant talocalcaneal overlap and medial displacement of the navicular on the talus. (E) Intraoperative stress lateral radiograph of the right foot. Gastrosoleus recession, radical plantar fascia release, and fractional lengthening of the abductor hallucis muscle have been performed. A valgus producing calcaneal slide osteotomy (held reduced by 2 pins), and a dorsiflexion osteotomy through the medial cuneiform (held reduced by the single pin) have been performed. Compensatory deformities have been created to improved foot segmental alignment. (F) Intraoperative stress anteroposterior radiograph of the right foot. Hindfoot, midfoot and forefoot alignment are greatly improved. (G) Postoperative clinical photograph of both feet 1 year after right-side skeletal surgery. Note the improved alignment of the hindfoot. (H) Postoperative pedobarograph of the right foot. The COPP is located in the central zone for each segment of the foot, indicating normalization of the loading pattern. (I) Postoperative lateral radiograph of the right foot. Compensatory deformities have been created to improve gross foot segmental alignment. (J) Postoperative anteroposterior radiograph of the right foot. Significant midfoot malalignment persists despite significant improvement in gross foot alignment and loading.

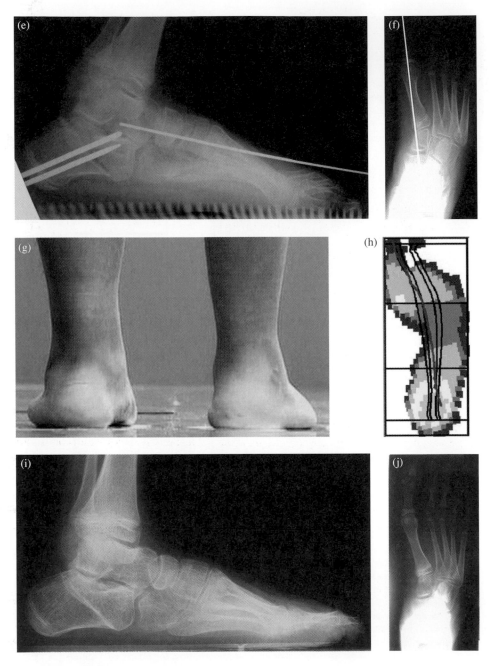

Fig. 5.8.6 continued

1. Correct hindfoot and midfoot soft-tissue contractures (Sutherland 1993, Mosca 2001). Fractional lengthening of the triceps surae muscle group and the tibialis posterior muscle are performed through a medial incision at the distal third of the calf. Fractional lengthening of the flexor hallucis longus and flexor digitorum longus muscles are rarely necessary, but may be performed through the same incision. Fractional lengthening of the abductor hallucis muscle is performed on the medial border of the foot, at the distal third of the great toe metatarsal. Finally, sequential release of the plantar fascia and the short intrinsic muscles of the foot may be performed through a plantar, medial or lateral approach.

   Split-tendon transfer of the posterior or anterior tibialis muscles is only appropriate for the management of mild equinocavovarus foot deformity, where the skeletal malalignment is purely dynamic, completely correctible on manipulation, and no fixed or myostatic shortening deformity of the muscle is present (Hoffer et al. 1985, Scott and Scarborough 2006). The result of complete tendon transfer of either of these muscles is unpredictable and should therefore be avoided when treating foot deformities in children with CP.

2. Restoration of normal skeletal segmental alignment in the presence of residual or fixed equinocavovarus deformity by osteotomy is usually not possible. However, gross alignment and dynamic loading of the foot may be greatly improved by performing sequential osteotomies to create deformities that compensate for segmental malalignments (Rathjen and Mubarak 1998). Sequential correction proceeds from proximal (the hindfoot) to distal (the forefoot). Residual hindfoot varus malalignment may be corrected by calcaneal slide or laterally based closing wedge osteotomies (or a combination of both techniques) (Koman et al. 1993). Residual midfoot supination deformity may be corrected by lateral column shortening through the cuboid (i.e. dorsolaterally based closing wedge osteotomy). Residual forefoot valgus deformity may be corrected by dorsiflexion osteotomy of the medial column (dorsally based closing wedge osteotomy of the medial cuneiform, or great toe metatarsal when the proximal physis has closed).

3. In the most extreme cases of equinocavovarus segmental malalignment, arthrodesis of the subtalar, calcaneocuboid and talonavicular joints (i.e. triple arthrodesis) is required to achieve optimal foot alignment. Triple arthrodesis for equinocavovarus foot segmental malalignment is best performed through a lateral incision, which usually provides adequate exposure of all three joints. Segmental alignment is restored from proximal to distal. Hindfoot varus alignment is corrected by subtalar arthrodesis. Midfoot supination deformity is then corrected by calcaneocubiod arthrodesis. Finally, forefoot valgus (or occasionally varus) deformity is corrected by talonavicular arthrodesis.

REFERENCES

Danko A, Allen B Jr, Pugh L, Stasikelis P (2004) Early graft failure in lateral column lengthening. *J Pediatr Orthop* **24**: 716–20.

Davids JR (2006) Quantitative gait analysis in the treatment of children with cerebral palsy. *J Pediatr Orthop* **26**: 557–9.

Davids JR, Foti T, Dabelstein J, Blackhurst DW, Bagley A (1999) Objective assessment of dyskinesia in children with cerebral palsy. *J Pediatr Orthop* **19**: 211–14.

Davids JR, Õunpuu S, DeLuca PA, Davis RB 3rd (2004) Optimization of walking ability of children with cerebral palsy. *Instr Course Lect* **53**: 511–22.

Davids JR, Gibson TW, Pugh LI (2005) Quantitative segmental analysis of weight-bearing radiographs of the foot and ankle for children: normal alignment. *J Pediatr Orthop* **25**: 769–76.

Davids JR, Rowan F, Davis RB (2007) Indications for orthoses to improve gait in children with cerebral palsy. *J Am Acad Orthop Surg* **15**: 178–88.

Davis RB Õunpuu S, Tyburski D, Gage JR (1991) A gait analysis data collection and reduction technique. *Hum Mov Sci* **10**: 575–87.

Davis RB, Jameson EG, Davids JR, Christopher LM, Rogozinski BM, Anderson JP (2007) The design, development, and initial evaluation of a multisegment foot model for routine clinical gait analysis. In: Harris GF, Smith P, Marks R, editors. *Foot and Ankle Motion Analysis: Clinical Treatment and Technology*. Boca Raton, FL: CRC Press. p 425–44.

Foran JR, Steinman S, Barash I, Chambers HG, Lieber RL (2005) Structural and mechanical alterations in spastic skeletal muscle. *Dev Med Child Neurol* **47**: 713–17.

Gage JR (1995) The clinical use of kinetics for evaluation of pathologic gait in cerebral palsy. *Instr Course Lect* **44**: 507–15.

Gage JR, Novacheck TF (2001) An update on the treatment of gait problems in cerebral palsy. *J Pediatr Orthop B* **10**: 265–74.

Gage JR, DeLuca PA, Renshaw TS (1996) Gait analysis: principle and applications with emphasis on its use in cerebral palsy. *Instr Course Lect* **45**: 491–507.

Hoffer MM, Barakat G, Koffman M (1985) 10-year follow-up of split anterior tibial tendon transfer in cerebral palsied patients with spastic equinovarus deformity. *J Pediatr Orthop* **5**: 432–4.

Horton GA, Olney BW (1995) Triple arthrodesis with lateral column lengthening for treatment of severe planovalgus deformity. *Foot Ankle Int* **16**: 395–400.

Inman VT, Ralston HJ, Todd F (1981) *Human Walking*. Baltimore, MD: Williams & Wilkins.

Jameson EG, Davids JR, Anderson JP, Davis RB 3rd, Blackhurst DW, Christopher LM (2008) Dynamic pedobarography for children: use of the center of pressure progression. *J Pediatr Orthop* **28**: 254–8.

Koman LA, Mooney JF 3rd, Goodman A (1993) Management of valgus hindfoot deformity in pediatric cerebral palsy patients by medial displacement osteotomy. *J Pediatr Orthop* **13**: 180–3.

Lieber RL (1986) Skeletal muscle adaptability. I: Review of basic properties. *Dev Med Child Neurol* **28**: 390–7.

MacWilliams BA, Cowley M, Nicholson DE (2003) Foot kinematics and kinetics during adolescent gait. *Gait Posture* **17**: 214–24.

Mosca VS (1995) Calcaneal lengthening for valgus deformity of the hindfoot. Results in children who had severe, symptomatic flatfoot and skewfoot. *J Bone Joint Surg Am* **77**: 500–12.

Mosca VS (1996) Flexible flatfoot and skewfoot. *Instr Course Lect* **45**: 347–54.

Mosca VS (1998) The child's foot: Principles of management. *J Pediatr Orthop* **18**: 281–2.

Mosca VS (2001) The cavus foot. *J Pediatr Orthop* **21**: 423–4.

Perry J (1992) *Gait Analysis: Normal and Pathologic Function*. Thorofare, NJ: Slack.

Rang M, Wright J (1989) What have 30 years of medical progress done for cerebral palsy? *Clin Orthop Relat Res* **247**: 55–60.

Rathjen KE, Mubarak SJ (1998) Calcaneal-cuboid-cuneiform osteotomy for the correction of valgus foot deformities in children. *J Pediatr Orthop* **18**: 775–82.

Rose SA, DeLuca PA, Davis RB 3rd, Õunpuu S, Gage JR (1993) Kinematic and kinetic evaluation of the ankle after lengthening of the gastrocnemius fascia in children with cerebral palsy. *J Pediatr Orthop* **13**: 727–32.

Sangeorzan BJ, Mosca V, Hansen ST Jr (1993) Effect of calcaneal lengthening on relationships among the hindfoot, midfoot, and forefoot. *Foot Ankle* **14**: 136–41.

Schaff PS (1993) An overview of foot pressure measurement systems. *Clin Podiatr Med Surg* **10**: 403–15.

Scott AC, Scarborough N (2006) The use of dynamic emg in predicting the outcome of split posterior tibial tendon transfers in spastic hemiplegia. *J Pediatr Orthop* **26**: 777–80.

Sutherland DH (1993) Varus foot in cerebral palsy: an overview. *Instr Course Lect* **42**: 539–43.

Sutherland DH, Cooper L, Daniel D (1980) The role of the ankle plantar flexors in normal walking. *J Bone Joint Surg Am* **62**: 354–63.

Yoo WJ, Chung CY, Choi IH, Cho TJ, Kim DH (2005) Calcaneal lengthening for the planovalgus foot deformity in children with cerebral palsy. *J Pediatr Orthop* **25**: 781–5.

5.9
POSTOPERATIVE CARE AND REHABILITATION

Steven E. Koop and Susan Murr

Key points
- Preoperative planning improves understanding of the proposed procedure by family and the care team
- Surgery and immediate postoperative care require close attention to many details
- Maximum improvement in function requires extensive therapy and may not be reached for more than a year.

Preoperative planning

A surgical intervention is considered when parents, therapists and physicians believe a child's function could improve and other interventions are no longer effective. It is important to ask parents and therapists to describe the problems they see and list their goals. The goal of surgical interventions may be to improve function in children classified as Gross Motor Function Classification System (GMFCS) levels I–IV or to prevent further secondary complications in children in level V (Palisano et al. 1997). Careful physical examination, radiographs, and a motion analysis study will yield a problem list and a list of possible interventions.

When the physician and family meet to discuss surgery, they should agree on the outcome they are seeking. The importance of this discussion cannot be overstated. Both long-term and short-term functional goals of the child and family should be discussed. Measures of preferred activity and participation such as the Children's Assessment of Participation and Enjoyment (CAPE) or the Activities Scale for Kids (ASK) may be helpful (Young et al. 2000, King et al. 2004). Adolescents should be involved in the surgery recommendation, including an honest discussion of the amount of effort that will be needed postoperatively and timelines for returning to their preoperative level of function. Preoperative and postoperative videos of other patients with similar problems and conversations with families who have gone through similar surgeries can help parents significantly. The physician should give a detailed description of the surgery (including risks and complications) and the hospital stay, and discuss the rehabilitation program that will be needed to achieve the best outcome. It is difficult for parents to remember every detail of this conversation and it is common for them to have additional questions once they have gone home and discussed what they have heard. Many families later report that they simply did not understand the magnitude of the surgery. They also report that they underestimated the complexity and duration of recovery and rehabilitation. A second meeting with the surgeon, and perhaps other families, will help them.

Visits with a physical therapist and a child life specialist are important. The physical therapist can assess the child's muscle strength, functional level, cognitive ability and behavioral aspects that may impact postoperative care. This information may affirm or modify the goals of treatment. Strength is typically measured using manual muscle testing, but may be more accurately measured using a hand-held dynamometer (Taylor et al. 2004, van der Linden et al. 2004). A tool such as the Gross Motor Function Measure may be used to determine motor function, with emphasis on one specific dimension or the whole measure (Russell et al. 1989). The Functional Mobility Scale (FMS), an evaluative measure of mobility in children with cerebral palsy, could also be used to determine a baseline record of the child's mobility at home, school and the community, or at 5, 50 and 500 meters (Graham et al. 2004). The FMS has been found to be a clinically useful tool for measuring changes after single-event multilevel surgery in children with cerebral palsy (Harvey et al. 2007). Factors such as motor planning and the ability to follow directions and cooperate with therapy should be discussed to determine the best option for postoperative rehabilitation. Crutches or a walker can be fit and postoperative therapy activities rehearsed when there is no pain.

A visit to the hospital with a child life specialist will allow the child and family to encounter elements of the hospital environment and meet personnel who may be involved in the child's care. At Gillette Children's, a manual has been created to serve as a resource for parents as they prepare for surgery. It helps them think of the care their child will need after leaving the hospital, the changes that may be needed at home to provide care during the early weeks of recovery, and the impact on the child's educational activities.

The child's pediatrician and neurologist have important roles. A careful preoperative examination is needed to address health concerns that could affect surgery. It is imperative that a child's nutrition be evaluated since poor nutrition will diminish early wound healing, bone and muscle healing, and rehabilitation outcomes. Medications should be reviewed as some may be affected by surgery. In the days after surgery there is often nausea, abdominal discomfort, or a general disinterest in eating. Baclofen, when taken as an oral medication, requires a gradual dosage tapering to avoid withdrawal symptoms. Most often it is best to discontinue baclofen before surgery to avoid this problem. Some antiepileptic medications, notably valproic acid, have been associated with greater hemorrhage from bone surgeries. No single preoperative laboratory test has been found to detect the multifocal effects on clotting associated with valproic acid. It is common to ask the child's neurologist to replace valproic acid with another medication in the weeks before surgery if adequate seizure control can be maintained.

The surgeon also must help the hospital prepare for the surgery and simply listing the proposed procedures is inadequate. Surgical planning documents should include information about equipment, bone graft material, intraoperative brace models, postoperative immobilization, length of the procedure, and other surgeons involved in the work. This allows operating room personnel to create an environment fully ready for surgery and it allows the nursing staff who will receive the child after the procedure to be effective in their work.

Surgery and the hospital stay

It is most common for children to come to the hospital on the day of surgery rather than being admitted the night before the procedure. This means that the hour or two in the preoperative area can be very busy. Operating-room personnel introduce themselves and explain how the environment works and how they will communicate with the family. The anesthesia team reviews pertinent records, explains the anesthesia process and final decisions are made about methods of pain management. The surgeon and family make a final review of the procedures that will be performed and the surgeon completes the surgical site marking protocol, a method by which every surgical site is identified and marked so that the correct procedure is done in the correct anatomic location.

Many children are accompanied to the operating room by a parent, who can then be present during the administration of anesthesia. If epidural analgesia is to be used, the anesthesiologist places the catheter after anesthesia has been administered and before the surgery starts. During this time the surgeon should review the entire procedure with the operating room team and answer questions. An anatomic drawing is a useful way to map the proposed right- and left-side procedures and whether they will be done when the child is prone or supine. Such a device allows the team to track the progress of the surgery and be certain that the preoperative plan is being followed or changes are appropriate. When two surgical teams are working at multiple sites it is imperative to maintain a clear understanding of the work being done.

Recovery from surgery occurs in three phases. The first phase includes management of fluid and electrolytes, blood loss, limb swelling and pain. Immediate postoperative limb immobilization is done with Robert Jones dressings, well padded plaster-reinforced bandages designed to accommodate swelling. Casts are almost never used for immediate immobilization. Control of limb rotation can be achieved by incorporating a Denis–Browne bar in the dressing. Overt efforts to reduce pain should start in the operating room. Pain management options include caudal blocks, epidural analgesia, wound infiltration with analgesic agents, patient or nurse controlled intravenous analgesia pumps, and intravenous anti-inflammatories such as ketorolac. Preoperative placement of botulinum toxin A may reduce postoperative spasms and simplify pain management (Barwood et al. 2000).

Epidural analgesia is a safe and effective method for managing postoperative pain in the majority of patients undergoing simultaneous multiple lower-extremity procedures. The catheter is placed in the lower lumbar spine unless the anatomy is altered by prior surgeries such as selective dorsal lumbar rhizotomy or spine fusion (Fig. 5.9.1). In such cases or in young children caudal insertion may be easier and safer and may facilitate proximal passage of the catheter. Ropivicaine (0.1%–0.25%) is the most common drug, in combination with clonidine, and after an initial bolus is delivered by a computer-controlled pump. A higher dosage is used during longer surgeries to reduce the need for other anesthetic agents, allowing more rapid emergence from anesthesia and earlier assessment of limb neurovascular function.

Concerns have been expressed about the safety of epidural analgesia. These concerns have centered on catheter site infections, drug toxicity, and masking of neurovascular changes including impending compartment syndrome. Catheter infections are extremely

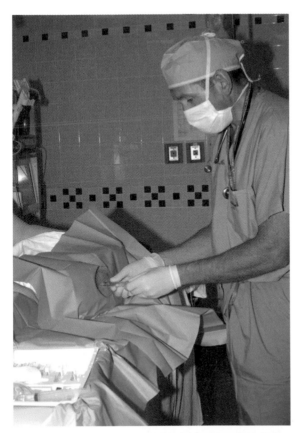

Fig. 5.9.1 (a) After the patient is anesthetized, the anesthesiologist places the epidural catheter. (b) The insertion needle has been withdrawn and the catheter taped into place. We routinely use continuous epidural anesthesia with clonidine 2µg/ml in conjunction with a 0.1% solution of ropivacaine delivered at a rate of 0.2–0.3 ml per kg per hour for 72 hours after surgery.

(b)

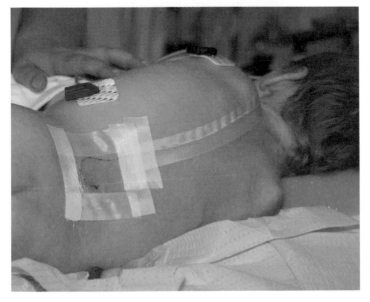

rare. The insertion site is prepared and draped like any surgical site and the catheter is protected by a sterile adherent plastic dressing that permits inspection. An indwelling catheter collects urine and bowel movements are uncommon in the first days after surgery. The pain management goal is to achieve analgesia while preserving light touch sensation and basic motor function. Bupivacaine is widely used for epidural analgesia due to its long duration and ability to spare motor function. However, equipotent doses of bupivacaine are more cardiotoxic than lidocaine. Careful placement of catheters and careful dosing will reduce the incidence and severity of bupivacaine toxicity.

Ropivacaine, a newer amide local anesthetic agent, has less cardiotoxicity and spares motor function better than bupivacaine. It is our preferred medication for epidural analgesia. For continuous infusions via epidural catheters a 0.1% solution of ropivacaine or bupivacaine is delivered at a rate of 0.2–0.3 ml per kg per hour. For many years we supplemented the local anesthetic effect of the epidural solution with analgesia provided by fentanyl in a dose of 1–2 µg per milliliter. This has been discontinued due to sedation, respiratory suppression, itching, and nausea and vomiting. Fentanyl has been replaced by clonidine. The analgesic effect is obtained with less sedation and respiratory compromise. Hypotension and bradycardia are side effects of clonidine and may necessitate reduction or elimination from the epidural solution.

For those patients who are not candidates for epidural delivery of analgesics, or those who do not consent to placement of an epidural catheter, a continuous infusion of narcotic medication is a good alternative. If the patient is alert and physically able to press a button the infusion can be administered by a patient-controlled analgesia (PCA) pump. If the patient is not capable the nurse at the bedside can give supplemental bolus doses as needed. There are several narcotics that can be used effectively in a PCA. Ketorolac (Toradol), a nonsteroidal anti-inflammatory drug administered intravenously or intramuscularly, can provide significant pain relief. In adults there are concerns that this class of anti-inflammatory drugs inhibit bone formation but we have not noted any impact on the healing of osteotomies in children and adolescents. If there has been substantial intraoperative blood loss or if there is a concern before surgery about a child's clotting function this medicine should not be used. Because of the potential for gastric ulceration ketorolac should not be used for more than 72 hours after surgery. See Table 5.9.1 for common intravenous pain and spasm controlling medications.

Epidural analgesia, in combination with intravenous spasm control and supplementary intravenous pain medications, is extremely effective. Conscientious monitoring of neuro-vascular function is imperative when this pain management technique is used. A clear

TABLE 5.9.1
Common intravenous pain and spasm controlling medications

Medication	Pediatric dose range
Ketorolac	0.25–0.5 mg/kg/dose IV every 6 hrs (maximum 3 days)
Morphine	0.1–0.2 mg/kg/dose IV every 2 hrs
Diazepam	0.04–0.15 mg/kg/dose IV every 2 hrs (maximum 0.6 mg/kg in 8 hrs)

understanding of a child's sensation and voluntary motor control must be established in order to understand whether the pain control is appropriate. Epidural analgesia should not remove all sensation or all voluntary motor control. If that occurs then the epidural should be turned off until motor and sensory function recovers to a degree that permits accurate understanding of neurovascular function. An assessment protocol should be established and assiduously applied to every patient. A responsive physician should always be available to examine the child, modify medications, and open postoperative bandages to inspect limbs and relieve pressure. This will help avoid compartment syndromes and nerve deficits.

The second phase of recovery starts approximately 3 days after surgery. A general sense of well-being starts to return. Severe pain and spasms abate and permit a transition to oral medications. The decrease in surgical site swelling makes it safe to remove Robert Jones dressings and apply casts. Casts are kept to minimum. Proximal femoral osteotomies, and most pelvic osteotomies, can be managed by applying two short leg casts with a removable Denis–Browne bar on the anterior surface just above the ankle between the casts for rotational control. Knee-immobilizers can be used intermittently to maintain knee extension and assist with transfers. With a hip-flexion restriction of 70° in the first 4 weeks after surgery to reduce stress at the proximal femur children can sit in a reclining wheelchair with elevating leg-rests. Hip spica casts are reserved for special circumstances and often can be removed at 3–4 weeks to start careful movement. Distal femoral extension osteotomies with advancement of the patella can be managed in the same manner with early use of a continuous passive motion machine (Fig. 5.9.2). Tenuous femoral or tibial tubercle fixation

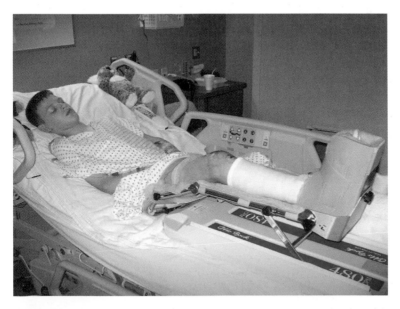

Fig. 5.9.2 During the inpatient postoperative stage, a continuous passive motion (CPM) machine is initiated to assist with gentle and limited knee flexion and extension. When not using the CPM, the patient is positioned in full extension with a knee-immobilizer. Prone positioning at least three times per day is encouraged to maintain full hip extension.

may necessitate a long leg cast until early bone healing is established. Tibial osteotomies and foot and ankle procedures are protected by a short leg cast.

The last phase of recovery before leaving the hospital is dedicated to early physical therapy and preparing the parents to take care of their child. The nature of the surgery will determine the limb movement and general activity that will be permitted while waiting for sufficient bone healing to remove casts and start more intense therapy work (Fig. 5.9.3).

Postoperative rehabilitation
When the early weeks of bone and muscle healing are finished many children and families do well with outpatient physical therapy. Others benefit from more intense therapy on an inpatient rehabilitation unit. During inpatient care adaptive equipment and braces can be fitted and adjusted, occupational therapy can address activities of daily living and upper-extremity strengthening, psychologists and child life specialists can help with anxiety and

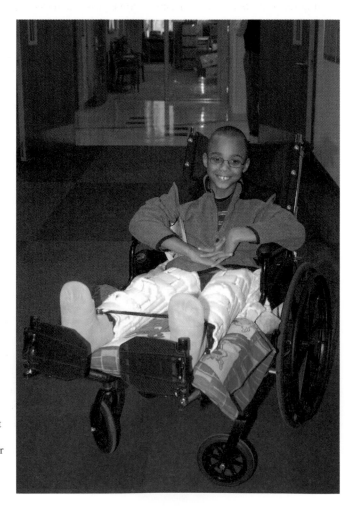

Fig. 5.9.3 By the time of discharge, the patient is typically casted with a Denis–Browne bar controlling rotation and knee immobilizers to maintain full knee extension. The child can sit with up to 70° of hip flexion. A rental wheelchair is ordered and sent home with the family for as long as needed.

540

motivation, and the family can be introduced to therapeutic recreation activities that will increase endurance and cardiovascular fitness. Principles of motor learning, which support periods of intensity for learning new patterns of movement, can be applied to this population (Damiano 2006). Although this can be decided after the surgery has occurred, it is helpful to discuss and plan for it at the time of the surgical recommendation, so that the child and family can prepare for a second admission and funding can be investigated.

Much like immediate recovery from surgery, long-term recovery occurs in three broad stages. The first stage, approximately 6 weeks, involves the healing of soft tissues and bone. The second stage, from 12 to 24 weeks, includes strengthening, and the third stage is regaining and refining of functional movement and gait and lasts up to 12 months.

Postoperative physical therapy goals can be grouped according to levels on the GMFCS, with the two broad groupings of levels I–III and IV–V. When bony procedures have been performed in either group, the first stage of healing requires the child to be non-weight bearing for some weeks. The caregivers are instructed in transfer training and passive range of motion to prevent stiffness or the introduction of soft-tissue contractures due to postoperative positioning. If knee surgery has been performed, a continuous passive motion (CPM) machine may be used which allows more comfortable achievement of knee range of motion. If the child is able to assist with transfers and positioning s/he is encouraged to do so, in order to give him/her some sense of control and participation with the caregiver. It is difficult for children to prepare for the feelings of complete dependency that often occur after this level of surgery. Additional help may be required to safely care for the child at home after discharge.

Surgery recommendations for adolescents and young adults are often limited to one-sided procedures. This preserves the opposite side for active motion and weightbearing, to enable transfers with less or no assistance and the ability to be upright and ambulatory if the patient can maintain a non-weightbearing status on the surgical side. This is often more acceptable to the patient, even if s/he anticipates having the second side operated on in the future. It may also impact the postoperative rehabilitation, more easily allowing the patient to be cared for at home and with an outpatient therapy program.

At 3–4 weeks radiographs are used to determine if bone healing will permit weightbearing. For children in levels I–III, supported standing and ambulation begin with an appropriate assistive device, typically a reverse walker to encourage upright posture. Support is needed at this time as the child learns to stand and move with new alignment. A new gait pattern will be developed based upon a significant amount of practice, verbal cueing and physical prompting. Body support devices that allow partial weightbearing such as the Lite-Gait can be of assistance for children who do well with temporary unloading of body weight during the re-learning stage (Fig. 5.9.4). This can be used on a gym floor surface or over a treadmill (Dodd and Foley 2007). The child's weight can gradually be increased until s/he is assuming full weight and is comfortable with a new gait pattern. Children in levels IV–V can often resume their program of passive standing with improved alignment and potentially less pain. Caregivers for children in these groups should be reminded that bone density may have been reduced and that fractures are possible. Transfer training is reviewed, with special attention to the risk of distal femur fractures.

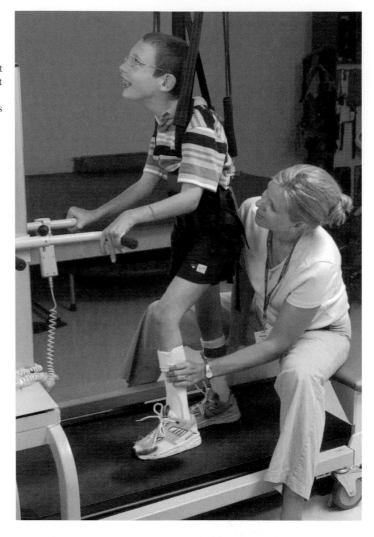

Fig. 5.9.4 The use of the Lite-Gait (for partial support weightbearing) and the treadmill can assist in the re-establishment of a gait pattern in children who have less selective motor control and greater fears of falling.

Muscle strength is reduced after muscle lengthening, although this has not been well studied (Seniorou et al. 2007). Those authors found that strength was significantly decreased in all lower-extremity muscle groups at 6 months postoperatively as was motor function measured using the GMFM. Harvey et al. (2007) demonstrated that children showed significant deterioration in their mobility on the FMS at all three levels (5, 50 and 500 meters) at 3 and 6 months postoperatively. For these reasons strengthening and functional activities are added to the therapy program 3 weeks after surgery. Strengthening may be in the form of progressive resistive exercise with free weights or a weight machine, especially in children in GMFCS levels I–III. Children who do not have the ability to isolate specific muscle groups and joint motions, typically GMFCS levels IV and V, can use their body weight and functional mobility activities to strengthen.

At 6 weeks bone and muscle healing have advanced sufficiently to remove casts and lift restrictions on therapeutic activities. At this point, an outpatient therapy plan may consist of three times per week, with a home exercise program of stretching, strengthening and functional activities to increase endurance (Fig. 5.9.5). If an inpatient admission has been suggested, this may be the optimal time, with a 2- to 4-week time-frame considered. Children and their caregivers should be actively involved in setting goals during this active period of rehabilitation. The Canadian Occupational Performance Measure (COPM) or the Goal Attainment Scaling (GAS) can be helpful in measuring progress towards goals (Law et al. 1990, King et al. 1999). The therapists should be able to assist with clarifying realistic goals without eroding long-term hopes. The child's functional mobility can be monitored using the Functional Mobility Scale at 3-month intervals.

The child may still be prevented from standing and walking without the support of orthoses, but could begin an aquatic program, benefiting from the buoyancy of the water

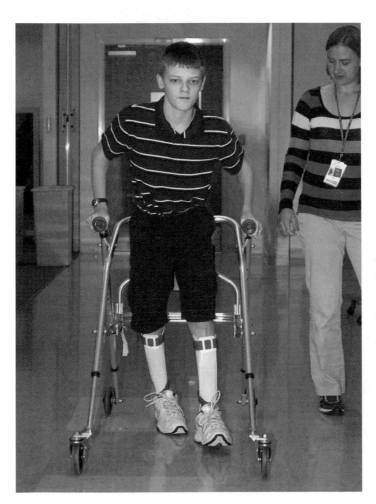

Fig. 5.9.5
Weightbearing in new orthoses typically occurs at 6 weeks, and a reverse walker is used to encourage an upright posture. Progressive ambulation may include transitioning to Lofstrand/forearm crutches or go directly to walking without assistance depending upon the patient's strength, balance and fear of falling.

and possibly an underwater treadmill to practice the new ambulation pattern (Fig. 5.9.6). Continued emphasis on walking in a variety of settings, with the addition of stair climbing, will reinforce the new pattern and build endurance. Good posture and alignment should be stressed, and the manner of reinforcement should match the child's chosen/identified style of learning. Typically, children at GMFCS levels I and II progress from the support of a reverse walker to Lofstrand crutches and then walk without an assistive device. Full range of motion at all lower-extremity joints should be encouraged, both passively and active. Pain should be minimal at this time. Strengthening must continue and can include greater resistance (Seniorou et al. 2007). Neuromuscular electrical stimulation may help some children with muscle re-education and muscle co-contraction.

For children at levels I–III, functional activities should be a focus of physical therapy at this time, with attention to transitions such as the activities in dimensions C (crawling and kneeling) and D (standing) of the GMFM. Children at levels IV and V also will benefit from being moved through functional activities, even if they are fully dependent. If they are able to direct their care they can work with their therapist to guide their movement or initiate activities. Once these children are comfortable resuming their sitting and standing programs, they may not require any additional therapy, but will continue to benefit from a home program of stretching and possibly the use of nighttime splinting to maintain muscle length.

The frequency and duration of an outpatient therapy program will depend upon many factors, most significant of which is the child's return to his/her preoperative function. Since Harvey et al. (2007) demonstrated that baseline functional level does not return to baseline

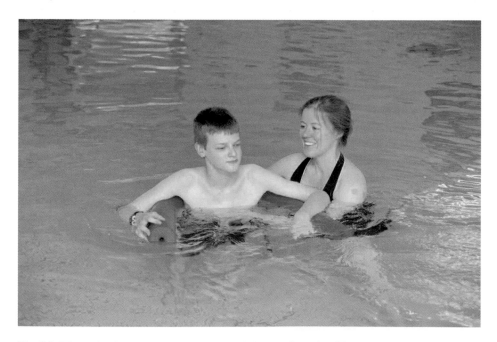

Fig. 5.9.6 Strengthening and progression in ambulation can be assisted in an aquatic environment, with attention to foot placement and full hip and knee extension.

until 6 months and exceed baseline until 9–12 months after surgery an active physical therapy program should be in place for at least the first 6 months. The program should be modified and tailored to the circumstances of each child, pursuing the preoperative goals whenever practical. Long-term therapy is an area requiring more careful study. The full benefit of a major surgical intervention may not be reached for up to 2 years after the procedure.

REFERENCES

Barwood S, Baillieu C, Boyd R, Brereton K, Low J, Nattrass G, Graham HK (2000) Analgesic effects of botulinum toxin A: a randomized, placebo-controlled clinical trial. *Dev Med Child Neurol* **42**: 116–21.

Damiano DL (2006) Activity, activity, activity: rethinking our physical therapy approach to cerebral palsy. *Phys Ther* **86**: 1534–40.

Dodd KJ, Foley S (2007) Partial body-weight-supported treadmill training can improve walking in children with cerebral palsy: a clinical controlled trial. *Dev Med Child Neurol* **49**: 101–5.

Graham HK, Harvey A, Rodda J, Nattrass GR, Pirpiris M (2004) The Functional Mobility Scale (FMS). *J Pediatr Orthop* **24**: 514–20.

Harvey A, Graham HK, Morris ME, Baker R, Wolfe R (2007) The Functional Mobility Scale: ability to detect change following single event multilevel surgery. *Dev Med Child Neurol* **49**: 603–7.

King G, McDougall J, Palisano R, Gritzan J, Tucker MA (1999) Goal attainment scaling: its use in evaluating pediatric therapy programs. *Phys Occup Ther Pediatr* **19**: 31–52.

King G, Law M, King S, Hurley P, Hanna S, Kertoy M, Rosenbaum P, Young N (2004) *Children's Assessment of Participation and Enjoyment (CAPE) and Preferences for Activities of Children (PAC).* San Antonio, TX: Harcourt Assessment.

Law M, Baptiste S, McColl M, Opzoomer A, Pollock N, Polatajko H (1990) The Canadian Occupational Performance Measure: an outcome measurement protocol for occupational therapy. *Can J Occup Ther* **57**: 82–7.

Palisano R, Rosenbaum P, Walter S, Russell D, Wood E, Galuppi B (1997) Development and reliability of a system to classify gross motor function in children with cerebral palsy. *Dev Med Child Neurol* **39**: 214–23.

Russell DJ, Rosenbaum PL, Cadman DT, Gowland C, Hardy S, Jarvis S (1989) The gross motor function measure: a means to evaluate the effects of physical therapy. *Dev Med Child Neurol* **31**: 341–52.

Seniorou M, Thompson N, Harrington M, Theologis T (2007) Recovery of muscle strength multi-level orthopaedic surgery in diplegic cerebral palsy. *Gait Posture* **26**: 475–81.

Taylor NF, Dodd KJ, Graham HK (2004) Test–retest reliability of hand-held dynamometric strength testing in young people with cerebral palsy. *Arch Phys Med Rehabil* **85**: 77–80.

van der Linden ML, Aitchison AM, Hazlewood ME, Hillman SJ, Robb JE (2004) Test–retest repeatability of gluteus maximus strength testing using a fixed digital dynamometer in children with cerebral palsy. *Arch Phys Med Rehabil* **85**: 2058–63.

Young NL, Williams JI, Yoshida KK, Wright JG (2000) Measurement properties of the Activities Scale for Kids. *J Clin Epidemiol* **53**: 125–37.

5.10
GENERAL ISSUES OF RECURRENCE WITH GROWTH

James R. Gage

Key points
- Adolescence is a time of rapid changes that include growth acceleration, hormonal changes, problems relating to socialization, and psychological issues
- Many of the issues relating to recurrent deformity can be avoided or minimized if the patient and his/her family have been forewarned. Problems that occur in adolescence require vigilance on the part of all concerned, as they may significantly alter the final outcome
- If surgery is required in an adolescent child or young adult, accommodations have to be made to allow him/her maximum mobility and independence during the period of recovery.

Figure 5.10.1 demonstrates the treatment timeline of a typical patient with spastic diplegia, GMFCS I or II at our institution. From birth until early childhood, management usually is non-operative with emphasis on therapy to maximize function, maintenance of range-of-motion, and strengthening. Appropriate daytime orthoses are used to maximize function and nighttime orthoses are useful to minimize growth deformity. If spasticity is a problem in mid-childhood (ages ≈ 5–8 years), surgical spasticity reduction is often carried out by means of selective dorsal rhizotomy or, in the case of mixed tone, an intrathecal baclofen pump. Residual orthopaedic deformities such as lever-arm dysfunction (e.g. foot deformities and long-bone torsions) and/or fixed muscle contractures are generally corrected a year or two following spasticity reduction. Ideally, this should complete the child's surgical treatment prior to the onset of puberty.

Recall that bones grow plastically and that the forces acting upon them guide their growth. If the forces on a growing bone are appropriate, its final shape will be correct. If the forces are abnormal, however, those abnormal forces will affect the final shape of the bone. The degree of the bone deformity present at maturity will be proportional to three factors: (1) the magnitude of the deforming forces, (2) the duration of time those forces are acting, and (3) the rate of growth.

Although the described interventions may have lessened the total disability significantly, the primary problems produced by the neurological injury (impairments in selective motor control, balance difficulties and abnormal tone) are still present. As such, the child's gait may be improved but it is still not normal. Because of this, if recurrence of deformity is to

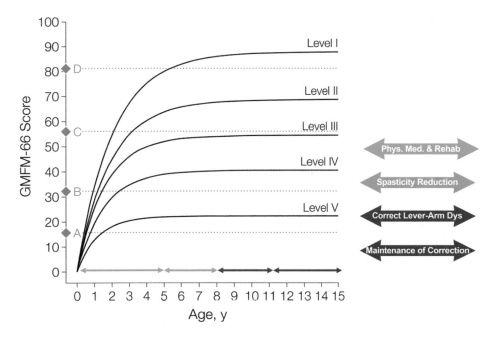

Fig. 5.10.1 The usual treatment timeline at our institution. In general, early treatment (up to age 5) is with physical therapy and bracing; spasticity reduction (if indicated) is generally done between the ages of 5 and 8 years; and correction of lever-arm dysfunction is done between age 8 and the onset of puberty. From that point on we attempt to maintain correction until the child has reached maturity.

be prevented, ongoing maintenance of correction will be required until maturity. Recurrence of deformity in cerebral palsy during childhood might be likened to rolling a bowling ball down an endless alley. Although the ball may start in the center, with enough time and distance traveled it will invariably drift into one or the other of the two gutters. Similarly, because muscle imbalance and abnormal motor control persist, a valgus foot that has been corrected may eventually drift back into valgus, or might even go into varus, if it is not adequately supported. Consequently, appropriate orthotic support and maintenance therapy in conjunction with a good home program of strengthening and stretching is necessary in all of these children until growth is complete.

What happens at adolescence?

The onset of adolescence is problematic for many reasons, but with respect to growth deformity two issues come to the fore: (1) the growth rate accelerates, and (2) body mass starts to increase rapidly, which in turn increases the magnitude of the ground reaction and torsional forces acting on the bone. Furthermore, since strength increases proportionally to cross-sectional area of the muscle (πr^2) and mass increases in proportion to volume (r^3), with the onset of the adolescent growth spurt the strength-to-mass ratio starts to fall dramatically. We refer to this phenomenon as 'the law of magnitude' (J.M. Cary, personal communication). Consequently, when a child with a high-energy cost of ambulation enters

547

adolescence, s/he may be further hindered by increased fatigue and limitations in ambulation (Fig. 5.10.2).

Because of the increase in body mass, latent muscle weakness also may become apparent. For example, many young children with spastic diplegia undergo heel-cord lengthening, but Delp et al. (1995) showed that a 1 cm tendo-Achilles lengthening will diminish soleus strength by 50%. The soleus is the driving force of the plantarflexion/knee-extension couple, which contributes half of the total extension torque required for erect posture. Consequently, the underlying weakness of the soleus coupled with the dramatic increase in body mass, which begins with puberty, may well contribute to a crouch gait. Furthermore, minor deformities of bone, which were largely static prior to puberty, are often amplified by rapid growth such that these deformities now also contribute to symptomatic gait deviations.

Balance invariably is compromised to some degree in children with cerebral palsy as well (Burtner et al. 1998, 1999, Wolff et al. 1998, Rose et al. 2002, Horstmann and Bleck 2007). As the child grows the body mass increases and the center of that mass gets further from the floor. Consequently with the onset of adolescence, children who were marginal walkers at a GMFCS II level, may move down to a GMFCS III level and begin using balance aids such as Loftstrand crutches or a walker.

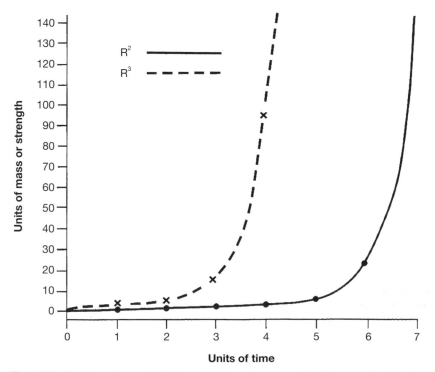

Fig. 5.10.2 The 'law of magnitude'. A graph of muscle power, which is proportional to its cross-sectional area (πr^2), is plotted versus mass which is cubic (r^3). It is apparent that with time and growth, mass will increase at a much faster rate than strength.

Any older parent who has seen his/her children through the teenage years, however, will tell you that adolescence brings a host of other issues with it. As adolescents enter puberty and start to pull away from their parents, peer pressure becomes much more significant. During the teenage years, behavior is often more dependent on acceptance by their peers than approval of their parents. Hormonal changes associated with puberty bring on some degree of behavioral change in all teens, but children who have a poor self-image because of their disability may be particularly vulnerable. If a child's physical disability prevents her/him from keeping up with peers, s/he may choose to fill her/his leisure hours with more sedentary activities in which they can compete, such as computer games. However, since muscle stretch is the impetus to muscle growth, failure to participate in activities which adequately stretch growing muscles during the adolescent growth spurt is a recipe for weakness and muscle contracture (Ziv et al. 1984). Unfortunately, in my personal experience, children in their teenage years often are much less compliant with exercise and strengthening programs. Couple that with the onset of rapid growth and the accumulation of body mass and it is easy to see why lever-arm dysfunction and muscle contractures often worsen rapidly during adolescence. Before puberty begins, therefore, it is important to forewarn both the parents and the child of the possible problems that may lie just beyond the horizon, and stress the importance of activity and exercise. If those issues are not addressed, recurrence of growth deformities is the likely outcome. Gillette Children's Specialty Healthcare has initiated a bicycle program for children with disability in which voluntary contributions from employees and friends of the hospital are used to assist parents in purchasing appropriate mobility devices for their children. Since many of these youngsters are unable to balance a standard bicycle, commercial recumbent tricycles have proved to be ideal in allowing many of these children to ride in the community with their non-disabled friends (Fig. 5.10.3).

The psychosocial changes that occur in adolescence can also be a source of problems. In an extensive review of the literature on health and well-being of adults with cerebral palsy, Liptak (2008) pointed out that as children with cerebral palsy transition into adulthood, they have a high prevalence of comorbid and secondary conditions like pain. He also pointed out that as children move into adulthood they have regression in several areas of functioning, which include mobility. The review also indicated that when individuals with cerebral palsy reach adulthood, they are less likely to be employed, marry, live independently, and/or participate in other areas of social interaction than the population at large. A Norwegian study based on a questionnaire indicated that adults with cerebral palsy reported significantly more physical fatigue than the general population (Jahnsen et al. 2003). The strongest predictors associated with fatigue were pain, deterioration of functional skills, and low life-satisfaction. They state that fatigue and factors related to fatigue should be addressed specifically in follow-up programs for persons with cerebral palsy. Schenker et al. (2005) also demonstrated that participation and activity performance increase as motor disability and/or additional neurological impairments decrease.

One might expect that the psychosocial problems would be related to the extent of the individual's disability, but Pirpiris et al. (2006) pointed out that in children with mild cerebral palsy the psychosocial effect on their well-being was greater than would be predicted by

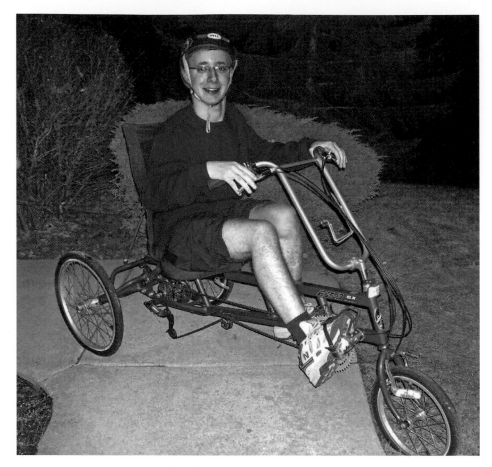

Fig. 5.10.3 For a child or adolescent with balance impairments, recumbent tricycles, such as the one pictured here, provide an excellent means to participate fully with friends. They are stable, have multiple gears, and can be ridden nearly as fast as a bicycle.

their functional disability. They indicated that functional measures were good at predicting the functional well-being but were weak at predicting the psychosocial arm of well-being.

Response to treatments/intervention
It would seem logical that the combination of reducing spasticity and fully correcting pre-existent orthopaedic deformity (lever-arm dysfunction and muscle contractures) prior to puberty would act to minimize the rate of recurrence of problems in adolescence. In my personal experience, I believe this to be true. Wren et al. (2005) have confirmed that growth deformity increases with time. Furthermore, many articles have been published, which indicate that rhizotomy and/or orthopaedic surgeries have long-term benefits on outcome (Õunpuu et al. 2002, O'Brien et al. 2004, Rodda et al. 2006, Harvey et al. 2007, Langerak et al. 2008). However, O'Brien et al. (2005) were the only authors to deal specifically with

rate of recurrence of deformity following spasticity reduction. Their study indicated that orthopaedic procedures were more likely to be needed in children who were destined to be non-ambulators, and that children who had rhizotomy done at a younger age needed fewer orthopaedic procedures than those who had the rhizotomy when they were older. They also found that children who walked independently at the time of selective dorsal rhizotomy (SDR) underwent fewer orthopaedic procedures than did children who required assistance ambulating, but this finding might be explained on the basis of their GMFCS level alone.

For years, therapists were advised not to attempt to strengthen spastic muscles for fear of worsening the spasticity. However, this has been proven to be fallacious and the benefit of strengthening programs in individuals with cerebral palsy has now been well proven (Dodd et al. 2002, Shinohara et al. 2002, Williams and Pountney 2007, Verschuren et al. 2008). It also is important for both the parents and the child to be aware of the excessive burden that excessive weight gain places on an individual with cerebral palsy. The decline in the strength to mass ratio with growth was discussed earlier in this chapter. If one recalls that kinetic energy is equal to one-half mass times velocity-squared (KE = $\frac{1}{2}$ MV^2), it will be apparent that excessive body mass will increase the magnitude of the disability exponentially. Hurvitz et al. (2008) pointed out that about 29% of children with cerebral palsy are overweight, although it is interesting to note that the percentage of obesity is higher in ambulators than in non-ambulators. It should be evident, however, that the results of a sedentary lifestyle (muscle weakness, contractures, weight gain, osteopenia, etc.) all act to generate a downward spiral that will compound the individual's difficulties with ambulation.

Correction of recurrent deformity in adolescence

Ideally one would like to finish up with a child's surgical interventions prior to puberty and then maintain the result until growth is complete. Because of the issues that have been discussed, however, this is not always achievable. Consequently, when surgery to correct recurrent deformity is necessary during adolescence, several things must be kept in mind.

(1) In an adolescent, who is rapidly acquiring size and weight, recovery following surgery is slower and more difficult than in a younger child. Even in a prepubertal child, however, it has been shown that recovery to preoperative strength level may take as long as a year (Harvey et al. 2007, Seniorou et al. 2007).

(2) Because of the enormous psychosocial problems imposed by limitations of mobility and loss of ADL skills such as toileting following surgery, it is important to get the adolescent back up on his/her feet as soon as possible. If possible bilateral correction of deformity, which is routinely done in the prepubertal child, should be avoided in the adolescent and young adult. Leaving one limb for weightbearing and transfer activities allows the individual maximal activity and independence. In my personal experience this approach makes for a much faster and easier recovery.

(3) Mobility must be maximized to minimize stiffness and loss of strength. Casting should be minimized, or if possible, avoided altogether. Short leg casts are acceptable if they are required to stabilize the foot or tibia for transfers, but long leg casts should be avoided so that the therapist can begin range-of-motion and strengthening as soon as possible post-

surgery. Modern methods of internal fixation are adequate to maintain position if procedures such as a femoral osteotomy and/or a tibial tubercle advancement have been done. Following surgery a soft-sided knee-immobilizer is usually adequate to keep the patient comfortable between sessions of therapy.

(4) Weightbearing on the operated limb should be resumed as soon as possible. At 3 weeks post-surgery, the postoperative short leg cast is replaced with snugly molded short leg walking cast and weightbearing is begun. With good internal fixation of the femoral osteotomy, this is possible without loss of correction (Fig. 5.10.4). To allow range-of-motion exercises to begin, casts should be removed and, if necessary, replaced by removable immobilization devices such as a CAM walker as soon as possible

Fig. 5.10.4 Anteroposterior radiograph of the pelvis of a child who has undergone bilateral intertrochanteric osteotomies with AO plate fixation prior to surgery (top) and 5 weeks later (below). These internal fixation devices are sufficient to maintain position of the osteotomies without resorting to a spica cast and will allow weightbearing as early as 3 weeks post-surgery. At our institution we generally discharge these children about 5 days post-surgery in bilateral, short-leg casts tied together with a Denis–Browne bar. Passive range-of-motion of the hips and knees is usually started 2–3 days post-surgery. Notice that if the osteotomy is made proximal to the trochanter with solid internal fixation, the osteotomy heals with very little external callus.

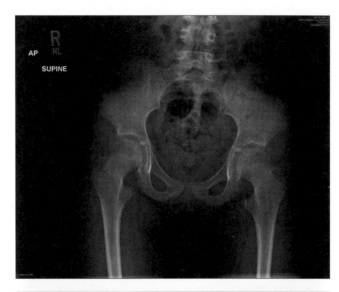

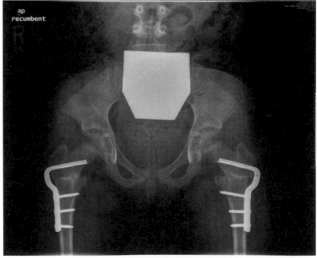

In summary, it is best to finish the treatment program prior to adolescence and, if possible, avoid corrective surgery during the adolescent growth spurt. Nevertheless, functional problems relating to growth, such as muscle contractures and/or bone deformity, will be amplified by the adolescent growth spurt. Once recognized, therefore, they should be addressed promptly before they impose significant functional loss on a growing child.

REFERENCES

Burtner PA, Qualls C, Woollacott MH (1998) Muscle activation characteristics of stance balance control in children with spastic cerebral palsy. *Gait Posture* **8**: 163–74.

Burtner PA, Woollacott MH, Qualls C (1999) Stance balance control with orthoses in a group of children with spastic cerebral palsy. *Dev Med Child Neurol* **41**: 748–57.

Delp SL, Statler K, Carroll NC (1995) Preserving plantar flexion strength after surgical treatment for contracture of the triceps surae: a computer simulation study. *J Orthop Res* **13**: 96–104.

Dodd KJ, Taylor NF, Damiano DL (2002) A systematic review of the effectiveness of strength-training programs for people with cerebral palsy. *Arch Phys Med Rehabil* **83**: 1157–64.

Harvey A, Graham HK, Morris ME, Baker R, Wolfe R (2007) The Functional Mobility Scale: ability to detect change following single event multilevel surgery. *Dev Med Child Neurol* **49**: 603–7.

Horstmann HM, Bleck EE (2007) *Orthopaedic Management in Cerebral Palsy*, 2nd edn. London: Mac Keith Press. p 26–7.

Hurvitz EA, Green LB, Hornyak JE, Khurana SR, Koch LG (2008) Body mass index measures in children with cerebral palsy related to Gross Motor Function Classification: a clinic-based study. *Am J Phys Med Rehabil* **87**: 395–403.

Jahnsen R, Villien L, Stanghelle JK, Holm I (2003) Fatigue in adults with cerebral palsy in Norway compared with the general population. *Dev Med Child Neurol* **45**: 296–303.

Langerak NG, Lamberts RP, Fieggen AG, Peter JC, van der Merwe L, Vaughan CL (2008) A prospective gait analysis study in patients with diplegic cerebral palsy 20 years after selective dorsal rhizotomy. *J Neurosurg Pediatr* **1**: 180–6.

Liptak GS (2008) Health and well being of adults with cerebral palsy. *Curr Opin Neurol* **21**: 136–42.

O'Brien DF, Park TS, Puglisi JA, Collins DR, Leuthardt EC (2004) Effect of selective dorsal rhizotomy on need for orthopedic surgery for spastic quadriplegic cerebral palsy: long-term outcome analysis in relation to age. *J Neurosurg* **101** (1 Suppl): 59–63.

O'Brien DF, Park TS, Puglisi JA, Collins DR, Leuthardt EC (2005) Orthopedic surgery after selective dorsal rhizotomy for spastic diplegia in relation to ambulatory status and age. *J Neurosurg* **103** (1 Suppl): 5–9.

Õunpuu S, DeLuca P, Davis R, Romness M (2002) Long-term effects of femoral derotation osteotomies: an evaluation using three-dimensional gait analysis. *J Pediatr Orthop* **22**: 139–45.

Pirpiris M, Gates PE, McCarthy JJ, D'Astous J, Tylkowksi C, Sanders JO, Dorey FJ, Ostendorff S, Robles G, Caron C, Otsuka NY (2006) Function and well-being in ambulatory children with cerebral palsy. *J Pediatr Orthop* **26**: 119–24.

Rodda JM, Graham HK, Nattrass GR, Galea MP, Baker R, Wolfe R (2006) Correction of severe crouch gait in patients with spastic diplegia with use of multilevel orthopaedic surgery. *J Bone Joint Surg Am* **88**: 2653–64.

Rose J, Wolff DR, Jones VK, Bloch DA, Oehlert JW, Gamble JG (2002) Postural balance in children with cerebral palsy. *Dev Med Child Neurol* **44**: 58–63.

Schenker R, Coster WJ, Parush S (2005) Neuroimpairments, activity performance, and participation in children with cerebral palsy mainstreamed in elementary schools. *Dev Med Child Neurol* **47**: 808–14.

Seniorou M, Thompson N, Harrington M, Theologis T (2007) Recovery of muscle strength following multi-level orthopaedic surgery in diplegic cerebral palsy. *Gait Posture* **26**: 475–81.

Shinohara TA, Suzuki N, Oba M, Kawasumi M, Kimizuka M, Mita K (2002) Effect of exercise at the AT point for children with cerebral palsy. *Bull Hosp Joint Dis* **61**: 63–7.

Verschuren OBSPT, Ketelaar M, Takken T, Helders PJMPCS, Gorter JW (2008) Exercise programs for children with cerebral palsy: a systematic review of the literature. *Am J Phys Med Rehabil* **87**: 404–17.

Williams H, Pountney T (2007) Effects of a static bicycling programme on the functional ability of young people with cerebral palsy who are non-ambulant. *Dev Med Child Neurol* **49**: 522–7.

Wolff DR, Rose J, Jones VK, Bloch DA, Oehlert JW, Gamble JG (1998) Postural balance measurements for children and adolescents. *J Orthop Res* **16**: 271–5.

Wren TAL, Rethlefsen S Kay RM (2005) Prevalence of specific gait abnormalities in children with cerebral palsy: influence of cerebral palsy subtype, age, and previous surgery. *J Pediat Orthop* **25**: 79–83.

Ziv I, Blackburn N, Rang M, Koreska J (1984) Muscle growth in normal and spastic mice. *Dev Med Child Neurol* **26**: 94–9.

5.11
TREATMENT OF CROUCH GAIT

Jean L. Stout, Tom F. Novacheck, James R. Gage and Michael H. Schwartz

Key points
- Crouch gait is one of the most serious and worrisome 'families' of gait patterns in cerebral palsy
- Crouch gait tends to be progressive, and if left untreated, often limits independence
- Crouch gait can be iatrogenic in nature
- Appropriate treatment of mild to moderate crouch gait involves a combination of the treatment principles outlined earlier (torsion, contracture, spasticity, etc.)
- Chronic/severe crouch gait can be effectively treated with procedures which address the quadriceps insufficiency (patellar tendon advancement) and joint contracture (distal femoral extension osteotomy).

Review of relevant pathophysiology
Crouch gait is a term that is often used generically to describe a gait pattern characterized by increased knee-flexion during the stance phase of the gait cycle, and is one of the most prevalent gait pathologies in children and adolescents with cerebral palsy (Wren et al. 2005). Without intervention, the pattern typically worsens with time and often leads to pain, gait deterioration, and decreasing (or loss) of walking ability (Rosenthal and Levine 1977, Sutherland and Cooper 1978, Lloyd-Roberts et al. 1985, Murphy et al. 1995, Bell et al. 2002). Intervention strategies are complex, because although the primary description of crouch gait is in the sagittal plane, lever-arm dysfunction in the transverse or coronal planes and issues of weakness are commonly present (Gage 2004). To best understand the complexities of treatment it is important to understand what is known about the mechanisms and risk factors that may contribute to development of the pattern.

Crouch gait should be thought as a continuum of deformity from mild to severe. The definition of what is considered 'crouch gait' varies in the literature, but most include a criterion at initial contact of $\geq 20°$ (Rozumalski and Schwartz 2008), a criterion at initial contact and mid-stance (Sutherland and Davids 1993, Arnold et al. 2006, Hicks et al. 2008), or a description that includes dorsiflexion at the ankle (Rodda et al. 2004). From a clinical perspective, a continuous knee-extensor moment is typical and sometimes is included in the definition (Gage 2004), as is a component of quadriceps insufficiency. The continuum of crouch likely encompasses all these definitions (see Videos 3.6.8–10 in the Patient Assessment section on the Interactive Disc). For the purposes of this chapter, the primary crouch gait pattern discussed is at the severe end of the spectrum: category 5 of Rozumalski and Schwartz's (2008) classification, and what Rodda et al. (2004) termed 'severe crouch'.

555

Regardless of definition, the key is to discover and treat the underlying mechanisms in order to restore erect posture, reduce pain, and maintain walking ability at any point in the continuum.

As discussed in Chapter 2.4, the biarticular muscles are involved primarily and more severely than are the monoarticular muscles in cerebral palsy. Biarticular muscles (e.g. psoas, hamstrings, rectus femoris, and gastrocnemius) have more spasticity and become relatively short, while the monoarticular muscles (e.g. iliacus, gluteus maximus, vasti, and soleus) are excessively elongated and weak. This principle has implications for the ultimate pathology in severe crouch gait in cerebral palsy.

One of the fundamental mechanisms of an erect posture during gait is the ability of numerous muscles to extend the knee and the hip through action at adjacent or distant joints (Kimmel and Schwartz 2006, Hicks et al. 2008). An example of this mechanism is the dynamic coupling between hip extension and knee extension, which works via the gluteus maximus. Clinicians are most aware of the plantarflexion/knee-extension (PF/KE) couple. Previously described in the section on typical gait, the hallmark of the PF/KE couple is the eccentric action of the plantar flexors (principally the soleus) during the first part of midstance which controls the progression of the ground reaction force (GRF) over the stationary foot (see Chapter 1.3). That is, it resists the external flexion moment produced by the GRF, which at this point in the gait cycle is behind the knee, by creating an acceleration in the opposite direction which works to extend the knee. The eccentric action of the soleus continues until the GRF is in front of the knee and the external moment becomes a knee-extensor moment (see Fig. 1.3.4). Any factor that reduces the effectiveness of the PF/KE couple will contribute to knee-flexion during the midstance phase of the gait cycle, and potentially lead to a crouch gait. For the child with cerebral palsy this may include hamstring tightness (Sutherland and Cooper 1978, Hoffinger et al. 1993), weakness and impaired balance (DeLuca et al. 1998, Gage 2004), and lever-arm dysfunction (Schwartz and Lakin 2003, Gage and Schwartz 2004, Hicks et al. 2007).

If the GRF remains behind the knee, it generates a strong external flexion moment that must be resisted by the quadriceps. Furthermore, since the GRF now passes in front of the hip, it also generates an external hip-flexor moment which must be resisted by the hip-extensors. The secondary effects of these moments can include increased patellofemoral pressures with resultant knee pain, and increased energy requirements (Fig. 5.11.1).

RISK FACTORS
The primary risk factors for crouch gait which will be discussed include (1) plantarflexor weakness, (2) lever-arm dysfunction including foot deformity, (3) knee-flexion contracture, and (4) hamstring contracture.

Of all the risk factors, soleus weakness has perhaps the greatest impact. Its contribution to support in normal walking has been corroborated both by forward dynamic simulation and induced acceleration techniques (Anderson and Pandy 2001, Kimmel and Schwartz 2006). An informal review of a large number of patients from our center indicated that the absolute risk of being in crouch gait was nearly 50% if plantarflexor strength was less than antigravity. Many factors can contribute to plantarflexor weakness including (1) lower

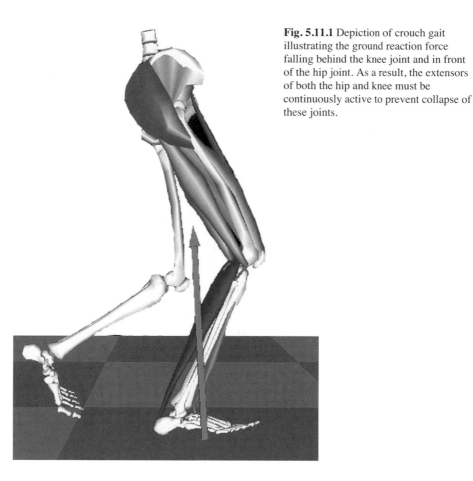

Fig. 5.11.1 Depiction of crouch gait illustrating the ground reaction force falling behind the knee joint and in front of the hip joint. As a result, the extensors of both the hip and knee must be continuously active to prevent collapse of these joints.

motor neuron loss, for example children with myelomeningocele; (2) inability to selectively activate the muscle; (3) the loss of a muscle's ability to generate force secondary to brain damage that occurs in children with cerebral palsy (CP). Unfortunately, however, loss of plantarflexor strength can also be iatrogenic in children with CP secondary to heel cord lengthening surgery (Borton et al. 2001, Gage 2004, Wren et al. 2005, Dietz et al. 2006). Adolescents in crouch have a greater likelihood to have had heelcord lengthening than those not in crouch (Morias Filho et al. 2008a). In a recent study of adolescents and young adults in persistent crouch gait, over 87% of the subjects who had undergone previous surgery had heel cord lengthening (Stout et al. 2008).

Lever-arm dysfunction, particularly external tibial torsion, has been identified as another primary risk factor for crouch gait (Schwartz and Lakin 2003, Hicks et al. 2007). Loss of typical bony alignment reduces knee extension acceleration during single-limb stance. That is, it diminishes the internal moment that restrains the forward motion of the tibia. Tibial torsion reduces the capacity of the soleus to extend the hip and knee by more than 50%, but does not change the moment arm of the muscle (Hicks et al. 2007) (see Chapter 3.6 for more detail). Other types of lever-arm dysfunction such as pes valgus foot deformity may also influence crouch gait, but have not been studied as rigorously. Observations at our center suggest that femoral anteversion does not increase the risk of crouch.

The presence of true knee-flexion contractures increases the absolute risk of crouch gait. Children with knee-flexion contractures (defined as ≥10° lack of extension) have an extremely high risk of walking in crouch gait.

What is less clear is the role of hamstring contracture and its influence on crouch gait. A growing body of evidence suggests that there may be an overestimation by the clinical community of the hamstring contracture–crouch gait relationship. Historically, hamstring tightness or contracture (short muscle length), hamstring spasticity (resistance of the hamstring to stretch, i.e. slow muscle velocity), or prolonged stance phase hamstring activity have been considered primary causes of crouch gait. Clinical examination of the knee by measurement of the conventional popliteal angle has not been found to be a reliable way of assessing or predicting the severity or degree of crouch gait (Thompson et al. 2001, Louis et al. 2008). Assessment of the dynamic length of the hamstring muscles by use of musculoskeletal models has demonstrated that not all individuals who walk in crouch walk with hamstrings that are shorter or slower than normal (Hoffinger et al. 1993, Delp et al. 1996, Arnold et al. 2006). In a study of 152 subjects walking in crouch, Arnold et al. (2006) reported that 34% of the subjects walked with hamstrings of typical length and velocity. Their action and ability to extend the hip is critical, but this capacity is diminished as crouch increases (Hicks et al. 2008).

What remains most unclear relative to the pathophysiology of crouch gait is the role of balance, proprioception, neurologic motor control and weakness. While there has been some work related to postural sway mechanisms in children with cerebral palsy (Nashner et al. 1983, Woollacott and Shumway-Cook 2005, Burtner et al. 2007, Chen and Woollacott 2007), only one study has investigated walking in a crouch posture (Burtner 1996). Because children with CP have difficulties with balance, they often walk with a foot flat gait and/or increased knee flexion to gain stability. However, because this posture greatly reduces the magnitude of the extension moment generated by the plantarflexion/knee-extension couple, with time and growth this walking pattern in itself may lead to a progressive crouch gait.

PROGRESSIVE CROUCH GAIT
The progressive nature of crouch was first described by Sutherland and Cooper (1978). Whatever the precipitating mechanisms for a crouched walking pattern, a cascade of events leads to progressive crouch. Once in a crouch pattern, the external flexion moment produced by the GRF at the knee must be resisted by the quadriceps (including the rectus femoris), and the external flexion moment at the hip must be resisted by the hip-extensors (including the hamstrings). Greater demand is placed on the muscles to resist the moments. If activity of the biarticular hamstrings and rectus femoris results in an increase in knee and or hip flexion, the ground reaction force will move even further anterior to the hip and posterior to the knee, thereby increasing the external lever arm and magnitude of the flexion moments at each joint. The result is a cycle in which the hip- and knee-flexion moments progressively increase and the extension moments become more inadequate. The progres-

sive nature of crouch is an example of positional lever-arm dysfunction as described by Gage and Schwartz (2004).

Once thought to create a situation where the hamstrings become more powerful knee flexors, recent evidence suggests that it is the loss of the gluteals', hamstrings' and the quadriceps' ability to extend the hip and knee that contributes to the cascade (Hicks et al. 2008, Stewart et al. 2008). The extension capacities of muscles working to extend the knee or the hip in severe crouch gait were all less than 50% of normal. This includes the extension capacity of the rectus femoris which was completely lost. Hicks and colleagues (2008) also demonstrated a progressive reduction in the extension capacities of the muscles with more severe crouch.

The implications for the progressive nature of crouch are far-reaching. Energy-requirements increase due to the extra demand placed on the quadriceps to stabilize the flexed knee joint in addition to spasticity. Knee pain is related to increased patellofemoral compressive forces, and/or eventual distal patellar pole or tibial tubercle stress fracture (Perry et al. 1975, Rosenthal and Levine 1977, Lloyd-Roberts et al. 1985). If stress fractures of the distal pole of the patella or tibial tubercle develop, quadriceps insufficiency, level of crouch, and knee pain can all increase. Loss of the extensor moment arm at the hip places an increased demand on the hamstrings to stabilize the hip joint. Hamstring overactivity may lead to muscle contracture and/or development of knee-flexion contractures.

Previously, little attention has been directed to the contributing influence of patella alta and quadriceps insufficiency (extensor lag) to the progressive and persistent nature of crouch gait (Chandler 1933, Lotman 1976, Lloyd-Roberts et al. 1985). Elongation of the patellar tendon results in the inability of the quadriceps to function appropriately in the last few degrees of knee extension.

Historical perspectives

Before the age of computers, muscle models, and gait analysis, treatment of crouch gait in cerebral palsy was confined to physical therapy, bracing, and soft-tissue surgery. Because of the high rate of infection, delayed healing, and limited internal fixation, bony surgery was reserved for the most extreme cases. Tone management was not available, so repeated tendon lengthenings with growth were common. Surgery in general included muscle-tendon lengthening including the tendo-Achilles, but traditional treatment specific to crouch gait focused on hamstring lengthening. Crouch gait treatment typically had two levels – the first stage included soft tissue tenotomy or lengthening or transfer of the hamstrings to the distal femur (Eggers 1950). A second level of treatment for long-standing knee-flexion deformities included hamstring lengthening and advancement of the patellar tendon. The complication of genu recurvatum from excessive hamstring lengthening was recognized. The first description of the patellar tendon transfer technique was by Chandler (1933). The need for a proximal rectus release was also advised, but never specifically reported (Cleveland and Bosworth 1936, Chandler 1940, Roberts and Adams 1953, Baker 1956, Keats and Kambin 1962). After this time little mention of patella alta or quadriceps insufficiency is noted until relatively recently (Lotman 1976, Beals 2001). We started to treat patella alta and quadriceps insufficiency surgically in 1995.

Indications from patient assessment

The complexity of crouch gait demands attention to numerous factors in order to understand it and to develop an appropriate treatment plan. Specific indications will be provided where possible; otherwise, general considerations will also be listed.

HISTORY

The history should consist of the following.

(1) Patient's current age and when the crouch gait began.
(2) A complete chronology of previous physical therapy, focal spasticity, neurosurgical, and orthopaedic treatment.
(3) The rate of progression of crouch in the previous 2 years.
(4) Endurance changes in walking over the previous 2 years; changes in ability to keep up with peers.
(5) History, location, intensity, duration and frequency of knee joint or patellofemoral pain – specific emphasis on anterior knee pain. Are there exacerbating factors for pain such as prolonged walking or standing, stair climbing, walking on uneven terrain? Other joint pain?
(6) Increased dependence on assistive devices.
(7) Loss or changes in function.

PHYSICAL EXAMINATION

Physical examination methods are described in Chapter 3.1. The importance of a finding is found in parentheses following the statement. For indications and management of specific soft-tissue or bony issues, please see Chapters 5.5 and 5.6 respectively.

(1) Presence or absence of knee-flexion contracture (management may include stretching casts, night splints, guided growth vs extension osteotomy of the distal femur).
(2) Presence of musculotendinous/contracture (see Chapter 5.5).
(3) Plantarflexor, gluteal, hamstring, quadriceps, abdominal, and abductor strength and selective motor control (strength relative to antigravity provides information about contributing factors to crouch, potential benefit of strengthening program, or ability to strengthen after surgery).
(4) Presence or absence of hip-flexor, rectus femoris, adductor, hamstring and gastro-cnemius spasticity (may require focal or global spasticity management).
(5) Presence of patella alta and knee-extensor lag (indicates quadriceps insufficiency, which may require compensation with floor reaction and ankle–foot orthosis or correction with patellar advancement).
(6) Point tenderness at the distal pole of the patella or tibial tubercle (requires radiograph to confirm or rule out stress injuries).
(7) Lever-arm malalignment including excessive femoral anteversion, tibial torsion, and foot deformity (see Chapters 5.6 and 5.8).

(8) Standing posture and balance: can they stand more erect? (Provides insight into whether postural mechanisms motor control are adequate to allow upright standing/walking following treatment.)

IMAGING STUDIES

Imaging studies identify lever-arm dysfunction, patella alta, distal pole patellar fracture, or tibial tubercle stress.

(1) Anteroposterior (AP) pelvis radiograph to rule out hip subluxation and/or severe anterior pelvic tilt.
(2) Standing AP and lateral radiographs of both feet to assess their ability to function as effective levers.
(3) Supine lateral knee(s) radiography in maximum extension to evaluate the magnitude of the knee-flexion contracture, measure patella alta, and stress fracture of the patella/tibial tubercle.

OBSERVATIONAL GAIT ANALYSIS

If crouch gait is defined as a persistent knee-flexed gait, it can take many forms. Ankle position can vary from true equinus in jump gait to apparent equinus gait to excessive ankle dorsiflexion in more severe crouch gait. The magnitude of knee flexion may vary depending on severity. The transverse plane may or may not include rotational deviation at the femurs, tibia, or feet. In the coronal plane one may observe a lateral trunk sway during loading response. Apparent adduction is commonly produced if crouch occurs with internal thigh rotation from femoral anteversion. The adductors themselves may or may not be tight.

QUANTITATIVE GAIT ANALYSIS

As stated previously, lever-arm dysfunction and soft-tissue or fixed joint contractures are common findings in individuals with crouch gait. For discussion of findings in individuals with lever-arm dysfunction (particularly femoral anteversion, tibial torsion and foot deformity) please refer to Chapters 5.6 and 5.8, and for soft-tissue or fixed joint contractures refer to Chapter 5.5.

The kinematic findings specific to crouch gait include persistent knee flexed position in midstance. Limited total knee range of motion is also common. Ankle kinematics may be variable depending on the level of crouch being evaluated. Severe crouch will include excessive dorsiflexion in midstance (excessive second rocker) which may be occurring through the ankle joint or midfoot. Kinetic data in severe crouch typically include a continuous knee-extensor moment in stance phase (Gage 2004). Decreased terminal stance hip extension is common across all levels of crouch. Hip-joint range of motion is typically not compromised, but a shift of the entire hip curve into flexion is noted. Pelvic tilt can vary from anterior to posterior depending upon the complex interactions between the hip-flexors and hip-extensors, balance, posture, and/or gait cluster identified (Rodda et al. 2004, Rozumalski and Schwartz 2008, Stout et al. 2008).

Origin to insertion muscle length and velocity data for individuals in crouch vary. Arnold et al. (2006) found that of the 152 subjects in their study, there was nearly equal

561

distribution of individuals with short and slow hamstrings (27%), slow only (30%), neither short nor slow hamstrings (34%). A limited number (9%) were found to be short only.

Goals of treatment

The ultimate goals for treatment of crouch gait include reduction or elimination of pain and restoration of walking function to the greatest extent possible. Treatment may also be initiated to interrupt a cascade of events that may lead to more severe crouch gait and loss of walking ability. It may include numerous modalities such as physical therapy, stretch casting, injectable medications such as botulinum toxin, bracing, tone management, and/or orthopaedic surgery. Any or all of these modalities may be used at any given time and may be dependent upon the severity of crouch encountered. Specific goals for each of these modalities can be found in previous chapters (4.1, 4.2, 4.4, 5.1, 5.2, 5.5–5.8). All aim to restore knee extension and erect posture.

Treatment options

Generally, treatment protocols can be divided into three categories based on the severity of crouch and to some extent, the length of time the child, adolescent or young adult has been walking in crouch. Even though the treatments themselves may vary, and regardless of crouch severity, the treatment principles are the same: (1) management of spasticity or tone, (2) correction of lever arm dysfunction, (3) restoration of length of contracted muscles, (4) restoration of length (relative shortening) of muscles or tendons that are excessively long, and (5) correction of fixed joint contractures. The specifics of each of these principles have been discussed in previous chapters, and the reader is referred the chapters on non-operative treatment, tone management, lever-arm dysfunction, and soft-tissue surgeries for information. Disorders of the knee in ambulatory cerebral palsy have often been categorized with treatment regimens outlined for a particular characteristic pattern (Sutherland and Davids 1993, Chambers 2001). The concept of single-event multilevel surgery has been embraced, and typically, comprehensive treatment programs have yielded good results (Kay et al. 2002, Gough et al. 2004, Schwartz et al. 2004, Rodda et al. 2006).

MILD CROUCH

Mild crouch is typically seen in the younger child, and may be referred to as 'jump gait', 'apparent equinus gait', or a particular cluster, but the knee is in some degree of persistent flexion (Sutherland and Davids 1993, Rodda et al. 2004, Rozumalski and Schwartz 2008). At Gillette, initial treatment would include conservative measures for management of spasticity such as the use of botulinum toxin, physical therapy, and orthoses. Eventually, this may lead to more permanent reduction of tone through selective dorsal rhizotomy or implantation of an intrathecal baclogen pump, if appropriate. The guiding principle of management of spasticity or tone is employed. If the child continues to walk in crouch post-tone management, a single-event multilevel surgery will be undertaken to address lever-arm dysfunction and residual soft-tissue tightness. Even though femoral anteversion is not a risk factor for development of crouch per se, correction of femoral anteversion restores the lever-arm for important muscles of extension such as the gluteus medius, and avoids potential development of compensatory external tibial torsion (Arnold et al. 1997).

MODERATE CROUCH

Moderate crouch is present in the peri-adolescent child who has been walking in this posture longer and hamstring contracture may have developed. In this scenario, focal spasticity management is typically less effective. A history of previous surgery is common. The treatment plan depends on the specific clinical and gait analysis findings. If lever-arm dysfunction is identified, this is corrected. Additional soft tissue procedures including appropriate muscle lengthenings may be considered. Biarticular muscles (e.g. psoas, hamstrings, rectus femoris, and gastrocnemius) have become relatively short while the monoarticular muscles (e.g. iliacus, gluteus maximus, vasti and soleus) are excessively elongated and weak. The triceps surae is made up of a monoarticular muscle (the soleus) and a pair of biarticular muscles (the medial and lateral gastrocnemii). The biarticular gastrocnemius is more severely involved than the monoarticular soleus, and in fact, this has been shown to be true (Rose et al. 1993, Delp et al. 1995). Yet tendo-Achilles lengthening (TAL), the procedure most commonly done to correct contracture of this muscle, lengthens both equally – often to the great detriment of the patient. Intramuscular psoas lengthening at the pelvic brim has been shown to be effective (Novacheck et al. 2002) while other surgeries such as tentomy of the iliopsoas tendon off the trochanter or transfer to the capsule excessively weaken hip flexion (Bleck 1971). Recession of the tendon is essentially a TAL of the hip, and so lengthens the iliacus, which is weak and not contracted, along with the psoas, which is short and needs to be elongated. The triceps surae and the iliopsoas are anatomically similar (in both cases a monoarticular and a biarticular muscle come together on a common tendon).

Gait analysis guides this treatment plan since not all individuals who walk in crouch do so because of contracted or spastic hamstrings. This was confirmed in the study by Arnold et al. (2006) where over one third of the subjects who walked in crouch gait did not have identifiable muscle-tendon length or velocity pathology. Additionally, it was noted that when hamstring surgery was performed consistent with muscle length velocity data, the majority had improved length and velocity and improved stance knee extension post-surgery. Results are less satisfactory for those who undergo hamstring surgery without first determining muscle-tendon length or velocity pathology. Muscle length data (not solely clinical indications of popliteal angle or knee-flexion contracture) determine the need for hamstring lengthenings (Thompson et al. 2001, Arnold et al. 2006, Louis et al. 2008).

SEVERE CROUCH

Severe or persistent crouch is a more challenging issue, as often the children are older, and again have had previous surgical intervention. They may or may not have fixed knee-flexion deformities and often have lever-arm dysfunction. Most have patella alta and elongation of the patellar tendon. Some present with distal pole patellar or tibial tubercle fractures and knee pain resulting in limited endurance for walking (Lloyd-Roberts et al. 1985, Stout et al. 2008). Previous surgery alone results in greater odds of developing a crouch gait pattern (Wren et al. 2005). Over-elongated triceps surae or lever arm dysfunction (external tibial torsion or pes valgus foot deformity) are frequent findings (Gage 2004, Morais Filho et al. 2008b).

Multiple options for treatment are noted in the literature. Rodda and colleagues (2006) describe success of a comprehensive treatment program of single-event multilevel surgery in conjunction with rehabilitation and orthotics for 10 individuals with severe crouch gait guided by gait analysis. Results indicated maintenance of improved gait at 5-year outcome and increased function and independence in the community. The only previous surgery in this small cohort was previous calf or heel-cord lengthening procedures. When more extensive previous surgery has been performed alternative methods may need to be considered. Westberry and colleagues describe a serial casting protocol for patients with resistant or persistent fixed knee-flexion deformities after adequate hamstring lengthening (Westberry et al. 2006) with good results.

Two current methods of treatment create an extension deformity in the femur to compensate for a fixed knee-flexion deformity. Anterior physeal arrest using stapling (Kramer and Stevens 2001) and more recently tension-band 8-plates (Klatt and Stevens 2008) across an open epiphysis to guide remaining growth in the distal femur into extension. Their series included eight patients with cerebral palsy and demonstrated largely positive improvements in knee-flexion deformity alone, but no information is provided on functional knee flexion during gait.

Distal femoral extension osteotomy is the second method that employs creating an extension deformity in the femur to compensate for a fixed knee-flexion deformity. Patellar tendon advancement with or without distal femoral extension osteotomy has been used for treatment of severe crouch gait at Gillette for the last 13 years (Stout et al. 2008). Our experience suggests correction of both the knee-flexion contractures and the elongation of the patellar tendon is necessary to restore upright posture in this population. These procedures are considered for the adolescent or young adult in crouch despite prior treatment. The specific indication for distal femoral extension osteotomy is a fixed knee-flexion contracture in the range of 10°–30° based on clinical examination. The indication for patellar tendon advancement is quadriceps insufficiency as indicated by an extensor lag ≥10° on physical examination or if a distal femoral extension osteotomy is performed.

The correction of patella alta typically represents an overcorrection not only to restore the function of the quadriceps but also to compensate for ankle plantar flexor insufficiency. Distal femoral extension osteotomy alone typically improved knee-flexion contracture, but most individuals continued to walk in crouch subsequent to the procedure (Morais Filho et al. 2008, Stout et al. 2008). As a result, we recommend that it no longer be done in isolation, but always in conjunction with patellar advancement.

TECHNIQUE (STOUT ET AL. 2008)

Distal femoral extension osteotomy (see Instructional Video 'Distal femoral extension osteotomy' on Interactive Disc)
A lateral approach to the distal femur posterior to the vastus lateralis is used. The chisel for a 90° blade-plate is inserted just proximal to a guide wire placed at a 90° to the femoral shaft just proximal to the physis (or physeal scar) with the angle guide of the chisel parallel to the tibia. This helps to avoid varus or valgus displacement of the osteotomy. The angle

between the guide and the femoral shaft is equal to the degree of extension achieved by the osteotomy. The distal osteotomy plane is parallel to the chisel and the second (proximal) is perpendicular to the femoral shaft. The two meet at the posterior cortex. An anterior triangular wedge of bone is removed. This should be no more than 25°–30° (Fig. 5.11.2). The osteotomy is displaced by extending the leg, closing the anterior opening. Malrotation (up to approximately 25°) and coronal-plane deformity can be corrected if indicated. The chisel is replaced with the 90° AO blade plate (typically with a small offset) and secured in the typical fashion. Any posterior bone prominence should be removed from the distal fragment (Fig. 5.11.3). A hemovac drain should be considered to avoid postoperative hematoma that could compromise neurovascular function.

Patellar tendon advancement (see Instructional Video 'Patellar tendon advancement', on Interactive Disc)
Two different methods are employed for patellar advancement depending skeletal maturity.

Prior to skeletal maturity an anterior longitudinal incision is made from the distal pole of the patella, exposing the patellar tendon and tibial tubercle apophysis. Dividing the medial and lateral retinaculum isolates the patellar tendon. Dissecting between the patellar tendon and the retropatellar fat pad avoids entry into the joint. The patellar tendon is shaved off its insertion on the growth cartilage of the epiphysis. The tendon is divided above the palpable apophysis. The periosteum is opened with a 'T-shaped' incision distal to the apophysis

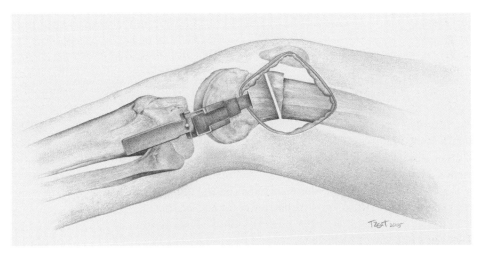

Fig. 5.11.2 Approach, exposure, and technique for the distal femoral extension osteotomy procedure. The chisel is inserted parallel and just proximal to a guide wire placed at a 90° angle to the femoral shaft just above the growth plate or physeal scar. Note that the angle guide on the chisel is parallel to the tibia. The angle between the guide on the chisel and the longitudinal axis of the femoral shaft is equal to the degree of extension achieved by the osteotomy. An oscillating saw is used to perform the osteotomy, with the planes of the osteotomy meeting at the posterior cortex. A triangle segment of the anterior cortex is removed and the osteotomy is displaced by extending the leg. Derotation can be incorporated into the osteotomy if desired.

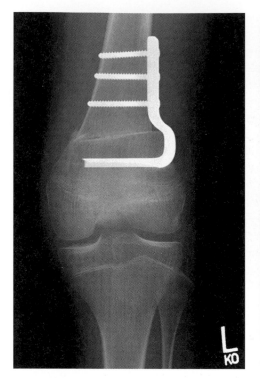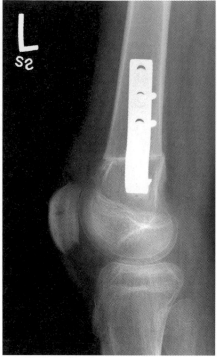

Fig. 5.11.3 Anterior–posterior (left) and lateral (right) radiograph of the knee in maximum extension post distal femoral extension osteotomy. The position of the AO blade plate is seen. The phalange of the plate is aligned parallel to the lateral border of the femoral shaft using C-arm fluoroscopy at the time of surgery (left). This placement helps to avoid varus or valgus displacement of the osteotomy. Any posterior bone protrusion on the distal fragment is removed (right). FiberTape was used for tension-band fixation of the patellar tendon advancement and is therefore not visible on either view.

exposing the tibia sub-periosteally (Fig. 5.11.4). The patella is advanced distally (until the inferior pole is at the joint line). Then the patellar tendon is repaired under the periosteal flaps. A tension band of FiberTape (Arthrex, Naples FL) is placed transversely through the patella (typically percutaneously through stab incisions) and then passed subcutaneously to the surgical wound. The tension band is then passed through a transverse drill hole in the tibia and tightened until there is slight slack in the advanced tendon (Fig. 5.11.5). Mobility is assessed to ensure at least 70° knee flexion. Further division of the retinaculum is performed if flexion is limited.

After skeletal maturity a bone block (with patellar tendon attached) approximately 1.5 cm wide × 2 cm long is created with an oscillating saw and completed with an osteotome. A receptacle site is created distally for the tibial tubercle. This piece is typically transposed proximally to the original site of the tibial tubercle and impacted into position. The tubercle is advanced (again, until the distal pole of the patella is at the joint line). A single 4.5 mm AO cortical lag screw is placed through the middle of the bone block (Fig. 5.11.6). The tension-band is placed as described above.

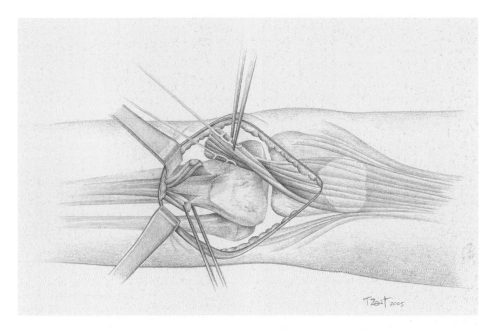

Fig. 5.11.4 Approach, exposure, and technique for patellar tendon advancement. Proximally, the medial and lateral retinaculum of the patella has been divided to isolate the patellar tendon. Distally, the patellar tendon has been shaved off its insertion on the growth cartilage of the epiphysis of the tibial tubercle. The periosteum of the tibial distal to the apophysis has been divided in a T-shaped fashion to expose the tibia.

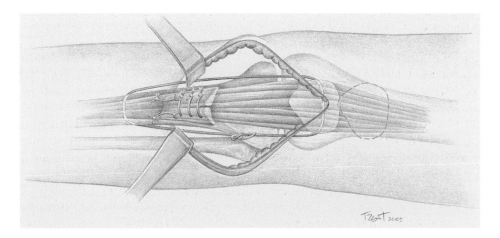

Fig. 5.11.5 The patellar tendon is advanced until the inferior pole of the patella is at the joint line. It is repaired with non-resorbable sutures under the periosteal flaps. The flaps are then closed over the end of the patellar tendon. A lag screw with/without a washer is used if the tendon is advanced with a block of bone. A tension band of FiberTape is used to protect the repair.

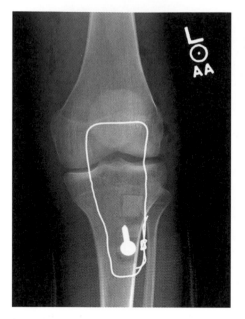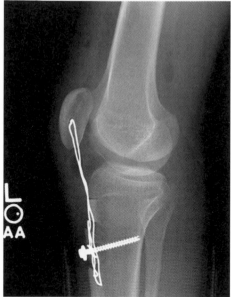

Fig. 5.11.6 Anterior–posterior (left) and lateral (right) radiograph of the knee in maximum extension post-patellar tendon and tibial tubercle advancement. The distal advancement of the tibial tubercle on a block of bone fixed by a cortical lag screw is noted. The transposed block from the distal site to the original site can also be seen. The entire repair in this case is protected by a 16 gauge stainless steel Luque wire tension-band.

For further details of both the patellar tendon advancement and distal femoral extension osteotomies, see the Interactive Disc that accompanies this book.

POTENTIAL PITFALLS

(1) Distal femoral extension osteotomy should not be performed as an isolated procedure without patellar tendon advancement. These procedures are part of a program which includes correction of all factors that contribute to the crouch condition including lever-arm dysfunction, appropriate lengthening of contracted muscles, and tone management.

(2) Correction of knee-flexion contractures greater than 30° alters the weightbearing position of the knee. This may have long-term consequences.

(3) It is difficult to correct more than 25°–30° malrotation correction through osteotomy site. Greater deformity requires consideration of proximal and distal femoral osteotomies.

(4) Performing distal femoral extension osteotomies too far proximally or inserting the chisel for the blade plate too posteriorly leads to anterior translation of the distal fragment and angular deformity putting the sciatic nerve in a position of stretch. To improve the rate of healing, avoid posterior angular deformity, and minimize the risk of neurovascular stretch, the chisel should be as close to the physis (or the physeal scar in mature patients) as possible.

(5) Excessive retraction for exposure can place excessive stretch on the neurovascular bundle.

(6) Care must be taken to avoid disrupting the proximal tibial physis in a growing child. Tibial tubercle transfer is done in the skeletally mature patient, but patellar tendon advancement surgery is preferred in skeletally immature patients.

(7) Patellar tendon advancement procedure without tension-band stabilization has a high risk of failure.

(8) If selective dorsal rhizotomy or rectus femoris transfer have not been performed previously, concurrent rectus femoris transfer is indicated to avoid stiff knee gait following patellar tendon advancement.

(9) Isolated patellar tendon advancement in the presence of minor knee-flexion contractures appears to pose a risk to patellar tendon fixation. Correction of contractures by distal femoral extension osteotomy is advised.

Avoiding Postoperative Complications

(1) Immobilization of the knee in 20°–30° of flexion for the first 3 days post-surgery with the use of a Robert Jones dressing reduces the stretch on the neurovascular structures.

(2) Continuous epidural analgesia is typically used for postoperative pain management for the first 3 days postoperatively. Because the epidural can mask neurovascular compromise, initial management at the first sign of neurovascular compromise is to reduce or turn off the epidural for a period of time until sensation returns.

(3) A continuous passive motion (CPM) program is initiated beginning day 3 for a minimum of 6 weeks or until 90° of knee flexion is obtained. Early mobilization is both a source of comfort as well as a benefit to regaining range of motion.

(4) A knee-immobilizer or a flexion-stop hinged knee brace is used at rest for the first 6–8 weeks.

(5) Weightbearing is initiated 3–4 weeks postoperatively.

Complications

The total complication rate in our distal femoral extension osteotomy (DFEO) series was 19% and 18% with patellar tendon advancement procedures (Stout et al. 2008). The type and frequency of complications differ between the two procedures. Stretch palsy and neuropathy accounted for the largest percentage of the total complications in the DFEO series. While knee pain (lasting more than 6 months) was the most frequent complication for patellar tendon advancement in the reported series, a broader look at all the complications (from the first procedure in 1994 through 2005) indicated that loss of fixation was the most frequent. When the rate of complication was assessed relative to consecutive procedures performed, a definite learning curve was identified, with a stabilization of complications for DFEO after approximately the first 40 procedures. The learning curve for the patellar tendon advancement series was found to be more gradual with the complication rate stabilizing after approximately 60 procedures (Fig. 5.11.7). The rate of fixation failure dropped significantly once use of a tension-band was instituted to protect the repair. Six fixation failures occurred

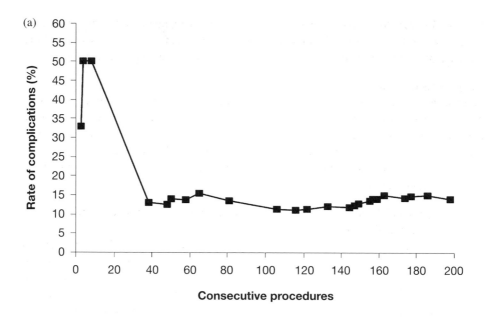

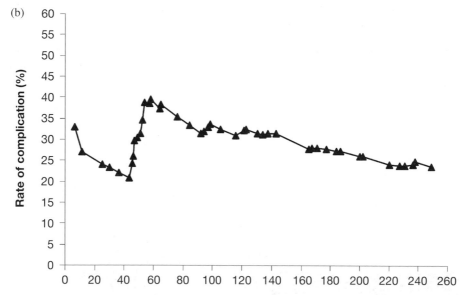

Fig. 5.11.7 Complication rate from 200 consecutive distal femoral extension osteotomy and 250 consecutive patellar tendon advancement procedures. (a) Rate of complication of distal femoral extension osteotomy relative to consecutive procedures performed is displayed. A stabilization of complications is noted after approximately 40 procedures at a rate of approximately 14%. (b) Rate of complication of patellar tendon advancement relative to consecutive procedures performed. A gradual decrease in the complication rate is noted after approximately 60 procedures through the remainder of the series. A rise in the complication rate occurred between 40 and 60 procedures when a series of fixation complications were encountered.

among 153 procedures when a tension band was used for a rate of 4%. Three of the six failures were related to loss of fixation of the tension-band itself. The rate of fixation failures when a tension-band was not used was 22% (20 failures among 96 procedures).

Supporting evidence
Patellar tendon advancement separately or in conjunction with distal femoral extension osteotomy can restore erect posture. As with most procedures to optimize gait, these are commonly performed with other procedures that are necessary to restore erect posture. Function is improved or maintained as evidenced by relief of pain, restoration of preoperative levels of strength, and improvements in skills that require complex knee function (Stout et al. 2008).

Case study: distal femoral extension osteotomy and patellar tendon advancement (Case 8 on Interactive Disc)
MK is a 13-year-old boy with spastic diplegic cerebral palsy, GMFCS level II, who was referred for gait analysis in 2003 for treatment advice regarding a persistent crouch gait pattern. He has a history of selective dorsal rhizotomy (SDR) in 1994 and three episodes of single event multilevel surgery in 1997, 2000, and 2002. As he entered adolescence, he developed a crouch gait and more limited endurance (Fig. 5.11.8). MK had a previous gait study in 1997 prior to his first orthopaedic intervention. Subsequent to that initial gait study, surgery at another institution included the following.

• *1997*: bilateral rectus femoris to semitendinosus muscle transfers; bilateral medial and lateral hamstring lengthening; bilateral Strayer-type gastrocnemius recessions; bilateral os-calcis lengthenings.

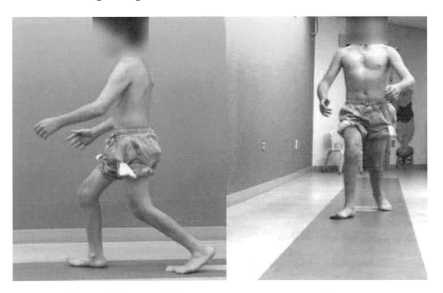

Fig. 5.11.8 MK in 2003 illustrating a severe crouch gait and associated external tibial torsion. See pro-op video in Case 8 on Interactive Disc for a dynamic illustration.

571

- *2000*: bilateral psoas lengthenings; right posterior tibialis to peroneus brevis transfer.
- *2002*: left foot soft-tissue procedures.

Physical examination findings in 2003 included (1) bilateral fixed knee-flexion contractures (15°L, 20°R); (2) bilateral hip-flexion contractures (15°); (3) bilateral patella alta with 20° knee extensor lags; (4) bilateral increased unilateral popliteal angle (60°); (5) bilateral external tibial torsion (25°–30° bimalleolar axis); (6) bilateral femoral anteversion (40°–50°); and (7) bilateral plantarflexor weakness (3-/5 Kendall). Radiographs show bilateral patella alta without distal pole patellar fractures, but the tibial tubercle apophysis show signs of excessive stress bilaterally.

A persistent knee flexed gait in the range of 50° during stance, excessive dorsiflexion, and bilateral continuous knee-extensor moments is identified in his gait analysis data (Fig. 5.11.9). The hamstrings achieve appropriate length and velocity in terminal swing bilaterally (Fig. 5.11.10). His net energy expenditure is more than 2 × normal at a typical walking velocity (Fig. 5.11.11).

Interpretation: MK's data are consistent with someone in severe crouch. Numerous contributing factors include lever arm dysfunction, plantarflexor weakness, knee-flexion contractures and quadriceps insufficiency.

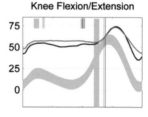

Knee Flexion/Extension

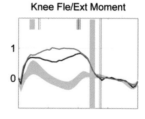

Knee Fle/Ext Moment

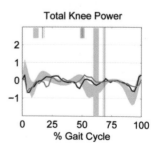

Total Knee Power

Fig. 5.11.9 Sagittal-plane right (green) and left (red) knee kinematic and kinetic graphs for case MK (control – gray band). 50° of stance phase knee flexion is noted bilaterally along with continuous knee-extensor moments. Swing phase knee range of motion is limited, but appropriate peak knee flexion is achieved.

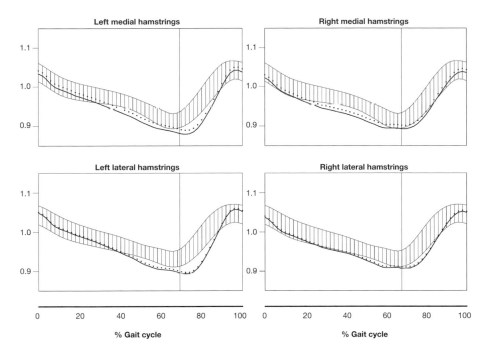

Fig. 5.11.10 Muscle length graphs for the medial and lateral hamstrings for case MK. The hatched area of the graph indicates the typical mean ± 1 SD. Percentage of gait cycle is displayed on the abscissa and normalized origin to insertion distance on the ordinate. Solid line depicts muscle length calculated with a generic model, dashed line depicts muscle length with a model that represents patient's anteversion (45° left and 40° right). Terminal swing phase data demonstrate appropriate muscle length and velocity on each side despite the crouch position. This indicates the hamstrings are functioning with appropriate length and velocity.

Treatment options: MK has already had global tone management via SDR. His muscle length data indicate his hamstrings are functioning normally (appropriate length and velocity) despite his knee-flexed posture. Repeat hamstring lengthening would be inappropriate considering their normal function. Because he has fixed knee-flexion contractures he is a candidate for distal femoral extension osteotomy and therefore patellar tendon advancement. Because he is not yet skeletally mature, this would be a tendon advancement without tibial tubercle osteotomy. Correction of external tibial torsion is also necessary to correct lever arm dysfunction. The need for treatment of his bilateral hip-flexion contractures is less clear. They may be compensatory to his crouch posture. He has had previous SDR and psoas lengthening.

Results: MK underwent bilateral distal femoral extension osteotomies with external rotation of the distal segments, patellar tendon advancements, correction of bilateral external tibial torsion and bilateral medial hamstring botulinum toxin type A injections in late 2003. Postoperative gait analysis in 2004 demonstrates complete resolution of crouch (Figs 5.11.12, 13a, b). MK's case is representative of someone walking in crouch with multiple causes. Upright gait can be restored with treatment guided by sound principles.

573

Fig. 5.11.11 Net energy expenditure for case MK. Non-dimensional normalized velocity is on the abscissa and net non-dimensional normalized rate of oxygen consumption (movement – resting) on the ordinate. Dashed vertical lines represent the 95% confidence interval of typical walking velocity. The solid line of the graph indicates typical net oxygen consumption at a given walking velocity. Dashed lines indicate the 95% confidence interval for net oxygen consumption by velocity. Solid dot displays case data plus error bars. Data indicate net energy expenditure is × 2.3 higher than typical at a velocity at the slower end of typical velocity.

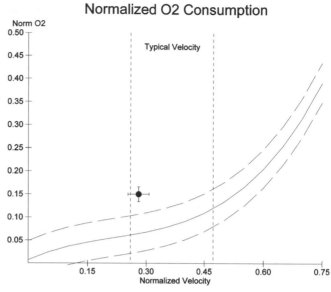

Normalized O2 Consumption

Norm O2

Typical Velocity

Normalized Velocity

● 17-Sep-2003 (13+0) B-None; B-None NetO2=0.15@0.28 (231%)

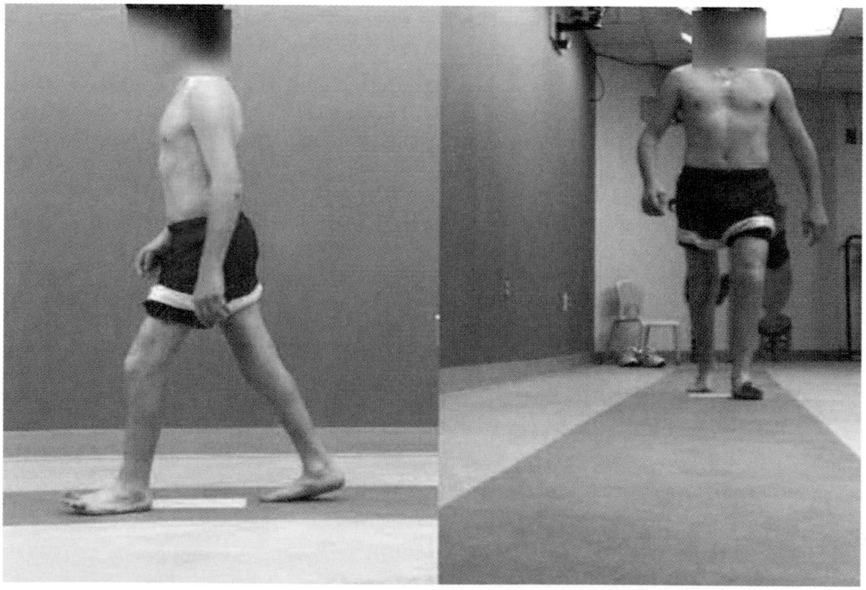

Fig. 5.11.12 MK in 2004 illustrating a resolution of crouch and restoration of an upright posture. See post-op video in Case 8 on Interactive Disc for a dynamic illustration.

574

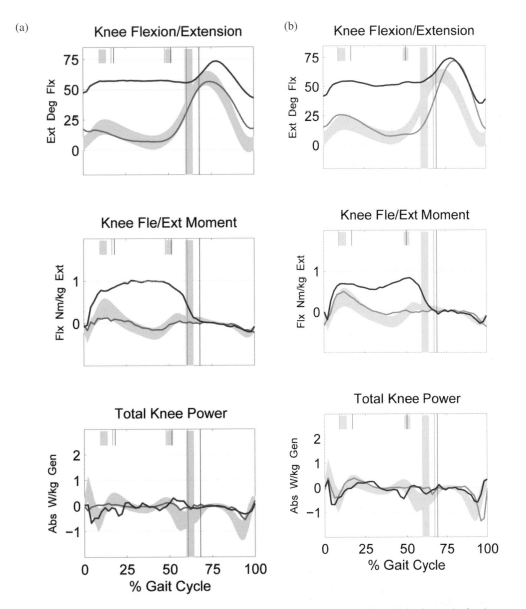

Fig. 5.11.13 Preoperative and postoperative sagittal plane knee kinematic and kinetic graphs for the right (a) and left (b) sides. Preoperative data (2003) are represented in blue in each case. Postoperative data (2004) are depicted in green on the right (a) and red on the left (b). Control data are depicted in gray on each graph. The stance-phase knee-flexion kinematic and knee moment have been restored to within typical limits bilaterally.

Treatment of crouch gait is complex. Many, but not all causative factors have been identified. A better understanding of the neural mechanisms of balance, motor control, proprioception, and weakness will lead to more effective treatments. However, current advances have been made that will allow children and young adults to remain ambulatory into adulthood.

REFERENCES

Anderson FC, Pandy MG (2001) Dynamic optimization of human walking. *J Biomech Eng* **123**: 381–90.

Arnold AS, Komattu AV, Delp SL (1997) Internal rotation gait: a compensatory mechanism to restore abduction capacity decreased by bone deformity. *Dev Med Child Neurol* **39**: 40–4.

Arnold AS, Liu MQ, Schwartz MH, Õunpuu S, Delp SL (2006) The role of estimating muscle–tendon lengths and velocities of the hamstrings in the evaluation and treatment of crouch gait. *Gait Posture* **23**: 273–81.

Baker LD (1956) A rational approach to the needs of the cerebral palsy patient. *J Bone Joint Surg Am* **38**: 313–23.

Beals RK (2001) Treatment of knee contracture in cerebral palsy by hamstring lengthening, posterior capsulotomy, and quadriceps mechanism shortening. *Dev Med Child Neurol* **43**: 802–5.

Bell KJ, Õunpuu S, DeLuca PA, Romness MJ (2002) Natural progression of gait in children with cerebral palsy. *J Pediatr Orthop* **22**: 677–82.

Bleck, E (1971) Postural and gait abnormalities caused by hip-flexion deformity in spastic cerebral palsy. Treatment by iliopsoas recession. *J Bone Joint Surg Am* **53**: 1468–88.

Borton DC, Walker K, Pirpiris M, Nattrass GR, Graham HK (2001) Isolated calf lengthening in cerebral palsy: outcome analysis of risk factors. *J Bone Joint Surg Br* **83**: 364–70.

Burtner PA (1996) *Mechanical and muscle activation characteristics during crouch stance balance in children with spastic cerebral palsy*. Dissertation, University of Oregon.

Burtner PA, Woollacott MH, Craft GL, Roncesvalles MN (2007) The capacity to adapt to changing balance threats: a comparison of children with cerebral palsy and typically developing children. *Dev Neurorehabil* **10**: 249–60.

Chambers HG (2001) Treatment of functional limitations at the knee in ambulatory children with cerebral palsy. *Eur J Neurol* **8** (Suppl 5): 59–74.

Chandler FA (1933) Re-establishment of normal leverage of the patella in knee flexion deformity in spastic paralysis. *Surg Gynecol Obstet* **57**: 523–7.

Chandler FA (1940) Patellar advancement operation: a revised technique. *J Int Coll Surg* **3**: 433–7.

Chen J, Woollacott MH (2007) Lower extremity kinetics for balance control in children with cerebral palsy. *J Mot Behav* **39**: 306–13.

Cleveland M, Bosworth DM (1936) Surgical correction of flexion deformity of knees due to spastic paralysis. *Surg Gynecol Obstet* **63**: 659–64.

Delp SL, Statler K, Carroll NC (1995) Preserving plantar flexion strength after surgical treatment for contracture of the triceps surae: a computer simulation study. *J Orthop Res* **13**: 96–104.

Delp SL, Arnold AS, Speers RA, Moore CA (1996) Hamstrings and psoas lengths during normal and crouch gait: implications for muscle-tendon surgery. *J Orthop Res* **14**: 144–51.

DeLuca PA, Õunpuu S, Davis RB, Walsh JH (1998) Effect of hamstring and psoas lengthening on pelvic tilt in patient with spastic diplegia cerebral palsy. *J Pediatr Orthop* **18**: 712–8.

Dietz FR, Albright JC, Dolan L (2006) Medium term follow-up of achilles tendon lengthening in the treatment of ankle equinus in cerebral palsy. *Iowa Med J* **26**: 27–31.

Eggers GW (1950) Surgical division of the patellar retinacula to improve extension of the knee joint in cerebral spastic paralysis. *J Bone Joint Surg Am* **32**: 80–6.

Gage JR (2004) *The Treatment of Gait Problems in Cerebral Palsy*. London: Mac Keith Press. p 382–97.

Gage JR, Schwartz MH (2004) Pathological gait and lever arm dysfunction. In: Gage JR editor. *The Treatment of Gait Problems in Cerebral Palsy*. London: Mac Keith Press. p 180–204.

Gough M, Eve LC, Robinson RO, Shortland AP (2004) Short-term outcome of multi-level surgical intervention in spastic diplegic cerebral palsy compared with natural history. *Dev Med Child Neurol* **46**: 91–7.

Hicks J, Arnold A, Anderson, F, Schwartz M, Delp S (2007) The effect of tibial torsion on the capacity of muscles to extend the hip and knee during single-limb stance. *Gait Posture* **26**: 546–52.

Hicks JL, Schwartz MH, Arnold AS, Delp SL (2008) Crouch postures reduce the capacity of muscles to extend the hip and knee during single-limb stance phase of gait. *J Biomech* **41**: 960–7.

Hoffinger SA, Rab GT, Abou-Ghaida H (1993) Hamstrings in cerebral palsy crouch gait. *J Pediatr Orthop* **13**: 722–6.

Kay RM, Rethlefsen SA, Skaggs D, Leet A (2002) Outcome of medial versus lateral hamstring lengthening surgery in cerebral palsy. *J Pediatr Orthop* **22**: 169–72.

Keats S, Kambin P (1962) An evaluation of surgery for the correction of knee-flexion contracture in children with cerebral spastic paralysis. *J Bone Joint Surg Am* **44**: 1146–54.

Kimmel SA, Schwartz, MH (2006) A baseline of dynamic muscle function during gait. *Gait Posture* **23**: 211–21.

Klatt J, Stevens PM (2008) Guided growth for fixed knee flexion deformity. *J Pediatr Orthop* **28**: 626–31.

Kramer A, Stevens PM (2001) Anterior femoral stapling. *J Pediatr Orthop* **21**: 804–7.

Lloyd-Roberts GC, Jackson AM, Albert JS (1985) Avulsion of the distal pole of the patella in cerebral palsy: a cause of deteriorating gait. *J Bone Joint Surg Br* **67**: 252–4.

Lotman DB (1976) Knee flexion deformity and patella alta in spastic cerebral palsy. *Dev Med Child Neurol* **18**: 315–19.

Louis ML, Viehweger E, Launay F, Loundou AD, Pomero V, Jacquemier M, Jouve JL, Bollini G (2008) Informative value of the popliteal angle in walking cerebral palsy children. *Rev Chir Orthop Reparatrice Appar Mot* **94**: 443–8.

Morais Filho MC, Kawamura C, Kanaji P, Juliano Y (2008a) Relation between triceps surae lengthening and crouch gait in patients with cerebral palsy. *Presented at the American Academy for Cerebral Palsy and Developmental Medicine, Atlanta, GA, Sept 2008.*

Morais Filho MC, Neves DL, Abreu FB, Juliano Y, Guimaraes L (2008b) Treatment of fixed knee flexion deformity and crouch gait using distal femoral extension osteotomy in cerebral palsy. *J Child Orthop* **2**: 37–43.

Murphy KP, Molnar GE, Lankasky K (1995) Medical and functional status of adults with cerebral palsy. *Dev Med Child Neurol* **37**: 1075–84.

Nashner LM, Shumway-Cook A, Marin O (1983) Stance postural control in select groups of children with cerebral palsy: Deficits in sensory organization and muscular organization. *Exp Brain Res* **49**: 393–409.

Novacheck T, Trost J, Schwartz M (2002) Intramuscular psoas lengthening improves dynamic hip function in children with cerebral palsy. *J Pediatr Orthop* **22**: 158–64.

Perry J, Antonelli D, Ford W (1975) Analysis of knee joint forces during flexed knee stance. *J Bone Joint Surg Am* **57**: 961–7.

Roberts WM, Adams JP (1953) The patellar-advancement operation in cerebral palsy. *J Bone Joint Surg Am* **35**: 958–66.

Rodda JM, Graham HK, Carlson L, Galea MP, Wolfe R (2004) Sagittal gait patterns in spastic diplegia. *J Bone Joint Surg Br* **86**: 251–8.

Rodda JM, Graham HK, Nattrass GR, Galea MP, Baker R, Wolfe R (2006) Correction of severe crouch gait in patients with spastic diplegia with use of multilevel orthopaedic surgery. *J Bone Joint Surg Am* **88**: 2653–64.

Rose SA, DeLuca PA, Davis RB 3rd, Õunpuu S, Gage JR (1993) Kinematic and kinetic evaluation of the ankle after lengthening of the gastrocnemius fascia in children with cerebral palsy. *J Pediatr Orthop* **13**: 727–32.

Rosenthal RK, Levine DB (1977) Fragmentation of the distal pole of the patella in spastic cerebral palsy. *J Bone Joint Surg Am* **59**: 934–9.

Rozumalski A, Schwartz MH (2008) Naturally arising crouch groups reflect clinical differences. *Presented at the European Society of Movement for Adults and Children, Antalya, Turkey, Sept 2008.*

Schwartz MH, Lakin G (2003) The effect of tibial torsion on the dynamic function of the soleus during gait. *Gait Posture* **17**: 113–18.

Schwartz MH, Viehweger E, Stout J, Novacheck TF, Gage JR (2004) Comprehensive treatment of ambulatory children with cerebral palsy: an outcome assessment. *J Pediatr Orthop* **24**: 45–53.

Stewart C, Postans N, Schwartz MH, Rozumalski A, Roberts AP (2008) An investigation of the action of the hamstring muscles during standing in crouch using functional electrical stimulation (FES). *Gait Posture* **28**: 372–7.

Stout JL, Gage JR, Schwartz, MH, Novacheck TF (2008) Distal femoral extension osteotomy and patellar tendon advancement to treat persistent crouch gait in cerebral palsy. *J Bone Joint Surg Am* **90**: 2470–84.

Sutherland DH, Cooper L (1978) The pathomechanics of progressive crouch gait in spastic diplegia. *Orthop Clin N Am* **9**: 143–54.

Sutherland DH, Davids JR (1993). Common gait abnormalities of the knee in cerebral palsy. *Clin Orthop Relat Res* **288**: 139–47.

Thompson NS, Baker RJ, Cosgrove AP, Saunders JL, Taylor TC (2001) Relevance of the popliteal angle to hamstring length in cerebral palsy crouch gait. *J Pediatr Orthop* **21**: 383–7.

Westberry DE, Davids JR, Jacobs JM, Pugh LI, Tanner SL (2006) Effectiveness of serial stretch casting for resistant or recurrent knee flexion contractures following hamstring lengthening in children with cerebral palsy. *J Pediatr Orthop* **26**: 109–14.

Woollacott MH, Shumway-Cook A (2005) Postural dysfunction during standing and walking in children with cerebral palsy: what are the underlying problems and what new therapies might improve balance? *Neural Plast* **12**: 211–19.

Wren TAL, Rethlefsen S, Kay RM (2005) Prevalence of specific gait abnormalities in children with cerebral palsy. *J Pediatr Orthop* **25**: 79–83.

Section 6
ASSESSMENT OF OUTCOME

6.1
MEASUREMENT TOOLS AND METHODS

Pam Thomason, Adrienne Harvey and H. Kerr Graham

In order to obtain a comprehensive picture of the child with cerebral palsy (CP) it is helpful to classify function and the presenting gait pattern, especially during assessments prior to major interventions. It can also be helpful to measure various aspects of body structures and functions, activities and participation, using where possible valid, reliable and responsive measurement tools. Classification categorizes individuals into groups which permits description of the level of disability or impairment, encourages clear communication, the prediction of future status and the ability to compare both series of cases and the evaluation of change in individuals at different points in time (Rosenbaum et al. 2007). The most commonly used classification of gross motor function in children with CP is the Gross Motor Function Classification System (GMFCS) (Palisano et al. 1997).

In the past, many outcome studies focused on the impairment rather than the functional limitations that may result from the impairment (Majnemer and Mazer 2004). The focus in disability research has now shifted to the measurement of relevant aspects of the International Classification Model of Functioning, Disability and Health (ICF), by the World Health Organization (2001), which includes an emphasis on both activities and participation. Health status measures can be categorized into discriminative, predictive and evaluative measures (Kirshner and Guyatt 1985). Most measures used to assess the outcomes of interventions are evaluative, because they measure the magnitude of change over time.

In recent years there has been extensive progress in the understanding of measurement of gait dysfunction and the development of an increasing range of appropriate tools with varying degrees of validity, reliability and practicality. Much work remains to be done in the area of responsiveness. In this regard it may be appropriate to consider that significant differences in natural history exist across the CP spectrum, even within the children who are usually described as 'ambulant' (GMFCS levels I–III). Measurements which may be appropriate and tools which may be responsive at GMFCS level I may not be as appropriate or as responsive at GMFCS level III, and vice versa.

Measurement frameworks in cerebral palsy
A number of approaches have been described in the past decade for the measurement and evaluation of the child with CP including the Health Care Compass, the framework promoted by the National Center for Medical Rehabilitation Research (NCMRR) (1993)

Fig. 6.1.1 ICF model, WHO 2001.

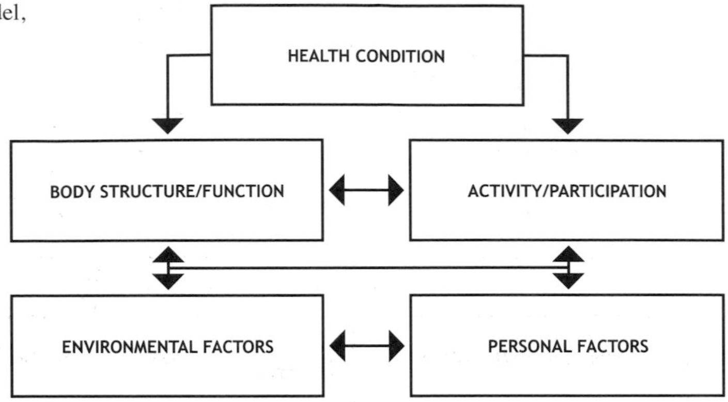

and the ICF by the World Health Organization (2001) (Fig. 6.1.1). The ICF is the most recent framework and is rapidly becoming the most popular.

In the ICF, the health condition is considered in a number of domains including 'body structure and function', 'activity limitations' and 'participation restrictions'. These are modified by the contextual factors of environmental and personal factors which may impact on a person's health state. While it can be readily appreciated that the ICF is the most comprehensive, flexible and embracing of the contemporary frameworks for the evaluation of the child with CP in gait problems, it is not yet fully established which existing measures fit within which domain and in which domains new measurement tools need to be developed. Measures that assess body structure and function include radiology, range of motion, strength measurement and spasticity measures. Measures that assess activity include the Gross Motor Function Measure (GMFM) and the Functional Mobility Scale (FMS). A systematic review has recently been published analyzing the available measures of activity limitation in children with CP (Harvey et al. 2008). It is often difficult to separate participation from activity. Tools that focus specifically on participation are becoming more available and are summarized in two reviews (Morris et al. 2005, Sakzewski et al. 2007). In a recent randomized clinical trial of multilevel surgery for children with gait problems in CP, we have used existing measures, and developed new measures and located these within the domains of the ICF as shown in Figure 6.1.2.

Classification and measurement of gross motor function in cerebral palsy

THE GROSS MOTOR FUNCTION MEASURE AND GROSS MOTOR FUNCTION CLASSIFICATION SYSTEM
The details of the Gross Motor Function Measure (GMFM) and Gross Motor Function Classification System (GMFCS) are discussed in Chapters 2.6 and 2.7. The descriptors for children aged 6–12 years and young people aged 12–18 years have recently been expanded and revised. It should be noted that the gross motor curves (Rosenbaum et al. 2002) include GMFM data up to the age of 15 years. There is much less information regarding changes in gross motor function in the 15–20 age group and beyond. However, the descriptors for

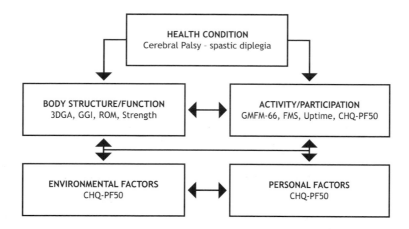

Fig. 6.1.2 Outcome measures according to ICF. GGI, Gillette gait index; ROM, range of motion, GMFM, Gross Motor Function Measure; FMS, Functional Mobility Scale; CHQ-PF50, Child Health Questionnaire.

the GMFCS, at ages 12–18, imply deterioration in gross motor function as evidenced by the need for assistive devices or increased use of wheeled mobility.

The descriptors and accompanying illustrations are found in Figure 6.1.3 and 6.1.4. These combined descriptors and illustrations are the most relevant for the age group in which most surgical management of gait problems in CP occur. Although GMFCS levels are considered to be stable over time, the descriptors for young people aged 12–18 years allow for deterioration in gross motor function at the time of the adolescent growth spurt, a decrease in independent walking abilities and an increase in the need for both assistive devices and wheeled mobility. This is particularly true at GMFCS levels II, III and IV (McCormick et al. 2007).

Baseline and serial recording of GMFCS levels is essential for initial assessment and longitudinal monitoring of children and young people with CP. It is expected that a child will remain within the same GMFCS level throughout their childhood, growth and development; or, to put it another way, that they will follow a specific gross motor curve. However, a number of children change GMFCS levels; and when this appears to have occurred, it is appropriate to check whether in fact the recorded levels were accurate. In our longitudinal studies of gait and function, it is more common for a child to demonstrate a decrease in gross motor function and to go down a GMFCS level, especially around the time of the pubertal growth spurt. We have noted numerous examples of children with spastic diplegia, GMFCS level II, who were managed with bilateral tendo-Achilles lengthening (TAL) for equinus gait, and who developed progressive crouch gait, anterior knee pain and patella fractures. At the time of the adolescent growth spurt, it is not uncommon for a child who has been functioning at GMFCS level II to lose independent walking and become reliant on an assistive device such as crutches, and to be reclassified as GMFCS level III. It is more difficult for a child to move up a GMFCS level but given the categorical nature of the classification, this is occasionally noted.

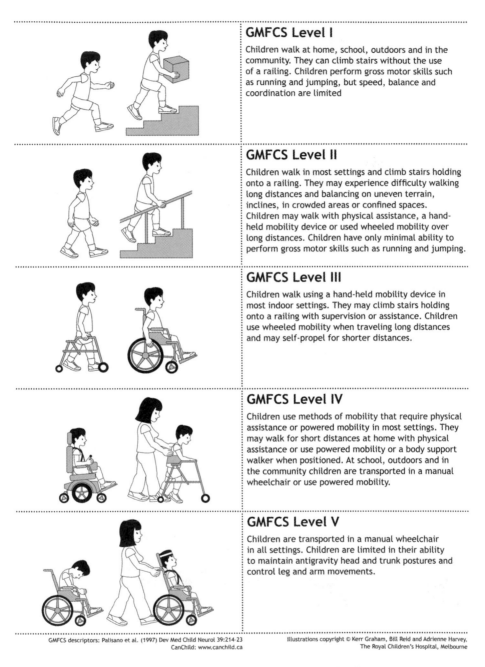

GMFCS Level I

Children walk at home, school, outdoors and in the community. They can climb stairs without the use of a railing. Children perform gross motor skills such as running and jumping, but speed, balance and coordination are limited

GMFCS Level II

Children walk in most settings and climb stairs holding onto a railing. They may experience difficulty walking long distances and balancing on uneven terrain, inclines, in crowded areas or confined spaces. Children may walk with physical assistance, a hand-held mobility device or used wheeled mobility over long distances. Children have only minimal ability to perform gross motor skills such as running and jumping.

GMFCS Level III

Children walk using a hand-held mobility device in most indoor settings. They may climb stairs holding onto a railing with supervision or assistance. Children use wheeled mobility when traveling long distances and may self-propel for shorter distances.

GMFCS Level IV

Children use methods of mobility that require physical assistance or powered mobility in most settings. They may walk for short distances at home with physical assistance or use powered mobility or a body support walker when positioned. At school, outdoors and in the community children are transported in a manual wheelchair or use powered mobility.

GMFCS Level V

Children are transported in a manual wheelchair in all settings. Children are limited in their ability to maintain antigravity head and trunk postures and control leg and arm movements.

GMFCS descriptors: Palisano et al. (1997) Dev Med Child Neurol 39:214-23
CanChild: www.canchild.ca

Illustrations copyright © Kerr Graham, Bill Reid and Adrienne Harvey,
The Royal Children's Hospital, Melbourne

Fig. 6.1.3 Gross Motor Function Classification System Expanded and Revised, 6–12 years.

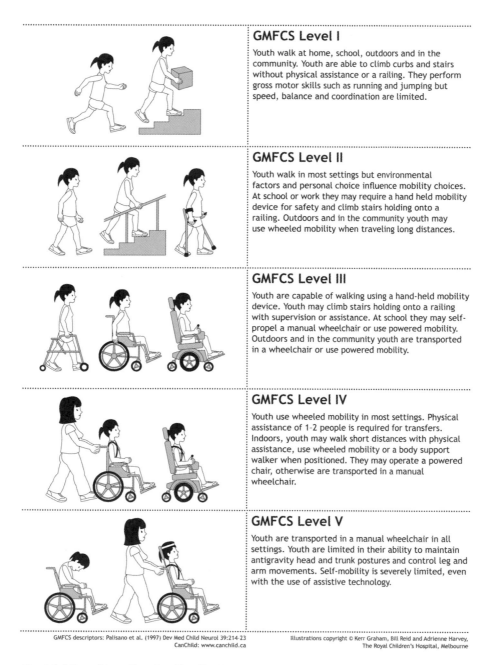

GMFCS Level I

Youth walk at home, school, outdoors and in the community. Youth are able to climb curbs and stairs without physical assistance or a railing. They perform gross motor skills such as running and jumping but speed, balance and coordination are limited.

GMFCS Level II

Youth walk in most settings but environmental factors and personal choice influence mobility choices. At school or work they may require a hand held mobility device for safety and climb stairs holding onto a railing. Outdoors and in the community youth may use wheeled mobility when traveling long distances.

GMFCS Level III

Youth are capable of walking using a hand-held mobility device. Youth may climb stairs holding onto a railing with supervision or assistance. At school they may self-propel a manual wheelchair or use powered mobility. Outdoors and in the community youth are transported in a wheelchair or use powered mobility.

GMFCS Level IV

Youth use wheeled mobility in most settings. Physical assistance of 1-2 people is required for transfers. Indoors, youth may walk short distances with physical assistance, use wheeled mobility or a body support walker when positioned. They may operate a powered chair, otherwise are transported in a manual wheelchair.

GMFCS Level V

Youth are transported in a manual wheelchair in all settings. Youth are limited in their ability to maintain antigravity head and trunk postures and control leg and arm movements. Self-mobility is severely limited, even with the use of assistive technology.

GMFCS descriptors: Palisano et al. (1997) Dev Med Child Neurol 39:214-23
CanChild: www.canchild.ca

Illustrations copyright © Kerr Graham, Bill Reid and Adrienne Harvey,
The Royal Children's Hospital, Melbourne

Fig. 6.1.4 Gross Motor Function Classification System Expanded and Revised, 12–18 years.

OM is a boy with spastic diplegia associated with preterm birth (Fig. 6.1.5). He presented to our gait laboratory age 12 for evaluation of knee pain and deteriorating gait and function. The key features on his assessment were that he required Canadian crutches for walking in the community and was classified as GMFCS level III. He had moderately severe bilateral anterior knee pain and walked in severe 'crouch gait'. Instrumented gait analysis confirmed that he walked with both ankles dorsiflexed in the calcaneus range and both knees flexed about 60° throughout the gait cycle. His joint kinetics showed a large knee extensor moment throughout the stance phase of gait. Radiographs revealed transverse fractures through the inferior pole of both patellae.

OM underwent a program of multilevel surgery which included bilateral lengthening of the iliopsoas at the brim of the pelvis, bilateral hamstring lengthening and rotational osteotomies and foot stabilization surgery. He was supplied with ground reaction ankle–foot orthoses (AFOs) and 12 months after multilevel surgery was able to walk independently. He no longer required the use of a wheelchair or crutches and a repeat gait analysis confirmed a stable correction of his gait pattern. He no longer needed his ground reaction AFOs. He returned for follow up at 5 and 12 years after multilevel surgery. Evaluation at that time confirmed healing of the patella fractures, complete relief of knee pain, and the ability to walk with extended knees and hips, without the use of aids or orthoses. By definition OM was then functioning at GMFCS level II having been originally graded at GMFCS level III prior to multilevel surgery. However, at long-term evaluation, another video recording of

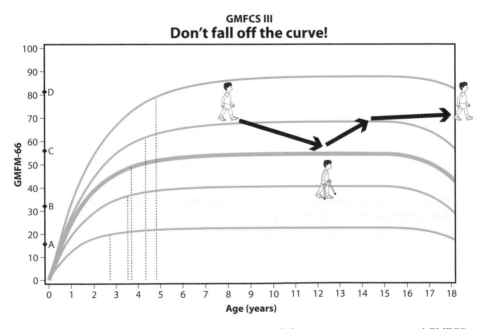

Fig. 6.1.5 Case study OM. Progress of motor function in relation to gross motor curves and GMFCS.

gait was reviewed which indicated that OM had walked independently between the ages of 3 and 6 years, when he was first managed with bilateral TALs. This was followed by deterioration in function which accelerated at age 8 years when he had a second TAL. By age 10 years he had become reliant on the use of crutches and a wheelchair for longer distances. OM was part of a prospective study into the surgical correction of severe crouch gait reported by Rodda et al. (2006).

PROGRESS OF MOTOR FUNCTION IN RELATION TO GROSS MOTOR CURVES AND GMFCS

This case illustrates a number of important points. It is possible, in exceptional circumstances, for a child to move up a GMFCS level after an intervention such as multilevel surgery. However this occurs infrequently and is usually the regaining of a level of function which has previously been lost either through the effects of natural history or an unhelpful intervention such as isolated TALs. However following optimum biomechanical realignment, and a successful rehabilitation program, the correction achieved at multilevel surgery, and the consequent improvement in gross motor function, is sustainable through the pubertal growth spurt and into adult life.

The relative stability of the GMFCS means that this is not an outcome measure and was never meant to be one. However, we think that the GMFCS is the essential baseline tool for communication about gross motor function in the child with CP in the multidisciplinary team and to guide our thoughts about long-term prognosis and the selection of appropriate management strategies. For example the child at GMFCS level I will have either spastic hemiplegia or mild spastic diplegia. Spasticity is usually mild and musculoskeletal deformities are also mild. In our center, this group of children is most often managed by injections of botulinum toxin type A in early childhood followed by an episode of single event multilevel surgery (SEMLS) between the ages of 6 and 10 years. For the majority this results in an excellent long term correction of gait pattern which remains stable throughout the teenage years and early adult life. In contrast, children at GMFCS level IV in the 6–12 age range have very limited walking abilities. Our surgical goals for these children are to maintain flexible, enlocated hips, because they have a very high incidence of spastic hip displacement. We also try to maintain extensibility of the hip and knees for standing transfers and limited ambulation. The majority require foot stabilization surgery so that their feet can be braced and standing transfers maintained. However, long-term functional ambulation is not a goal at GMFCS level IV and we will therefore not choose to perform procedures such as transfer of the rectus femoris, an operation which improves swing-phase gait problems. We concentrate on improving stance phase to maintain limited ambulation and standing transfers for as long as possible. Despite our best efforts, the majority of teenagers at GMFCS level IV lose their walking abilities and it can be a struggle just to maintain standing transfers. At both GMFCS level I and level IV, the GMFCS provides an excellent guide to long term prognosis and is directly influential in our decision making as to the choice of management strategy.

THE FUNCTIONAL MOBILITY SCALE AND FUNCTIONAL ASSESSMENT
QUESTIONNAIRE (SEE CASES 10, 11 AND 12 ON INTERACTIVE DISC)
The FMS (Functional Mobility Scale) and the Functional Assessment Questionnaire (FAQ)
were discussed in the Classification Chapter (2.6) (Novacheck et al. 2000, Graham et al.
2004). The former is a 6-level ordinal scale that rates the mobility of children with CP over
three distances according to their need for assistive devices. The latter is a 10-level parent-
report of walking that encompasses a range of walking abilities. These were designed to be
responsive to change and can be used to document the attainment of mobility and function,
the deterioration or improvement in these skills after intervention, or other changes
consequent on growth and development. The FAQ is a good measure of parental perspective
but unlike the FMS does not consider the assistive devices required for mobility. However,
it is a good indicator of how the child is functioning in the community.

Classification of the child using the GMFCS and measures of function using the FMS
and FAQ provides a very clear picture of the gross motor function and mobility level of a
child with CP. The three together provide valuable information of the functional abilities
of the child. The FMS and the FAQ can be completed quickly by a physical therapist and
parents respectively during visits to the gait laboratory and are useful tools for both clinical
management and clinical research.

The FMS and FAQ for three children pre-SEMLS and at 3 months, 6 months, 9 months,
1 year and 2 years post-SEMLS are displayed in Table 6.1.1. These data highlight the
sensitivity and utility of these measures. In the cases of DB and MP we can see that both
measures demonstrate deterioration in functional mobility initially postoperatively with a
return in mobility seen over time.

The case of HM is interesting as these measures show some counterintuitive results. HM
initially was classified as a GMFCS level III using a walker for mobility and we can see the
FAQ results were quite high and showed that she was functioning very well in the
community with the walker. Postoperatively, however, as her function has improved, she
has chosen to walk without a mobility aid and is now rated as at FMS 5,5,5 and at GMFCS
level II. We can see that her FAQ score for community ambulation is lower, because she
has chosen to walk independently. To function in the community at the same FAQ score,
she would have to use balance aids, which would then put her on a GMFCS III level.
This highlights that these measures, though measuring similar aspects of mobility, are
not measuring the exact same construct and should be used in conjunction with each other
to give a full overall picture of the child's functional mobility. You can have children at the
same GMFCS level but with quite different scores on the FMS, and children who are using
a walking device of some kind can still function as highly in the community – as is shown
by the FAQ score – as children who are walking independently without assistive devices.

SELF-REPORTED MEASURES OF FUNCTION AND HEALTH-RELATED QUALITY
OF LIFE IN CHILDREN AND YOUNG PEOPLE WITH CEREBRAL PALSY
In recent years the assessment of quality of life has become a major goal in health management including children with CP. A number of generic and specific instruments have been
developed which address aspects of health, functioning and quality of life. The Child

TABLE 6.1.1
Functional Mobility Scale (FMS) and Functional Assessment Questionnaire (FAQ) scores for three children before and after single-event multilevel surgery

Clinical cases		FMS			FAQ
		5 m	50 m	500 m	
DB (Video Case 10)					
GMFCS III	Pre-SEMLS	4	2	1	6
	3 months	4	1	1	5
	6 months	4	2	1	6
	9 months	4	2	1	6
	1 year	4	2	1	6
	2 years	5	2	1	6
HM (Video Case 11)					
GMFCS II	Pre-SEMLS	C	2	1	8
	3 months	2	2	1	8
	6 months	2	2	1	8
	9 months	5	5	1	6
	1 year	5	5	1	6
	2 years	5	5	5	7
MP HM (Video Case 12)					
GMFCS II	Pre-SEMLS	5	5	5	9
	3 months	4	2	1	6
	6 months	5	5	5	7
	9 months	5	5	5	8
	1 year	5	5	5	9
	2 years	5	5	5	9

Health Questionnaire (CHQ) is a widely used tool and is not disease specific (Waters et al. 2000a, b, 2006). It has the advantage that the scores of children with CP can be compared to children with normal health or with other disease conditions in which data have been gathered. The Pediatric Outcomes Data Collection Instrument (PODCI) (Daltroy et al. 1998) has a more musculoskeletal focus and contains several domains directly relevant to children with CP and gait problems. Although some information exists on the use of both of these instruments in children with CP, the responsiveness to change and the value of using these as outcome instruments is not yet fully established. It is also the case that neither can be considered to be a true quality of life measure. In addition the perception of chronic physical disability varies from family to family in terms of its impact on health. This may lead to anomalous responses when the parents of a child with spastic diplegia complete the physical functioning domains of both the CHQ and the PODCI.

CLINICAL CASE: DB (CASE 10 ON INTERACTIVE DISC)
DB, an 8-year-old boy with severe spastic diplegia, was at GMFCS level III. He ambulated using a posterior walker, had severe contractures at the hip, knee and ankle/foot level bilaterally. His mobility was very limited, and he had pain and discomfort in his knees and feet.

He was enrolled at our center in a trial of multilevel surgery in which we used the CHQ as part of our outcome measures. At baseline, his parents reported that his physical functioning was 100. After a successful program of multilevel surgery in which he was able to walk for short distances independently, he no longer required a posterior walker but used sticks for community distances. His parents reported at 12-month follow-up that his physical functioning was now 72.

Our experience with the use of these measures is that some parents and children have adjusted to physical disability, limitations in gross motor function and gait dysfunction so successfully that they no longer consider it to be a 'health problem'. Their responses when using self-reported measures such as the CHQ and PODCI may be at variance with the responses of other parents and children who view their physical disability in a different light.

Neither the CHQ nor the PODCI are true quality-of-life measures. Recently developed and reported tools include the Pediatric Quality of Life Inventory (PedsQL) and the Cerebral Palsy Quality of Life Questionnaire for Children (CPQoL-Child). The CPQoL-Child is a specific quality-of-life measure developed for children with cerebral palsy and is showing promise in initial testing. However its responsiveness to physical interventions such as gait improvement surgery is not yet known.

In summary, we found that the FMS and FAQ are extremely useful and practical tools in the longitudinal assessment of ambulant children with CP. We use these tools routinely in both clinical management and clinical research. Questionnaires such as the CHQ, PODCI and CPQoL-Child (Waters et al. 2006) are being used in our outcome studies. At this point the responsiveness and the correlation with other objective measures of gait and function are not fully established.

The diagnostic matrix

Having established the context of the natural history of gross motor function by the gross motor curves and GMFCS, it is now appropriate to consider how these tools may be incorporated with other forms of assessment especially in relation to major interventions such as gait improvement surgery. Major interventions, such as selective dorsal rhizotomy and multilevel orthopaedic surgery, are designed to improve gait and functioning in children with cerebral palsy. Ideally these major interventions are most appropriately conducted following the most comprehensive and objective assessment possible. This should include instrumented gait analysis because clinical assessments do not offer sufficient objectivity, validity, reliability or the volume of information which instrumented gait analysis can offer. However we recognize that not all children in all centers have access to IGA although we believe this to be the gold standard for evaluation. In addition, some children are unable to complete instrumented gait analysis because of reasons such as intellectual disability, behavioral disturbance or severe physical impairment. In such cases, we believe VGA to be a useful substitute although clearly inferior to instrumented gait analysis.

Neither IGA nor VGA stand in isolation but are best considered to be part of a 'diagnostic matrix' as described by Davids and colleagues (2003). They described a diagnostic matrix consisting of clinical history, physical examination, diagnostic imaging,

IGA and examination under anesthesia as five components of a diagnostic matrix useful in clinical decision-making, in relation to gait correction surgery in children with CP. We have added the routine use of the GMFCS, FMS, FAQ and sagittal gait pattern classification as part of the diagnostic matrix in our center. Each of the modalities described by Davids and colleagues (2003) and those utilized in the Hugh Williamson Gait Laboratory contributes a different but key component of the understanding of gait dysfunction. This type of comprehensive evaluation is able to generate a list of gait abnormalities, suggest underlying causative factors and point towards management strategies. The systematic application of the same tools at intervals following multilevel surgery is able to objectively describe outcomes and contribute to outcome studies and clinical research findings.

CLINICAL HISTORY AND STANDARDIZED PHYSICAL EXAMINATION (Fig. 6.1.6)
The necessities of a careful, complete clinical history and thorough, standardized physical examination, employing both standard and instrumented methods of measuring strength, were discussed in detail in Chapter 3.1, and will not be reiterated here. Parental expectations were discussed briefly there as well. It is worth noting, however, that although the majority of children who undergo multilevel surgery will have significant improvement in gait patterns and measures of physical functioning, it is likely that their GMFCS level will remain

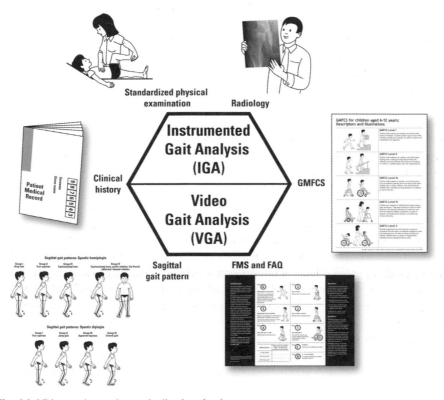

Fig. 6.1.6 Diagnostic matrix standardized evaluation.

stable. Consequently, if there is an unspoken expectation that a child at GMFCS level III or IV will become an independent ambulator, the scene is set for disappointment and failure. The specific expectations of the child and family can be formalized in the context of goal attainment scaling.

In summary the clinical history is obtained by a careful review of all current and previous medical records complemented by an up to date interview of the child in the context of his family or care providers. Associated medical comorbidities and the response to previous interventions are also crucial to the planning of gait correction surgery. Given the arduous and prolonged nature of rehabilitation after multilevel surgery, sensitive investigation of the social history and family dynamics is crucial to the planning of a successful gait multilevel surgery program. An explicit dialogue in relation to goals and expectations committed to a written record to be shared with the family and referring agency is also extremely valuable.

Prior to the physical examination, it is important to observe the patient's gait in a systematic manner. This can be done as either a purely clinical observation of gait or as part of VGA. The observed gait pattern can be classified on purely visual grounds using the classifications for gait patterns in hemiplegia or diplegia. If this is done prior to the physical examination, it is likely that the examination will be more targeted and possibly more reliable. For example, if the child with hemiplegia is observed to have a type IV pattern, a key part of the physical examination will be to assess the presence of fixed deformities around the hip including asymmetry of femoral neck anteversion. Although this should be detected in a good-quality routine physical examination, it is certainly helpful to know which areas are worth concentrating on.

Gross Motor Function Classification System
The importance of the GMFCS has been described above and is repeated here as part of the diagnostic matrix. In our application of the diagnostic matrix the GMFCS is considered twice. It is part of the clinical history where it is often included in the documentation as part of the child's referral. It is also recorded after gait and gross motor function have been observed and VGA has been completed. There is usually a good agreement between the GMFCS level as part of the gait laboratory referral and that recorded by the physical therapist evaluating the patient. However this is not always the case and cannot be taken for granted.

Functional Mobility Scale and Functional Assessment Questionnaire
We record FMS and FAQ at every visit to the gait laboratory irrespective of whether the child is having a full IGA prior to surgery or a VGA at intervals following intervention. The information from FMS and FAQ are complementary and very useful in tracking progress of children through the rehabilitation process especially in the first year after major interventions such as selective dorsal rhizotomy, intrathecal baclofen pumps and multilevel orthopaedic surgery.

Sagittal gait patterns
We believe that classification of sagittal gait patterns initially from VGA and then from the information from IGA (sagittal gait kinematics) to be very important. The amount of

information from IGA is extensive and prior to the consideration of the details of each kinematic and kinetic plot, we think it is helpful to consider which broad category the child's gait pattern is part of. The classification of sagittal gait patterns in spastic hemiplegia (Winters et al. 1987) is a valid and reliable tool which helps in framing logical management strategies. The sagittal gait classification described by Rodda and Graham (2004) can be useful in planning interventions in spastic diplegia. Both gait patterns suggest common patterns of musculoskeletal deformity, target muscles which are likely to be contracted and may need correction. In addition there are suggested correlations with the use of orthoses, e.g. a posterior leaf spring or hinged ankle–foot orthosis (AFO) in true equinus versus a ground reaction AFO in crouch gait.

Standardized radiography

Radiography is important in the diagnostic matrix as high proportions of children with CP have skeletal deformities including torsional deformities of long bones and instability of the hip and foot specifically the subtalar and mid tarsal joints. Radiology of the hips, including plain radiographs, supplemented by computed tomography measurements of femoral torsion and tibial torsion can be very useful as additional information in the planning of multilevel surgery. The assessment of foot deformity by analysis of weight bearing radiographs is also particularly important. Weight bearing radiographs can be analyzed by the measurement of a series of key radiological indices which can help identify segmental malalignments in the hindfoot, midfoot and forefoot in a systematic manner. This contributes greatly to the analysis of segmental foot deformity and the planning of intervention. Instrumented gait analysis most typically interprets the foot as a rigid segment and does not provide detailed information on segmental malalignments within the foot. Until better foot models are in routine use, standardized weightbearing radiographs remain the cornerstone of analysis of deformities within the foot. This information can be augmented by dynamic pedobarography which is in use in a number of laboratories. Pedobarography provides detailed information on the force distribution on the plantar aspect of the foot during gait. In conjunction with the other components of IGA and weightbearing radiographs, this can augment the assessment of deformities of the foot and ankle at presentation and also provide supplementary methods of evaluation of the outcome after corrective and reconstructive surgery to the foot and ankle.

Video gait analysis

VGA is a component of IGA and can also be used when IGA is either not appropriate or not available. VGA can therefore be considered as the core objective modality of the diagnostic matrix in the absence of IGA. We found VGA to be particularly useful for the objective documentation of younger children commencing botulinum toxin type A therapy. At this stage they are too small, too young and uncooperative for IGA. It is also useful for the selection and monitoring of the use of AFOs and for the monitoring of children after major intervention such as selective dorsal rhizotomy (SDR) or multilevel surgery.

Serial VGA recordings provide an objective measure of gait and functioning. It is useful in confirming GMFCS levels, changes in FMS and FAQ responses and the confirmation of sagittal gait patterns. Testing of the reliability of sagittal gait pattern classification using video gait analysis confirms satisfactory reliability. However, the reliability is not as high as when instrumented gait analysis and sagittal plane kinematics are available.

We do not consider VGA an adequate substitute for IGA when decisions regarding major intervention such as selective dorsal rhizotomy or multilevel surgery have to be made. Nor is VGA adequate for outcome measurement in clinical trials of gait correction surgery.

Instrumented gait analysis

Techniques of measurement during IGA have been covered extensively elsewhere in this book and will only be summarized here. The capture of 3-dimensional kinematics, kinetics and dynamic electromyography is the core of IGA and provides a comprehensive description of joint movements, moments and powers and muscle timing, all of which are highly relevant to decision making in the management of gait disorders in children with CP. The extensive information retrieved from IGA is interpreted in the light of physical examination as well as examination under anesthetic.

The objectivity and relative freedom from bias of IGA is a factor of major importance in establishing objective outcomes. We strongly support the use of instrumented gait analysis, and a composite measure of gait such as the Gillette Gait Index (GGI) (Schutte et al. 2000), or the newly developed Gait Deviation Index, as the most convenient method to describe outcomes, of prospective cohort studies as well as randomized trials of multilevel surgery in children with CP. At our center colleagues have developed the Movement Analysis Profile (MAP, Fig. 6.1.7) and overall Gait Profile Score (GPS) (Baker et al. 2008). The MAP has been developed to summarize much of the complex information contained within the kinematic data arising from 3-dimensional gait analysis. It is a bar chart in which each column represents the root mean square (RMS) difference between each clinically relevant kinematic variable for a particular subject and the average values of that variable from people without pathology calculated over the gait cycle.

This represents a clinical meaningful measure of differences in gait variables as it measures difference in degrees and may be of value both clinically and in the research setting to evaluate change following surgery.

These measures evaluate the quality of gait in relation to normal gait. However, they do not give us information regarding how functional the gait pattern is. The use of temporospatial measures such as walking speed and stride length in conjunction with these measures may give more information regarding functional walking (Baker et al. 2008, Thomason et al. 2008).

The following case study illustrates the use of outcome measures in an integrated approach using the diagnostic matrix to evaluate a child's function both at baseline and after intervention.

CASE STUDY: MH (CASE 13 ON INTERACTIVE DISC)
MH, a boy with spastic diplegia, GMFCS level II, was referred to the gait laboratory for the evaluation of gait and function prior to multilevel surgery at age 7 years 8 months.

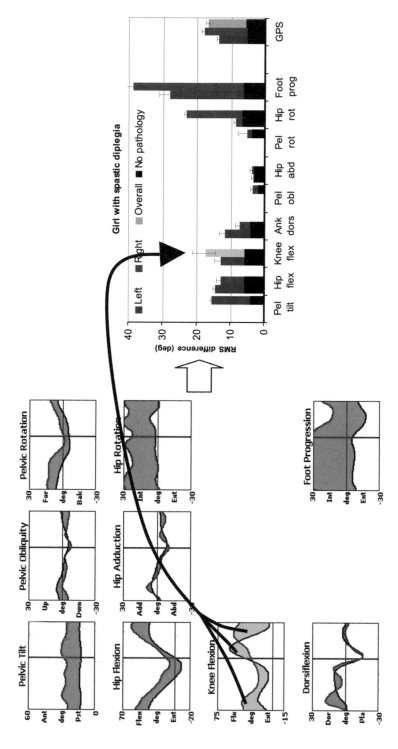

Fig. 6.1.7 Movement Analysis Profile.

His parents' stated concerns were intoed gait, twisted legs, inability to wear AFOs and deteriorating function. There were concerns about increasing falls at school, requiring use of a posterior walker for safety reasons. Although he was recorded as functioning at GMFCS level II, his FMS score was 5,2,5 and his FAQ score was 8.

The principal findings on physical examination were

- increased internal rotation and decreased external rotation at both hips, left hip worse than right hip
- increased femoral neck anteversion, bilaterally
- reduced left hip abduction
- bilateral equinus contractures, left worse than right, affecting mainly gastrocnemius
- reduced popliteal angles and hamstring tightness bilaterally, right worse than left.
- hip-extensor and hip-abductor weakness
- height 119.2 cm, weight 20.8 kg.

MH underwent instrumented gait analysis and his three dimensional kinematics are displayed in Figure 6.1.8.

Following a discussion with MH and his parents, a multilevel surgery program was recommended to include the following procedures:

- bilateral varus derotation osteotomies of the proximal femur with greater rotational correction on the left compared to the right
- bilateral psoas lengthening over the brim of the pelvis
- bilateral adductor longus lengthening
- bilateral Strayer calf-lengthening plus soleal fascial lengthening on the left side only.

Concern was expressed regarding MH's weight and on discussion with his family it was decided to refer him to a developmental pediatrician and pediatric gastroenterologist to assess his nutritional status and to see if he could gain weight prior to surgery. The delay in proceeding with multilevel surgery was also used to institute a program of progressive resistance strength training. MH had a further comprehensive gait laboratory evaluation 12 months later. At this time his parents expressed concern regarding further deterioration in function with MH needing to use a posterior walker for the majority of the time, especially at school. His FMS score had deteriorated to 5, 2, N but FAQ was still 8. Further physical examination revealed the following problems:

- fixed flexion deformity at both hips
- further increase in hip internal rotation and reduction in external rotation at both hips, left more than right
- a further reduction in the range of hip abduction bilaterally
- height 123.4 cm, weight 22.85 kg.

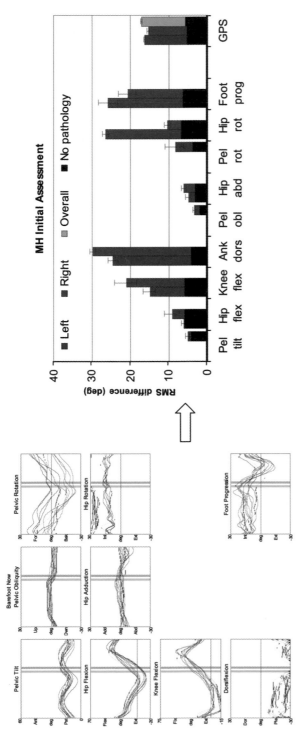

Fig. 6.1.8 MH: kinematic data and Movement Analysis Profile – initial assessment.

His gait kinematics showed a substantial deterioration in sagittal kinematics affecting the left lower limb with cross-plane involvement to both coronal and transverse planes. Figure 6.1.9 shows the measures used in his evaluation prior to surgery.

Radiography. An anteroposterior radiograph of the hips showed mild uncovering and interruption of Shenton's arch bilaterally, left worse than right. Weightbearing radiographs of the feet showed a fixed equinovarus contracture of the left foot and a relatively normal right foot. These images are displayed in Figure 6.1.10.

The surgical prescription following the second evaluation was as follows:

- bilateral proximal femoral varus derotation osteotomies
- bilateral psoas lengthening over the brim of the pelvis
- bilateral percutaneous lengthening of adductor longus
- left medial hamstring lengthening with transfer of semitendinosus to the adductor tubercle
- left gastrocsoleus lengthening (Strayer plus soleal fascial lengthening) combined with intramuscular lengthening of tibialis posterior
- right gastrocnemius lengthening.

MH spent 5 days in hospital after his multilevel surgery and made a satisfactory initial postoperative recovery. He was discharged in below knee plaster-casts and with removable knee-immobilizers. He commenced weightbearing as tolerated 3 weeks after surgery, and 6 weeks after surgery his plaster-casts were removed and AFOs were fitted. He attended the gait laboratory at 3, 6, 9, 12 and 24 months postoperatively. The assessments at 3, 6 and 9 months included VGA as well as the other components of the diagnostic matrix. At 12 and 24 months postoperatively he had IGA (Figs 6.1.11, 12). The serial measurements made at 3 monthly intervals following surgery were an important guide to orthotic and rehabilitation management. At the 12 month review after multilevel surgery MH's gait pattern was noted to have improved considerably but a mild persistent knee flexion deformity was noted on the right side which was corrected by right medial hamstring lengthening and transfer of semitendinosus to the adductor tubercle at the time of blade plate removal. This resulted in a further improvement in gait parameters at 24 months after multilevel surgery.

Serial changes in physical function (FMS), strength (leg press), gross motor function (GMFM) and self-reported physical functioning (CHQ) are shown in Figure 6.1.13. The FMS shows the deterioration in gait in the 12-month interval between initial assessment and multilevel surgery. A further deterioration is noted at 3, 6 and 9 months after multilevel surgery with a return to pre-surgery status by 12 months and a significant improvement at both 18 and 24 months after multilevel surgery. The leg press results show that strength improved during the progressive resistance strength training program in the year before multilevel surgery, deteriorated after multilevel surgery, returning to baseline at 9 months postoperatively. There was a further deterioration at 12 months before an improvement to better than before noted at 24 months. GMFM showed little change until 24 months postoperatively when a significant gain of 6% was found. Self-reported physical function using the CHQ showed a progressive improvement at each interval.

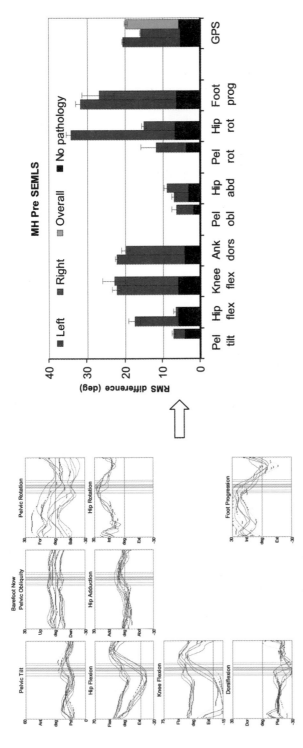

Fig. 6.1.9 MH: before single-event multilevel surgery (SEMLS). RMS, root mean square; GPS, Gait Profile Score.

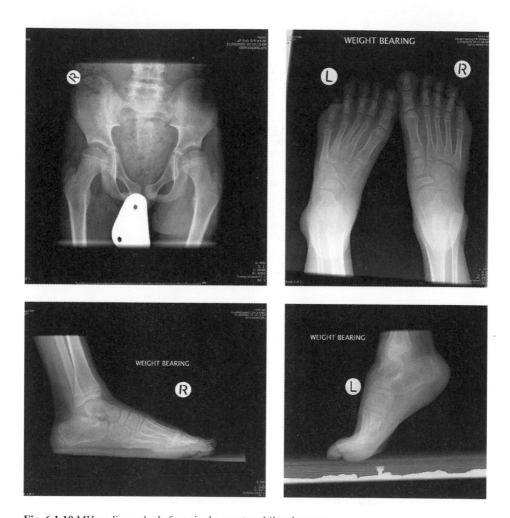

Fig. 6.1.10 MH: radiography before single-event multilevel surgery.

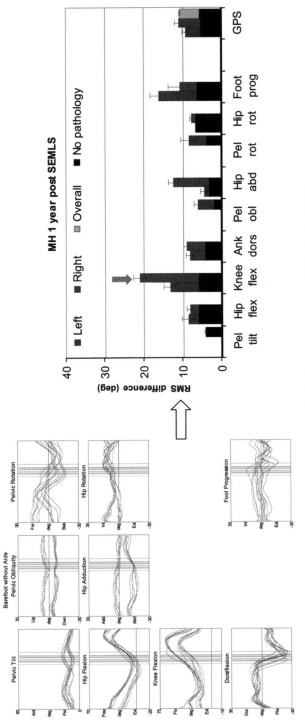

Fig. 6.1.11 MH: 1 year after single-event multilevel surgery (SEMLS). RMS, root mean square; GPS, Gait Profile Score.

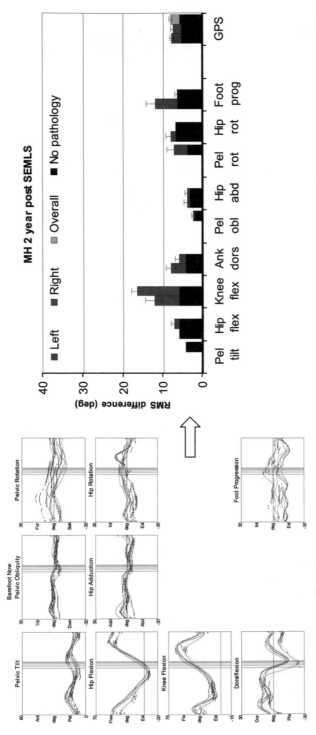

Fig. 6.1.12 MH: 2 years after single-event multilevel surgery (SEMLS). RMS, root mean square; GPS, Gait Profile Score.

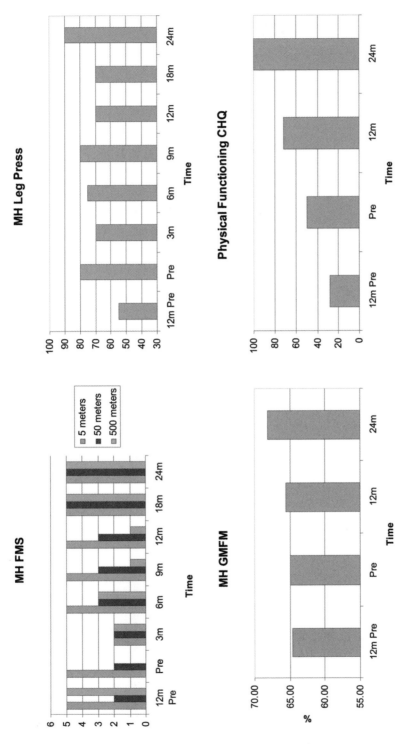

Fig. 6.1.13 MH: serial measurements of function before and after single-event multilevel surgery. FMS, Functional Mobility Scale; GMFM, Gross Motor Function Measure; CHQ, Child Health Questionnaire

603

REFERENCES

Baker R, Tirosh O, McGinley J, Graham K (2008) The Movement Analysis Profile (MAP) and the Gait Profile Score (GPS). *Gait Posture* **28** (Suppl 2): S7.

Daltroy LH, Liang MH, Fossel AH, Goldberg M (1998) The POSNA Pediatric Musculoskeletal Functional Health Questionnaire: report on reliability, validity and sensitivity to change. The Pediatric Outcomes Instrument Development Group. *J Pediatr Orthop* **18**: 561–71.

Davids JR, Õunpuu S, DeLuca PA, Davis RB (2003) Optimization of walking ability of children with cerebral palsy. *J Bone Joint Surg Am* **85**: 2224–34.

Graham HK, Harvey A, Rodda J, Nattrass GR, Pirpiris M (2004) The Functional Mobility Scale (FMS). *J Pediatr Orthop* **24**: 514–20.

Harvey A, Robin J, Morris ME, Graham HK, Baker R (2008) A systematic review of measures of activity limitation for children with cerebral palsy. *Dev Med Child Neurol* **50**: 190–8.

Kirshner B, Guyatt G (1985) A methodological framework for assessing health indices. *J Chron Dis* **38**: 26–7.

McCormick A, Brien M, Plourde J, Wood E, Rosenbaum P, McLean J (2007) Stability of the Gross Motor Function Classification System in adults with cerebral palsy. *Dev Med Child Neurol* **49**: 265–9.

Majnemer A, Mazer B (2004) New directions in the outcome evaluation of children with cerebral palsy. *Semin Pediatr Neurol* **11**: 11–17.

Morris C, Kurinczuk JJ, Fitzpatrick R (2005) Child or family assessed measures of activity performance and participation for children with cerebral palsy: a structured review. *Child Care Health Dev* **31**: 397–407.

NCMRR (1993) *Research Plan for the Center for Medical Rehabilitation.* NIH Publication Nos 93–3509, p 23–26. US Department of Health and Human Services, Public Health Service, National Institutes of Health, National Institute of Child Health and Human Development.

Novacheck TF, Stout JL, Tervo R (2000) Reliability and validity of the Gillette Functional Assessment Questionnaire as an outcome measure in children with walking disabilities. *J Pediatr Orthop* **20**: 75–81.

Palisano R, Rosenbaum P, Walter S, Russell D, Wood E, Galuppi B (1997) Development and reliability of a system to classify gross motor function in children with cerebral palsy. *Dev Med Child Neurol* **39**: 214–23.

Rodda JM, Graham HK, Carson L, Galea MP, Wolfe R (2004). Sagittal gait patterns in spastic diplegia. *J Bone Joint Surg Br* **86**: 251–8.

Rodda JM, Graham HK, Nattrass GR, Galea MP, Baker R, Wolfe R (2006) Correction of severe crouch gait in patients with spastic diplegia with use of multilevel orthopaedic surgery. *J Bone Joint Surg Am* **88**: 2653–64.

Rosenbaum PL, Walter SD, Hanna SE, Palisano RJ, Russell DJ, Raina P, Wood E, Bartlett DJ, Galuppi BE (2002) Prognosis for gross motor function in cerebral palsy: Creation of motor development curves. *JAMA* **288**: 1357–63.

Rosenbaum PL, Livingston MH, Palisano RJ, Galuppi BE, Russell DJ (2007) Quality of life and health-related quality of life of adolescents with cerebral palsy. *Dev Med Child Neurol* **49**: 516–21.

Sakzewski L, Boyd R, Ziviani J (2007) Clinimetric properties of participation measures for 5 to 13 year old children with cerebral palsy: a systematic review. *Dev Med Child Neurol* **49**: 232–40.

Schutte LM, Narayanan U, Stout JL, Selber P, Gage JR, Schwartz MH (2000) An index for quantifying deviations from normal gait. *Gait Posture* **11**: 25–31.

Thomason P, Yu X, Baker R, Graham HK (2008) Evaluating the outcome of single event multilevel surgery: find the way use the MAP (movement analysis profile). *Gait Posture* **28** *(Suppl 2): S86–7.*

Waters E, Salmon L, Wake M, Hesketh K, Wright M (2000a) The Child Health Questionnaire in Australia: reliability, validity and population means. *Aust NZ J Publ Health* **24**: 207–10.

Waters E, Salmon L, Wake M (2000b) The parent-form child health questionnaire in Australia: comparison of reliability, validity, structure, and norms. *J Ped Psychol* **25**: 381–91.

Waters E, Davis E, Boyd R, Reddihough D, Mackinnon A, Graham HK, Lo SK, Wolfe R, Stevenson R, Bjornson K, Blair E, Ravens-Sieberer U (2006) *Cerebral Palsy Quality of Life Questionnaire for Children (CP QOL-Child) Manual.* Melbourne: Deakin University.

Winters TF, Gage JR, Hicks R (1987) Gait patterns in spastic hemiplegia in children and young adults. *J Bone Joint Surg Am* **69**: 437–41.

World Health Organization (2001) *International Classification of Functioning, Disability and Health. (Short Version).* Geneva: World Health Organization p 121–60.

6.2
CONSEQUENCES OF INTERVENTIONS

Pam Thomason and H. Kerr Graham

Interventions to improve gait and functioning in children with cerebral palsy (CP) are inevitably followed by consequences which include both intended outcomes and unintended outcomes. These include complications and adverse events following surgery which may be noted acutely in the postoperative period as well as more subtle long term effects on musculoskeletal health and functioning. Physical interventions can be considered in three principal domains: spasticity interventions, orthopaedic surgery and strengthening (Fig. 6.2.1).

The effects of these interventions occur against the background of a changing natural history. An understanding of the natural history is important because if the individual patient's baseline is changing, the consequences of an intervention have to be understood in the light of that changing natural history. The natural history can also be usefully considered in three main domains: growth and development, gross motor function and gait.

Growth and development
The majority of our surgical interventions to improve gait and function in children with CP are performed between the ages of 6 and 12 years. Our standard postoperative monitoring program is a video gait assessment (VGA) in the Gait Laboratory at 3, 6 and 9 months after multilevel surgery. Instrumented gait analysis (IGA) and a full biomechanical assessment are performed at 12 months after single-event multilevel surgery (SEMLS). We then revert to a VGA 2, 3 and 4 years postoperatively, with a further IGA 5 and 10 years post-SEMLS. The majority of children who have a 5-year assessment will have been through the pubertal growth spurt and undergone dramatic changes in body proportions, height and weight between their 1- and 5-year post-multilevel surgery assessments. An understanding of these changes and their implications for gait, musculoskeletal health and functioning is important. Dramatic increases in height and weight may heighten the impact of underlying weakness. Post multilevel surgery interventions to correct leg-length inequality, angular deformity or residual flexion deformity around the knee must be carefully timed in respect of the pubertal growth spurt. The pubertal growth spurt, in effect, represents a 'last chance' to employ growth plate surgery in children with CP who have residual musculoskeletal deformities amenable to this type of intervention. Our understandings of the magnitude and timing of changes in body proportions and their relationship to

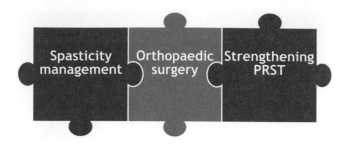

Fig. 6.2.1 The principal domains of physical interventions for cerebral palsy. PRST, progressive resistance strength training.

the pubertal growth spurt and skeletal maturation have been enhanced by many studies. Dimeglio (2005) has synthesized this material and added much original material to enhance our understanding of growth and its relevance to orthopaedic issues.

Systematic, accurate measurements of height, weight and bone age are important in the systematic follow-up of children with CP before and after intervention.

Standing height is the global marker of growth and is the most valuable index in the gait laboratory. Bodyweight is also important in the assessment of the child with CP. Children with spastic diplegia associated with preterm birth are often underweight in comparison to their typically developing peers. Hyperkinetic movement disorders may result in more calories being consumed and children with CP may follow quite different growth trajectories. Identification of significant nutritional deficiencies before surgical interventions may be very important. Nutritional supplementation may allow improvements in children who are underweight, promoting better healing and function postoperatively. However, the CP population is also being affected by the obesity epidemic in developed countries. The identification of excess weight gain and its impact on gait and function in individuals with significant motor deficits is also very important. We collect these data routinely in the gait laboratory at each of the major intervals outlined above.

Skeletal maturity and the pubertal growth spurt in children with CP
In children with CP, as in pediatric orthopaedic conditions in general, chronological age is of limited usefulness and everything depends on bone age. About 50% of children with normal motor development have a bone age that is significantly different from their chronologic age. In CP, variations are even more frequent, more marked and probably related to Gross Motor Function Classification System (GMFCS) level. In addition children with CP are often bone age mosaics, that is, bone age determined from different skeletal sites (for example the wrist, elbow and pelvis) may show differing results. Given the importance of knowing where a child is on the ascending limb of the pubertal growth spurt, the closure of the triradiate cartilage and the olecranon epiphysis are more useful than the progression of the Risser sign, which occurs in the descending limb of the pubertal growth spurt (Figs 6.2.2, 3).

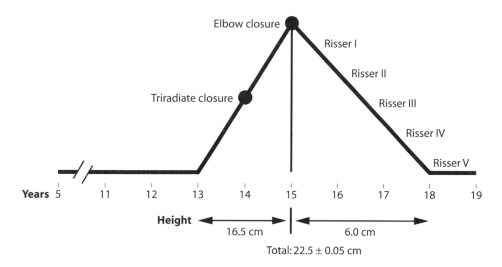

Fig. 6.2.2 The pubertal growth spurt and skeletal maturation in typically developing boys.

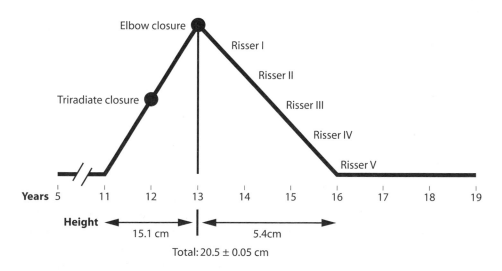

Fig. 6.2.3 The pubertal growth spurt and skeletal maturation in typically developing girls.

Given the wide variation noted in the onset of puberty and its relationship to skeletal maturation in children with CP, systematic measurements of height, weight, and bone age and the involvement of colleagues with expertise is strongly recommended.

Natural history: gait

In typically developing children, independent walking is achieved around the age of 12 months but there is a wide variation. The toddler's gait is typically immature and develops progressively to the normal adult pattern at about age 5 years. There is then a long period of relative stability in gait parameters before age-related changes in old age. The development of gait in children with CP is substantially different. In early childhood, delay in achieving gross motor milestones is one of the most common features of CP and often the principal finding leading to diagnosis. In general, the development of gait relates to both the topographical type of CP and the gross motor function level. Children with hemiplegia have relatively mild delay in gaining independent walking unless they are compromised by severe intellectual disability or uncontrolled epilepsy. Children with mild spastic diplegia typically gain independent walking between the ages of 2 and 4 years. These children will function at GMFCS level I or II. Children at GMFCS level III do not attain independent walking except for very short distances and remain dependent on an assistive device throughout their lives (Palisano et al. 1997).

Less is known about the maturation of gait in children with CP but it is clear that gait maturation is delayed and variable across GMFCS levels. However, once the early childhood plateau of gross motor function has been achieved, a number of studies using IGA have found that there is a measurable deterioration in gait parameters without intervention (Bell et al. 2002). Some of the trends which have been noted include decrease in walking velocity, increasing time spent in double support, decreased range of motion in the sagittal plane with increasing stiffness at the hip and knee and a gradual shift from equinus through neutral to calcaneus at the ankle. It is therefore very important for parents, therapist and surgeons to realize that the child with CP who is being considered for multilevel surgery is already on a slow downward trajectory. Against this background, maintenance of gait at the current level might be considered to be an improvement over natural history. Improvements in gait parameters compared to baseline may be an even greater gain.

Natural history: gross motor function

As noted previously, the extensive studies by Rosenbaum and colleagues (2002), with the generation of gross motor curves, have given vital information illustrating the rapid progression of gross motor development in younger children with CP, followed by a plateau in childhood. Much less information is known and little has been published concerning changes in gross motor function in later childhood, adolescence and adult life. However, it is of significance that the recently developed descriptors in the GMFCS for the age band 12–18 years allows deterioration in gross motor function, especially at GMFCS levels II, III and IV. This is illustrated in Figure 6.2.4 where the gross motor curves have been extended to age 18 years and the descriptors for GMFCS at age 6–12 and 12–18 have been

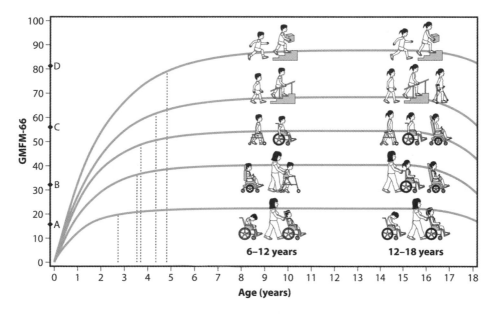

Fig. 6.2.4 Gross-motor curves for GMFCS level extended to 18 years.

added in conjunction with extrapolation of the gross motor curves to a postulated deterioration after the pubertal growth spurt.

The understanding of gross motor curves has the potential to transform communication, the understanding of locomotor prognosis and the counseling of children and adolescents with CP and their families. Again as noted in the discussion of the natural history of gait, if the natural history of gross motor function is a trend downwards, then maintenance of gross motor function at a baseline level can be considered an improvement over natural history. At this time, the benefits of SEMLS in relation to the natural history of deterioration have not been established. As we continue to gather 5- and 10-year follow-up data, we note a trend suggesting that children with optimal biomechanical alignment after multilevel surgery tend to show stability of GMFCS levels as well as Functional Mobility Scale (FMS) levels.

Consequences of musculoskeletal surgery
The consequences of musculoskeletal surgery, in particular multilevel surgery, can be considered along temporal lines as acute, intermediate and long term.

ACUTE CONSEQUENCES OF MULTILEVEL SURGERY
The acute postoperative management of multilevel surgery requires a highly skilled multidisciplinary team in which clear communication and role delineation are important.

Good postoperative management may set the scene for rapid healing, early recovery of function, avoidance of anxiety and depression and a long-term successful functional

609

outcome. Failures in acute postoperative management, including inadequate pain management and acute postoperative complications, may result in high levels of stress and anxiety in the patient and the immediate family. This may set the scene for delayed recovery of function and long term suboptimal outcomes. A detailed discussion of perioperative management is outside of the scope of this discussion but the principles include optimal pain management (including routine use of epidural infusions), maintenance of lower limb alignment and muscle length, early weightbearing and an individually structured program to regain function and independence.

Adverse events related to surgery include superficial and deep wound infections, delayed union or malunion of osteotomies, inadequate correction, or overcorrection of fixed musculoskeletal deformities.

THE FIRST YEAR AFTER MULTILEVEL SURGERY

Management of children through the first year following multilevel surgery is crucial to long-term outcomes. Management in this period relates to GMFCS level, the surgical program and the goals of the intervention. It is much easier to conduct and monitor the rehabilitation program when the intervention has been preceded by a comprehensive evaluation of gait and function and explicit goal setting. Take the example of a child at GMFCS level III who ambulates only with the use of a posterior walker, with hip sub-luxation and fixed equinus deformities precluding the use of ankle–foot orthoses (AFOs). Specific goals may be graduation to a lower level of support, stabilization of hip subluxation and reconstructive surgery to the foot and ankle to permit comfortable wearing of orthoses. The child and the family may have an unstated goal of achieving independent walking. This should be sensitively discussed and realistic resetting of goals achieved, i.e. better reduction in the level of support from a posterior walker to Canadian crutches or single point sticks may well be achievable but independent walking, except over very short distances, may not be an achievable goal.

The child, the family and the rehabilitation team must plan for increased dependency and decreased function in the first year after multilevel surgery. The increased dependency and subsequent return to presurgical functional levels vary specifically for the individual but more generally depending on GMFCS. Paradoxically the increase in dependency and decrease in function is more pronounced at the higher GMFCS levels. It is also greater after more extensive programs which include multiple bony procedures. This is not to denigrate the usefulness of bony reconstructive surgery. Rotational osteotomies are probably the most beneficial component of SEMLS in the long term. It is simply to point out that multilevel soft-tissue surgery can be accompanied by very early weight bearing and return of function. Multiple rotational osteotomies require a longer period of non-weightbearing and a slower recovery to full weightbearing and independence. Previous work from our center has shown that the level of support increases after surgery and recovers slowly back to baseline over the course of about 12 months.

Older children and adolescents at GMFCS levels I and II have a high level of function and independence. They have a greater loss of independence and increase in dependency after multilevel surgery than those at GMFCS level III.

Children functioning at GMFCS level III show greater improvement in function and mobility post-SEMLS and have shown large improvements by 12 months post-surgery and continued to improve at 24 months post-surgery. Children functioning at GMFCS level II generally take up to 24 months to show functional improvement.

At GMFCS level III children and adolescents are dependent on a walking device prior to surgery and are able to return to their baseline function faster than those at GMFCS levels I and II who prior to surgery walked without aids. Changes to assistive devices are best monitored by the FMS. Examples of changes in mobility following surgery for children functioning at GMFCS levels II and III are shown in Figure 6.2.5.

We have previously characterized the decrease in function and increase in dependency after multilevel surgery in a study in which we examined the need for assistive devices, walking speed and energy cost of walking at 3 monthly intervals in a group of children after multilevel surgery (Olesch 2003). In general, we found a marked increase in dependency

(a)

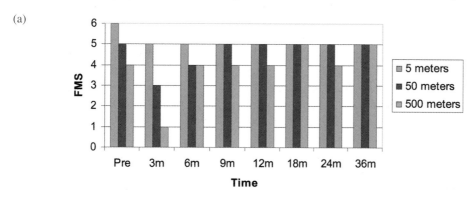

(b)

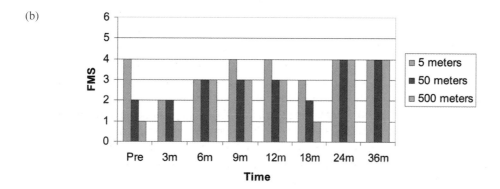

Fig. 6.2.5 Changes in Functional Mobility Scale (FMS) after multilevel surgery for a child at GMFCS levels II (a) and III (b).

noted by the need for assistive devices in the first 3–9 months after surgery. This was accompanied by a marked decrease in walking speed and a marked increase in the energy cost of walking. In the majority of children, walking speed and oxygen consumption followed a 'mirror image' pattern of change.

In the context of these findings we found 3-monthly assessments through the gait laboratory including a standardized physical examination, VGA and discussion with rehabilitation staff invaluable in monitoring recovery after multilevel surgery. Early identification of deviations from the expected recovery trajectory can be investigated and corrective action taken to prevent long term underachievement of preoperative goals and expectations.

THE 12-MONTH POSTOPERATIVE ASSESSMENT

Approximately 1 year after multilevel surgery, we conduct a more extensive evaluation of gait and functioning including IGA, energy cost of walking and the completion of functional outcome scores including the FMS and Functional Assessment Questionnaire (FAQ). Not all children will have reached a full recovery by 12 months, and many continue to improve into the 2nd and even 3rd year after multilevel surgery. However, the 12-month assessment is an excellent opportunity to compare postoperative status to baseline before the effects of growth, including major changes in height and weight at the time of puberty, interfere with the preoperative to postoperative assessments. In addition, the 12-month assessment includes an evaluation of the need for additional procedures which might be conducted at the time of implant removal which is frequently scheduled soon after the 12-month evaluation. We prefer to remove most metal fixation devices in growing children because they are frequently a source of discomfort and pose a risk of peri-prosthetic fracture in active children. The scheduling of implant removal provides an opportunity to 'fine-tune' residual recurrent deformities. In particular residual knee-flexion contractures may benefit from growth plate surgery with either stapling or '8' plates to the anterior aspect of the distal femoral growth plate. At 12–24 months after multilevel surgery it may also be an appropriate time to conduct research based investigations using functional questionnaires and quality of life measures or remote activity monitoring. The use of the Child Health Questionnaire (CHQ) in our center has shown changes in the physical functioning domain similar to changes seen on functional measures. It is difficult to interpret results from other domains as the influence of changes relating to other factors such as the social and emotional changes of puberty may influence the result. However, it is important not to discount the major impact that the intensive program of SEMLS followed by rehabilitation has both on the child and their family.

TRAJECTORY OF CHANGE AFTER MULTILEVEL SURGERY

An important issue in understanding the consequences of multilevel surgery, which has a direct bearing on the design of clinical trials, is the trajectory of change in outcome parameters. This has already been referred to above where a number of studies have established that the pattern of change is quite different following multilevel soft tissue surgery compared to combined bony and soft tissue surgery (Nene et al. 1993, Abel et al. 1999, Saraph et al. 2002, Gough et al. 2004, Kondo et al. 2004, Adolfsen et al. 2007, Graham and Harvey 2007). The baseline GMFCS level may also influence the trajectory of change, as may the age of the patient. Younger children heal more quickly, are more resilient and return to baseline function much faster than older children and adolescents. Children at GMFCS level III return to assisted walking faster than children at GMFCS levels I and II return to independent walking. In a preliminary analysis of a randomized clinical trial of 19 children undergoing multilevel surgery at our hospital, robust improvements in gait parameters as measured by the Gillette Gait Index (GGI) (Schutte et al. 2000) are found at 12 months after SEMLS but significant improvements in gross motor function (GMFM) and self reported quality of life (CHQ) may not be seen until 2 years or more after multilevel surgery (Fig. 6.2.6).

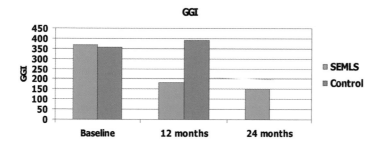

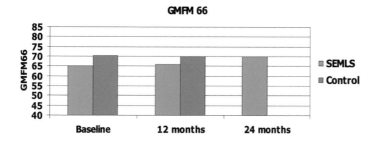

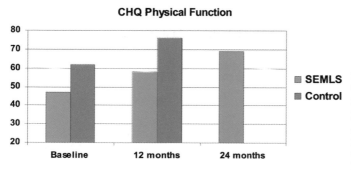

Fig. 6.2.6 Preliminary results of a randomized controlled trial of 19 children who underwent multilevel surgery. GGI, Gillette Gait Index; CHQ, Child Health Questionnaire; SEMLS, single-event multilevel surgery; GMFM, Gross Motor Function Measure.

These findings are very important in the concept, planning and design of trials of multilevel surgery. It may be ethically acceptable and practically possible to recruit children for a trial of multilevel surgery in which the control group defers progression to surgery for a year. However, it would be in both ethical and practical terms very difficult to consider assigning patients to a control group for periods of longer than a year given that the natural history of gait and function in the surgical age group is for deterioration in both.

Strengthening: progressive resistance strength training (PRST)

The third major physical intervention which may be relevant to children, adolescents and adults with CP is strengthening programs. The role of strength training and in particular progressive resistance strength training (PRST) in children with CP has recently been reported in cohort studies, clinical trials and review articles (MacPhail and Kramer 1995, Damiano and Abel 1998, Dodd et al. 2002, 2003). Evidence is growing that PRST is feasible, safe and has some efficacy in improving gait, function, self esteem and quality of life in children with CP. Although the majority of reports favor PRST, other forms of strengthening including aerobic exercise using therapeutic horse riding (Davis et al. 2009) and treadmill training (Dodd and Foley 2007) have also been advocated. PRST employs specific principles drawn from established exercise physiology (American College of Sports Medicine 2002) and applies them to children, adolescents and adults with CP. The design and implementation of such programs requires creativity and ingenuity. It is not yet known with certainty whether it is better to employ short bursts of strengthening or more prolonged and continuous programs. The benefit of PRST in relation to the timing of multilevel surgery and spasticity interventions has also not been established and is worthy of further study. For example, it has now been clearly established from a number of studies that multilevel surgery results in temporary but profound weakness and de-conditioning (Nene et al. 1993, Gage and Novacheck 2001, Gough et al. 2004). Strength changes seen in one repetition maximum (1 RM) leg press in our study demonstrate this (Fig. 6.2.7).

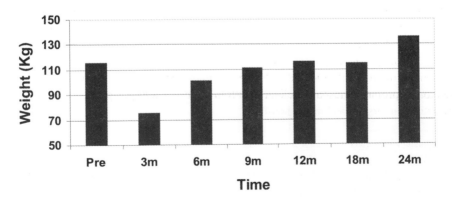

Fig. 6.2.7 Changes in leg strength measured by one repetition maximum leg press in 19 children following multilevel surgery.

Should PRST be used as a program to prepare children for SEMLS? Would PRST be better employed as part of the post-SEMLS rehabilitation program? It is our impression that children and adolescents respond more favorably to PRST following optimum musculoskeletal alignment achieved through a SEMLS program. In addition, many children and adolescents show signs of 'burnout' from involvement in more traditional physical therapy programs throughout their childhood. Following SEMLS, many of them are ready for something different and the challenges of an individually tailored PRST program have been beneficial for many. It is clear that gait and function are related much more closely to weakness than to spasticity in adolescents and adults. We think there is much to support a logical sequence of management which commences with spasticity interventions (combined with physical therapy and the use of orthoses) in early childhood, progressing to SEMLS when appropriate. There is clearly much scope for further research into the most effective combination of these interventions. Our preliminary work in 5- to 10-year follow-up studies of adolescents and young adults following SEMLS suggest that optimum biomechanical realignment results in maintenance and stability of gait and gross motor function well into adult life. An additional benefit may be an alteration in the otherwise premature ageing of the skeleton which many individuals with CP experience as they age. Residual deformity and biomechanical impairment of the skeleton, at the hip, knee and ankle/foot levels, seem to be associated with premature aging of the skeleton, the early onset of symptoms of fatigue and degenerative arthritis and further impairment of health-related quality of life in young adults with CP. For example, mild residual hip displacement which is asymptomatic in the teenager may cause a relatively rapid onset of premature degenerative arthritis and the need for additional reconstructive surgery including joint arthroplasty. Residual knee-flexion deformity and patella alta is associated with a constant overloading of the knee during gait because of the need to continuously use the quadriceps throughout the stance phase of gait. Recurrent anterior knee pain, patella femoral arthritis and arthritis of the knee joint itself may result in early adult life if crouch gait has not been fully corrected. Residual deformities in the foot including external tibial torsion and pes plano–abducto–valgus are often asymptomatic in teenagers but in early adult life are associated with degenerative changes in the subtalar and mid-tarsal joints as well as symptomatic hallux valgus and forefoot deformities. Orthopaedic surgery for adults is often organized on an anatomic basis with surgeons practicing elective reconstructive surgery at the hip, the knee or the ankle/foot. The pediatric orthopaedic surgeon is one of the few last generalists. Multilevel surgery may be the last opportunity for a child with CP to have optimum biomechanical realignment of the skeleton to promote musculoskeletal health in adult life and postpone the need for reconstructive surgery for as long as possible.

Case presentation: HW (Fig. 6.2.8, Case 14 on Interactive Disc)

HW is a 9-year-old boy with spastic diplegic CP who presented to the gait laboratory for assessment and planning of SEMLS. At that time he was classified as level III according to the GMFCS and used a posterior walker for ambulation in all settings. According to the FMS he was rated as FMS 2,2,2. He was known to have bilateral hip dysplasia with a migration percentage of 40% on the right and 30% on the left. These had been noted to be

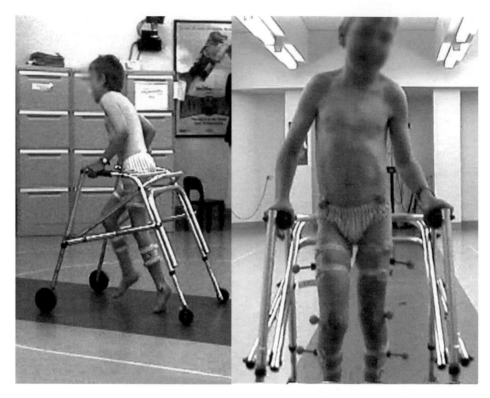

Fig. 6.2.8 Video capture image of HW pre-surgery. (See pre-op video in Case 14 on Interactive Disc.)

slowly increasing with time. Previous interventions had included injections of botulinum toxin type A to the calf muscles and hamstrings on two previous occasions, with limited benefit.

Following comprehensive assessment according to the diagnostic matrix, the following procedures were recommended:

- bilateral varus derotation osteotomies of the proximal femur, to stabilize the hips and to improve gait
- bilateral percutaneous lengthening of adductor longus
- bilateral distal hamstring lengthening with transfer of rectus femoris to semitendinosus
- bilateral gastrocnemius recession, Strayer type (no surgery to soleus).

Postoperatively he was managed in below knee plasters with removable knee-immobilizers and mobilized using a wheelchair.

At 5 weeks postoperatively, his plaster casts were removed and solid AFOs were fitted. At 3 months postoperatively HW was walking independently using his posterior walker. He appeared to have good biomechanical alignment on VGA and on physical examination muscle length and rotational alignment were noted to be very satisfactory. He was then recommended to move from the posterior walker to the use of Canadian crutches and the hinges on his solid AFOs were opened. Six months post-SEMLS he was able to progress to a lesser level of support, and ambulate with single-point sticks. Figure 6.2.9 illustrates the changes in his mobility status following multilevel surgery.

Figure 6.2.10 shows his pre-SEMLS kinematic data and movement analysis profile (MAP). The principal gait deviations are highlighted on the MAP with arrows. At 1 year post-SEMLS there had been a significant improvement in gait as noted by the reduction in overall Gait Profile Score (GPS) (Figs. 6.2.11, 12) with good correction of his equinus and knee in the sagittal plane and correction of hip rotations and foot progression in the transverse plane. However, there was some overcorrection of right hip rotation and under correction of left hip rotation as noted on the MAP scores (Fig. 6.2.11, 12).

At the full biomechanical evaluation at 5-year follow-up (Fig. 6.2.13) new problems were noted particularly on the left side with increasing external foot progression, increasing hip and knee flexion during gait and an increase in leg-length discrepancy, now noted to be 2 cm short on the left both clinically and confirmed by computed tomography. There was also increased dorsiflexion into a calcaneus range at the ankle bilaterally, related to increasing plano–abducto–valgus foot deformities. These deformities were both noted clinically and confirmed radiographically on standardized weight bearing radiographs of the feet.

In relation to growth and skeletal maturation, it was felt that this was the ideal time to intervene to correct his lever arm deformities, and equalize his leg length by growth-plate surgery. His surgical prescription at this time included bilateral subtalar fusions and percutaneous drill epiphysiodesis of the left distal femoral physis.

At the 5-year follow up no change had been noted on a pelvic radiograph but as he went into the adolescent growth spurt, during the next follow up, he was noted on VGA to have increased trunk shift over the right hip in single leg stance and a further radiograph confirmed

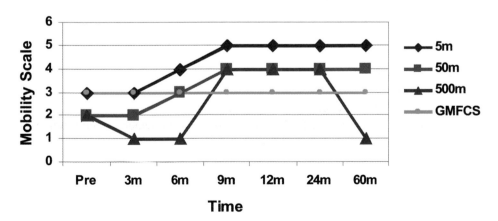

Fig. 6.2.9 HW: changes in mobility before single-event multilevel surgery and up to 5 years follow-up according to Functional Mobility Scale.

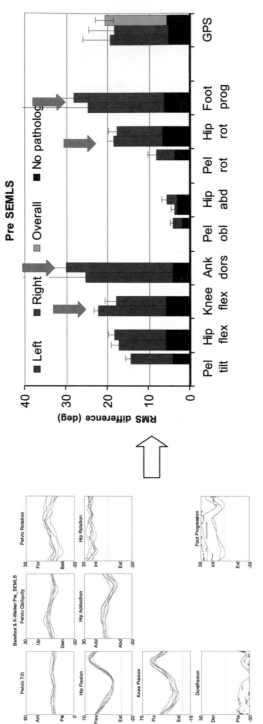

Fig. 6.2.10 HW: kinetic data and Movement Analysis Profile before single-event multilevel surgery (SEMLS). Arrows highlight most important gait deviations. RMS, root mean square; GPS, Gait Profile Score.

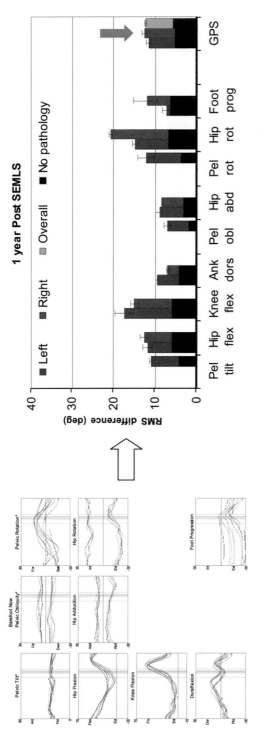

Fig. 6.2.11 HW: kinematic data and Movement Analysis Profile 1 year after single-event multilevel surgery (SEMLS). RMS, root mean square; GPS, Gait Profile Score.

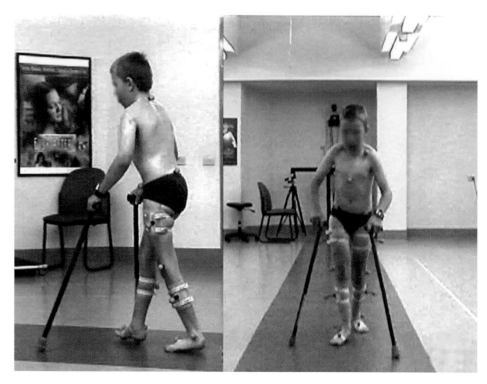

Fig. 6.2.12 Video capture image of HW 1 year post-surgery. (See one-year post-op video in Case 14 on Interactive Disc for gait index of this patient.)

recurrent progressive right hip subluxation. Following a further evaluation, a revision right proximal femoral osteotomy incorporating varus derotation and extension was performed to stabilize the right hip subluxation (Fig. 6.2.14).

The lessons from this boy's management are pertinent. First, population-based studies from our center indicate that approximately 50% of children with CP at GMFCS level III will develop significant hip subluxation. Appropriate management of these children requires an approach which will deal with their hip displacement as well as their gait deviations. In general this usually requires varus derotation osteotomies of the proximal femora combined with adductor lengthening. If this is performed early enough, acetabular dysplasia is unlikely to develop. We think it is very important to try to avoid the need for pelvic osteotomy in these children because the hip-abductors are already substantially weaker than normal. Most approaches to pelvic osteotomy for the management of acetabular dysplasia require the mobilization of the hip abductors which can result in further substantial weakening and impairment of rehabilitation.

Asymmetric hip displacement is often associated with both asymmetric neurological involvement and a real and apparent leg length discrepancy. Identification of leg-length discrepancy and correction by growth plate surgery (percutaneous epiphysiodesis) at the appropriate time can be a substantial help in maintaining gait symmetry. Finally, despite a

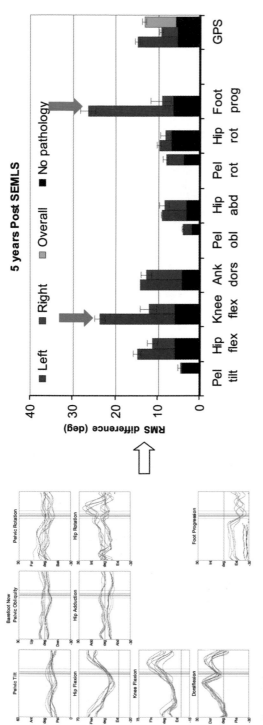

Fig. 6.2.13 HW: 5 years after single-event multilevel surgery (SEMLS). Arrows highlight marked problems since the 1-year analysis. RMS, root mean square; GPS, Gait Profile Score.

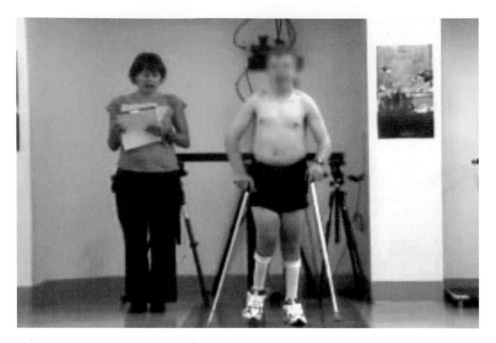

Fig. 6.2.14 Video capture image of HW 5 years post-surgery. (See five-year post-op video in Case 14 on Interactive Disc for gait video of this patient.)

good outcome from his index multilevel surgery, progressive and recurrent lever arm deformities occurred during the pubertal growth spurt requiring further correction to prevent progressive crouch gait. The need for systematic objective follow up from initial presentation to skeletal maturity using the tools and measures outlined is confirmed.

REFERENCES

Abel MF, Damiano DL, Pannunzio M, Bush J (1999) Muscle-tendon surgery in diplegic cerebral palsy: functional and mechanical changes. *J Pediatr Orthop* **19**: 366–75.

Adolfsen SE, Õunpuu S, Bell KJ, DeLuca PA (2007) Kinematic and kinetic outcomes after identical multilevel soft tissue surgery in children with cerebral palsy. *J Pediatr Orthop* **27**: 658–67.

American College of Sports Medicine (2002) Progression models in resistance training for healthy adults. *Med Sci Sports Exerc* **34**: 364–80.

Bell KJ, Õunpuu S, DeLuca PA, Romness MJ (2002) Natural progression of gait in children with cerebral palsy. *J Pediatr Orthop* **22**: 677–82.

Damiano DL, Abel MF (1998) Functional outcomes of strength training in spastic cerebral palsy. *Arch Phys Med Rehabil* **79**: 119–25.

Davis E, Davies B, Wolfe R, Raadsveld R, Heine B, Thomason P, Dobson F, Graham HK (2009) A randomised controlled trial of the impact of therapeutic horse riding on the quality of life, health and function of children with cerebral palsy. *Dev Med Child Neurol* **51**: 111–19.

Dimeglio A (2005) Growth in pediatric orthopaedics. In: Morrissy T, Weinstein SL, editors. *Lovell and Winter's Paediatric Orthopaedics*, 6th edn, vol. 1. Philadelphia, PA: Lippincott William and Wilkins. p 35–65.

Dodd KJ, Taylor NF, Damiano DL (2002) A systematic review of the effectivness of strength-training programs for people with cerebral palsy. *Arch Phys Med Rehabil* **83**: 1157–64.

Dodd KJ, Taylor NF, Graham HK (2003) A randomized clinical trial of strength training in young people with cerebral palsy. *Dev Med Child Neurol* **45**: 652–7.

Dodd KJ, Foley S (2007) Partial body-weight-supported treadmill training can improve walking in children with cerebral palsy: a clinical controlled trial. *Dev Med Child Neurol* **49**: 101–5.

Gage JR, Novacheck TF (2001) An update on the treatment of gait problems in cerebral palsy. *J Pediatr Orthop B* **10**: 265–74.

Gough M, Eve LC, Robinson RO, Shortland AP (2004) Short-term outcome of multilevel surgical intervention in spastic diplegic cerebral palsy compared with the natural history. *Dev Med Child Neurol* **46**: 91–7.

Graham HK, Harvey A (2007) Assessment of mobility after multi-level surgery for cerebral palsy. *J Bone Joint Surg Br* **89**: 993–4.

Kondo I, Hosokawa K, Iwata M, Oda A, Nomura T, Ikeda K, Asagai Y, Kohzaki T, Nishimura H (2004) Effectiveness of selective muscle-release surgery for children with cerebral palsy: longitudinal and stratified analysis. *Dev Med Child Neurol* **46**: 540–7.

MacPhail HE, Kramer JF (1995) Effect of isokinetic strength-training on functional ability and walking efficiency in adolescents with cerebral palsy. *Dev Med Child Neurol* **37**: 763–75.

Nene AV, Evans GA, Patrick JH (1993) Simultaneous multiple operations for spastic diplegia. Outcome and functional assessment of walking in 18 patients. *J Bone Joint Surg Br* **75**: 488–94.

Olesch CA (2003) *Single event multilevel surgery: its influence on walking speed and oxygen cost during a 10-minute walk in children with cerebral palsy.* D. Phil. thesis, University of Melbourne.

Palisano R, Rosenbaum P, Walter S, Russell D, Wood E, Galuppi B (1997) Development and reliability of a system to classify gross motor function in children with cerebral palsy. *Dev Med Child Neurol* **39**: 214–23.

Rosenbaum P, Walter SD, Hanna SE, Palisano RJ, Russell DJ, Raina P, Wood E, Bartlett DJ, Galuppi BE (2002) Prognosis for gross motor function in cerebral palsy: creation of motor development curves. *J Am Med Assoc* **288**: 1357–63.

Saraph V, Zwick EB, Zwick G, Steinwender C, Steinwender G, Linhart W (2002) Multilevel surgery in spastic diplegia: Evaluation by physical examination and gait analysis in 25 children. *J Pediatr Orthop* **22**: 150–7.

Schutte LM, Narayanan U, Stout JL, Selber P, Gage JR, Schwartz MH (2000) An index for quantifying deviations from normal gait. *Gait Posture* **11**: 25–31.

EPILOGUE

James R. Gage

In this text, we have discussed normal function and pathophysiology of cerebral palsy, reviewed methods and means of evaluation and treatment, and outlined the range of treatment methods as they currently exist. Now that we have completed that exercise it is time to switch from the realm of science to the realm of philosophy – to look back and reflect upon the road we've traveled, and then look forward and contemplate the final destination to which it leads.

Until the advent of clinical gait analysis laboratories, the treatment of cerebral palsy was an art, not a science. Physicians tended to treat patients in the way they had been taught to treat them by their mentors without questioning why. In general, beyond the clinical examination, there was no attempt to precisely define the pathology; very little thought about how the treatments would affect the dynamics of that pathology in either the short or long term; and little effort to assess the outcome of the intervention. Since the priorities of normal gait were not well understood, treatments were not aimed at reestablishing those priorities. The importance of muscles as prime movers in gait and bones as the levers upon which they act was known only in a general way, and little effort was made to define and preserve muscles or to restore their lever arms. As a result, iatrogenic injury was often added to the physiologic burden inflicted by the cerebral palsy, with the result that often the child was worse off after the intervention than before. Prolonged immobilization after surgery added further damage, which left the child weak and stiff. And finally, frequent surgical interventions converted childhood from a time of play to a perpetual state of recovery. Our physical therapy colleagues recognized this and often argued long and hard against surgical treatment.

A. Bruce Gill, an orthopaedist of an earlier era, said: 'Study principles not methods. If one understands the principle, he can devise his own methods' (Gill 1928). In this book we have sought to pursue principles and then determine optimal treatment using today's best methods. It is our expectation that by the time the next edition of this book is published, we will have better and more sophisticated methods of treatment. I suspect, however, that the principles of treatment will have changed very little.

What are the general principles of treatment?
For the first one, we have to back to the Hippocratic Oath, 'Primum non nocere!' – First, do no harm!

From there, we could go on to Dr James Cary's principles, outlined in the introduction to Section 4, which were: (1) define the long-term goal, (2) precisely identify the patient's problem, (3) predict the effects of growth on the patient with and without the proposed treatment, (4) consider valid treatment alternatives, and (5) treat the whole child, not just his motor–skeletal parts (Cary 1976).

The principles outlined in Niebuhr's Serenity Prayer also are worth restating: (1) accept what can't be changed, (2) change the things that can be changed (with intelligent thought, innovation, and courage), and (3) have the wisdom (knowledge/insight) to know the difference.

Finally, we can add the principle of careful, precise, and comprehensive assessment of outcome, which allows us to learn from the mistakes of the past and then apply that knowledge to the future treatment of others. The Gross Motor Functional Classification System, which was discussed in Chapters 2.6, 2.7 and 6.1, has helped us a great deal in defining the ultimate musculo–skeletal potential of children with cerebral palsy, which in turn allows us to set realistic long-term goals.

In essence, then, one should approach the treatment of these children as one would a math problem. By that I mean carefully define the elements of the problem and then logically solve it. Even in math, one applies general methods of solution to a particular set of problems, but the unique solution to a specific problem depends upon the particular elements of that problem. It is no different when one sets about to minimize the disabilities of gait in a child with cerebral palsy.

REFERENCES

Gill AB (1928) Operation for old or irreducible congenital dislocation of the hip. *J Bone Joint Surg* **10**: 696.
Cary JM (1976) *Principles for Caring for a Handicapped Child*. Resident Lectures. Newington Children's Hospital, Newington, Connecticut, USA.

INDEX

Illustrations are comprehensively referred to from the text. Therefore, significant material in illustrations has only been given a page reference in the absence of their concomitant mention in the text referring to that illustration.

627

643